Mental health care

FIFTH EDITION

Catherine Hungerford

Donna Hodgson

Richard Clancy

Gillian Murphy

Kerrie Doyle

Maree Bernoth

Michelle Cleary

Fifth edition published 2024 by
John Wiley & Sons Australia, Ltd
310 Edward Street, Brisbane, Qld, 4000
First edition published 2012

© John Wiley & Sons Australia, Ltd 2024, 2021, 2018, 2015, 2012

Typeset in Times LT Std Roman 10/12pt

The moral rights of the authors have been asserted.

Authorised adaptation of *Mental health care for nurses: Applying mental health skills in the general hospital* (ISBN 978 1 405 12455 3), published by Blackwell Publishing Ltd, Oxford, United Kingdom. © 2006 in the United Kingdom by Blackwell Publishing Ltd.

A catalogue record for this book is available from the National Library of Australia.

The authors and publisher would like to thank the copyright holders, organisations and individuals for their permission to reproduce copyright material in this book.

Every effort has been made to trace the ownership of copyright material. Information that will enable the publisher to rectify any error or omission in subsequent editions will be welcome. In such cases, please contact the Permissions Section of John Wiley & Sons Australia, Ltd.

Wiley acknowledges the Traditional Custodians of the land on which we operate, live and gather as employees, and recognise their continuing connection to land, water and community. We pay respect to Elders past, present and emerging.

Creators/Contributors
Hungerford, Catherine (Author), Hodson, Donna (Author), Clancy, Richard (Author), Murphy, Gilian (Author), Doyle, Kerrie (Author), Bernoth, Maree (Author), Cleary, Michele (Author), Bostwick, Richard (Author), Ngune, Irene (Author) and de Jong, Gideon (Author).

Wiley
Mark Levings (Publishing Manager), David Hobson (Product Manager), Jess Carr (Manager, Higher Education Content Management), Emily Echlin (Production Editor), Tara Seeto (Senior Publishing Coordinator), Renee Bryon (Copyright & Image Research), Delia Sala (Cover Design), Carly Slater (Copyeditor)

Cover: © Laure F / Adobe Stock

Typeset in India by diacriTech

Printed in Singapore
M WEP262639 090224

BRIEF CONTENTS

CONTENTS

ABOUT THE AUTHORS

Dr Catherine Hungerford

Dr Catherine Hungerford is a registered nurse, credentialed mental health nurse and endorsed nurse practitioner. She is also an Associate Professor of Mental Health Nursing at Central Queensland University and an Adjunct Professor at Federation University. Catherine has extensive experience as a clinician, educator (clinical and academic), manager (front-line management, project management, area management, policy, executive management) and researcher. In addition, she has written widely on mental health recovery, the scope of practice of mental health nurses and other mental health topics, including leadership, health care models, health service evaluation, cultural issues and workforce issues.

Donna Hodgson

Donna Hodgson is a registered nurse who has held a credential to practice with the Australian College of Mental Health Nurses since 2003.

After several years of general nursing, Donna transferred to mental health nursing and commenced postgraduate studies. Enjoying research and new initiatives, Donna was the first Australian nurse Clozapine Co-ordinator appointed under the First National Mental Health Plan. Since then, she has worked in numerous clinical roles, including as the Clinical Nurse Consultant in the acute adult inpatient unit, and as a Clinical Manager in the community.

Donna is enthusiastic about professional development activities, and ensuring a connection exists between evidence-based theory and the practice of mental health nursing. Given this, Donna has a long history of educating and mentoring undergraduate and postgraduate nurses in the field of mental health, and passionately worked as the coordinator of mental health nursing education programs for more than 20 years.

In recent years, Donna has enjoyed participating with like-minded colleagues on research and mental health nursing practice projects, and is the co-author of a number of papers related to mental health nursing, scope of practice, disability and educational frameworks. Donna is currently a Clinical Nurse Consultant in Adult Community Mental Health Services.

Associate Prof. Richard Clancy

Richard Clancy is a Conjoint Associate Professor with the University of Newcastle and an affiliate with the Hunter Medical Research Institute. He has over 40 years' experience as a registered nurse, including 20 years as a clinical nurse consultant in mental health, and has worked in a variety of mental health settings, including over 20 years in the specialty of comorbid mental health and substance use. His research and associated publications have focused on implementation science in areas of comorbid mental health, substance use, physical health and motivational interviewing. Richard has delivered numerous comorbidity workshops in Australia over the past 25 years, as well as a number of Australian and international conference presentations. Richard has qualifications in epidemiology and the social sciences as well as his hospital-based nursing certificates.

Dr Gillian Murphy

Gillian Murphy is a Senior Lecturer with the School of Nursing and Midwifery, Western Sydney University. Gill has worked as a mental health nurse for 25 years, with experience in forensic, in-patient, community and emergency mental health services. She has worked in both UK and Australian clinical mental health services.

Gill is actively engaged with mental health research. Her PhD study generated parenting narratives of adults who had experienced childhood parental mental illness. Her past research include an international study which focused on health outcomes for people diagnosed with schizophrenia; supporting people with personality disorder using a clinical network; familial experiences of bereavement as a result of suicide and childhood parental death. Gill's current research program focuses on mental illness; loss and recovery. Gill has published in the area of mental illness in international journals, and is a peer reviewer for mental health and nursing-related publications.

Gill is also a qualified nurse educator and Senior Fellow, Advance HE (SFHEA). She is currently engaging with undergraduate students as they embark on their nursing careers. Sheis also a supervisor for higher degree research candidates engaging in a range of mental health related studies.

Aunty Kerrie Doyle

Aunty Kerrie is the inaugural Professor of Indigenous Health in the School of Medicine at Western Sydney University, and leader of the Aboriginal and Torres Strait Islander Clinical Academic Group at Maridulu Budyari Gumal (SPHERE). A social scientist and mental health clinician, she has over 40 years' experience working in Indigenous health and communities, and has various research interests, including as a collaborator in the Global Burden of Disease project. She is married to a chiefly Maori, and they have two sons, two grandchildren and two poodles.

Associate Professor Maree Bernoth

Associate Professor Maree Bernoth is an academic at Charles Sturt University. She has worked as a registered nurse in aged care for over 30 years and moved into the academy after completing her PhD Professor Bernoth has an extensive research history in aged care and is a strong advocate for ensuring partnerships with older people and their carers. Professor Bernoth has had collaborative grants with aged care organisations to develop teaching strategies for aged care workers, evaluated service delivery models in community-based services and has completed a report on strategies to prevent the unnecessary admission of older people to emergency departments. Professor Bernoth has co-edited an aged care text, *Healthy Ageing and Aged Care* which is a collaboration of academics and clinicians working in aged care aimed at engaging students in learning about ageing. Maree is the Chair of the Murrumbidgee Primary Health Network Aged Care Consortium and works closely with aged care facilities and services in this role.

Professor Michelle Cleary

Professor Michelle Cleary is a Professor of Nursing at Central Queensland University, with adjunct professorial positions at Charles Darwin University and the University of Adelaide. Michelle has led research in several areas of mental health and health care generally, aiming to improve professional practice, consumer care and translating research programs to strengthen health service delivery. Michelle is widely published and holds editorial positions on multiple peer review journals. In addition to supervising higher-degree research students, Michelle provides advice and consultation to a variety of departments and organisations in relation to policies, guidelines and program development.

CHAPTER 1

Mental health care in Australia

LEARNING OBJECTIVES

This chapter will:

1.1 define the major terms and concepts used in the delivery of mental health care in Australia

1.2 describe the effects of stigma on people with mental health problems

1.3 explain the notions of 'care' and 'trauma-informed care'

1.4 discuss the context of care in Australia

1.5 outline the prevalence and impact of mental illness in Australia

1.6 identify the most common mental health issues that health professionals in Australia will encounter.

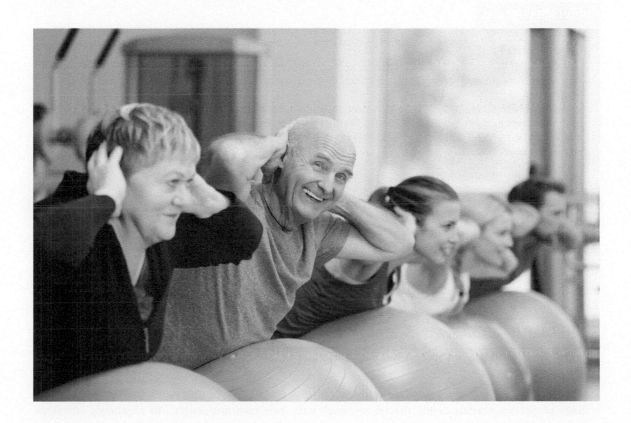

Introduction

All **health professionals** in Australia will encounter people with mental health issues, no matter where they work. Around 46 per cent of Australians aged between 16 and 85 years will experience a mental health problem in their lifetime (Australian Institute of Health and Welfare [AIHW], 2020a). Mental illness and substance use disorders account for 12 per cent of Australia's total **burden of disease**, ranking fourth for **morbidity** and **mortality** after cancer, cardiovascular disease and musculoskeletal conditions (AIHW, 2020b). Suicide and self-inflicted injuries were the leading cause of disease burden in younger people aged 15–24 and adults aged 25–44 (AIHW, 2020b). Therefore, all health professionals must understand how to help the person who experiences symptoms of mental illness.

This text introduces health professionals to the mental health field and describes how mental health services are delivered in Australia today. The text also gives an overview of the core skills and knowledge required by health professionals to support people affected by mental illness. While there are differences between the states and territories in mental health policy frameworks, legislation, practice approaches and terminology, there are enough similarities to enable health professionals to work together to improve mental health outcomes nationwide.

The focus of this chapter includes the frameworks that guide the delivery of mental health services in Australia. The chapter commences with definitions of the terms 'health professional', 'mental health', 'mental ill-health', 'mental illness' and other key terms used when supporting people with a mental illness. Following this, the power of language and the impact of stigma on people affected by mental health problems are considered. Another focus of the chapter is the notion of care, including trauma-informed care, and the contexts of care in Australia — a discussion that sets the scene for an outline of the prevalence of mental illness in Australia and descriptions of the most common mental health problems encountered by health professionals in all settings.

UPON REFLECTION

Need help?

Mental Health Australia is the peak national non-government organisation promoting the interests of the Australian mental health sector. The organisation is committed to achieving better mental health for all Australians.

Mental Health Australia provides a list of resources that people in the community and health professionals can access to learn more about mental health, mental illness, and the services that can be accessed by those who need help. Read the list of resources on the Mental Health Australia website: https://mhaustralia.org/need-help.

....

QUESTIONS

1. What are two organisations a person could contact if they were feeling suicidal?
2. What are two websites a person could access if they wanted to find out about a particular mental health condition?
3. What resources are available for specific groups of people, such as people who have experienced childhood trauma, people with an eating disorder, people with gambling problems, Aboriginal and Torres Strait Islander peoples, men, veterans, parents and LGBTQIA+ people?

1.1 Definitions

LEARNING OBJECTIVE 1.1 Define the major terms and concepts used in the delivery of mental health care in Australia.

Health professionals often work in **multidisciplinary teams**. The multidisciplinary team in health settings comprises various health disciplines, each with their own professional or regulatory standards and requirements, working together to deliver systematic and comprehensive health care to those in need (Williams & Smith, 2019). This health care encompasses all aspects of what it means to be a person, including the behavioural, biological, cultural, educational, emotional, environmental, financial, functional, mental, occupational, physical, recreational, sexual, spiritual and social aspects of who we are. The disciplines or fields of health that focus on these different aspects of humanity include:

- ambulance officers and **paramedics**
- counsellors and psychotherapists

- dietitians and nutritionists
- Aboriginal and Torres Strait Islander health workers
- medical practitioners
- midwives
- nurses, including enrolled and registered nurses, and nurse practitioners
- occupational therapists
- pastoral workers and chaplains
- pharmacists
- physiotherapists
- psychologists, including clinical psychologists
- social workers.

Each of these disciplines has a vital role in delivering health care. For example, paramedics are frontline health professionals who provide emergency or life-saving health care and other unscheduled care that occurs out-of-hospital and in the community. Such situations most often involve stabilising a person's health condition for or during transport to hospital. Paramedics work with ambulance officers and specialise in medical emergencies and the short-term management of high acuity patients.

Another group of health professionals is social workers, who are committed to pursuing social justice, enhancing the quality of life and developing the full potential of individuals, groups and communities. Given the importance of the social determinants of health in influencing the health outcomes of people and communities, the role of **social workers** in the multidisciplinary team is crucial.

Occupational therapists support the person to attend to their everyday needs and preferences (often referred to as 'functional needs and preferences') and to participate in meaningful activities. Enabling people to be independent and self-sufficient is integral to supporting good health in our society. Occupational therapists also work with families, groups and communities to address the effects of social, political and environmental factors that contribute to the exclusion of people from employment and facilitate the personal, social and recreational activities in which a person would like to become involved.

Other health professionals include counsellors, dietitians or nutritionists, Aboriginal and Torres Strait Islander health workers, pastoral workers and chaplains, pharmacists and physiotherapists. Each of these health professionals plays a significant role in delivering health care to people with mental health issues. The specific roles of these health professionals will vary according to the scope of practice of each profession, and can range from crisis or emergency care, to brief consultation or ongoing support. Regardless of their scope of practice, all health professionals must understand what is required to help the person affected by symptoms of mental illness.

In the mental health sector, there are several health professionals with similar roles, which can be confusing. For example, people may be uncertain about the difference between a **psychiatrist** and a **psychologist**. A psychiatrist is a medical practitioner who has undertaken additional studies and acquired a high level of expertise in diagnosing and treating mental illness. A particular focus of the care and treatment provided by a psychiatrist — like all medical practitioners — is the physical or biological aspects of a person's illness. A psychiatrist can prescribe medications and admit a person to hospital. Some psychiatrists have been trained to provide psychotherapy or other forms of psychological therapy.

In contrast, psychologists and clinical psychologists have been trained to provide psychological interventions or therapies for people. Psychologists and clinical psychologists focus on a person's cognition and behaviours. While both the psychologist and clinical psychologist can provide psychological therapy, the clinical psychologist holds a master's degree in clinical psychology, which means that they can provide more complex interventions. However, neither the psychologist nor clinical psychologist can prescribe medication or admit a person to hospital.

Nurses are the most common health professional in public mental health services. People may feel confused by the different types of nurses or nursing roles — assistants in nursing, enrolled nurses, registered nurses and nurse practitioners. Each of these categories of nurses or nursing roles has diverse educational requirements and scopes of practice. Moreover, registered nurses undertake countless roles across various specialty areas, including nurse researchers, clinical educators, clinical specialists, health service managers, clinical coordinators and care coordinators. Regardless of the role or function, however, nurses are defined by the type of care they provide — person-centred care, often around the clock, to help address the full range of needs and preferences of the individual and their families. The nurse's approach is defined by holism, encompassing all aspects of what it means to be a person, not just the physical needs.

The term 'mental health nurse' is often used to describe the nurse, enrolled or registered, who works in a mental health-related field. Occasionally these nurses are called psychiatric nurses; however, 'mental health nurse' is the preferred terminology because 'psychiatric' has biomedical connotations and a nurse's scope of practice is far broader than biomedicine alone. Also, the Nursing and Midwifery Board of Australia (NMBA), the regulatory authority for nurses and midwives that is part of the Australian Health Practitioner Regulation Agency (AHPRA), has no specific category for 'mental health' or 'psychiatric' nurse. Instead, the Australian College of Mental Health Nurses, the national professional body for mental health nursing, administers a credential for registered nurses with relevant specialist postgraduate qualifications who can demonstrate substantial, current experience in the mental health sector and ongoing professional development. Credentialed mental health nurses are often leaders in the public mental health services, as well as the defence health and justice health systems, and can work as autonomous practitioners in the primary health care context, providing care to people with complex symptoms of mental illness.

Key to the multidisciplinary team are support workers, including peer workers employed by community-managed organisations to provide ongoing support to people with mental illness. Such support includes counselling or psychotherapy, social and recreational support, housing and accommodation support, assistance to obtain employment, and educational opportunities. With one in five Australians experiencing symptoms of mental illness at some stage in their lives, delivering high-quality mental health and support services has become an increasing focus for governments and communities alike. There is a need, then, for health professionals, regardless of discipline or specialty, to develop a greater understanding of mental health and illness, together with the different types of mental health services available for those in need.

Mental health and mental illness

The term '**mental health**' has different meanings for different people. In health settings, mental health describes an area of health care that focuses on the population's psychological, emotional and behavioural wellbeing. The National Mental Health Strategy in Australia was first endorsed in the early 1990s to guide mental health reform and has been reaffirmed several times since. Originally, mental health was defined as the capacity of individuals and groups to interact with one another and their environment in ways that promote subjective wellbeing and the optimal development and use of mental abilities (cognitive, affective and relational), to achieve individual and collective goals consistent with justice (Australian Health Ministers, 1991). This definition has remained unchanged over the years.

Mental ill-health is most commonly referred to as **mental illness or disorder** in Australia. According to the Australian government, a mental illness is a health problem that significantly affects how a person feels, thinks, behaves and interacts with other people (Department of Health, n.d.). Mental illness is diagnosed according to standardised criteria, such as those provided by the DSM-5 or ICD-11 (the chapter on assessment in the mental health context has further information on assessment and diagnosis). One reason the term 'mental illness' is so commonly used to describe a mental health problem is because the **biomedical approach** to treatment and care continues to dominate the Australian health system.

A **mental health problem** interferes with how a person thinks, feels and behaves, but to a lesser extent than a mental illness (Benton, 2018). Mental health problems are more common and less severe than mental illnesses or disorders, and include the concerns experienced temporarily in response to the stresses of life. A person with a mental health problem may develop a mental illness if they are not supported effectively (Williams, 2019).

First responders, trauma and mental health

Most first responders (including people who work in the ambulance and paramedical services, fire and rescue services, police forces and state emergency services) are involved in or witness traumatic events.

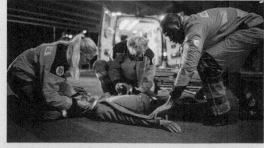

Over time, these traumatic events may affect the first responders' mental health, with many of them reporting experiences of depression, anxiety, post-traumatic stress disorder, relationship difficulties, alcohol or substance misuse and suicidal thoughts as a result of their work (Szeto et al., 2019).

Heads Up, or the Mentally Healthy Workplace Alliance (www.headsup.org.au), sponsored by organisations such as the Australian Government and Beyond Blue (www.beyondblue.org.au), supports the development of mentally healthy workplaces across Australia. This work includes helping managers develop action plans to support employees' mental health, enabling employees to take responsibility for their own mental health and support colleagues who may be struggling. Beyond Blue (2017) have also developed the *Good practice framework for mental health and wellbeing in first responder organisations*. All health professionals are encouraged to read this handbook and consider how they can better help first responders manage their stress levels.

The Black Dog Institute (www.blackdoginstitute.org.au) has developed guidelines for first responders. This Australian not-for-profit organisation has become a leader in research on the diagnosis, treatment and prevention of mood disorders such as depression and bipolar disorder. The Black Dog Institute joined forces with several universities, as well as Phoenix Australia — Centre for Posttraumatic Mental Health and St John of God Hospital, to produce A Clinician's Summary of the Expert Guidelines in the Diagnosis and Treatment of Post-traumatic Stress Disorder in Emergency Service Workers (Harvey et al., 2018). These guidelines aim to improve the support given to emergency workers who report ongoing psychological consequences from exposure to trauma.

Resources such as these are essential for health professionals who support the health of first responders or who experience traumatic events at work.

Biomedical approaches to health care

The biomedical perspective evolved after the Age of Enlightenment, a period that began in the late seventeenth century and ended one hundred years later, characterised by the advancement of scientific knowledge. Supported by the theories of the French philosopher René Descartes, the Age of Enlightenment saw the development of the 'rational' explanation of health and illness. The human body was viewed as a material object that could be understood only by scientific study and physical examination (Urban, 2018). In contrast, the mind was posited as part of a higher order and understood through introspection. The body and mind were separated into two distinct entities, with illness considered as either somatic (physical) or psychic (mental) (Maung, 2019). This philosophy paved the way for the development of an area of science known as biomedicine, with its primary focus on the somatic or physical aspects of illness (Derkatch, 2016).

Today, the biomedical approach to the treatment of illness is viewed by some as a paternalistic or vertical approach to health care. It involves 'expert' health professionals assessing a person's symptoms, making a diagnosis and devising treatment based on their scientific knowledge of the disease process. In turn, the unwell person follows the directions provided by the expert health professional to reduce the severity of their symptoms (Ferry-Danini, 2018). The biomedical approach focuses on the cause (disease or condition), effect (illness or deficiency), treatment (pharmacological, surgical and rehabilitative) and outcome (cure or disability) of illness (Ibeneme et al., 2017).

Psychiatry is the branch of biomedicine that specialises in treating mental illness. A psychiatrist diagnoses a person according to the reported or observed symptoms that fit a set of predetermined criteria (e.g. DSM-5 or ICD-11). Diagnoses range in type and degree of severity, and can include depression, anxiety, substance use disorder, psychosis, schizophrenia and dementia. Upon diagnosis, the person is prescribed medication and often advised to engage in a psychological therapy. In addition, if appropriate, electroconvulsive therapy or transcranial magnetic stimulation may be recommended. Once the person responds to this treatment regimen, they are discharged from care.

The biomedical model's dominance in the field of mental health has given rise to terminology that is likewise dominated by notions of disease or pathology. Consequently, the concepts of health and wellness can take second place to those of 'disorder', 'dysfunction', 'illness', 'deviancy' or 'abnormality'. Legislative frameworks influence language use in mental health settings across Australia. For example, the terms 'mental illness', 'mental disorder' and 'mental dysfunction' are defined in different ways, according to the mental health legislation of each state and territory. This legislation creates tension for health professionals committed to working within a health and wellness framework, and who find themselves moving between the notions of health and illness or wellbeing and dysfunction. The inconsistent language use also explains a common misunderstanding that the term 'mental health' now replaces or is synonymous with 'mental illness'. Frequent errors in using the term 'mental health' include the following.

- 'The person has mental health; she is hearing voices', rather than the more appropriate 'The person may have a mental health problem; she is hearing voices'.
- 'The consumer has been diagnosed with mental health', rather than the more appropriate 'The consumer has been diagnosed with a mental illness'.

Health professionals are encouraged to familiarise themselves with the most appropriate and current usage of relevant terms in the mental health sector. Appropriate language use will help health professionals maintain their authenticity and show their awareness of the substantial power and influence of language in today's society.

The power of language

In the past, numerous philosophers have discussed how language plays a crucial role in framing, informing, developing and maintaining social relations (e.g. Fairclough, 1989; Foucault, 1961; Goffman, 1967). Language shapes and interprets the way people see the world; language is also used to define or describe personal experiences or situations. Language has the power to persuade, control and even manipulate the way people think, act and react (Nguyen, 2019). Language, then, must be used carefully.

Health professionals who work within a health and wellness framework aim to inspire hope in others (Elsegood et al., 2018). Such approaches include helping a person to focus on their strengths and abilities, rather than their deficiencies or disabilities. One way to inspire hope is to employ language that empowers rather than disempowers. Health professionals must make the conscious choice to use one word over another.

For example, the word 'patient' has a long association with medical practitioners and hospitals and signifies a person being attended to by a health professional. Notions of 'patient' have been connected with ideas of passivity (i.e. a patient is a diseased or disabled person who is being treated by an active and expert health professional). In this way, the word 'patient' sets up ideas of disempowerment, with health professionals positioning themselves as authorities and the patients taking a more subordinate role. This unequal relationship that has led to the development of alternative terms, including 'client', 'consumer', 'service user' or, quite simply, 'person', when referring to individuals who seek assistance from a health professional.

In this text, the word 'person' is preferred when referring to someone who is being cared for by a health professional. Addtionally, the terms 'patient', 'consumer', 'service user' or 'client' are used occasionally due to their common occurrence in clinical settings.

Similarly, health professionals are referred to in various ways throughout the text. The term 'health professional' has already been defined. Other similar terms employed in this text may include 'clinician', 'health care professional', 'personnel', 'practitioner', 'staff member' or 'person'. The use of different names reflects our health system's diversity, which is inclusive and avoids labels.

Indeed, health professionals are encouraged to examine how language can be utilised to label or stereotype people. Such stereotypes are often derived from misperceptions or 'myths' about a particular (often minority) group of people. The most common myths about people with mental illness that are encountered in Australian society are outlined in table 1.1.

TABLE 1.1   Myths about mental illness

Myth: Mental illness is a life sentence.

Facts
- There are many interventions available to support people with mental illness, including medications. Other interventions focus on helping the person to address the psychological, social or other personal issues they may be experiencing.
- The earlier a person receives help for a mental health problem, the better their outcomes.
- There is no reason why people with mental health problems cannot live full and productive lives.
- People experiencing mental health problems may delay seeking help because they fear stigma and discrimination. Reducing stigma will encourage more people to seek help early.
- Most people with mental illness are treated in the community by their general practitioners (GPs).

Myth: Mental illnesses are all the same.

Facts
- There mental health problems are diverse, each with different symptoms.
- Each mental illness has its own set of symptoms, but not every person will experience all of these; for example, some people with a diagnosis of schizophrenia may hear voices, while others may not.
- Knowing a person has a mental illness will not tell you about their own unique experiences of that illness.
- Mental health problems are not just 'psychological' or 'all in the mind'. While a mental health problem may affect a person's thinking and emotions, it can also have physical effects such as insomnia, weight gain or loss, increase or loss of energy, chest pain and nausea.

Myth: Some cultural groups are more likely than others to experience mental illness.

Facts
- Anyone can develop a mental health problem; no-one is immune to experiencing a mental illness.
- Indigenous Australians experience significantly higher rates of mental illness, such as suicide, anxiety and depression, than non-Indigenous Australians. Reasons include loss of identity and culture, land and connections to Country, leading to unresolved grief; intergenerational trauma; discrimination and racism; fewer economic opportunities and poorer physical health.
- People from culturally and linguistically diverse and refugee backgrounds may have experienced torture, trauma and enormous loss before coming to Australia. Such experiences can cause substantial psychological distress, predisposing people with diverse backgrounds to developing mental health problems.
- Cultural background affects how people experience mental health problems and how they understand and interpret their symptoms.

Myth: People with a mental illness are violent.

Facts
- Research indicates that people who receive treatment for a mental illness are no more violent or dangerous than the general population.
- People living with a mental illness are more likely to be victims of violence (including self-harm).
- There is an association between violence and alcohol misuse or violence and being a young male between 15 and 25 years of age.

Source: Adapted from Mindframe (2019).

In the mental health sector, stereotyping or labelling can have quite negative consequences. It is necessary to acknowledge that those who experience symptoms of mental illness are people first, and their symptoms or conditions are of secondary importance. Outdated descriptors such as 'schizophrenic', 'the mentally ill', 'mentally ill person' or 'mental institution' are unhelpful, even counterproductive. Instead, health professionals are encouraged to use language such as:
- a person who is experiencing symptoms of schizophrenia
- a person with schizophrenia or living with schizophrenia
- a person who is receiving help for their mental health issue
- a mental health facility or unit.

Fostering constructive language is one way that health professionals can help manage the stigma experienced by people with mental health issues. Stigma and its outcomes are the focus of the next section of this chapter.

LIVED EXPERIENCE

Stigma hurts

I had some good experiences as a child, growing up. Most of these occurred when I was with my grandparents — my brothers and sister and I stayed with them during the school holidays. It was good to get away from home. Other than the holidays, my memories are not so good.

My mother was always busy and tired, working hard to hold down a job and keep the family together. My father went from job to job. He was unemployed more than he was working. This was never his fault, or so he would say. It was always someone else's problem that he had to leave. Then he would come home and make it our problem.

We lived in a regional town where everyone knew everyone else. We went to a church where we were taught about loving and supporting one another, but the reality was all about fear, control and punishment. I found the hypocrisy hard to deal with and often felt angry. Mum and I had heaps of arguments about the church.

When I was around 16, I began to experience dark thoughts about myself, my life and my future. I started seeing things — small movements, out of the corner of my eye or the floor warping around me. I felt scared by this; I had no idea what was happening. After a while, the dark thoughts became voices, telling me to do bad things to myself. So I started cutting myself. Watching the bleeding and feeling the pain gave me a passing sense of release and relief, so I did it again, until suddenly I found myself being transferred to a locked psychiatric unit for adolescents in the city.

I don't remember much about my time there, except that my grandparents visited me a lot, my mother visited me when she could, I started taking medication and the hallucinations settled. Then, when I was discharged back home, my father had moved out, and we were going to a different church — apparently, the 'love' and 'support' given by the old church didn't stretch to helping a person with a mental illness.

But things didn't improve. Everyone at school seemed to know what had happened and I started getting names thrown at me: 'looney', 'psycho', 'attention seeker'. Like there wasn't easier ways of getting attention?! Sure, a few friends stuck by me — I wouldn't have survived without them. But the names hurt me like nothing else before or after; so I left school early and found a job, which really affected my recovery. Not only was I trying to manage my life on the medication, I was trying to adapt to being part of the workforce. That was hard because the negative attitudes were everywhere. While my colleagues didn't resort to name-calling, they were clearly uncomfortable when I mentioned my experiences. I floundered for a long time, trying to work through the social stigma attached to my illness. It was over a decade before I was stable enough to decide to use my experiences to change social perceptions of mental illness. I enrolled in a social work degree at the university as a mature aged student.

1.2 Stigma

LEARNING OBJECTIVE 1.2 Describe the effects of stigma on people with mental health problems.

Seminal philosopher Goffman (1967) defined social stigma as the social disapproval, overt or covert, of personal characteristics, beliefs, behaviours or conditions that a society perceives to be at odds with social or cultural norms. **Stigma** works to discriminate between those who are accepted as 'insiders' and those who are rejected as 'outsiders' by making a clear distinction between 'us' as 'normal' and 'them' as 'deviant' — with the latter marginalised or ostracised accordingly (Jackson-Best & Edwards, 2018).

There are many examples of groups that have experienced social stigma over the centuries. These examples include those who belong to a minority cultural group or ethnicity, have diverse sexual preferences or expressions of gender, or have a mental illness or a disability (Benz et al., 2019). Other social differences that can lead to social marginalisation include contagious or transmittable diseases (e.g. leprosy, HIV/AIDS), a criminal conviction, an unemployed status, an eating disorder, or an addiction to alcohol or illicit drugs (Andersen & Kessing, 2019).

There is evidence globally that some progress has been made to reduce social stigma and change how people who experience symptoms of mental illness are perceived (Rai et al., 2018). These changes are partly due to developments in pharmacology and other treatment interventions that have brought about a marked improvement in outcomes for people with a mental illness. Changed attitudes have also been achieved through the progress made by the global human rights movement and evolving socio-cultural perceptions of how minority groups should be treated. In Australia, improved community perceptions have resulted from work that has been undertaken by primary health care organisations such as Beyond Blue, SANE Australia and the National Youth Mental Health Foundation, known as 'headspace'. The roles of these community-managed organisations include supporting people with mental health issues to live in the community and educating the community about mental illness. (The chapter on mental health service delivery has further information about the role of community-managed organisations.)

Although such progress and associated community initiatives play a central role in reducing social stigma, there is always room for improvement (Kinson et al., 2018; McCann et al., 2018). Questions for health professionals include: 'Which is the more socially acceptable diagnosis in Australia, depression that results from physical pain or illness or depression caused by emotional concerns?' 'Which condition is viewed as the more acceptable, depression or psychosis?' 'Psychosis with no known cause or psychosis linked to the misuse of illicit drugs and alcohol?'. Considering the answers to these questions will help health professionals to support a reduction in the levels of social stigma in the community (SANE, 2019).

Community attitudes

People with mental health problems continue to be stigmatised in and by the community through their misrepresentation in the news and entertainment media (Ma, 2017). Perhaps most concerning is the suggestion that people experiencing symptoms of mental illness are the main perpetrators of violent crime. This representation is statistically inaccurate (Saleh, 2020), with the major determinants of violence linked to social and economic status, and substance misuse (Kleissl-Muir et al., 2018). Questions must be asked, then, about the Hollywood caricature of people with a mental illness as, for example, a maniac on a killing spree, a free-spirited rebel, a narcissistic parasite or victims of mind games played by psychopaths (e.g. *Psycho, One Flew Over the Cuckoo's Nest, Silence of the Lambs, Shutter Island*). Certainly, there are exceptions to such representations. For instance, in the movie, *A Beautiful Mind*, a man with a serious mental illness is portrayed sympathetically. However, a feature of this and similar movies is that the protagonists have genius-like attributes in addition to their mental illness, thereby suggesting that mental illness is acceptable only if the person has other exceptional qualities to compensate.

Media representations reflect and perpetuate community values and attitudes: journalists construct the community in a particular way, and community members generally understand media representations as 'the way things are' (Röhm et al., 2017). Such understanding has ramifications for people diagnosed with mental illness. For example, misrepresentations work to dehumanise, marginalise and isolate people with mental health issues. Although changes in community attitudes are evident, it would seem the fundamental problem remains — that is, people with mental health issues continue to be stigmatised by the community.

IN PRACTICE

StigmaWatch: Keeping an eye on the media

SANE Australia is a national charity working for a better life for people affected by mental illness through campaigning, education and research.

SANE's StigmaWatch program (www.sane.org/about-sane/advocacy/stigmawatch) responds to community concerns about media stories, advertisements and other representations that may stigmatise people with mental illness or inadvertently promote ideas of self-harm or suicide. StigmaWatch provides positive feedback to the media, where they have produced accurate and responsible portrayals of mental illness and suicide.

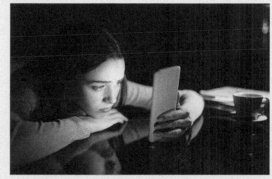

StigmaWatch follows up on reports submitted by hundreds of 'StigmaWatchers' — ordinary Australians, people with mental health problems and their families, as well as health professionals — who are concerned about how the media depict mental illness and suicide.

StigmaWatch reviews these reports against the Mindframe Media Guidelines and the Australian Press Council Standards. If StigmaWatch finds that a media story is stigmatising, inaccurate or irresponsible, it will raise concerns with the media outlet or journalist responsible and encourage them to revise or withdraw the article. StigmaWatch also provides advice on safeguarding against future media coverage that may stigmatise mental illness and suicide. This is essential in light of the changing media landscape, including online resources and entertainment, and social media channels.

QUESTIONS

1. The terms 'fruitcake', 'nutter', 'psycho' or 'mad' are often used colloquially to describe people who experience mental health problems. Discuss the effects of labels on people with mental illness, their families and communities as a whole.
2. Over the next week, record the number of times you hear family members, partners, friends, colleagues, people in the community or people on television or in films using words with a negative connotation to describe mental illness. As a health professional, what can you do to discourage this kind of communication?

The impact of the stigma associated with mental illness is considerable — it includes reduced options for employment, accommodation and socialising, as well as personal distress and low self-esteem (Kirsh et al., 2018). Self-stigma, where people with mental health issues view themselves negatively, leads to diminished self-esteem and self-efficacy (Crowe et al., 2018). Moreover, stigma can give rise to reluctance in people with mental health problems to disclose their symptoms or postpone seeking help.

To support the reduction of stigmatising attitudes in our community, the Australian government has legislated to protect the rights of minority groups. When stigma is acted upon, and a person is mistreated because they have a mental illness or other disability, they are experiencing discrimination. In Australia, such **discrimination** is unlawful under the *Disability Discrimination Act 1992* (DDA). Even so, discrimination against people with a mental illness is one of the biggest obstacles to feeling supported and receiving effective care and treatment (Morgan et al., 2017). Health professionals are therefore encouraged to familiarise themselves with the DDA and model its principles.

Indeed, health professionals are in a prime position to assist with reducing social stigma. Reducations are best achieved by understanding the impact of social stigma on a person's life, including their level of education, employment, income, housing, community involvement and, ultimately, health. By speaking out against stigma, educating the community, and advocating for the person with mental health issues, health professionals can assist in breaking down the barriers. These barriers include the stigma that is evident within the health professions themselves.

Attitudes of health professionals

Sadly, the negative attitudes towards people who experience symptoms of mental illness are evident in health professionals who, as community members, may view people with mental illness as 'dangerous' or 'not really sick' (Giandinoto et al., 2018). Other negative attitudes that are evident include 'guilt by association', where mental health professionals experience stigma (Ebsworth & Foster, 2017; Happell et al., 2019). For example, non-mental health professionals may express negative attitudes through statements such as 'Everyone who works in mental health gets assaulted!', 'You have to be mad to work in mental health' or 'Don't go and work in mental health, you'll lose your clinical skills!' These kinds of comments are based on stereotypes rather than research evidence and provide one possible reason for the difficulty experienced nationally in recruiting health professionals to work in the mental health sector (Gibbs et al., 2018).

Also concerning are the attitudes and behaviours of a few health professionals when interacting directly with people with a mental illness. These attitudes and behaviours can include:

- talking about consumers rather than to consumers
- putting down and ridiculing consumers
- failing to provide information to consumers to enable them to make informed decisions
- failing to provide appropriate or respectful services
- failing to respect the information shared with the service by family members
- perpetuating negative stereotypes (Schiavo, 2018).

It is essential, then, that health professionals understand the issues involved, particularly how stigmatising attitudes and behaviours influence the **empowerment** and disempowerment of people with a mental illness (De Ruysscher et al., 2019).

Some health professionals feel doubtful about the notion of empowerment for consumers (Juntanamalaga et al., 2019). This can lead health professionals to:

- removing the personal freedoms of the individuals with mental illness who present to health services
- forcing people with a mental illness to take medication against their will
- deciding which aspects of treatment and care will or will not be provided to the person without consulting them
- making decisions about a person's 'best interests' without consulting them
- using language and terminology that alienates or excludes the person experiencing symptoms of mental illness (Beckett et al., 2017).

Instead, health professionals must self-examine and reflect on their personal attitudes towards, or perceptions of, people with mental health problems. This process of self-examination and reflection must include consideration of the value placed by people with mental illness on respectful and inclusive approaches to care (Priddis & Rogers, 2018). Such approaches include:

- considering the unique situation of each consumer
- being aware of the insidious, even seductive nature of the power that health professionals can wield over vulnerable people
- adapting and adjusting professional responses to people with a mental illness based on the person's individual needs and preferences.

Health professionals may ask themselves as they reflect, 'How do I view people with a mental illness?' and 'How do these attitudes and perceptions impact my professional practice?' Answering these questions honestly will assist the health professional in becoming a practitioner with high levels of self-awareness.

Indeed, fostering self-awareness is necessary for all health professionals. It is only through self-awareness that health professionals can address issues that may impede their capacity to:

- build and maintain an effective therapeutic alliance or relationship
- collaborate with consumers and their carers or families
- support the development of coping strategies for people with mental health issues
- facilitate the Recovery journey and positive long-term outcomes for mental health consumers.

Reflective practice

Critical reflection is the examination of thoughts and actions. Health professionals can reflect on their practice by focusing on how they interact with their colleagues and their work environment. Reflective practice is a process by which health professionals can develop higher levels of self-awareness, build on their strengths, focus on areas of development and take action to change the future. Health professionals from different disciplines participate in reflective practice, including allied health professionals, first responders, medical practitioners, midwives and nurses (Delport et al., 2018; Priddis & Rogers, 2018).

QUESTIONS

1. Reflection-in-action involves considering events that have occurred in the past. Identify an event you were a part of where a person with a mental illness was stigmatised. What could you have done differently?
2. Reflection-in-action involves considering events, including your own behaviour(s) and the behaviour of others, as they occur. As a health professional, what techniques could you use to develop reflection-in-action?
3. Critical reflection involves uncovering our assumptions about ourselves, other people and the workplace. What techniques could you use to critically reflect on your assumptions and attitudes towards people with a mental illness?

1.3 A focus on caring

LEARNING OBJECTIVE 1.3 Explain the notions of 'care' and 'trauma-informed care'.

In a context characterised by negative attitudes towards people with a mental illness, what does it mean for a health professional to 'care'? With the advancements made in science and technology, as well as research and evidence-based practice, is 'caring' still relevant to the delivery of health services today? These are important questions for health professionals working in settings that seem to place more emphasis on meeting **key performance indicators** (**KPIs**) and collecting **empirical data** to inform **evidence-based practice**, than on care and caring (Jeffs et al., 2018).

Interestingly, precise definitions of the terms 'care' and 'caring' are lacking in the health context. For example, care is both a noun and a verb — it is a feeling or attitude, such as concern, and it involves action or activity, such as attending to a person. This means that care and caring can be understood as both a way of being and a way of behaving (Ray, 2019).

The lack of precise definitions also results from the presumptions that understanding the notion of caring 'comes naturally' to health professionals (Freshwater et al., 2017). For example, by choosing to work in the field of health, a health professional may be described as a caring person. However, the nature of health care in the twenty-first century means that health professionals will practise, intervene, treat, manage, assist and support, engage in therapy or deliver a service (Ackerman, 2019). Efficiency and effectiveness are the names of the game. This raises the question, where do care and caring fit? Answers to this question lie partly in the history of caring.

History of caring

Different disciplines have developed different knowledge bases to explain what it means to provide care. For example, nurses have a long tradition of providing care, developed from the work undertaken as far back as Florence Nightingale in the mid 1800s. Caring theorists Peplau (1952, 1991) and, more recently, Leininger (1981), Watson (1988), Barker (2004), and Sitzman and Watson (2018) have built on this work, describing the notion of caring as both a science and an art; that is, caring comprises a set of evidence-based technical skills as well as personal qualities such as sensitivity, giving respect and accepting others.

From a multidisciplinary perspective, the seminal philosopher Heidegger (1962) described 'caring' as a **universal phenomenon** that influences the way people think, feel and behave. Almost 30 years later in the health context, Morse and colleagues (1991) went on to suggest five categories of caring:
1. a human trait
2. a **moral imperative**
3. an effect or outcome

4. an interpersonal interaction
5. a therapeutic intervention.

Caring is much more than demonstrating concern for a person or even attending to that person. Caring involves knowledge, thinking, planning, implementation and evidence of effectiveness. At the same time, the categories of interpersonal interaction and therapeutic intervention suggest that caring has a personal focus.

These ideas were highlighted by Watson (1988), a nursing theorist who conceptualised care and caring as an interpersonal process between two people that protects, enhances and preserves the person's dignity, and enables the survival, development and growth of all those involved. Caring, then, is a construct that is both theoretical and practical, as well as procedural and personal.

The differences noted by Leininger (1981) between general or generic caring and professional caring are particularly important. General or **generic caring** is learned as part of a person's ongoing growth and development, through upbringing, family background, cultural values and life experiences. **Professional caring** has a more conscious and comprehensive focus, and encompasses each dimension of personhood. For example, health professionals care for a person's physical and mental health, and social, spiritual and emotional wellbeing.

Over the years, other researchers have supported this view. While feelings of concern and the act of attending to a person hold a central place in the delivery of health services, they are unlikely to be therapeutic unless the person providing the care is competent or proficient (Chambers, 2017; Leininger, 2012; Walker, 2017). For health professionals, health care and caring involves specific knowledge, skills, attitudes and actions, with proficient and professional care and caring having a context and purpose to support better health outcomes for all.

Definitions of 'care' and 'trauma-informed care'

In light of the history, context and purposes of delivering health care, in this text, the terms 'care' and 'caring' are understood as a collaborative process between health professionals and a person or persons to achieve mutually agreed objectives. Health services deliver care and caring systematically to support people and improve health outcomes. Care and caring are also attitudes and sets of actions demonstrated by competent health professionals in their work (Tierney et al., 2017). The best **health care** and caring is consumer-centred and person-focused; it is delivered according to each person's individual needs, preferences and choices (Australian Commission on Safety and Quality in Health Care [ACSQHC] 2019a).

Interestingly, research has identified a marked difference between the activities that consumers identify as the most important to them when they receive care, and the caring activities health professionals identify as the most important to consumers (Habib et al., 2019; Roberts et al., 2019). For example, consumers often report that they remember the kindness exhibited by a health professional, while health professionals focus on providing effective clinical interventions as efficiently as possible. Such differences suggest health professionals must always allow consumers to express their preferences and make their own choices, negotiating care in a process that involves caring *with* and caring *for* the person (Ackerman, 2019).

Trauma-informed care

According to the Australian Institute of Health and Welfare (AIHW) (2020c):
- 57–75 per cent of Australians will experience a potentially traumatic event at some point in their lives
- 62–68 per cent of young people will have been exposed to at least one traumatic event by the age of 17
- 2 per cent of Australians experience PTSD in their life (lifetime prevalence), with women being at almost twice the risk of men (15.8 per cent and 8.6 per cent respectively)
- 1.7 per cent of women and 1.3 per cent of men reported that they had been told by a doctor, nurse or health professional that they have PTSD.

Trauma exposure is more common among specific groups such as:
- people who experience homelessness
- young people in out-of-home care or under youth justice supervision
- refugees
- women and children experiencing family and domestic violence
- LGBTQIA+ people
- Aboriginal and Torres Strait Islander peoples
- certain occupation groups (e.g., emergency services, defence personnel and veterans).

In addition to this, historical and current trauma experience resulting from separation from family, land and cultural identity, has seriously impacted the social and emotional wellbeing of Aboriginal and Torres Strait Islander peoples.

Trauma usually results from a single event and/or a series of events over a period of time, including childhood abuse, interpersonal violence at any age, the experience of an accident or natural disaster, and/or experiencing distressing or terrifying events in war zones, military campaigns, emergency services work or police work (Cleary & Hungerford, 2015). Such traumatic events and experiences can impact a person physically, psychologically, emotionally, interpersonally, culturally, spiritually as well as other aspects of what it means to be a person (Hales et al., 2019). Physiologically, these experiences give rise to autonomic nervous system responses which, depending on numerous factors, can result in mental health problems such as flashbacks, heightened arousal (e.g. sleep difficulties and irritability) and avoidance of the stimuli that they associate with the trauma (Chang et al., 2021; Regan, 2020).

Past traumatic experiences can affect how a person engages with health professionals or the services offered (Middleton et al., 2019). For example, some health settings may perpetuate the trauma or reignite the physiological responses related to the trauma for the person seeking help, creating barriers to the person receiving care.

In response to this, trauma-informed care has become a widely accepted strengths-based approach that supports health professionals in delivering health services that support people who have been affected by trauma (Adams Hillard, 2019). According to the Mental Health Coordinating Council (n.d.), trauma-informed care is 'a strengths-based framework that is responsive to the impact of trauma, emphasising physical, psychological and emotional safety for both service providers and survivors; and creates opportunities for survivors to rebuild a sense of control and empowerment'.

Trauma-informed care involves shifting of the focus from 'labelling' or 'pathologising' to enabling the health professional and the person to articulate their concerns and overcome the challenges as they present themselves (Bailey et al., 2019).

While organisations can implement policies and procedures to ensure the services they provide are trauma-informed, health professionals often struggle to know what is meant by trauma-informed care. This is because trauma-informed care is principles based, involving:
- understanding trauma and the effect it can have on people
- recognising the signs of trauma in people and responding accordingly
- making sure the person in need of help is and feels safe, and will not be re-traumatised from their current experiences accessing health services
- focusing on the interpersonal relationship with the person and building trust
- collaborating with and advocating for the person and helping them to feel that they have choices
- inspiring hope and supporting recovery for the person
- empowering the person to access a range of services (Complex Trauma WA, 2022).

Trauma-informed care, then, is the care given to a person, by a health professional, that is informed by an understanding that trauma — whatever that traumatic experience may have been — will affect how the person acts and reacts (Bailey et al., 2019).

In mental health settings, trauma-informed approaches are critical. Nine out of ten people with symptoms of mental illness or who misuse substances and access services have experienced a traumatic event at one stage or another. Moreover, two out of three people presenting at emergency, inpatient or outpatient mental health settings have experienced underlying complex trauma secondary to childhood physical or sexual abuse (Agency for Clinical Innovation, 2019). These links between mental illness and trauma suggest the need for trauma-informed care when supporting people with mental health issues (Niimura et al., 2019).

While trauma-informed care is principles based, it also involves **competencies** that the health professional must learn. These competencies include specific knowledge, clinical skills and communication skills to:
- engage with the person
- actively listen to the person
- build a relationship with the person.

Further, trauma-informed care requires health professionals to demonstrate compassion and sensitivity, a giving of self, as well as honesty and sincerity (Brown & Bright, 2017). While some of these attributes are personal, health professionals must nevertheless take the practical steps needed to develop these competencies, so that they can provide trauma-informed care regardless of the situation. Remember, when competent care and caring are delivered and people connect to and with one another, the health outcomes will speak for themselves (Fagerström, 2021).

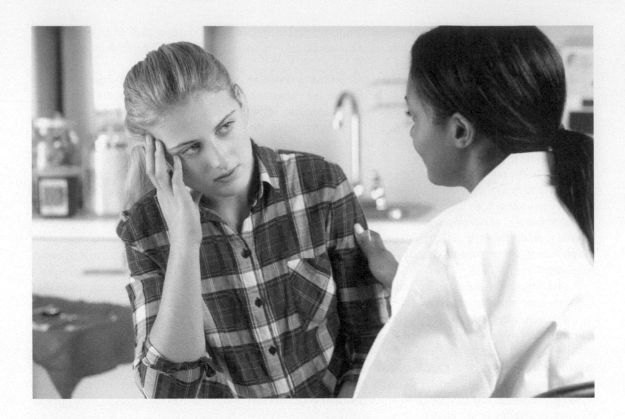

Aims of care and trauma-informed care

Broadly speaking, health care and health services aim to improve health outcomes (World Health Organization [WHO], 1986). Another aim of health services in Australia is to ensure consumer participation (ACSQHC, 2019a). This aim aligns with the national strategic direction for mental health services (Department of Health, 2015) and the growing influence of the consumer movement (Consumers Health Forum of Australia [CHF], 2019).

Care and caring in the professional sense will always be influenced by their delivery aims, which will depend upon the context of the care and caring. The health care context is complex and comprises many relational and environmental factors (Jangland et al., 2018). This includes the structures and settings created by organisations that provide services, the type of service delivery, the knowledge base and approach of the health professional providing the service, together with the needs and preferences of the person(s) receiving the care.

In turn, each of these contextual aspects is multifaceted. For example, the context of the individual receiving care comprises the multiple aspects of what it means to be a person. For this reason, health professionals must change or adapt their practice to meet the specific needs and preferences of the individuals they support. There is no **one-size-fits-all approach** to the delivery of care. Instead, the type of care delivered must be flexible enough to fit the needs and preferences of the person it serves.

UPON REFLECTION

The effects of childhood trauma

People with complex histories of childhood abuse, neglect, or insecure attachment commonly exhibit behavioural patterns, such as substance misuse, dissociation, intentional self-injury, risky or compulsive sexual behaviours, food bingeing and purging, compulsive gambling, compulsive shoplifting, reaction aggression, thrill- or sensation-seeking behaviours, compulsive skin picking and hair pulling, fire-setting or extensive preoccupation with internet activities (Briere, 2019, pp.7–8)

Health professionals must understand the correlations between complex trauma and self-destructive behaviours to minimise the risk of stigmatising or 'labelling' the person, and reducing the person's risk of harm or risk of entering the criminal justice system. Understanding such correlations will enable health professionals to give the person the best possible support and care.

1.4 Caring in the health context

LEARNING OBJECTIVE 1.4 Discuss the context of care in Australia.

Multiple historical factors have shaped the current context of mental health care in Australia. In early colonial times, people with a mental illness were locked away from the community in 'lunatic' asylums. The first 'mental institution' in Australia was located at Castle Hill, New South Wales, from 1811 to 1825 (Raeburn et al., 2018). Before this, 'the insane' were housed at either Parramatta Gaol or, in some cases, Bedlam Point at Gladesville. In the years that followed, other asylums were established in each of the new colonies around Australia (Vrklevski et al., 2017).

Over the years, endeavours were made to improve humane treatment, with numerous commissions and inquiries into the reported abuses. Even so, overcrowding in institutions across Australia meant that a predominantly custodial approach was taken to care of those who were 'committed' (Sutton, 2017). Moreover, the limited treatment options provided were mostly physical, including straitjackets and cold baths (Raeburn et al., 2018).

After the Second World War, scientific advancement gave rise to new pharmacological interventions that enabled better outcomes for people with a mental illness (Kassianos, 2016). In turn, with improved knowledge and better outcomes came changes to how people and societies viewed mental health and mental illness. Such perceptions included recognising that people with mental health issues had the right to live freely in the community, and that the previously common practice of locking people away from mainstream society with no right of reply was unethical.

In response, Western governments began to examine how health care was delivered to people with a mental illness. In Australia, the inquiries and reports that were most influential in questioning the ethics and practices of the day included the:

- Richmond Report (1983)
- Barclay Report (1988)
- Burdekin, Guilfoyle and Hall Report (1993).

Detailed information about these reports can be found on the websites of relevant state and territory health departments, or the University of Sydney Index of Australian Parliamentary Reports.

The implementation of recommendations made by these and similar reports and inquiries gave rise to considerable changes to how mental health care was delivered in Australia (Richmond, 1983). These changes have included:

- the **deinstitutionalisation** of mental health services
- a decrease in the size and number of psychiatric hospitals
- the separation of developmental disability services from mental health services
- support for consumers to live in the community
- the development and expansion of **integrated community services** or networks, including health services, accommodation services and other social services
- changes in funding arrangements to support the new era in mental health service delivery (Milton & Garton, 2017).

The process of deinstitutionalisation also saw the development and implementation of new mental health legislation in each of the Australian states and territories. While there are clear differences in how this legislation is enacted, the fundamental principles are the same. These principles include:

- protecting the human rights of people with mental health problems
- guarding the safety of people with mental health problems, and the safety of the community
- ensuring that people with mental health problems are treated in the least restrictive environment
- promoting individual choice of lifestyle for consumers.

By upholding these principles, health professionals will effectively support the spirit of the legislation, regardless of location.

In addition to mental health legislation, each state and territory developed its own legal frameworks to protect the rights of people with disabilities. This legislation was distinct from mental health legislation, but reflected many of the same principles. With the passing of the *National Disability Insurance Scheme (NDIS) Act* in 2013, followed by the roll-out of the NDIS nationally, there has been an increasing cross-over in the services and/or funding that people with a mental illness and/or a disability can access. The health services available for people with both mental illness and intellectual disability are outlined in the chapter focusing on mental health service delivery. Health professionals are encouraged to seek out information on this critical aspect of health service delivery, especially as people with a disability have a higher incidence of mental illness than the general population.

In addition, the advent of deinstitutionalisation saw the development and implementation of new approaches to delivering care and treatment to people with mental illness and/or a disability. For example, **mainstreaming** was introduced to reduce the health inequalities and stigma experienced by people with mental health issues. Today, people who present to health services with symptoms of mental illness are no longer sent to separate campuses at 'other' locations. Instead, mental health services have been integrated into the mainstream health system (AIHW, 2022a; Atkinson et al., 2018).

Not only that, the traditional custodial function of those who treated or cared for people with mental health issues has now been replaced by a therapeutic function. Today, it is the role of health professionals to enable consumers to live in the community as contributing members of that community. To do this, health professionals work with government departments and agencies, such as social and housing services, to facilitate comprehensive, integrated, trauma-informed care that addresses all aspects of the person's life (Benjamin et al., 2019).

The evolution of current policy directions

At the national and state or territory levels, mental health policy in Australia has developed over time and in response to the United Nations and the **World Health Organization (WHO)** directives. Also important has been the ongoing lobbying of governments by human rights groups and members of the consumer movement.

In 1991, the United Nations (UN) established the *Principles for the Protection of Persons with Mental Illness and the Improvement of Mental Health Care*. This document commences with a statement upholding the fundamental freedoms and basic rights of those who experience symptoms of mental illness. The remaining 24 principles guide how these freedoms and rights are upheld. They include enabling people with mental health problems to live in the community, and ensuring that care is readily accessible, has the least number of restrictions on the person's freedom and rights, and is appropriate for the person's specific needs and preferences.

In 2009, Australia was reviewed by the UN Special Rapporteur for its human rights performance, as part of a regular process for all UN member states. The Human Rights Council made over a hundred recommendations to the Australian government for change, including how people with mental illness were treated. For example, the UN recommended that the Australian Government:

- allocate adequate resources for mental health services and other support measures for persons with mental health problems, in line with the UN *Principles for the Protection of Persons with Mental Illness and the Improvement of Mental Health Care*
- reduce the high rate of incarceration of people with mental illness
- ensure that all prisoners receive adequate and appropriate mental health treatment when needed (Parliament of Australia, 2006).

Today, many of these recommendations have been implemented so that Australia delivers mental health services better aligned with the framework provided by the UN.

No less important is the guidance provided by WHO at the turn of the century, including the recommendation that all mental health policies are anchored by the following four guiding principles:

1. access
2. equity
3. effectiveness
4. efficiency (WHO, 2001).

Services that are accessible allow people to seek treatment sooner rather than later. In Australia, providing accessible and equitable services can be challenging when considering the population's cultural and linguistic diversity, together with the vast distances between rural and remote communities (Arat et al., 2019; Enticott et al., 2018). Even so, access and equity remain two of several cornerstones of mental health service delivery in Australia today. Indeed, Australians pride themselves on the fact that quality mental health services are universally made available to all, regardless of distance, cultural background, religion or ability of the person to pay (Fisher et al., 2017).

Likewise, the Australian Government is committed to supporting the delivery of appropriate, timely, effective and efficient mental health care that aligns with the best available, contemporary, evidence-based research (Department of Health, 2019). Services are comprehensive, integrated and facilitate the timely treatment of those needing help (National Mental Health Commission, 2017). As with access and equity, effectiveness and efficiency are core tenets that guide the delivery of all health services in Australia, including mental health services.

Since the early 1990s, the national and state or territory governments have developed numerous mental health strategies, plans and policies to reflect UN and WHO principles and recommendations. For example, the National Mental Health Strategy provides direction to state and territory governments across Australia to improve the quality of life of people living with symptoms of mental illness. This Strategy was first endorsed in April 1992 by the Australian Health Ministers' Conference (1992a, 1992b) as a framework to guide mental health reform.

According to the Department of Health website (www.health.gov.au), the National Mental Health Strategy aims to:
- promote the mental health of the Australian community
- prevent the development of mental health problems
- reduce the impact of mental health problems on individuals, families and the community
- assure the rights of people with a mental illness.

Milestones for developing the National Mental Health Strategy are outlined in the various documents that mark the evolution of the Strategy. These include the:
- National Mental Health Policy (1992, 2008)
- National Mental Health Plan(s) (1992–1997, 1998–2003, 2003–2008, 2009–2014, 2017–2022)
- National Mental Health Standards (2010)
- Mental Health: Statements of Rights and Responsibilities (1991, 2012)
- E-Mental Health Strategy for Australia (2012)
- National Roadmap for National Mental Health Reform (2012–2022)
- Establishment of the National Mental Health Commission (2012)
- Contributing Lives, Thriving Communities — Report of the National Review of Mental Health Programmes and Services (2014)
- Australian health care agreements.

The National Mental Health Strategy and ongoing developments are significant for all health professionals across Australia. All health professionals are responsible for familiarising themselves with and abiding by the principles and policies outlined in the Strategy. An A–Z listing of mental health publications to support health professionals in this work is available on the national Department of Health website (www.health.gov.au).

UPON REFLECTION

Australia's E-Mental Health Strategy

Australia's national E-Mental Health Strategy was established in 2012 to help embed e-mental health into the primary mental health care system. The progress made was hastened by the isolation of people in Australia during the COVID-19 pandemic in 2020–2021, including the development of digital mental health services online (via desktops, mobile devices and apps) or phones (via calls or texts). Today, digital services include:
- crisis support and counselling for those with mental health problems
- telehealth, enabling people to access medical or other consultations, assessment and treatment, including electronic prescriptions
- recovery support and staying connected with other people (Australian Digital Health Agency, 2022).

Many of the digital services commenced during the pandemic lockdowns continued afterwards due to the benefits experienced by consumers, including high levels of accessibility and convenience.

QUESTIONS

1. What do you see as the benefits of digital health services?
2. What do you see are the challenges of digital health services?

▶

Current service frameworks

There is a need for health professionals to understand the frameworks within which they provide health care. Such understanding enables health professionals to see the high-level impact of their everyday work. This section provides a brief overview of the principles that guide health care delivery in Australia. The information will help health professionals to contextualise the information provided throughout this text.

The overarching framework within which health care is delivered to people with mental health issues in Australia is the same as that which guides all health care and treatment. This framework is called the **public health framework** or approach.

Public health framework

'**Public health**' relates to the population as a whole. This term is not to be confused with the **public health care system**, which, in Australia, includes Medicare funding that supports the government's **universal health coverage** for all Australians and permanent residents. Instead, by examining the health trends in populations, communities or groups, and recommending or overseeing appropriate interventions, the public health framework in Australia aims to:

- prevent disease
- promote good health practices
- prolong life.

Public health includes epidemiology, the study of patterns of health and illness in populations or groups, which involves statistical analysis of data generated to provide an evidence base that shapes strategic direction (Centers for Disease Control and Prevention, 2016). Some health professionals would know this approach as 'population health', which identifies groups of people that are particularly vulnerable to health issues because of their demographic characteristics (e.g. age or cultural background) or past experiences (e.g. exposure to trauma or abuse) (AIHW, 2021a). For example, the statistics cited earlier about the mental health status of the Australian population, fall into the population health category and provide a basis upon which Australian governments develop strategic direction and shape services (e.g. the Fifth National Mental Health and Suicide Prevention Plan, 2017–2022). The public health framework also incorporates services such as prevention and promotion, environmental health, occupational health and safety services, and other services that enable self-determination, self-care and self-help for all communities and people. These services form an integral part of the Australian primary health care agenda.

Primary health care agenda

Primary health care is an integral part of the public health framework. The WHO defines primary health care:

> Essential health care made universally accessible to individuals and families in the community by means acceptable to them, through their full participation and at a cost that the community and country can afford. It forms an integral part both of the country's health system of which it is the nucleus and of the overall social and economic development of the community (WHO, 1978).

Primary health care is essential care because it supports people, families and communities (AIHW, 2019a). It focuses on physical, mental and social wellbeing. It is people-centred rather than disease-centred (WHO, 2019), concentrating on health rather than illness, prevention rather than cure and communities rather than hospitals.

An essential aspect of all the primary health care services in Australia is the delivery of resources and information to promote healthy lifestyles within communities, by communities and to support communities (Randall & Crawford, 2018). Other areas of attention include equity in health care; research-based methods; accessible, acceptable and affordable technology; promotion of health; prevention of illness; early intervention; and continuity of care. In short, primary health care is 'community-centric'.

Primary care — a subset of primary health care — is accessible, affordable and enables people or groups to participate individually and/or collectively in the planning and implementation of their health care (Henderson et al., 2018). Australia has tended to position 'primary care' within the biomedical model and the domain of GPs who operate small businesses in the community. Consequently, the term is often construed as the 'first point of contact' in the health care system (Hills et al., 2019). However, primary care is much bigger than this. All health professionals can provide primary care, regardless of setting, because this type of care enables them to:

- acknowledge diversity in the culture, values and belief systems of the person while promoting their dignity as a person and right to self-determine
- establish collaborative partnerships with the person, together with their family or significant others, ensuring open channels of communication and active participation in all aspects of their care
- engage therapeutically with the person, together with their family or significant others, in a way that is respectful of the person's choices, experiences and circumstances; building on the strengths of the person, enhancing the person's resilience and promoting health and wellness
- collaboratively plan and provide health care options to the person (including the coordination of these options) and ascertain that these options are consistent with the person's mental, physical, spiritual, emotional, social, cultural, functional and other needs
- actively value the contributions of other health professionals, health services, agencies and stakeholders, ensuring the collaborative and coordinated delivery of holistic or comprehensive evidence-based health care
- pursue opportunities to participate in health promotion and illness prevention activities with and for the person, including health education and support of social inclusion and community participation (WHO, 2019).

It is easy for health professionals to overlook the essential role played by primary health care services, such as prevention and promotion services, because these services tend to be staffed by the 'unsung heroes' who work behind the scenes. Similarly, health professionals who work as first responders or in busy **secondary health care** and **tertiary health care** sectors may lack understanding of the critical and ongoing health-related work carried out by non-government or community-managed organisations, or small medical or allied health practices. Although primary health services do not ordinarily provide emergency or acute services, they are a necessary means by which people, especially those with mental health issues, are supported to live meaningfully in the community. More information about the primary health care agenda, primary care and the primary health care services that are delivered in Australia is provided in the chapter that focuses on mental health service delivery.

Current service approaches

All health systems will take a particular approach to how they deliver their services, with different approaches taken at the different levels of health care. For example, one approach may be used when providing a service to the individual and their family or carers, whereas a different approach may be used when supporting communities as a whole. The best approach to take will depend on many factors, including infrastructure, service linkages, workforce and other resources (Sayers et al., 2017).

In Australia, the national government has identified person-centred and family-centred care as the first principle for guiding health care delivery (ACSQHC, 2019b). These approaches to care are responsive to the individual differences and preferences of care recipients. The approaches involve health professionals focusing on the needs, preferences and aspirations of people as individuals; together with the needs, preferences and aspirations of the families who support these individuals, in the process of planning and delivering care (Dowrick, 2017; Lukersmith et al., 2017). Person-centred and family-centred care are partly achieved by facilitating a range of service options or health care choices. For health professionals, the principles for delivering person-centred and family-centred care include being accessible and flexible, respecting the person and their significant others as someone who shares in the decision making around the health services they utilise, and ensuring health care is comprehensive and well-coordinated (McCormack & McCance, 2017).

Another common approach to care is the strengths-based approach. This approach focuses on the strengths of the person, their family or significant others, and their community. The approach features health professionals building on the abilities and resilience of the person, their family, and community (Kilcullen et al., 2018) and aims to assist the person (or community) to develop their strengths so they can self-manage their circumstances (Kiwanuka et al., 2019).

These approaches, however, have been developed by health professionals and tend to feature health professionals playing a central role in the process of service delivery. For example, it is the health professional who works to know the patient as a person; it is the health professional who is accessible and flexible to meet the needs of the person; it is the health professional who empowers the person. Essentially, these approaches maintain the position of the health professional at the centre of delivering health services. In so doing, such approaches maintain the health professional's position of power.

In contrast, consumer-centred approaches place the person with a health need at the centre of the care they receive (CHF, n.d.). **Consumer-centred care** is becoming an increasingly common approach by health services located in Western countries such as Australia (Happell et al., 2019). The participation of consumers and carers in the planning, development and delivery of mental health services is now an expectation of Australian governments at national and state or territory levels (Blignault et al., 2017; National Mental Health Commission, 2017). Consumer and carer participation in mental health service delivery is said to increase adherence to, and the effectiveness of treatment programs, facilitate consumer satisfaction and promote best-evidence practice (Cook et al., 2019; Minshal et al., 2021).

Consumer-centred approaches grew out of the 'patients' rights' movement in the United States, which was part of the wider civil rights movement of the late 1960s, that advocated for the rights of women, African Americans, people with diverse sexualities, and other minority groups. This rights' movement eventually gave rise to postmodern notions of multiple realities, including the varied individually con-structed meanings of experiences of health and ill-health (Davidson et al., 2021). Consequently, there are now several different consumer-centred approaches to delivering health care. At the heart of each of these approaches are the principles of consumer participation, with consumers involved with — even driving — the development of health services and treatment approaches, as well as the individual health care they receive (National Mental Health Commission, 2017). As noted by Deegan (1996, p. 92), an internationally renowned mental health consumer peer advocate and researcher who advocated strongly for consumer-centred care in the 1990s, 'those of us who have been diagnosed are not objects to be acted upon. We are fully human subjects who can act and in acting, change our situation'. Consumer-centred approaches, then, position the consumer as the person who determines how they respond to the challenges of their lives, not the health professional. Consumer-centred approaches are characterised by an active consumer rather than a passive patient, and health professionals act as co-workers in identifying and addressing the person's health needs.

Recovery

Derived from consumer-centred care, Recovery approaches position consumers as the experts in their own lived experience of mental illness who collaborate or work in partnership with health professionals to make choices about the health care they receive (De Ruysscher et al., 2019). Recovery for people with a mental illness involves a whole-of-life journey of transformation, as they move from a position of disempowerment to one of self-determination and autonomy, with health professionals enabling consumers to move beyond the challenges of their ill-health.

The Australian government is firmly committed to Recovery-oriented mental health services (Depart-ment of Health — Health Direct, 2019). This commitment is demonstrated in several ways, and includes the government's definition of Recovery:

> Recovery-oriented approaches recognise the value of this lived experience and bring it together with the expertise, knowledge and skills of mental health practitioners, many of whom have experienced mental health issues in their own lives or in their close relationships. Recovery approaches challenge traditional notions of professional power and expertise by helping to break down the conventional demarcation between consumers and staff. Within recovery paradigms all people are respected for the experience, expertise and strengths they contribute. Recovery-oriented approaches focus on the needs of the people who use services rather than on organisational priorities (Australian Health Ministers' Advisory Council, 2013, p. 10).

The Principles of Recovery focus upon the concepts of:
- acceptance, hope, optimism, individual strengths and wellness
- meaning and purpose for the person and their life
- personal growth, self-confidence, empowerment and agency.

In summary, Recovery is viewed as a process more than an outcome, a journey rather than a destination.

There has been frequent confusion about how to integrate Recovery approaches to care into the practice of health professionals (Rosen & O'Halloran, 2014). One reason for this confusion is the more traditional understanding of the term 'recovery' in the context of the biomedical model of treatment and its focus on 'cure'. Another reason is the challenge involved in fitting a truly consumer-centred approach into health service organisations that are, firstly, dominated by the biomedical model and, secondly, restricted by the demands of clinical governance (such as the publicly funded health system in Australia). This challenge presents hurdles for the health professionals who work in or for state-run health services in Australia.

According to Australia's *National Standards for Mental Health Services* (Department of Health, 2010), which guide how health professionals care for people with a mental illness, Recovery-oriented practice is guided by six principles:

1. the uniqueness of the individual
2. real choices
3. attitudes and rights
4. dignity and respect
5. partnership and communication
6. evaluating Recovery.

Each of these principles is now discussed in turn.

The uniqueness of the individual

The health professional recognises that Recovery is not necessarily about cure, but rather the opportunity for people who experience symptoms of mental illness to live a meaningful, satisfying and purposeful life as valued community members. The health professional accepts that the outcomes of Recovery-oriented health care are personal and unique for each person, going beyond an exclusive health focus to include an emphasis on quality of life and social inclusion. Finally, this principle involves the health professional supporting empowerment of the person, with that person recognising that they are at the centre of the care received (Sellin et al., 2018).

Real choices

Consumers are supported to make their own decisions about their treatments and how they live. Consumers are encouraged to make meaningful choices and develop their strengths. Health professionals must balance their duty of care with supporting the person to take positive risks and embrace new opportunities (Coffey et al., 2019).

Attitudes and rights

This principle promotes the health professional as someone who listens to, learns from and acts upon communications received from the consumer and their partners, families or friends about what is important to them. The health professional respects each person's legal, citizenship and human rights. Finally, the health professional supports each person to 'maintain and develop meaningful social, recreational, occupational and vocational activities'; and instils hope into the person's future and ability to live meaningfully (Scott et al., 2018).

Dignity and respect

The health professional is courteous, respectful and honest in all interactions with the consumer and their partners, families or friends. This principle requires health professionals to be sensitive and respectful when dealing with values, beliefs and cultures that are different to their own. Finally, the principle of dignity and respect involves the health professional challenging discrimination and stigma wherever it exists, whether in their organisation or the broader community (Lindgren et al., 2019).

Partnership and communication

The health professional acknowledges that the person who experiences symptoms of mental illness is an expert in their own life and that Recovery involves working in partnership with the consumer, their partner and/or family members to support them as they choose. In addition, health professionals value sharing relevant information, communicating clearly, and working in positive and realistic ways to help people realise their hopes, goals and aspirations (Jørgensen & Rendtorff, 2018).

Evaluating Recovery

The health professional supports the continuous evaluation of Recovery-oriented practice at all levels, including supporting the person to track their own progress in their Recovery journey; as well as reporting key outcomes of Recovery that include (without being limited to) the social determinants of health, such as education, employment, housing, and social and family relationships (Bakračevič et al., 2022; Department of Health, 2010; Isobel, 2019).

When six principles frame the mental health care received by the consumers, there is every chance Recovery will be achieved.

Working towards this end, however, is no easy task. As historically noted by Deegan (1996), health professionals cannot force Recovery to happen — instead, they must work to create an environment in which the Recovery process is nurtured. This work is challenging when considered in light of the gap that remains between Recovery-in-policy and Recovery-in-practice (John, 2017). Even so, with time and effort, Recovery as a journey of hope and optimism building on a person's strengths can be achieved by people with mental illness when supported by committed health professionals.

Indigenous Australians: trauma-informed, recovery-oriented approaches in emergencies

Many health professionals have identified challenges to taking a Recovery approach during emergency situations. Such challenges are particularly evident when working with Aboriginal and Torres Strait Islander peoples who have trauma experiences, including childhood, intergenerational and transgenerational trauma.

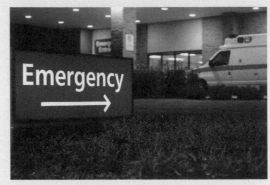

For example, Indigenous Australians are more likely to be brought into the Emergency Department (ED) of a hospital by emergency services personnel for mental health problems than non-Indigenous Australians (Australasian College for Emergency Medicine & Department of Policy, Research and Advocacy, 2018). Research also suggests that Indigenous Australian males with mental health issues are reluctant to use ambulance services for fear of being stigmatised (Ferguson et al., 2019). It is crucial, then, that those who work in the emergency services learn to work within trauma-informed, recovery-oriented frameworks when supporting Aboriginal and Torres Strait Islander peoples.

Take, for example, Shane, a 14-year-old Indigenous Australian living in an outer metropolitan area. He has a past history of childhood sexual abuse perpetrated by a community uncle when he was 9. The community uncle was arrested and incarcerated for five years, but has now returned to the community.

Shane was doing okay before the return of the uncle to the community. The reappearance of the uncle distressed Shane, so he decided to sit in the park with his friends. When they asked him if he was okay, he told them he felt ashamed and couldn't handle what was happening. He walked away. His friends wondered if they should call the emergency services for help, but they didn't want to make things worse for him. They followed him into a train station and were horrified when they saw him jump in front of a passing train.

When the emergency services personnel arrive, they found Shane's mother, Shane's friends and Indigenous Australlian community members on the scene. They were all upset and shouting. They blamed the legal system for allowing the uncle to return to the community and the emergency services personnel for being part of that system. They cried out that they could not get any support, and now Shane was dead.

QUESTIONS

1. What cultural considerations did the emergency services team need to consider when communicating with his mother and family members?
2. What trauma-informed, recovery-oriented approaches could be taken in this situation?
3. What short-term and long-term effects could this incident have on Shane's friends and the community?

1.5 The prevalence of mental illness in Australia

LEARNING OBJECTIVE 1.5 Outline the prevalence and impact of mental illness in Australia.

As noted earlier in this text, mental illness is one of Australia's leading contributors to the non-fatal burden of disease and injury in Australia (AIHW, 2019d). Mental illness is associated with increased exposure to health risk factors, higher rates of disability, poorer physical health and higher death rates (including suicide). Of concern, then, is that nearly 46 per cent of Australians aged between 16 and 85 years will experience a mental illness at some point in their lives, and one in five Australian adults will experience a mental illness in any given year (AIHW, 2020a). Figure 1.1 outlines the prevalence rates of anxiety, mood and substance use disorders across the lifespan in Australia. In particular, there are worrying trends for those aged 25–54 years, who are most likely to be raising families and working.

These statistics suggest Australia's widespread — even endemic — nature of mental illness. The statistics are even more worrying when considered in light of the effect of mental health problems on a person's ability to interact positively with their family members, friends, colleagues and/or the broader community. For example, people with mental health problems may find it more difficult to relate to others or maintain cohesive relationships. Further, mental illness has a financial cost. For example, the economic cost of serious mental illness in Australia, including opioid dependence, has been estimated at almost $100 billion annually, including losses in productivity and labour force participation (Royal Australian and New Zealand College of Psychiatrists, 2016). Additionally, the leading cause of the loss of healthy years of life due to disability has been identified as mental illness (Doran & Kinchin, 2019).

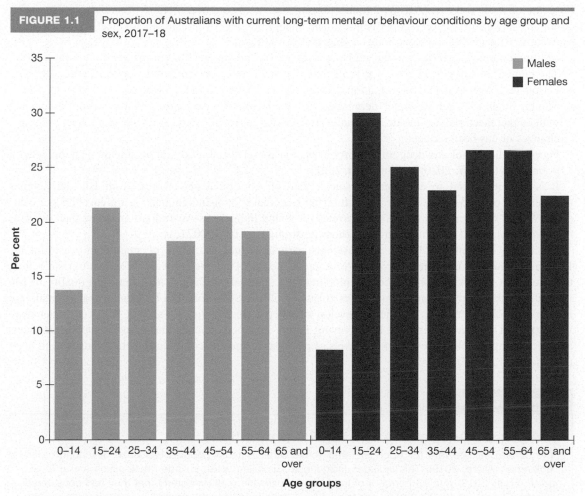

FIGURE 1.1 Proportion of Australians with current long-term mental or behaviour conditions by age group and sex, 2017–18

Note: Refers to individuals who reported having a current medical condition (at the time of interview) that has lasted, or is expected to last, for 6 months or more, unless otherwise stated.
Source: Australian Institute of Health and Welfare (2020a).

The prevalence of mental illness across Australia is an important motivating factor for health professionals to learn about the issues involved, and integrate quality mental health care into their everyday practice. Such motivation can be underscored by the many people currently seeing health professionals for a physical health problem who have mental health issues that have not yet been identified.

Indeed, there has been an increase in the number of people in Australia with physical illnesses or injuries who also have mental health problems. This means a large number of people who are seen by paramedics or who arrive at or are admitted to a hospital to be treated for a physical health problem will be experiencing symptoms of mental illness (Emond et al., 2019). Moreover, people in hospital or who have been recently discharged from hospital may go on to develop mental health issues. Of particular concern are those with a chronic physical illness (such as heart disease, stroke, cancer, diabetes, chronic pain), as they are more likely than those who are physically well to develop depression, anxiety or other forms of psychological distress (Hills et al., 2019). Research suggests that a substantial proportion of these people receive no treatment or interventions for their mental health problems (Parrish, 2018), indicating that health professionals are either not identifying mental health issues in the person with a chronic illness or they are unable to provide the care required (Young, 2018).

Prevalence of suicide in Australia

Suicide and other self-harming behaviours are discussed in detail in the chapter on caring for a person who has self-harmed. In this text, the prevalence of suicide in Australia is briefly reviewed as a means to introduce readers to this significant public health issue and establish a platform for further reading.

Suicide was the leading cause of death among people aged 15–44 in 2016–2018 (AIHW, 2020d). Over three-quarters of these deaths were males, with men aged between 40 and 44, 55 and 59, and over 85 years of most concern (AIHW, 2020d). Overall, the most common method of suicide was hanging, strangulation or suffocation (63 per cent of male and 49 per cent of female suicide deaths), followed by poisoning by drugs (8.2 per cent males and 29 per cent females).

Common themes derived from the statistics related to suicide include the following.

- The number of suicides in 2018 was more than two and a half times that of the national road toll.
- People with a previous history of attempted suicide are at greatest risk of suicide.
- Mental illnesses (such as major depression, psychotic illnesses and eating disorders) are associated with an increased risk of suicide, especially after discharge from hospital and when a treatment regimen changes or has been reduced.
- People with alcohol and drug misuse problems have a higher risk of dying by suicide than the general population (AIHW, 2020; Life in Mind, 2022).

It is also important to consider the suicide rate of Aboriginal and Torres Strait Islander peoples (5.5 per cent of all deaths), which is much higher than that of non-Indigenous Australians (1.9 per cent) (AIHW, 2022b). Significantly, the suicide rates for young Indigenous Australians are more than twice as high when compared to young non-Indigenous Australians (AIHW, 2021c).

Much can be done by health professionals to help reduce the rates of suicide in Australia for Indigenous and non-Indigenous groups. Preventative measures include early identification of risk factors; together with the promotion of social, emotional and spiritual wellbeing, and improved quality of life for individuals, families and communities (Cousins, 2017; Snowdon, 2017). Health professionals are in a prime position to help people to develop stronger protective factors so that they can better cope with stress. This can be achieved by involving family members, friends and relevant support services, and supporting people to develop high levels of personal resilience, community connectedness and hope (Hatcher et al., 2017).

UPON REFLECTION

Indigenous Australians and suicide prevention

The current suicide rate for Aboriginal and Torres Strait Islander peoples has been described as an 'epidemic' (Allam, 2019). This includes Indigenous Australian youth suicide rates, which are at 'crisis point' (Fryer, 2019) with 23 per cent of Indigenous Australian youth reporting that they had considered suicide (Skerrett et al., 2018). The risk factors for suicide in Indigenous Australian youth include racism, disadvantage and other social determinants of health. In Indigenous communities more broadly, there are many reports of intergenerational trauma, alongside feelings of disconnection to community and/or from Country (Wilson et al., 2018). Young Indigenous Australians who engage in self-harm practices, such as the misuse of substances, are at an even higher risk of suicide attempts (Kilian & Williamson, 2018). In some locations, suicide prevention shop fronts have been established, where Indigenous Australians can talk to a mental health professional or participate in group leisure activities. These services are open after-hours and are free of charge.

....

QUESTIONS

1. Aboriginal and Torres Strait Islander Elders can support community-driven responses, including suicide prevention initiatives, to youth suicide. Identify three reasons why the influence of Elders is so important in Indigenous communities.
2. What are the benefits and challenges to pop-up shop fronts that provide mental health services to Indigenous Australian communities?

Issues for young people

Adolescence is a time of great physical, emotional and social change. It is a time of life that brings with it new, adult-like challenges and associated stresses. How a young person reacts to stress will affect their ability to cope with life (Vohra et al., 2019). This is why it is crucial to support young people to develop personal coping skills and to become aware of how they may be affected by stress (Yoo, 2019). Stress can be a positive factor because it can motivate people and groups into action (see the chapter on common reactions to stressful situations for further information). Stress can also have a negative impact on people, especially young people who are already feeling insecure, confused or anxious. This, in turn, can give rise to mental health issues for the young person.

According to Mission Australia (Mission Australia, 2021) and the AIHW (2021b), one in four young people living in Australia have experienced mental health problems, with some expressing a reluctance to seek professional help. Anxiety disorders are the most commonly reported issues (7 per cent), followed by Attention Deficit Hyperactivity Disorder (ADHD) (just over 6 per cent), then major depressive disorder (5 per cent) (AIHW, 2020e). To compound this, around 11 per cent of adolescents (12–17 years) deliberately hurt or injure themselves (AIHW, 2020e). During the COVID-19 pandemic, the level of psychological distress in young people increased, with over one-third of Australian youth reporting high or very high levels of psychological distress (headspace, 2021).

While the prevalence of mental illness is relatively high in young people, they have a relatively low use of mental health services (MacDonald et al., 2018). For example, adolescents aged 13–17 years seeking services was around 30 per cent, with this percentage slightly higher for those with suicidality (Islam et al., 2020). Over half the young peoples accessed online services the most, while over half of parents sought help from health services, such as general practitioners and psychologists (Islam et al., 2020). Young people with a substance use disorder are the least likely to use mental health services (Orygen, 2016).

The main reason for this lack of utilisation of services is that most young people (85 per cent) do not feel the need to seek help (Calear et al., 2017). Another reason is that the current mental health system is not adequately resourced to deal with young people who have mild-to-moderate mental health issues (McGorry et al., 2022). As a consequence, young people may have difficulty finding a service that can meet their needs or preferences. This is concerning because it means young people are not receiving the support or health care they need.

There is a pressing need, then, for health professionals from across the disciplines to know what services are available and how these services can be accessed. Advising young people and their families of these services is crucial. Young people with mental health problems are more likely to experience issues with their physical wellbeing and educational, psychological and social development (Kirk & Hinton, 2019). In contrast, when the early signs of mental health issues are identified and addressed, outcomes for the young person are improved. More information about the early intervention strategies currently used to help young people with mental health problems, together with the services that are available for young people in Australia, are discussed in the chapter on mental health service delivery.

IN PRACTICE

Online mental health services for young people

Over the past two decades, there has been a massive growth in online mental health services for young people, including helplines, discussion forums, and online programs. These services are primary health services, as they are easily accessible by anyone without an assessment or referral from a health professional. They can be beneficial for young people who don't feel comfortable talking to people they know or face-to-face.

Examples of helplines for young people in Australia include Kids Helpline (1800 55 1800), Beyond Blue (1300 22 4636), and headspace (1800 650 890).

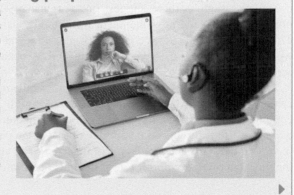

Examples of online counselling support, including chats, are: Counselling Online (https://counsellingonline.org.au); headspace (https://headspace.org.au); the Butterfly Foundation (https://thebutterflyfoundation.org.au) for people with eating disorders; and QLife (https://qlife.org.au) for LGBTQIA+ people.

Examples of online forums are Beyond Blue (www.beyondblue.org.au/get-support/online-forums) and Reach Out (https://au.reachout.com)

Websites with comprehensive information about mental health and the mental health problems experienced by young people are also provided by Reach Out (https://au.reachout.com), Kids Helpline (https://kidshelpline.com.au), headspace (https://headspace.org.au), and Emerging Minds (https://emergingminds.com.au) and Children of Parents with a Mental Illness (https://copmi.net.au).

Online programs and apps include Bite Back (https://biteback.org.au), Brave Program (https://brave4you.psy.uq.edu.au), and MoodGYM (https://moodgym.com.au).

Awareness of these services is essential for health professionals, who can then recommend the services to parents or young people with mental health problems.

For instance, consider the situation of Eric, a 15-year-old high school student. Eric is an only child with a Chinese background. He is also a high academic performer.

One day at school, Eric feels like he can't breathe, and the world is closing in on him. He feels scared by what is happening to him.

But Eric feels even more scared to tell his teachers in case they tell his parents. His parents moved to Australia to give Eric more opportunities, and they expect him to achieve top grades. He doesn't want to let them down.

Eric has noticed posters on the back of the toilet doors at school advertising phone numbers for young people who may be experiencing worrying thoughts. The poster says the phone calls are confidential. Eric decides to find a quiet place in a nearby park to ring headspace and ask for help.

QUESTIONS

1. Reflect on the mental health promotion and illness prevention posters or advertisements you have encountered. How likely is it that a young person would read them and act?
2. Whose responsibility is it to develop and post promotional material about mental health and illness?
3. Considering Eric's situation, what other options for help are available to him?

1.6 Common mental health issues

LEARNING OBJECTIVE 1.6 Identify the most common mental health issues that health professionals in Australia will encounter.

The most common mental health issues in Australia are anxiety disorders, including generalised anxiety disorder, social phobia, panic disorder and obsessive-compulsive disorder (14 per cent) (AIHW, 2020a). Affective or mood disorders, such as depression or bipolar disorder, are the next most common issue (6.2 per cent). Substance use disorders are also of concern (5.1 per cent). Other mental health conditions that health professionals may encounter in the emergency context include suicide attempts, self-harming and challenging behaviours due to psychosis or a mania. Health professionals may also interact with those who exhibit physical symptoms that have a psychological basis, often called **somatisation**.

Statistics such as these suggest one reason why the National Mental Health Strategy prioritises an improved understanding of mental health issues by all health professionals and members of the community. This prioritisation includes community education and the delivery of mental health education to frontline workers in health, emergency, welfare and associated sectors, ensuring coordination between these services.

At the same time, these statistics present a challenge to health professionals providing comprehensive care. When mental health issues go unrecognised, there are consequences for individuals, families, communities and health services. As noted in figure 1.2, these consequences can include a decrease in quality of life and reduced health outcomes for the person. It is essential, then, that health professionals recognise the signs and symptoms of mental illness; and have knowledge that will enable them to provide the most appropriate referral for, or treatment and care to, the person exhibiting these symptoms.

What happens if mental illness goes unrecognised or untreated?

- Worsening mental illness, leading to poor health outcomes and quality of life
- Increased burden on carers and families
- Somatic or physical illness, including pain, as the body expresses the psychic pain in other ways
- Unnecessary physical investigations in response to the somatic concerns
- Difficulty in coping with everyday life, including the personal and professional parts of life
- Social isolation
- Incarceration, with untreated mental illness sometimes leading to violence or anti-social behaviours
- Homelessness, with untreated mental illness leading to loss of employment and challenges in engaging with services
- Increased suicide risk
- Additional cost to the mental health system, in the long term

Source: Adapted from Grecco & Chambers (2019) and Mekonen et al. (2022).

A list of the mental health issues that health professionals are likely to encounter in a general health context is provided in table 1.2, together with a brief description of how the person experiencing these issues may present and the recommended interventions. Those who seek more detailed information are encouraged to access the range of sources from which the information was drawn. These sources include the diagnostic manuals DSM-5 and ICD-11, evidence-based clinical practice guidelines produced by organisations and institutions such as the Australian and New Zealand Academy for Eating Disorders (2015), Phoenix Australia — Centre for Posttraumatic Mental Health (2020), National Eating Disorders Collaboration (2018), National Institute for Health and Clinical Excellence (2019), the Royal Australian and New Zealand College of Psychiatrists (2019) and the Royal Australian College of General Practitioners (2019), alongside various textbooks, including Chambers (2017) and Sadock, Sadock and Ruiz (2017).

For health professionals working in the wider health context, the conditions outlined in table 1.2 may be experienced by the person as a **co-occurring** or co-associated condition, where people with mental health issues also have physical health conditions that require medical or other interventions or people with physical health conditions who develop a mental health problem. More comprehensive descriptions of co-occurring or co-associated conditions are provided in other chapters.

This list of common mental health issues in table 1.2 provides health professionals with a convenient means of categorising a person's experiences and thereby intervening in a more timely and appropriate way. At the same time, it is necessary to acknowledge that medically oriented, even reductive information about diagnoses, signs, symptoms and interventions, does not lead to better outcomes for the person. Table 1.2 aims to provide health professionals with an understanding of how mental illnesses are identified and addressed in mainstream Australian health systems. The categories are not meant to undermine the need for health professionals to take individualised, consumer-centred approaches to support mental health consumers, carers or family members. Many people view diagnoses as stigmatising (Ketchell, 2018). As explained throughout this chapter, what is most important is the quality of the care and caring a person receives.

High-quality health service delivery is achieved only through high-quality relationships between the person affected by mental health problems and the health professionals (Totura et al., 2018). Indeed, the therapeutic relationship has been identified as the most effective means of bringing about positive change in the health outcomes of people with a mental illness (Harris & Panozzo, 2019; Royal Australian and New Zealand College of Psychiatrists, 2019). Quality therapeutic relationships assist with problem solving, medication adherence and improving quality of life. They also promote positive personal growth and development, and increased levels of personal functioning and coping (Silverman, 2022). The therapeutic relationship is explored at length in the chapter focusing on assessment in the mental health context.

TABLE 1.2 Summary of the more common mental health issues

Mental health issue	Typical presentation	Recommended intervention
Acute stress reaction (ASR), also called acute stress disorder (ASD) (see also the chapter on common reactions to stressful situations)		
A transient psychological condition that develops in response to a traumatic event. The person does not need to have been physically involved in the traumatic event to experience this reaction. Traumatic events include any experience that threatens, or is perceived to threaten life or physical safety of the person or others around them and arouses feelings of intense fear, helplessness or horror.	Usually begins within minutes of the event and disappears after hours or days. Symptoms can be severe and distressing for the person, and may include: (i) initial state of 'daze' or other dissociative symptoms such as emotional detachment or an inward focus that reduces attention to and awareness of the person's surroundings; (ii) memory loss — especially for the traumatic event ('dissociative amnesia'), and depersonalisation (a perceived loss of contact with reality, feeling unreal); and (iii) altered levels of consciousness, agitation/overactivity or withdrawal, symptoms of anxiety (e.g. sweating, increased heart rate or flushing).	The condition is usually self-limiting, with most people recovering using their internal resources. In the short term, health professionals must (i) 'treat the symptoms' (e.g. if a person is shivering, provide them with a blanket) and (ii) provide verbal reassurance and normalise the experience for the person and their partner or family. These interventions include providing explanations and information about the condition, and social support if necessary. Structured psychological interventions such as debriefing should not be routinely offered as they are not ordinarily necessary. After two weeks, a person for whom ASR persists may be offered a comprehensive clinical assessment. Dependent upon the findings of this assessment, therapeutic interventions may include trauma-focused cognitive behavioural therapy, including exposure and/or cognitive techniques and/or other relevant psychological or social interventions.
Adjustment disorder (see also the chapter on common reactions to stressful situations)		
A maladaptive emotional or behavioural reaction to an identifiable stressful life event or life change. The reaction generally occurs one to three months after the initial stressor and tends to resolve within six months.	Associated symptoms fall on a continuum, from mild depression and/or anxiety, to traumatic stress, distress and, at times, suicidality. Impaired social or occupational functioning can occur, ranging from withdrawal from social or occupational activity to an inability to cope with these activities. The reaction generally resolves when the identified stressor(s) abates.	Initially, interventions can include: (i) reassurance; (ii) arousal reduction; (iii) addressing the cause of the person's stress or feelings of conflict; and (iv) skills and/or relaxation training. In the longer term, similar strategies are used, such as psychosocial support and psychological interventions.

Anxiety (see also the chapter on depression, anxiety and perinatal mental health)

Characterised by tension, worried thoughts and physical changes (including increased blood pressure). There may be recurring intrusive thoughts or concerns, avoidant behaviours and physical symptoms such as increased blood pressure, sweating, trembling, dizziness or rapid heartbeat. Six anxiety disorder subtypes are: (i) panic; (ii) generalised anxiety; (iii) social anxiety; (iv) specific phobias; (v) obsessive-compulsive; and (vi) post-traumatic stress.

Subjective symptoms include feelings that range from apprehension, discomfort and dread, up to the fearful impression of impending doom and panic.

Objective symptoms include palpitations, chest pain, diarrhoea, headache, nausea, urinary frequency, increased respiration rate and muscle spasm.

Initially, people with anxiety can be helped with reassurance and calming techniques such as using a soft measured voice and moving the person to a quiet space for de-stimulation.

In the longer term, interventions include: (i) psychological therapies such as cognitive behavioural therapy or anxiety management techniques, such as mindfulness or relaxation; and (ii) pharmacotherapy such as benzodiazepines and anti-depressant medications.

A combination of psychological therapy and pharmacotherapy is also beneficial.

Bipolar affective disorder (including manic/hypomanic and depressive phases)

A mood or 'affective' disorder that cycles between mania and depression.

For most people, bipolar affective disorder is a recurring and sometimes disabling condition. People often have difficulties in maintaining stable relationships and employment. Bipolar affective disorder accounts for 12 per cent of all Australian suicides annually.

The major ongoing Recovery issue is non-adherence to pharmacological treatment. This issue may result from the symptoms, or be due to difficulties with self-concept, self-esteem, or the social stigma attached to the disorder.

Lifetime misdiagnosis is not uncommon, with symptoms frequently ascribed to schizophrenia or a personality disorder.

Mania and hypomania (i.e. mania of a lesser intensity) are characterised by episodes of: (i) impaired insight and judgement; (ii) chaotic behaviour that can include irritability, aggression, disinhibition; (iii) disorganised cognition (e.g. grandiosity, tangentiality); and (iv) psychosis (e.g. delusions, hallucinations).

For depressive symptoms, see the separate entry for depression.

Initially, (i) ensure safety from harm to self or others; (ii) exclude underlying organic conditions (e.g. substance-induced mania, delirium); (iii) treat physical complications (e.g. dehydration); and (iv) keep the person safe.

The primary longer-term interventions are: (i) pharmacological (e.g. mood stabilisers); (ii) psychosocial support to help manage the symptoms; (iii) psychological interventions to help manage stress and other symptoms; and (iv) psychoeducation to help with levels of adherence with pharmacotherapy, suicide prevention and family therapy to manage the symptoms. Support groups can also achieve good outcomes.

Borderline Personality Disorder (BPD) (see also the chapters on deliberate self-harm and challenging behaviours)

A mental health condition that can severely impact a person's ability to regulate emotions. The condition can increase the person's impulse control, placing them at higher risk of harm to themselves and others; and impact their relationships with others.

People with BPD experience intense emotions or mood swings, view people and life in extreme terms (e.g. all good or all bad), and act impulsively.

Other symptoms that may be experienced include:
(i) behaviours aimed at avoiding real or perceived abandonment; (ii) a pattern of intense and unstable relationships with family and friends; (iii) a distorted and unstable self-image or sense of self; (iv) impulsive and often dangerous behaviours; (iii) self-harming behaviours, such as cutting; (iv) recurring thoughts of suicidal behaviours or threats; (v) intense and highly variable moods, including anger, with episodes lasting from a few hours to a few days; (vi) chronic feelings of emptiness; and (vii) feelings of dissociation.

People with BPD may also have a chronic post-traumatic disorder, often resulting from childhood trauma.

The best interventions for this condition are psychological. Pharmacological interventions are not ordinarily recommended but may be prescribed to help manage high-risk behaviours.

Psychological interventions include dialectical behavioural therapy or schema therapy which teaches the person new ways of interacting with people, of viewing themselves and the world around them.

Pharmacological interventions can include mood stabilises, anti-depressants and anxiolytics.

(continued)

TABLE 1.2 (continued)

Mental health issue	Typical presentation	Recommended intervention
Deliberate self-harm (DSH) (see also the chapter on caring for a person who has self-harmed)		
An acute, deliberate, non-fatal act that may or may not include suicidal intent. Often associated with other mental health conditions such as depression, substance use and anxiety disorders. There is a particular association with borderline personality disorder. Vulnerability to DSH may persist long-term for some people.	Self-injury includes a wide variety of behaviours: self-mutilation (e.g. self-cutting or self-burning), jumping from heights, attempted hanging and deliberate car crashes. Self-poisoning refers to an overdose of medicines or other drugs, or ingesting other substances.	Initially, (i) ensure safety from further self-harm; (ii) if injuries require medical attention, transport to an emergency department; and (iii) refer to the mental health specialist team. In the longer term, (i) cognitive behavioural therapy and problem-oriented approaches (especially dialectical behaviour therapy [DBT]); (ii) address underlying mental health concerns; and (iii) manage triggers/stress and enhance coping skills.
Delirium (see also the chapter on caring for an older person with mental illness)		
Delirium is a medical emergency: if left untreated, it can result in death. It is generally reversible when the underlying cause is treated. Delirium can be challenging to detect and is often undiagnosed, in (i) older people with co-occurring dementia and (ii) up to 20 per cent of younger hospitalised people, with many health professionals presuming only older people develop delirium. Delirium is also called acute brain syndrome, acute confused state or acute organic psychosis. It is generally caused by an underlying illness, or metabolic or chemical disturbance. It is sometimes caused by stress.	There are three main signs: (i) acute or swift onset and fluctuating course over hours to days, which tends to be worse at night ('Sundown syndrome'); (ii) inattention or erratic/disorganised thinking and behaviour (e.g. confusion, disorientation, paranoia, hallucinations, memory impairment); and (iii) altered levels of consciousness, from comatose (unable to be aroused), to lethargic (drowsy), to hyper-aroused (agitated), to a mixed presentation. Health professionals are advised to consider delirium if at least one of the following '5 Ps' are present. • Pus — an infected lesion. • Pills — including misuse, adverse reactions and drug interactions for over-the-counter medicines and prescribed medicines, illicit drugs and alcohol. • Pain — especially in people whose ability to communicate has been compromised. • Pee — urinary tract infections often go undetected, especially in older people who have become dehydrated. • Poo — constipation or diarrhoea (gastrointestinal problems).	In the short term, the underlying cause of the delirium must be treated. Psychosocial support and reassurance must also be given to reduce the distress of the person and their family members. In extreme cases, where the person is at risk of further harm, pharmacological interventions may be used.

Dementia (see also the chapter on caring for an older person with mental illness)

A cluster of symptoms that provide a label for behavioural, psychological, physical and social deficits. The incidence increases dramatically with age but tends to be rare in the under-55 age group. The most common form of dementia is Alzheimer's disease, which accounts for 50–70 per cent of all cases. The onset is insidious and irreversible. The disease progresses gradually but continuously and survival is approximately 8–11 years from the onset of symptoms.	Symptoms include: (i) slow cognitive decline exhibited through slowly increasing functional deficits such as memory loss, confusion, language disturbance, an increasing inability to self-care, and often depression and anxiety; and (ii) 'challenging behaviours' or behavioural and psychological symptoms of dementia, including wandering, pacing, hoarding, verbal and physical aggression, screaming, repetitive vocalisations, delusions and hallucinations, sexual disinhibition and faecal smearing. Typically dementia ends in permanent dependence on all aspects of care and, ultimately, death.	In the short term, (i) reassure the person and (ii) keep the person safe. In the longer-term interventions include: (i) person-centred approaches where health professionals respond to the immediate needs and preferences of the person and their carer; and (ii) pharmacological treatments (e.g. anticholinesterases).

Depression (see also the chapter on depression, anxiety and perinatal mental health)

Diagnosed when a person's mood is consistently sad or 'low' — they lose interest and pleasure in activities or events that ordinarily interest or please the person — for at least 2 weeks. Accompanied by four or more other symptoms from those listed under 'Typical presentation'. Physical illnesses such as cancer, respiratory and cardiovascular disease, diabetes, stroke and neurological conditions increase the risk of depression. Similarly, depression following a cerebral vascular accident, myocardial infarction or prolonged physical illness is associated with increased mortality.	Symptoms include: (i) feelings of worthlessness or guilt; (ii) impaired concentration; (iii) loss of energy/fatigue; (iv) suicidal thoughts; (v) appetite/weight change; (vi) altered sleep pattern; (vii) tearfulness; (viii) depressive body posture; (ix) agitation; (x) social withdrawal; and (xi) inability to be 'cheered up'. Symptoms of depression can be difficult to identify in people with a physically illness. This is because the symptoms may be mistaken for the side-effects of some treatments for physical illness, such as medicines, chemotherapy or radiotherapy (e.g. changes in sleep and appetite). It is therefore important to provide a comprehensive assessment to ensure an appropriate diagnosis.	Initially, (i) ensure the person is safe; (ii) provide psychosocial support; and (iii) refer the person to a mental health professional for a comprehensive health assessment. Longer-term, interventions include: (i) medication (antidepressants); (ii) psychological therapies (e.g. cognitive behavioural therapy or interpersonal therapy); (iii) social support and physical care if required; or (iv) a combination of (i), (ii) and (iii).

(continued)

TABLE 1.2   *(continued)*

Mental health issue	Typical presentation	Recommended intervention
Eating disorders (anorexia nervosa, bulimia nervosa) (see also the chapter on caring for a person who has self-harmed)		
Eating disorders are a group of serious, complex and potentially life-threatening mental disorders with variable causes and a high relapse rate that require specialist, multidisciplinary care. A person with an eating disorder requires appropriate therapeutic interventions as early as possible after diagnosis. Without this early intervention, the disorder is more likely to be long-term, lead to physical health conditions, reduce the person's quality of life and also their life expectancy. There are different types of eating disorders. The main diagnoses are anorexia nervosa and bulimia nervosa.	*Anorexia nervosa:* Deliberate weight loss and a refusal to eat. Hyperactivity is common. About 50 per cent of people with this condition also use purging and vomiting behaviours to lose weight. A common symptom is a preoccupation with body shape and size, including delusions (e.g. seeing self as fat even when severely underweight). Depression and obsessions are often found in people with an eating disorder, particularly in those with anorexia nervosa. Medical complications can be experienced from both conditions. These can affect all body systems but amenorrhoea, osteoporosis and hypometabolic symptoms are common in people with anorexia nervosa. *Bulimia nervosa:* People with this condition episodically binge on food (repeatedly over-eat to an extreme degree) and then take measures to prevent weight gain such as making themselves vomit, taking laxatives or starving themselves. Low self-esteem, impulsivity, problems with intimacy and dependency, and difficulty managing anger are common in people with bulimia nervosa. Common medical conditions for bulimia nervosa include gastrointestinal problems and electrolyte imbalances.	Initially, address any life-threatening symptoms (e.g. cardiac arrest, severe malnourishment). In the longer term, all eating disorders require complex, specialist multifactorial and multidisciplinary care across various settings including medical support, psychiatry, psychology, mental health nursing, dietetics and social work. People with eating disorders can be best supported with (i) access to treatment and support; and (ii) improved workforce knowledge and skill application of evidence-based clinical practice guidelines and strong family support preventative strategies.
Panic (see also the chapter on depression, anxiety and perinatal mental health)		
Panic is an intense form of anxiety. When a person experiences a panic attack, the intense symptoms develop abruptly and tend to peak within 10 minutes.	A panic disorder is diagnosed when the person experiences recurrent and unexpected panic attacks and at least one of the attacks has been followed by (i) at least one month of either persistent concern about having additional attacks; (ii) worry about the implications of the attack or its consequences; and/or (iii) a significant change in behaviour related to the attacks.	In the short term, (i) treat physical symptoms (e.g. hyperventilation); (ii) reassure the person; and (iii) keep the person safe. In the longer term, the aims of interventions include: (i) control and cessation of panic attacks; (ii) control and cessation of fear-driven avoidance; and (iii) reduction in vulnerability to relapse. Both psychological and pharmacological treatments can achieve the first two goals but there is no evidence that pharmacotherapy can reduce vulnerability to relapse. Cognitive behavioural therapy can help the person develop the skills to deal with panic attacks and reduce the probability of relapse.

Post-traumatic stress disorder (PTSD)

Classified as a trauma and stressor-related disorder in the DSM-5, PTSD occurs as a delayed psychological response (i.e. after 4 weeks) after an individual has been exposed to an extreme traumatic stressor involving actual or threatened death or serious injury or a threat to the physical integrity of self or others.

The individual will have experienced intense fear, helplessness or horror. Most people exposed to a traumatic event will adapt over time. For the 5 per cent of people who develop PTSD after experiencing a traumatic event, psychosocial functioning can be seriously impaired.

Primary signs and symptoms are evident for more than a month after the event and include: (i) reliving the trauma — such as through nightmares and intrusive memories, with associated physical reactions, anxiety and panic; (ii) hypervigilance, including trouble sleeping, irritability, difficulty concentrating, hyperarousal; (iii) avoidance of reminders of the trauma including people, places and activities; and (iv) feelings of unreality or emotional numbness (up to and including dissociation).

Initially, (i) keep the person safe; (ii) reassure the person that the condition is relatively common and very treatable; and (iii) refer the person for comprehensive health assessment.

In the longer term, preferred interventions are psychological therapies, including trauma-focused cognitive behavioural therapy or eye movement desensitisation and reprocessing with supervised, 'real life' exposure to the triggers.

Pharmacological interventions are not generally regarded as first-line interventions although antidepressants can usefully support psychotherapy.

Prevention is supported by psychological screening for vulnerability and providing information and emotional support, as needed, immediately post-trauma.

Psychosis

The causes of psychosis are not completely understood. About three in every hundred people will experience a psychotic episode in their lifetime.

Psychosis is generally understood to be the result of organic brain dysfunction.

A person experiencing psychosis has a reduced ability to distinguish what is real.

Psychosis is also associated with several organic conditions, including delirium, dementia and the use of alcohol or other drugs.

Not everyone who experiences psychosis will go on to be diagnosed with schizophrenia, schizoaffective disorder or bipolar affective disorder.

Some people only experience one or two episodes of psychosis, while others experience ongoing episodes and are diagnosed as having a serious mental illness.

The most common symptoms are (i) confused thinking (where thoughts are disorganised or nonsensical); (ii) delusions (beliefs not shared with others of the same cultural background); and (iii) hallucinations (visual, auditory — the most common), olfactory, tactile or taste sensations or representations that are not objectively real.

In the short term, (i) reassure the person; (ii) keep the person safe; (iii) reduce stimulation; and (iv) transport the person for a comprehensive health assessment. In the longer term, interventions are pharmacological and psychosocial: (i) antipsychotic medication; (ii) stress reduction, including a reduced-stimulus environment; (iii) support and reassurance; and (iv) lifestyle management.

(continued)

TABLE 1.2 *(continued)*

Mental health issue	Typical presentation	Recommended intervention
Schizophrenia		
Schizophrenia is a long-term and debilitating psychotic disorder that affects how a person thinks, feels and behaves. People are diagnosed with schizophrenia after being unwell for six months or more, including at least one month during which they experience active symptoms of psychosis. Schizophrenia is also associated with a reduced capacity to function as an active and contributing member of the community, leading to long-term disability.	Symptoms of schizophrenia are similar to those of psychosis, but they are experienced long-term. In addition, people with schizophrenia experience 'negative' symptoms, such as: (i) a lack of emotional expression; (ii) a lack of interest or enthusiasm in activities or life; and (iii) reduced ability to relate to others.	In the short term (i) reassure the person; (ii) keep the person safe; (iii) reduce stimulation; and (iv) transport the person for a comprehensive health assessment. In the longer term, to achieve the best outcome, people diagnosed with schizophrenia are treated with a combination of medication and community support. Interventions most commonly include: (i) pharmacological, including antipsychotics; (ii) psychological therapies, including family interventions and cognitive behavioural therapy; (iii) early interventions; and (iv) community support programs.
Somatisation		
The development of physical symptoms in response to psychosocial distress. There are three aspects: (i) physical symptoms with no pathophysiological cause; (ii) the person believes they are physically ill; and (iii) the person seeks the help of health professionals (usually GPs). In Western societies, somatisation is more common than depression and anxiety in general medical practices. Somatisation is found in around 20 per cent of people who seek the help of a GP and often, people found to be depressed or anxious will present first with somatic symptoms. Women are twice as likely to present with somatic complaints than men.	People who somatise symptoms are not feigning or 'putting on' symptoms but are genuinely convinced that they are physically unwell. The most common somatic complaints are: (i) throat problems; (ii) pregnancy; (iii) chest pain; and (iv) anxiety. Other common somatic problems are: (v) hypertension; (vi) depression; and (vii) oesophageal problems.	In the short term, as for anyone in distress, (i) reassure the person; (ii) make sure the person is safe; and (iii) transport person for comprehensive health assessment. Long-term interventions are psychological, including cognitive behavioural therapies, interpersonal psychotherapies and the technique of reattribution, where people are encouraged to move away from somatic concerns to consider their emotional issues.

SUMMARY

This chapter provided an overview of the frameworks that guide the delivery of mental health services in Australia. It defined key terms, such as 'mental health' and 'mental illness', and explained the need for health professionals to be careful about how they use language in the mental health context. This explanation led to a discussion about the effects of stigma on people with mental health issues. There was a particular focus on care, including trauma-informed care, together with how health professionals can foster a caring approach to helping people. Current policy directions, service frameworks and approaches were also examined, including the place of mental health Recovery. This section was followed by an explanation of the prevalence of mental illness in Australia, focusing on suicide and mental health issues for young people. Finally, the chapter outlined the most common mental health issues encountered by health professionals who work across various health settings.

KEY TERMS

biomedical approach The Western scientific approach to treating illness or disease. The causes of illness are viewed as biological. The health professional's role is to make a diagnosis, prescribe treatment interventions and achieve measurable outcomes.

burden of disease The overall impact of disease or injury on a society, including that which is beyond the immediate cost of treatment. Burden of disease incorporates individual, societal and economic costs.

competencies Capabilities, standards or levels of practice comprising knowledge, skills and attitudes that are measured by a set of valid and reliable items.

consumer-centred care An approach to care that involves the health professional 'working with' the consumer rather than 'acting upon' the patient. Consumer-centred care enables consumers to participate activley in their treatment and care.

co-occurring or co-associated conditions sometimes referred to as comorbid conditions, describe a disease, disorder or condition that occurs at the same time and/or is related to another unrelated disease, disorder or condition.

deinstitutionalisation The process of dismantling the asylum or mental institution network and rethinking the social position of people with a mental illness.

discrimination The unfair treatment of a person or group based on categories such as gender, age, class, relationship, ethnicity, culture, religion, health issue or disability.

empirical data Data gathered from observation or experiment, most often related to values that form part of the scientific method.

empowerment The process through which people become more able to influence the individuals and organisations that affect their lives.

evidence-based practice Relates to the health interventions or practices for which systematic research has provided evidence of effectiveness.

generic caring Learned as part of a person's ongoing growth and development, by way of upbringing, family background and life experiences.

health care A systematic and comprehensive service delivered in the health context; is person-centred, collaborative, supportive; and aims to improve health outcomes.

health professionals People who deliver competent, appropriate and effective health care systematically.

integrated community services Services located in the community that work in together, in partnership, to improve outcomes for consumers.

key performance indicators (KPIs) A set of quantifiable measures used by health services to gauge or compare performance in meeting strategic and operational goals.

mainstreaming The integration of mental health services with general health services.

mental health The capacity of individuals and groups to interact with one another and their environment in ways that promote subjective wellbeing, optimal personal development and use of their abilities to achieve individual and collective goals.

mental health problem A mental health issue that is less severe than a mental illness or disorder which, if not dealt with, can develop into a mental illness or disorder.

mental illness or disorder The terms commonly used in health care to describe the spectrum of cognitive, emotional and behavioural conditions that interfere with social and emotional wellbeing and the lives and productivity of people.

moral imperative Originally defined by the philosopher Kant, who described a principle of conscience and reason that compels a person to act.

morbidity The incidence of ill-health or disease.

mortality The incidence of death in a population.

multidisciplinary team A group of health professionals from multiple disciplines, with different skills or areas of expertise, who work together to provide systematic and comprehensive care and treatment to those in need.

nurse A health professional with a holistic and comprehensive or 'whole of person' approach to health care.

occupational therapist A health professional who supports and enables people to accomplish everyday tasks to achieve a maximum level of independence and safety.

one-size-fits-all approach An approach or intervention that does not take into consideration diversity or difference but rather demands a single, standardised approach or intervention meet the needs and preferences of all people.

paramedic A frontline health professional who provides emergency, life-saving, or other unscheduled health care, out-of-hospital and in the community.

primary care A subset of primary health care; it is accessible and affordable, enabling people or groups to participate individually or collectively in the planning and implementation of their health care.

primary health care Health care that focuses on the multiple determinants of health and the need for community control over health services.

professional caring Caring that is conscious, comprehensive, competent and context specific, and encompasses the physical, psychological, social and spiritual aspects of a person.

psychiatrist A medical practitioner who has specialised in the field of psychiatry with their focus often on the biological causes of illness and prescribing medication.

psychiatry The branch of medicine specialising in the treatment of mental illness.

psychologist A health professional who focuses on the cognitive and behavioural aspects of a person and their health. A clinical psychologist has a higher level of education and expertise in this area of health delivery than a psychologist.

public health The organised response by a society or nation to promote health, wellbeing, rehabilitation, recovery and disability support; and to prevent injury, illness and disability. Public health focuses on the health and wellbeing of populations rather than individuals.

public health care system Universal health care funded and administered by the national and state/territory governments in Australia. This system is subsidised by these governments through Medicare, and state and territory health departments, and can be accessed by all Australian citizens or permanent residents.

public health framework The overarching approach to health service delivery in Australia that focuses on population trends, illness prevention and health promotion of health.

secondary health care Health care that is generally accessed after referral by a health professional; it is typically delivered through hospitals or other related services funded by state or territory public health services.

social worker A health professional who intervenes to support those who are socially disadvantaged by providing psychological counselling, guidance and assistance with social services.

somatisation The experience of a person who feels, reports, or is preoccupied with physical symptoms that have no biological cause and/or are disproportionate to any actual physical disturbance.

stigma An attribute, behaviour or reputation that is perceived, constructed and/or represented by a group of people, society or culture in a negative way.

tertiary health care Health care that is delivered by highly specialised health professionals and services, often located in larger service centres.

trauma-informed practice A strengths-based approach to providing health care that includes understanding of the potential impact of trauma on the person. The health professional ensures physical, psychological and emotional safety for the person and actively supports or enables them to develop a sense of control in their current situation.

universal health coverage A health care system that provides health care and financial protection to all citizens of a country at little or no cost.

universal phenomenon A factor, feature, event, situation or dynamic that is not confined to any particular category, group, culture or population.

World Health Organization (WHO) An agency of the United Nations that is an overarching authority on international public health and coordinates international public health initiatives. Its headquarters are in Geneva, Switzerland.

REVIEW QUESTIONS

1 Define 'mental health' and 'mental illness'.
2 What is meant by 'stigma' and how does it affect people, groups and communities?
3 What is the difference between a psychologist and a psychiatrist?
4 List two common myths about mental illness and the facts that debunk these myths.
5 Describe at least four ways mental illness can affect a person and their family members.
6 What are the different ways in which people can experience trauma?
7 Define 'trauma-informed care'.
8 What are the differences between person-centred and consumer-centred approaches to helping people?
9 Identify the main principles of Recovery approaches to mental health service provision.
10 What is the mental illness that young people in Australia most likely to experience?
11 What intervention is most effective for helping young people with mental health problems?
12 What are the main indicators that someone is experiencing anxiety? Or depression?

DISCUSSION AND DEBATE

1 Consider the following scenario.

Sophie is studying nursing at university and is keen to work in the emergency department of a tertiary referral hospital after she graduates. In her view, this will be an exciting and varied job that will allow her to make a difference for acutely unwell people. Luca is studying paramedicine and is looking forward to using his knowledge and skills in emergencies that require quick thinking and fast action to save lives. Neither Sophie nor Luca can see the relevance in learning about mental health and illness, Recovery in mental health, consumer-centred approaches to helping people or even the most common mental health disorders. In their view, all they needed to know was how to 'stop the bleeding' while dealing with the occasional 'drunk' or 'madman' who may cross their paths.

Consider the points of view of Sophie and Luca in light of the article 'I was worried if I don't have a broken leg, they might not take it seriously' by Ferguson and colleagues (2019), which outlines the concerns of males with mental health issues and/or substance use problems who need to access emergency services.

2 'There is no way I would ever work in the mental health specialty, it is too dangerous. Also, I would lose my clinical skills.' This attitude is evident in most health professionals. Discuss this perspective in light of the many people with a physical illness who also have a mental health problem, and people with a mental illness who also have a physical illness.

3 One person may find an event traumatising and the next person may view the same event as something to shrug off. Discuss the subjective nature of traumatic experiences in health service delivery.

4 Discuss the difference between primary health care, secondary health care and tertiary health care. Why are these differences important?

5 Why is it necessary for all health professionals to understand current national and state/territory policy directions and the approaches to care utilised by mental health services?

6 Consider the alarming suicide rate of Aboriginal and Torres Strait Islander peoples. What do you see as the main contributors to this situation? What role does racism play? What more can all health professionals do to address the issues involved?

7 How does knowing the most common mental health problems, the signs and symptoms of these problems, and the main interventions to address the mental health problems, support health professionals in their caring role?

8 Why do health professionals continue to diagnose people with mental health problems, knowing such diagnoses can be stigmatising? What other options are there instead of a diagnosis?

PROJECT ACTIVITY

The Blue Knot Foundation is Australia's National Centre of Excellence for Complex Trauma. Read about trauma-informed care on their website www.blueknot.org.au. Find other resources about trauma-informed care, including academic journal articles and reputable websites and spend some time reading them. Once you have done this, answer the following questions.

1 What is the difference between health care and trauma-informed health care? Why is this difference important?

2 What steps can you take to ensure you 'become trauma-informed' and change how you practice as a health professional?

WEBSITES

1 The Australian Government's Mental Health Commission was established in 2012 to provide independent reports and advice to the community and government on what is working and not working in the mental health sector. The Mental Health Commission sees mental wellbeing as crucial to the individual, their family, support people and the community, employers and co-workers, health professionals, teachers and friends. The Mental Health Commission aims to support all people and groups to work together to improve mental wellbeing and a sense of a life well-lived: www.mentalhealthcommission.gov.au.

2 Emerging Minds actively promotes the mental health and wellbeing of infants, children, adolescents and their families/carers. This website is dedicated to advocating for the development and implementation of appropriate prevention, promotion and early mental health programs and services for children and their families. The level of mental health of infants, children and adolescents significant impact their future health and wellbeing. This website provides information on the programs and services available for children with mental health problems, and their families: www.emergingminds.com.au.

3 Mindframe is a national program that provides national leadership to help reduce stigma by encouraging safe media representation or reporting about suicide, mental illness and substance use. Mindframe is managed by the Australian government's Department of Health: www.mindframe.org.au.

4 The Australian Institute of Health and Welfare provides information about a range of the mental health services delivered in Australia. It also provides a statistical overview of the number and/or proportion of Australians who experience mental illness and access these services, each year: www.aihw.gov.au/reports-data/health-welfare-services/mental-health-services/overview.

5 Mental Health Australia is the peak, national non-government organisation representing and promoting the interests of the Australian mental health sector. Mental Health Australia is committed to achieving better mental health for all Australians. The organisation was established in 1997 as the first independent peak body in Australia to represent the full spectrum of mental health stakeholders and issues. Mental Health Australia members include national organisations representing consumers, carers, special needs groups, clinical service providers, public and private mental health service providers, researchers and state/territory community mental health peak bodies: www.mhaustralia.org.

6 Phoenix Australia — the Centre for Posttraumatic Mental Health is supported by the Australian government to improve the recognition and treatment of PTSD and related conditions in people affected by trauma. The organisation provides resources to help practitioners who work with people who have experienced trauma, including volunteers, peer workers, community workers and mental health practitioners: www.phoenixaustralia.org/for-practitioners/practitioner-resources.

7 Australian Indigenous Health InfoNet is a web resource for people working, studying or interested in addressing issues that influence Aboriginal and Torres Strait Islander peoples' social and emotional wellbeing (including mental health). The resources provided include research evidence and other knowledge that supports the work of practitioners and policy makers in the social and emotional wellbeing area: www.healthinfonet.ecu.edu.au/learn/health-topics/social-and-emotional-wellbeing.

8 The United Nations is an international organisation that works to develop friendly relations among nations and promote social progress and human rights. It guides how people with mental illness can expect to be treated in the health care system through its Principles for the Protection of Persons with Mental Illness and the Improvement of Mental Health Care: www.equalrightstrust.org/content/un-principles-protection-persons-mental-illness-and-improvement-mental-health-care.

9 The World Health Organization (WHO) is the public health arm of the United Nations. The primary role of WHO is to direct and coordinate international health within the countries that are part of the United Nations' system. The main areas of work of WHO are health systems, promoting health through the life-course, noncommunicable diseases, communicable diseases, corporate services, preparedness, surveillance and response. Information about mental health from a global point of view is also available: https://who.int/health-topics/mental-health.

REFERENCES

Ackerman, L. (2019). Caring science education: Measuring nurses' caring behaviors. *International Journal of Caring Sciences*, *12*(1), 572–583.

Adams Hillard, P. (2019). Why and how to perform trauma-informed care. *Contemporary OB/GYN*, *64*(8), 15–17.

Agency for Clinical Innovation. (2019). *Trauma-informed care and practice in mental health services*. NSW Government. www.aci.health.nsw.gov.au/networks/mental-health/trauma-informed-care-and-practice-in-mental-health-services

Allam, L. (2019, May 14). "Unspeakable": How can Australia stop the Indigenous suicide epidemic. *The Guardian*.

Andersen, D., & Kessing, M. (2019). Stigma, problem drug use, and welfare state encounters: Changing contours of stigmatization in the era of social investment. *Addiction Research & Theory*, *27*(4), 277–284. https://doi.org/10.1080/16066359.2018.1508568

Arat, A., Burström, B., Östberg, V., & Hjern, A. (2019). Social inequities in vaccination coverage among infants and pre-school children in Europe and Australia: A systematic review. *BMC Public Health*, *19*(290). https://doi.org/10.1186/s12889-019-6597-4

Atkinson, S., Collis, B., & Schneider, J. (2018). Mainstream education as a possible route to recovery and social inclusion: A review. *Mental Health Review Journal*, *23*(4), 246–252. https://doi.org/10.1108/MHRJ-03-2018-0008

Australasian College for Emergency Medicine & Department of Policy, Research and Advocacy. (2018). *Aboriginal and Torres Strait Islander and non-Indigenous presentations to Australian emergency departments report*. ACEM.

Australian and New Zealand Academy for Eating Disorders. (2015). *ANZAED position papers*. www.anzaed.org.au/position-statements

Australian Commission on Safety and Quality in Health Care. (2019a). *Australian charter of healthcare rights* (2nd ed.). ACSQHC. www.safetyandquality.gov.au/publications-and-resources/resource-library/australian-charter-healthcare-rights-second-edition-a4-accessible

Australian Commission on Safety and Quality in Health Care. (2019b). *Person-centred care*. ACSQHC. www.safetyandquality.gov.au/our-work/partnering-consumers/person-centred-care

Australian Digital Health Agency. (2022). *Connecting Australia to a healthier future*. Australian Government. www.digitalhealth.gov.au

Australian Health Ministers. (1991). *Mental Health statement of rights and responsibilities: Report of the Mental Health Consumer Outcomes Taskforce*. Australian Government Publishing Service.

Australian Health Ministers' Advisory Council. (2013). *A national framework for recovery-oriented mental health services: Guide for practitioners and providers*. Commonwealth of Australia.

Australian Health Ministers' Conference. (1992a). *National mental health plan 1992*. Australian Government.

Australian Health Ministers' Conference. (1992b). *National mental health policy*. Australian Government Publishing Service.

Australian Institute of Health and Welfare. (2019). *Primary health care in Australia*. AIHW. www.aihw.gov.au/reports/primary-health-care/primary-health-care-in-australia/contents/about-primary-health-care

Australian Institute of Health and Welfare. (2020a). *Mental health*. AIHW. www.aihw.gov.au/reports/australias-health/mental-health

Australian Institute of Health and Welfare. (2020b). *Burden of disease*. AIHW. www.aihw.gov.au/reports/australias-health/burden-of-disease

Australian Institute of Health and Welfare. (2020c). *Stress and trauma*. AIHW. www.aihw.gov.au/reports/australias-health/burden-of-disease

Australian Institute of Health and Welfare. (2020d). *Suicide and intentional self-harm*. AIHW. www.aihw.gov.au/reports/australias-health/suicide-and-intentional-self-harm

Australian Institute of Health and Welfare. (2020e). *Health of young people*. AIHW. www.aihw.gov.au/reports/australias-health/health-of-young-people

Australian Institute of Health and Welfare. (2021a). *Glossary*. AIHW. www.aihw.gov.au/reports-data/australias-welfare/australias-welfare-snapshots/glossary

Australian Institute of Health and Welfare. (2021b). *Mental illness*. AIHW. www.aihw.gov.au/reports/children-youth/mental-illness

Australian Institute of Health and Welfare. (2021c). *Suicide and self-harm monitoring: Deaths by suicide amongst Indigenous Australians*. AIHW. www.aihw.gov.au/suicide-self-harm-monitoring/data/populations-age-groups/suicide-indigenous-australians

Australian Institute of Health and Welfare. (2022a). *Mental health services in Australia*. AIHW. www.aihw.gov.au/reports/mental-health-services/mental-health-services-in-australia/report-content/about

Australian Institute of Health and Welfare. (2022b). *Mental health services in Australia: Prevalence, impact and burden of mental health*. AIHW. www.aihw.gov.au/reports/mental-health-services/mental-health-services-in-australia/report-content/prevalence-impact-and-burden-of-mental-health

Bailey, C., Klas, A., Cox, R., Bergmeier, H., Avery, J., & Skouteris, H. (2019). Systematic review of organisation-wide, trauma-informed care models in out-of-home care (OhHC) settings. *Health & Social Care in the Community*, *27*(3), e10–e22. https://doi.org/10.1111/hsc.12621

Bakračevič, K., Zorjan, S., Tement, S., Christie, L., & Musil, B. (2022). Emotions in our lives: The evaluation of a user-centered training course »living e-Motions« in the context of recovery of people with mental health challenges. *Mental Health Review Journal*, *27*(2), 137–145. https://doi.org/10.1007/s40737-022-00319-y

Barclay, W. (1988). *Report to the minister for health*. New South Wales Ministerial Implementation Committee on Mental Health and Developmental Disability.

Barker, P. (2004). The tidal model: The lived experience in person-centred mental health nursing care. *Nursing Philosophy*, *2*(3), 213–223. https://doi.org/10.1046/j.1365-2850.2001.00391.x

Beckett, P., Holmes, D., Phipps, M., Patton, D., & Molloy, L. (2017). Trauma-informed care and practice: Practice improvement strategies in an inpatient mental health ward. *Journal of Psychosocial Nursing and Mental Health Services*, *55*(10), 34–38. https://doi.org/10.3928/02793695-20170818-03

Benjamin, R., Haliburn, J., & King, S. (2019). *Humanising mental health care in Australia: A guide to trauma-informed approaches*. Taylor and Francis.

Benton, S. (2018). The difference between mental health and mental illness: It might not be what you think (blog post). *Psychology Today*. www.psychologytoday.com/au/blog/reaching-across-the-divide/201804/the-difference-between-mental-health-and-mental-illness

Benz, M., Palm Reed, K., & Bishop, L. (2019). Stigma and help-seeking: The interplay of substance use and gender and sexual minority identity. *Addictive Behaviors*, *97*, 63–69. https://doi.org/10.1016/j.addbeh.2019.05.023

Beyond Blue. (2017). *Good practice framework for mental health and wellbeing in first responder organisations*. www.beyondblue.org.au/docs/default-source/resources/bl2042_goodpracticeframework_a4.pdf

Blignault, I., Aspinall, D., Reay, L., & Hyman, K. (2017). Realisation of a joint consumer engagement strategy in the Nepean Blue Mountains region. *Australian Journal of Primary Health*, *23*(6), 531–535. https://doi.org/10.1071/PY16103

Briere, J. (2019). Chapter 2: An overview of specific distress reduction behaviours. In *Treating risky and compulsive behavior in trauma survivors* (pp. 22–43). The Guilford Press.

Brown, K., & Bright, L. (2017). Teaching caring and competence: Student transformation during an older adult focused service-learning course. *Nurse Education in Practice*, *27*, 29–35. https://doi.org/10.1016/j.nepr.2017.08.013

Burdekin, B., Guilfoyle, M., & Hall, D. (1993). *Report of the national inquiry into the human rights of people with mental illness: Vol. 1. Human rights and equal opportunities commission. Human rights and mental illness*. Australian Government Publishing Service.

Calear, A., Banfield, M., Batterham, P., Morse, A., Forbes, O., Carron-Arthur, B., & Fisk, M. (2017). Silence is deadly: A cluster-randomised controlled trial of a mental health help-seeking intervention for young men. *BMC Public Health*, *17*, 1–8. https://doi.org/10.1186/s12889-017-4845-z

Centers for Disease Control and Prevention. (2016). *What is epidemiology?*. US Department of Health & Human Sciences. www.cdc.gov/careerpaths/k12teacherroadmap/epidemiology.html

Chambers, M. (Ed.). (2017). *Psychiatric and mental health nursing: The craft of caring* (3rd ed.). Hodder Arnold.

Chang, H., Tang, J., & Feng, J. (2021). Implementation of trauma-informed healthcare. *Journal of Nursing*, *68*(3), 81–89. https://doi.org/10.6224/JN.202106_68(3).11

Cleary, M., & Hungerford, C. (2015). Trauma-informed mental health care: How can mental health nurses take the lead to support women who have survived sexual assault? *Issues in Mental Health Nursing*, *36*, 370–378. https://doi.org/10.3109/01612840.2015.1009661

Coffey, M., Hannigan, B., Meudell, A., Jones, M., Hunt, J., & Fitzsimmons, D. (2019). Quality of life, recovery and decision-making: A mixed methods study of mental health recovery in social care. *Social Psychiatry and Psychiatric Epidemiology*, *54*(6), 715–723. https://doi.org/10.1007/s00127-018-1635-6

Complex Trauma WA. (2022). *Our story*. COTWA. www.complextraumawa.org.au/about-cotwa

Consumers Health Forum of Australia. (n.d.). *What is consumer-centred care?* www.chf.org.au/real-people-real-data-toolkit/real-people-real-data/what-consumer-centred-care.

Consumers Health Forum of Australia. (2019). *National Health Plan opens way for reform*. www.chf.org.au/media-releases/national-health-plan-opens-way-reform

Cook, J., Shore, S., Burke-Miller, J., Jonikas, J., Hamilton, M., Ruckdeschel, B., Norris, W., Markowitz, A., Ferrara, M., & Bhaumik, D. (2019). Mental health self-directed care financing: Efficacy in improving outcomes and controlling costs for adults with serious mental illness. *Psychiatric Services*, *70*(3), 191–201. https://doi.org/10.1176/appi.ps.201800337

Cousins, S. (2017). Suicide in Indigenous Australians: A "catastrophic crisis". *The Lancet*, *389*(10066), 242–242. https://doi.org/10.1016/S0140-6736(17)30137-X

Crowe, A., Mullen, P., & Littlewood, K. (2018). Self-stigma, mental health literacy, and health outcomes in integrated care. *Journal of Counseling & Development*, *96*(3), 267–277. https://doi.org/10.1002/jcad.12155

Davidson, L., Rowe, M., DiLeo, P., Bellamy, C., & Delphin-Rittmon, M. (2021). Recovery-oriented systems of care: A perspective on the past, present and future. *Alcohol Research: Current Reviews*, *41*(1), 1–11. https://doi.org/10.35946/arcr.v41.1.09

De Ruysscher, C., Tomlinson, P., Vanheule, S., & Vandevelde, S. (2019). Questioning the professionalization of recovery: A collaborative exploration of a recovery process. *Disability & Society*, *34*(5), 797–818. https://doi.org/10.1080/09687599.2019.1588708

Deegan, P. (1996). Recovery as a journey of the heart. *Psychosocial Rehabilitation Journal*, *19*, 91–97. https://doi.org/10.1037/h0101301

Delport, S., Gyuran, J., Knox, S., & Batt, A. (2018). Implications for reflective practice and safer care in paramedicine: The Bawa-Garba case. *Journal of Paramedic Practice*, *10*(11), 462–462. https://doi.org/10.12968/jpar.2018.10.11.462

Department of Health. (n.d.). *Mental health and suicide prevention*. Australian Government. www.health.gov.au/health-topics/mental-health-and-suicide-prevention

Department of Health. (2009). *National mental health policy 2008*. Australian Government.

Department of Health. (2010). *National standards for mental health services*. Australian Government.

Department of Health. (2015). *National mental health strategy*. Victoria State Government. www.health.vic.gov.au/priorities-and-transformation/national-mental-health-strategy

Department of Health. (2019). *The Australian health system*. Australian Government. www.health.gov.au/about-us/the-australian-health-system

Department of Health and Ageing. (2013). *National Aboriginal and Torres Strait Islander suicide prevention strategy*. Australian Government. pp. 10–13

Department of Health, Health Direct. (2019). *Recovery and mental health*. Australian Government. www.healthdirect.gov.au/mental-health-recovery

Derkatch, C. (2016). *Bounding biomedicine: Evidence and rhetoric in the new science of alternative*. University of Chicago Press.

Doran, C., & Kinchin, I. (2019). A review of the economic impact of mental illness. *Australian Health Review*, *43*(1), 43–48. https://doi.org/10.1071/AH16115

Dowrick, C. (2017). *Person-centred primary care: Searching for self*. Routledge.

Ebsworth, S., & Foster, J. (2017). Public perceptions of mental health professionals: Stigma by association? *Journal of Mental Health*, *26*(5), 431–441. https://doi.org/10.1080/09638237.2016.1207228

Elsegood, K., Anderson, L., & Newton, R. (2018). Introducing the recovery inspiration group: Promoting hope for recovery with inspirational recovery stories. *Advances in Dual Diagnosis*, *11*(4), 137–146.

Emond, K., O'Meara, P., & Bish, M. (2019). Paramedic management of mental health related presentations: A scoping review. *Journal of Mental Health*, *28*(1), 89–96. https://doi.org/10.1080/09638237.2018.1487534

Enticott, J., Lin, E., Shawyer, F., Russell, G., Inder, B., Patten, S., & Meadows, G. (2018). Prevalence of psychological distress: How do Australia and Canada compare? *Australian and New Zealand Journal of Psychiatry*, *52*(3), 227–238. https://doi.org/10.1177/0004867417708612

Fagerström, L. (2021). The caring advanced practice nursing model. In L. Fagerström (Ed.), *A caring advanced practice nursing model: Theoretical perspectives and competency domains* (pp. 65–73). Springer.

Fairclough, N. (1989). *Language and power*. Longman.

Ferguson, N., Savic, M., Sandral, E., Lubman, D., McCann, T., Emond, K., Smith, K., Roberts, L., & Bosley, E. (2019). "I was worried if I don't have a broken leg they might not take it seriously": Experiences of men accessing ambulance services for mental health and/or alcohol and other drug problems. *Health Expectations*, *22*(3), 565–574. www.ncbi.nlm.nih.gov/pmc/articles/PMC6543159

Ferry-Danini, J. (2018). A new path for humanist medicine. *Theoretical Medicine and Bioethics*, *39*(1), 57–77. https://doi.org/10.1007/s11017-018-9433-4

Fisher, M., Baum, F., MacDougall, C., Newman, L., McDermott, D., & Phillips, C. (2017). Intersectoral action on SDH and equity in Australian health policy. *Health Promotion International*, *32*(6), 953–963. https://doi.org/10.1093/heapro/daw035

Foucault, M. (1961). *The history of madness* (J. Khalfa & J. Murphy, Trans.). Routledge.

Freshwater, D., Cahill, J., Esterhuizen, P., Muncey, T., & Smith, H. (2017). Rhetoric versus reality: The role of research in deconstructing concepts of caring. *Nursing Philosophy*, *18*(4). https://doi.org/10.3390/healthcare8020170

Fryer, B. (2019). Indigenous youth suicide at crisis point. *NITV News*. www.sbs.com.au/nitv/article/2019/01/15/indigenous-youth-suicide-crisis-point

Giandinoto, J., Stephenson, J., & Edward, K. (2018). General hospital health professionals' attitudes and perceived dangerousness towards patients with comorbid mental and physical health conditions: Systematic review and meta-analysis. *International Journal of Mental Health Nursing*, *27*(3), 942–955. https://doi.org/10.1111/inm.12433

Gibbs, C., Murphy, B., Hoppe, K., Ratnaike, D., & Lovelock, H. (2018). Improving collaborative mental health care across Australia: Development and evaluation of the Mental Health Professionals Network (MHPN) initiative. *International Journal of Integrated Care*, *18*(S2), A57, 1–8.

Goffman, E. (1967). *Interaction ritual: Essays on face-to-face behavior*. Penguin Books.

Grecco, G., & Chambers, A. (2019). The Penrose Effect and its acceleration by the war on drugs: A crisis of untranslated neuroscience and untreated addiction and mental illness. *Translational Psychiatry*, *9*(1), 320. https://doi.org/10.1038/s41398-019-0661-9

Habib, P., Killington, M., McNamara, A., Crotty, M., Fyfe, D., Kay, R., Patching, A., & Kochiyil, V. (2019). Rehabilitation environments: Service users' perspective. *Health Expectations*, *22*(3), 396–404.

Hales, T., Green, S., Bissonette, S., Warden, A., Diebold, J., Koury, S., & Nochajski, T. (2019), Trauma-informed care outcome study. *Research on Social Work Practice*, *29*(5), 529–539. https://doi.org/10.1177/1049731518766618

Happell, B., Platania-Phung, C., Bocking, J., Ewart, S., Scholz, B., & Stanton, R. (2019). Consumers at the centre: Interprofessional solutions for meeting mental health consumers' physical health needs. *Journal of Interprofessional Care*, *33*(2), 226–234. https://doi.org/10.1080/13561820.2018.1516201

Happell, B., Scholz, B., Bocking, J., & Platania-Phung, C. (2019). Promoting the value of mental health nursing: The contribution of a consumer academic. *Issues in Mental Health Nursing*, *40*(2), 140–147. https://doi.org/10.1080/01612840.2018.1490834

Harris, B., & Panozzo, G. (2019). Therapeutic alliance, relationship building and communication strategies for the schizophrenia population: An integrative review. *Archives of Psychiatric Nursing*, *33*(1), 104–111. https://doi.org/10.1016/j.apnu.2018.08.003

Harvey, S., Bryant, R., & Forbes, D. (2018). *A clinician's summary of the expert guidelines on the diagnosis and treatment of post-traumatic stress disorder in emergency service workers*. Black Dog Institute. www.blackdoginstitute.org.au/docs/default-source/research/ptsd_guidelines_2018.pdf

Hatcher, S., Crawford, A., & Coupe, N. (2017). Preventing suicide in indigenous communities. *Current Opinion in Psychiatry*, *30*(1), 21–25. https://doi.org/10.1097/YCO.0000000000000295

Headspace. (2021). *Insights: Headspace national youth mental health survey 2020*. Headspace National Youth Mental Health Foundation. www.headspace.org.au/assets/Uploads/Insights-youth-mental-health-and-wellbeing-over-time-headspace-National-Youth-Mental-Health-Survey-2020.pdf

Heidegger, M. (1962). *Being and time*. Harper and Row.

Henderson, J., Javanparast, S., MacKean, T., Freeman, T., Baum, F., & Ziersch, A. (2018). Commissioning and equity in primary care in Australia: Views from Primary Health Networks. *Health & Social Care in the Community*, *26*(1), 80–89. https://doi.org/10.1111/hsc.12464

Hills, D., Hills, S., Robinson, T., & Hungerford, C. (2019). Mental health nurses supporting the routine assessment of anxiety of older people in primary care settings: Insights from an Australian study. *Issues in Mental Health Nursing*, *40*(2), 118–123. https://doi.org/10.1080/01612840.2018.1517285

Ibeneme, S., Eni, G., Ezuma, A., & Fortwengel, G. (2017). Roads to health in development countries: Understanding intersection of culture and healing. *Current Therapeutic Research*, *86*, 13–18. https://doi.org/10.1016/j.curtheres.2017.03.001

Islam, I., Khanam, R., & Kabir, E. (2020). The use of mental health services by Australian adolescents with mental disorders and suicidality: Findings from a nationwide cross-sectional survey. *PLOS One*, *15*(4), e0231180. https://doi.org/10.1371/journal.pone.0231180

Isobel, S. (2019). "In some ways it all helps but in some ways it doesn't": The complexities of service users' experiences of inpatient mental health care in Australia. *International Journal of Mental Health Nursing*, *28*(1), 105–116. https://doi.org/10.1111/inm.12497

Jackson-Best, F., & Edwards, N. (2018). Stigma and intersectionality: A systematic review of systematic reviews across HIV/AIDS, mental illness, and physical disability. *BMC Public Health*, *18*(1), 919. https://doi.org/10.1186/s12889-018-5861-3

Jangland, E., Teodorsson, T., Molander, K., & Muntlin Athlin, A. (2018). Inadequate environment, resources and values lead to missed nursing care: A focused ethnographic study on the surgical ward using the Fundamentals of Care framework. *Journal of Clinical Nursing*, *27*(11–12), 2311–2321. https://doi.org/10.1111/jocn.14095

Jeffs, L., Muntlin Athlin, A., Needleman, J., Jackson, D., & Kitson, A. (2018). Building the foundation to generate a fundamental care standardised data set. *Journal of Clinical Nursing*, *27*(11–12), 2481–2488. https://doi.org/10.1111/jocn.14308

John, T. (2017). Setting up recovery clinics and promoting service user involvement. *British Journal of Nursing*, *26*(12), 671–676. https://doi.org/10.12968/bjon.2017.26.12.671

Jørgensen, K., & Rendtorff, J. (2018). Patient participation in mental health care—Perspectives of healthcare professionals: An integrative review. *Scandinavian Journal of Caring Sciences*, *32*(2), 490–501. https://doi.org/10.1111/scs.12531

Juntanamalaga, P., Scholz, B., Roper, C., & Happell, B. (2019). They can't empower us': The role of allies in the consumer movement. *International Journal of Mental Health Nursing*, *28*(4), 857–866. https://doi.org/10.1111/inm.12585

Kassianos, S. (2016). History of pharmacological treatments for mental health. In S. Boslaugh (Ed.), *SAGE encyclopedia of pharmacology and society* (pp. 699–704).

Ketchell, M. (2018, October 10). Diagnostic labels for mental health conditions are not always useful. *The Conversation*. www.theconversation.com/diagnostic-labels-for-mental-health-conditions-are-not-always-useful-102943

Kilcullen, M., Swinbourne, A., & Cadet-James, Y. (2018). Aboriginal and Torres Strait Islander health and wellbeing: Social emotional wellbeing and strengths-based psychology. *Clinical Psychologist*, *22*(1), 16–26. https://doi.org/10.1111/cp.12112

Kilian, A., & Williamson, A. (2018). What is known about pathways to mental health care for Australian Aboriginal young people?: A narrative review. *International Journal For Equity In Health*, *17*(1), 12–15. https://doi.org/10.1186/s12939-018-0727-y

Kinson, R., Hon, C., Lee, H., Abdin, E., & Verma, S. (2018). Stigma and discrimination in individuals with first episode psychosis; one year after first contact with psychiatric services. *Psychiatry Research*, *270*, 298–305. https://doi.org/10.1016/j.psychres.2018.09.044

Kirk, S., & Hinton, D. (2019). "I'm not what I used to be": A qualitative study exploring how young people experience being diagnosed with a chronic illness. *Child Care, Health and Development*, *45*(2), 216–226. https://doi.org/10.1111/cch.12638

Kirsh, B., Krupa, T., & Luong, D. (2018). How do supervisors perceive and manage employee mental health issues in their workplaces? *Work*, *59*(4), 547–555. https://doi.org/10.3233/WOR-182698

Kiwanuka, F., Rad, S., & Alemayehu, Y. (2019). Enhancing patient and family-centered care: A three-step strengths-based model. *International Journal of Caring Sciences*, *12*(1), 584–590. http://internationaljournalofcaringsciences.org/docs/65_kiwanuka12_1.pdf

Kleissl-Muir, S., Raymond, A., & Rahman, M. (2018). Incidence and factors associated with substance abuse and patient-related violence in the emergency department: A literature review. *Australasian Emergency Care*, *21*(4), 159–170. https://doi.org/10.1016/j.auec.2018.10.004

Leininger, M. (2012). The phenomenon of caring, part v: Caring: The essence and focus of nursing. *International Journal for Human Caring*, *16*(2), 57–58.

Leininger, M. (1981). Some philosophical, historical, and taxonomic aspects of nursing and caring in American culture. In M. Leininger (Ed.), *Caring, an essential human need. Proceedings of the Three National Caring Conferences* (pp. 133–143). Wayne State University Press.

Life in Mind. (2022). *The national suicide and self-harm monitoring system*. www.lifeinmind.org.au/about-suicide/suicide-data/the-national-suicide-and-self-harm-monitoring-system

Lindgren, B., Ringnér, A., Molin, J., & Graneheim, U. (2019). Patients' experiences of isolation in psychiatric inpatient care: Insights from a meta-ethnographic study. *International Journal of Mental Health Nursing*, *28*(1), 7–21. https://doi.org/10.1111/inm.12519

Lukersmith, S., Croker, D., Maclean, L., & Gleeson, R. (2017). My plan: A new meso to micro level building block to promote person-centred care planning. *International Journal of Integrated Care*, *17*(5), A60. www.ijic.org/articles/abstract/10.5334/ijic.3363

Ma, Z. (2017). How the media cover mental illnesses: A review. *Health Education*, *117*(1), 90–109. https://doi.org/10.1108/HE-01-2016-0004

MacDonald, K., Fainman-Adelman, N., Anderson, K., & Iyer, S. (2018). Pathways to mental health services for young people: A systematic review. *Social Psychiatry and Psychiatric Epidemiology*, *53*(10), 1005–1038. https://doi.org/10.1007/s00127-018-1578-y

Maung, H. (2019). Dualism and its place in a philosophical structure for psychiatry. *Medicine, Health Care and Philosophy*, *22*(1), 59–69. https://doi.org/10.1007/s11019-018-9841-2

McCann, T., Savic, M., Ferguson, N., Cheetham, A., Witt, K., Emond, K., Bosley, E., Smith, K., Roberts, L., & Lubman, D. (2018). Recognition of, and attitudes towards, people with depression and psychosis with/without alcohol and other drug problems: Results from a national survey of Australian paramedics. *BMJ Open*, *8*(12), e023860. https://bmjopen.bmj.com/content/8/12/e023860

McCormack, B., & McCance, T. (2017). *Person-centred practice in nursing and health care: Theory and practice*. Wiley Blackwell.

McGorry, P., Mei, C., Chanen, A., Hodges, C., Alvarez-Jimenez, M., & Killackey, E. (2022). Designing and scaling up integrated youth mental health care. *World Psychiatry*, *21*(1), 61–76. https://doi.org/10.1002/wps.20938

Mekonen, T., Ford, S., Chan, G., Hides, L., Connor, J., & Leung, J. (2022). What is the short-term remission rate for people with untreated depression? A systematic review and meta-analysis. *Journal of Affective Disorders*, *296*, 17–25.

Mental Health Coordinating Council. (n.d.). *Trauma-informed care and practice (TICP)*. https://mhcc.org.au/publication/trauma-informed-care-and-practice-ticp

Middleton, J., Bloom, S., Strolin-Goltzman, J., & Caringi, J. (2019). Trauma-informed care and the public child welfare system: The challenges of shifting paradigms: Introduction to the special issues on trauma-informed care. *Journal of Public Child Welfare*, *13*(3), 235–244. https://doi.org/10.1080/15548732.2019.1603602

Milton, M., & Garton, S. (2017). Mental health in Australia, 1788–2015: A history of responses to cultural and social challenges. In H. Minas & M. Lewis (Eds.), *Mental health in Asia and the Pacific: Historical and cultural perspectives* (pp. 289–313). Springer.

Mindframe. (2019). *Mindframe guidelines for communicating about mental ill-health*. www.mindframe.org.au

Minshall, C., Stubbs, J., Charleston, R., Van-Dunem, H., Wallace, A., & Hynan, C. (2021). What should guide cross-sector collaborations between mental health and alcohol and other drug services? A scoping review. *Advances in Mental Health*, *19*(1), 29–39. https://doi.org/10.1080/18387357.2019.1664309

Mission Australia. (2021). *1 in 4 young people facing psychological distress during pandemic: Media Release*. www.missionaustralia.com.au/media-centre/media-releases/1-in-4-young-people-facing-psychological-distress-during-pandemic

Morgan, A., Reavley, N., Jorm, A., & Beatson, R. (2017). Discrimination and support from friends and family members experienced by people with mental health problems: Findings from an Australian national survey. *Social Psychiatry & Psychiatric Epidemiology*, *52*(11), 1395–1403. https://doi.org/10.1007/s00127-017-1391-z

Morse, J., Bottorff, J., Anderson, G., O'Brien, B., & Solberg, S. (1991). Beyond empathy: Expanding expressions of caring. *Journal of Advanced Nursing*, *53*(1), 75–87. https://doi.org/10.1111/j.1365-2648.1992.tb02002.x

National Eating Disorders Collaboration. (2018). *National Practice Standards for eating disorders*. www.nedc.com.au/assets/NEDC-Resources/national-practice-standards-for-eating-disorders.pdf

National Institute for Health and Clinical Excellence. (2019). *Guidance and advice*. www.nice.org.uk

National Mental Health Commission. (2017). *The Fifth National Mental Health and Suicide Prevention Plan 2017–2022*. Australian Government.

Nguyen, D. (2019). Mapping knowledge domains of non-biomedical modalities: A large-scale co-word analysis of literature 1987–2017. *Social Science & Medicine*, *233*, 1–12. https://doi.org/10.1016/j.socscimed.2019.05.044

Niimura, J., Nakanishi, M., Okumura, Y., Kawano, M., & Nishida, A. (2019). Effectiveness of 1-day trauma-informed care training programme on attitudes in psychiatric hospitals: A pre-post study. *International Journal of Mental Health Nursing*, *28*(4), 980–988. https://doi.org/10.1111/inm.12603

Orygen. (2016). *Two at a time: Alcohol and other drug use by young people with a mental illness*. Orygen, the National Centre of Excellence in Youth Mental Health. www.orygen.org.au/Policy/Policy-Reports/Alcohol-and-other-drug-use/alcohol_and_other_drug_policy_paper_2016?ext

Parliament of Australia. (2006). *Chapter 3 — Mental health and human rights*. www.aph.gov.au/Parliamentary_Business/Committees/Senate/Former_Committees/mentalhealth/report/c03

Parrish, E. (2018). Comorbidity of mental illness and chronic physical illness: A diagnostic and treatment conundrum. *Perspectives in Psychiatric Care*, *54*(3), 339–340. https://doi.org/10.1111/ppc.12311

Peplau H. (1952, 1991). *Interpersonal relations in nursing*. MacMillan.

Phoenix Australia – Centre for Posttraumatic Mental Health. (2020). *Australian guidelines for the prevention and treatment of acute stress disorder, posttraumatic stress disorder and complex PTSD*. www.phoenixaustralia.org/australian-guidelines-for-ptsd

Priddis, L., & Rogers, S. (2018). Development of the reflective practice questionnaire: Preliminary findings. *Reflective Practice*, *19*(1), 89–104. https://doi.org/10.1080/14623943.2017.1379384

Raeburn, T., Liston, C., Hickmott, J., & Cleary, M. (2018). Life of Martha Entwistle: Australia's first convict mental health nurse. *International Journal of Mental Health Nursing*, *27*(1), 455–463. https://doi.org/10.1111/inm.12356

Rai, S., Gurung, D., Kaiser, BN., Sikkema, K., Dhakal, M., Bhardwaj, A., Tergesen, C., & Kohrt, D. (2018). A service user co-facilitated intervention to reduce mental illness stigma among primary healthcare workers: Utilizing perspectives of family members and caregivers. *Families, Systems and Health: The Journal of Collaborative Family Healthcare*, *36*(2), 198–209. https://doi.org/10.1037/fsh0000338

Randall, S., & Crawford, T. (2018). Hold on to primary healthcare nurses. *Community Practitioner*, *91*(8), 28–30.

Ray, M. (2019). Remembering: My Story of the founder of transcultural nursing, the late Madeleine, M. Leininger, PhD, LHD, DS, RN, CTN, FAAN, FRCNA (born: July 13, 1925; died: August 10, 2012). *Journal of Transcultural Nursing*, *30*(5), 429–433. https://doi.org/10.1177/1043659619863089

Regan, D. (2020). How the challenging behaviour of a traumatised child tells their trauma story and is a vital part of their recovery. *Journal of Social Work Practice*, *34*(1), 113–118. https://doi.org/10.1080/02650533.2019.1572081

Richmond, D. (1983). *Inquiry into health services for the psychiatrically ill and developmentally disabled (NSW)*. Department of Health.

Roberts, B., Roberts, M., Yao, J., Bosire, J., Mazzarelli, A., & Trzeciak, S. (2019). Development and validation of a tool to measure patient assessment of clinical compassion. *JAMA Network Open, 2*(5), e193976–e193976. https://doi.org/10.1001/jamanetworkopen.2019.3976

Röhm, A., Hastall, M., & Ritterfeld, U. (2017). How movies shape students' attitudes toward individuals with schizophrenia: An exploration of the relationships between entertainment experience and stigmatization. *Issues in Mental Health Nursing, 38*(3), 193–201. https://doi.org/10.1080/01612840.2016.1257672

Rosen, A., & O'Halloran, P. (2014). Recovery entails bridging the multiple realms of best practice: Towards a more integrated approach to evidence-based clinical treatment and psychosocial disability support for mental health recovery. *East Asian Archives of Psychiatry, 24*(3), 104–9.

Royal Australian and New Zealand College of Psychiatrists. (2016). *The economic cost of serious mental illness and comorbidities in Australia and New Zealand.* RANZCP.

Royal Australian and New Zealand College of Psychiatrists. (2019). *Guidelines and resources for practice.* www.ranzcp.org/Resources/Statements-Guidelines.aspx

Royal Australian College of General Practitioners. (2019). *Clinical guidelines.* www.racgp.org.au/your-practice/guidelines

Sadock, B., Sadock, V., & Ruiz, P. (2017). *Kaplan and Sadock's comprehensive textbook of psychiatry* (10th ed.). Wolters Kluwer.

Saleh, N. (2020). *How the stigma of mental health is spread by mass media.* Very Well Mind. www.verywellmind.com/mental-health-stigmas-in-mass-media-4153888

SANE. (2019). *Reducing stigma.* www.sane.org/information-and-resources/facts-and-guides/reducing-stigma#:~:text=Reducing%20stigma%20by%20recognising%20'Good,illness%20and%20sharing%20inspirational%20stories

Sayers, J., Cleary, M., Hunt, G., & Burmeister, O. (2019). Service and infrastructure needs to support recovery programmes for Indigenous community mental health consumers. International *Journal of Mental Health Nursing, 26*(2), 142–150. https://doi.org/10.1111/inm.12287

Schiavo, R. (2018). *Turning the tide on mental health: Communication professionals needed. Journal of Communication in Healthcare, 1*(1), 4–6. https://doi.org/10.1080/17538068.2018.1443716

Scott, A., Pope, K., Quick, D., Aitken, B., & Parkinson, A. (2018). What does "recovery" from mental illness and addiction mean? Perspectives from child protection social workers and from parents living with mental distress. *Children and Youth Services Review, 87,* 95–102. https://doi.org/10.1016/j.childyouth.2018.02.023

Sellin, L., Kumlin, T., Wallsten, T., & Gustin, L. (2018). Caring for the suicidal person: A Delphi study of what characterizes a recovery-oriented caring approach. *International Journal of Mental Health Nursing, 27*(6), 1756–1766. https://doi.org/10.1111/inm.12481

Silverman, M. (2022). The therapeutic relationship and alliance. In M. Silverman (Ed.), *Music therapy in mental health for illness management and recovery.* Oxford University Press.

Sitzman, K., & Watson, J. (2018). *Caring science, mindful practice: Implementing Watson's human caring theory* (2nd ed.). Springer.

Skerrett, DM., Gibson, M., Darwin, L., Lewis, S., Rallah, R., & De Leo, D. (2018). Closing the gap in aboriginal and Torres Strait Islander youth suicide: A social–emotional wellbeing service innovation project. *Australian Psychologist, 53*(1), 13–22. https://doi.org/10.1111/ap.12277

Snowdon, J. (2017). Should the recently reported increase in Australian suicide rates alarm us? *Australian and New Zealand Journal of Psychiatry, 51*(8), 766–769. https://doi.org/10.1177/0004867416681855

Sutton, A. (2017). Delineating the fine line between the mad and the bad: Victorian prisons and insane asylums, 1856–1914. *Australian and New Zealand Journal of Psychiatry, 51*(7), 741–742. https://doi.org/10.1177/0004867416682837

Szeto, A., Dobson, K., & Knaak, S. (2019). The road to mental readiness for first responders: A meta-analysis of program outcomes. *Canadian Journal of Psychiatry, 64*(1 Suppl.), 18S–29S. https://doi.org/10.1177/0706743719842562

Tierney, S., Seers, K., Tutton, E., & Reeve, J. (2017). Enabling the flow of compassionate care: A grounded theory study. *BMC Health Services Research, 17,* 1–12. https://doi.org/10.1186/s12913-017-2120-8

Totura, C., Fields, S., & Karver, M. (2018). The role of the therapeutic relationship in psychopharmacological treatment outcomes: A meta-analytical review. *Psychiatric Services, 69*(1), 41–47. https://doi.org/10.1176/appi.ps.201700114

Urban, E. (2018). On matters of mind and body: Regarding Descartes. *Journal of Analytical Psychology, 63*(2), 228–240. https://doi.org/10.1111/1468-5922.12395

Vohra, S., Punja, S., Sibinga, E., Baydala, L., Wikman, E., Singhal, A., Dolcos, F., & Van Vliet, K. (2019). Mindfulness-based stress reduction for mental health in youth: A cluster randomized controlled trial. *Child and Adolescent Mental Health, 24*(1), 29–35. https://doi.org/10.1111/camh.12302

Vrklevski, L., Eljiz, K., & Greenfield, D. (2017). The evolution and devolution of mental health Services in Australia. *Inquiries Journal, 24*(1), 29–35. http://www.inquiriesjournal.com/a?id=1654

Walker, N. (2017). Mental health nurse fails to provide competent care. *Kai Tiaki Nursing New Zealand, 23*(4), 44–45.

Watson, J. (1988). *Nursing: Human science and human care. A theory of nursing.* National League of Nursing.

Williams, T. (2019). Loneliness and social isolation: The consequences of being lonely. *DNA Reporter, 44*(3), 4.

Williams, T., & Smith, G. (2019). Laying new foundations for 21st century community mental health services: An Australian perspective. *International Journal of Mental Health Nursing, 28*(4), 1008–1101. https://doi.org/10.1111/inm.12590

Wilson, A., Reilly, R., & Mackean, T. (2018). Analysis of factors associated with Aboriginal and Torres Strait Islander suicide in Australia: A scoping review. *Transcultural Psychiatry.* (In press)

World Health Organization. (1978, September 6–12). *Primary health care: Report of the International Conference on Primary Health Care.* Alma-Ata, USSR.

World Health Organization. (1986). *Ottawa charter for health promotion.* First International Conference on Health Promotion: WHO/HPR/HEP/95.1.

World Health Organization. (2001). *The world health report 2001: Mental health, new understanding, new hope.* Author.

World Health Organization. (2019). *Primary health care.* www.who.int/health-topics/primary-health-care

Yoo, C. (2019). Stress coping and mental health among adolescents: Applying a multi-dimensional stress coping model. *Children and Youth Services Review*, *99*, 43–53.https://ideas.repec.org/a/eee/cysrev/v99y2019icp43-53.html

Young, N. (2018). How nurses can improve care for people with severe mental illness. *Nursing Times*, *114*(9), 1. www.nursingtimes.net/roles/mental-health-nurses/how-nurses-can-improve-care-for-people-with-severe-mental-illness-13-08-2018

ACKNOWLEDGEMENTS

Extract 1A: World Health Organization. (1978.) *Primary health care: Report of the International Conference On Primary Health Care.* Alma-Ata, USSR, 6–12 September.

Extract 1B: Australian Health Ministers' Advisory Council. (2013.) *A national framework for recovery-oriented mental health services: Guide for practitioners and providers.* Canberra: Commonwealth of Australia.

Figure 1.1: Adapted from Australian Institute of Health and Welfare, *Mental health services in Australia: Mental health: prevalence and impact, 2022.*

Photo 1A: racorn / Shutterstock.com

Photo 1B: Gorodenkoff / Adobe Stock

Photo 1C: Antonio Guillem / Shutterstock.com

Photo 1D: Monkey Business Images / Shutterstock.com

Photo 1E: Steve Shepard / Getty Images

Assessment in the mental health context

This chapter will:

2.1 justify the use of a biopsychosocial assessment framework

2.2 clarify contemporary approaches to assessment

2.3 explain the most common mental health assessments

2.4 outline the place of diagnostic manuals in mental health assessments

2.5 describe the risk and protective factors for young people with mental health concerns

2.6 highlight the importance of age-appropriate communication when assessing young people.

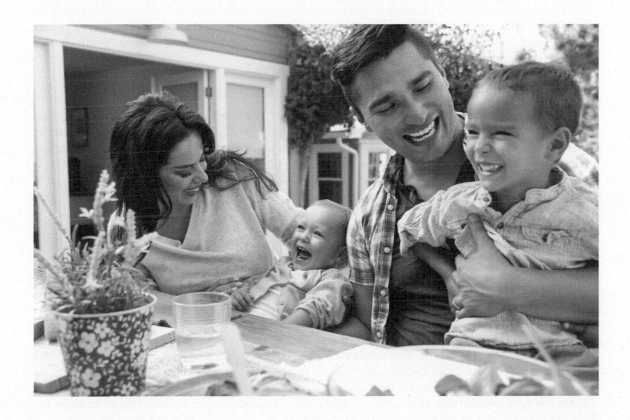

Introduction

Assessment is a key component of health care. Assessments are used to determine a person's level of health. Without assessment, a person cannot receive appropriate and targeted help.

Mental health assessments are just one part of the overall health assessment. Each person has physical, mental, social, emotional, functional or other issues that could be affecting them. Such complexity explains why this chapter begins with an introduction to the biopsychosocial framework, which provides a simple structure for approaching comprehensive health assessments. Contemporary approaches to assessment are also explained, including person-centred and recovery-oriented approaches that enable health professionals to meet the health needs and preferences of the person.

The chapter then examines the most common mental health assessments, including the mental state examination and suicide risk assessment. Following this, the ICD-11 and DSM-5 diagnostic frameworks are discussed.

The chapter concludes by exploring approaches to assessing young people with mental health concerns, including the use of age-appropriate communication and the need to obtain collaborative information from the young person's family, teachers and friends.

2.1 Biopsychosocial assessment

LEARNING OBJECTIVE 2.1 Justify the use of a biopsychosocial assessment framework.

According to the World Health Organization (WHO) constitution (1948), health is 'a state of complete physical, mental and social wellbeing and not merely the absence of disease or infirmity'. This definition suggests that health involves more than physical or mental considerations; it also includes social wellbeing, which is linked to relationships, happiness and life satisfaction.

With health a multifaceted concept, a comprehensive health assessment must likewise have multiple components. Biopsychosocial health assessment provides a structured and systematic way of collecting, analysing and documenting comprehensive information about a person's physical health, mental health, and social and emotional wellbeing (Lewis & Foley, 2020).

Biopsychosocial assessment frameworks

The term 'biopsychosocial' is generally credited to US psychiatrist George Engel (1977, 2012), who developed the biopsychosocial model as an alternative to the biomedical model assessment and treatment. Although the **biomedical model** dominates the provision of health services in contemporary Western settings, its focus can be reductive — that is, it tends to limit itself to the biological aspects of illness and disease (Burns et al., 2019). In contrast, the **biopsychosocial framework** considers the full range of a person's experience, with the term 'biopsychosocial' providing a shorthand means of encapsulating the many different aspects of **personhood** (Bolton & Gillet, 2019).

The biopsychosocial assessment framework includes the:

- biological or the physical or physiological health of the person
- psychological aspects or thoughts, feelings and behaviours of the person, including mental health and substance use
- social aspects of the person, including their cultural, environmental, functional, financial, occupational, sexual, spiritual and relational aspects.

Engel (1977, 2012) argued that these many aspects of personhood inter-connect, each influencing or impacting the other. Examples include a person with chronic physical pain impacted in the psychological and social spheres; or the person with substance misuse issues impacted physically, psychologically and socially by their choices. More specifically, there is a strong link between depression and various physical illnesses, including stroke, coronary heart disease, diabetes, cancer, chronic pain, dementia, Parkinson's disease and hypertension (Ma et al., 2021). Engel (1977, 2012) also suggested that mental health issues intersect at the biological, psychological and social level of a person's mental health, each a component of what it means to be a person.

Online health assessments

Conducting a comprehensive health assessment using the biopsychosocial framework in the online or virtual environment presents several challenges to consider and overcome. These challenges include the following.

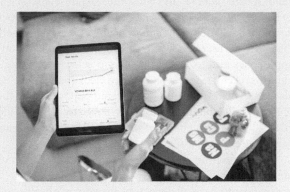

Physical and mental health challenges

While web-based assessments can be effective (Mirea et al., 2021), they can also present limitations when conducting a physical or mental health assessment. These limitations include hands-on physical examinations and accurately reading body language or the nuances in facial expressions, potentially leading to issues being missed or misidentified and inappropriate treatments recommended (Palmer et al., 2022).

Ethical challenges

Some online assessments are undertaken on health services or organisational equipment using software that ensures the safety of users. Other online assessments are conducted using software or programs owned by multinational organisations that harvest data to sell for profit. The safety and security of some online assessments cannot be guaranteed (Cummin & Schuller, 2020).

Social challenges

Health professionals have different levels of capability when using digital health solutions. At this point, inconsistent standards are guiding digital competencies for health professionals. Likewise, people with health issues have different levels of access and capacity to use the Internet. Such variables could impact the quality of an assessment, particularly for those with serious physical or mental illness or suicidal intent (Jarva et al., 2022).

QUESTIONS

1. What other challenges to conducting online biopsychosocial assessment have you encountered in your practise?
2. What steps can you take to conduct safe, ethical and effective online biopsychosocial assessments?

2.2 Approaches to assessment

LEARNING OBJECTIVE 2.2 Clarify contemporary approaches to assessment.

Alongside the biopsychosocial framework, health professionals can take various assessment approaches. This section clarifies the person-centred, recovery-oriented approaches commonly used in the mental health sector. It then explains the four Rs of assessment — reflection, relationship, recording and reporting.

Person-centred, recovery-oriented approaches

Health professionals developed person-centred approaches in response to the limitations that arose from biomedical approaches to health care (McCormack et al., 2020). **Person-centred care** aims to be more responsive to the individual's health needs and preferences (McKay et al., 2021). Person-centred approaches include:

1. valuing the individual for their intrinsic worth and promoting their rights and wellbeing
2. treating each person as a unique individual who has their own particular life experiences, history, culture and background
3. engaging the individual according to their needs, preferences and abilities
4. understanding the social nature of what it means to be human and providing for this to promote health and wellbeing (Stein-Parbury, 2021).

At the heart of person-centred care lies the person, their relationships and their communities (Rietkerk et al., 2021). A person has the potential to achieve the best possible outcomes when supported by their families, social networks and health professionals (McCormack et al., 2020). For this reason, person-centred care involves the consumer's spouse, partner, family or significant others.

Person-centred approaches align well with recovery-oriented approaches. These approaches were developed by mental health consumers who felt disempowered by conventional health systems, arguing that personal recovery was a subjective state rather than a medical outcome. For example, recovery-oriented approaches aim to support people to achieve meaning and purpose in their lives through personal growth, empowerment, agency and shared decision making (Coffey et al., 2019). Recovery-oriented approaches also recognise the value of the lived experience of the person who is being assessed, focusing on hope, optimism and building the individual strengths of the person (Standsfield & Shah, 2021; van Weeghel et al., 2019). You can read more about recovery-oriented approaches in the chapter introducing mental health care in Australia.

Working within a biopsychosocial framework, person-centred, recovery-oriented approaches to assessment enables the:
- consideration of all aspects of the person's health and wellbeing by the health professional, including the behavioural, biological, cultural, educational, emotional, environmental, financial, functional, mental, occupational, physical, recreational, sexual, spiritual and social aspects of a person
- a focus on the needs and preferences of the person rather than the preoccupations of health professionals
- empowerment of the person to self-determine, achieve their health goals and live a meaningful life.

UPON REFLECTION

How confident are you in conducting comprehensive health assessments?

Many health professionals will limit their assessments to the area of a person's health in which they feel most skilled, knowledgeable or comfortable. For example, medical practitioners tend to focus on the person's physical health, social workers on the person's social situation and psychologists on the person's psychological status. In the United Kingdom, paramedics reported low confidence in managing mental health calls, preferring to have specialist mental health professionals working with them for these call-outs (Briggs et al., 2021).

There are many good reasons for developing knowledge, skills and confidence in assessing a person's mental health concerns. Knowing the 'hows' and 'whats' of an assessment allows health professionals to address a person's anxieties about the assessment process. There may also be times when mental health specialists are not immediately available to conduct an assessment, with non-specialists required to determine the most appropriate way forward in the short term. Understanding what is involved when assessing a person's mental health concerns will ensure that the needs of the person are addressed.

QUESTIONS

1. Reflect on your assessment skills. How confident do you feel when conducting a comprehensive health assessment?
2. What practical steps can you take to develop your assessment skills in comprehensive assessments?

Working within a person-centred, recovery-oriented approach, the following four steps provide a practical guide to conducting an assessment:
1. *R*eflection
2. *R*elationship
3. *R*ecording
4. *R*eporting.

Using the 'four Rs' of assessment as a guide will enable health professionals to conduct thoughtful and thorough assessments. Each of these four Rs is now explained in turn.

Reflection

The first step in undertaking an assessment is reflection, including self-reflection and practice reflection. Both of these processes help health professionals develop self-awareness and realistically assess or evaluate their skills and performance as practitioners (Johns, 2022).

Self-reflection

Health professionals bring the many concerns and frustrations of life to their workplace (Wong & Vinsky, 2021). Indeed, to presume a health professional's personal life will not influence their practise would be to deny a health professional's personhood. For example, there is an expectation in many organisations that health professionals will provide effective, appropriate and competent care regardless of their levels of stress, circumstances or what is happening in their personal life (Raudenská et al., 2020). At times, such expectations can be unrealistic, particularly in long-term crisis situations. Many examples of this occurred during the COVID-19 pandemic, when some health professionals felt unable to cope and experienced physical and mental health issues as a result of their stress (Mollica & Fricchione, 2021).

As Socrates once suggested, self-examination and self-knowledge are the beginning of knowledge and wisdom. Likewise, self-reflection and self-awareness involve the conscious cultivation of personal and professional growth, learning, ethical development and caring for others (Delderfield & Bolton, 2018). For example, health professionals may need to assess the health of people with alternative lifestyles or hear the stories of those who have experienced horrendous trauma events. Self-reflection and self-awareness will enable the health professional to manage their reactions to such encounters and provide the person with the care they need.

The questions health professionals may ask themselves in the process of self-reflection could include the following.

- What are my own beliefs and values about maintaining positive mental health and wellbeing and preventing mental health concerns?
- What are my feelings about supporting people who are experiencing mental illness?
- What assumptions or preconceptions am I making that help maintain my beliefs and emotions in this situation?

The questions that health professionals may ask themselves about the people they are helping could include the following.

- Are the individual's experiences similar or different to my own? How does this influence my own thoughts and feelings?
- Can I better understand the person's presentation or behaviours in the context of their past experiences?
- How can more understanding of the person's experiences facilitate depth in our relationship?

Answers to such questions will help health professionals to understand their own beliefs and values, including how these beliefs and values may affect their attitudes, reactions and behaviours towards others.

Indeed, effective engagement with others can be challenging if health professionals have not critically reflected on their own values and attitudes (Watts, 2019). For example, difficulties can arise when a health professional's personal reactions to others becomes a barrier to meaningful interaction. It is only when health professionals are aware of what is behind or driving their reactions to people or events, that they will be able to manage their feelings. For more information on the need for self-awareness in health professionals, read the chapter discussing the common reactions to stressful situations.

Practise reflection

Just as self-reflection will help a health professional to develop self-awareness, leading to personal and professional growth and ethical development, practise reflection can improve how health professionals deliver health care. Practise reflection is a process by which a health professional first, identifies a workplace event or experience; second, closely considers their role in this event or experience, including their behaviour, thinking and feelings; and third, determines changes to their practice to improve their work.

Many different models can guide practice reflection, such as the Proctor, Heron, Kadushin and the Growth and Support Models. Perhaps the most commonly used model is the Gibbs' Reflective Cycle (1988), which provides a framework for examining practice experiences, including:

1. describing the experience
2. articulating your feelings and thoughts about the experience
3. evaluating the experience in terms of the benefits and challenges
4. analysing the situation to make sense of it
5. concluding what you have learned from the experience and what you could have done differently
6. developing an action plan for how to deal with similar situations in the future or general changes to practice that may be appropriate.

These steps, described in figure 2.1, can be used in single or repeated events or situations.

FIGURE 2.1   Gibbs' Reflective Cycle

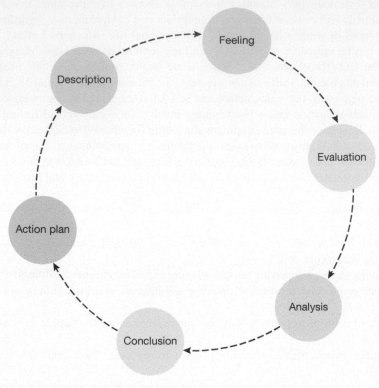

Source: Gibbs 1988.

To help them with the process of practice reflection, health professionals often find a clinical or professional supervisor with the knowledge, skills and abilities to support them through the process of reflection through constructive questioning (Lonergan et al., 2021) Regular clinical or professional supervision is beneficial for supporting health professionals to reflect on and improve their practice, including their skills in assessment (Davies et al., 2022). You can read more about clinical or professional supervision in the chapters on common reactions to stressful situations and the management of challenging behaviours.

IN PRACTICE

Reflective supervision

Many health professionals engage in regular reflective supervision, also known as 'professional supervision' or 'clinical supervision', a formal professional arrangement and process by which practitioners undertake practice reflection in a confidential setting (Driscoll et al., 2019). Active participation in professional or clinical supervision enables health professionals to: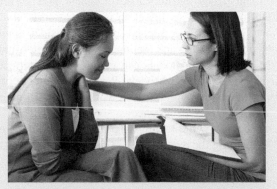

- enhance the safety of clients, consumers, patients and/or residents
- engage in professional development activities
- protect their own health and wellbeing (Snowdon et al., 2020).

For example, Duong works as a paramedic. One day, the team is called out to a person expressing suicidal ideation. His colleagues ask Duong to complete a suicide risk assessment. Duong has only learned about this type of assessment at university; he has never actually conducted this a suicide risk assessment. Duong does his best, but later, when he reflects on his work, he feels there is room for improvement. In particular, he wonders why he felt so stressed when conducting the assessment, but finds it difficult to unpack the issues.

Duong already engages in regular clinical supervision. He decides to make an additional appointment with his clinical supervisor to confidentially discuss what happened. During the session, he uses Gibbs' Reflective Cycle to describe what had happened on the day and then talks about his feelings. Duong then moves on to evaluate the outcome of his assessment and analyse the situation. Reflecting with his clinical supervisor helps Duong realise his lack of experience in conducting suicide risk assessments made him nervous on the day, and his diverse cultural background, including his religious beliefs about suicide and experiences in his country of origin, has affected his perceptions of mental illness. He works with his clinical supervisor to develop an action plan to help him move forward. Duong finds this clinical supervision session helpful for his personal and professional growth.

QUESTIONS

1. What are the benefits of regular professional or clinical supervision?

2. What are the challenges of engaging in regular professional or clinical supervision?

3. How can regular clinical supervision help health professionals to reflect more effectively on their practice?

Reflection on other factors

Together with engaging in self-reflection and practice reflection, health professionals must take the time to consider the factors that can affect assessments. For example, a person's context and culture will inevitably influence how they respond to health professionals, who must adapt their assessments accordingly.

Context

Assessments are always context-specific (Bor et al., 2017). The context of a health assessment includes its timing, urgency, location and setting. For example, assessments undertaken in clinical settings will be affected by the power imbalance between a health professional and the person with the health issue (Bhattacharya & Priya, 2022). The person may feel intimidated or unwilling to disclose information that could reflect badly on them. They may also fear what is happening to them or around them. Health professionals must therefore reflect on how they can support the person to be proactive during the assessment process.

Another contextual factor that can impact an assessment is privacy. While most clinical settings provide privacy, locations, such as the person's home or workplace, could present a range of distractions. Such contexts raise questions for health professionals about how they will manage these distractions or interruptions to maintain the privacy of the person they are assessing.

Different contexts can also give rise to unconscious bias in health professionals. For example, some health professionals may unnecessarily pathologise the behaviours of a person who presents in a dishevelled state, is angry or is from a minority culture. While health professionals must consider what has led to the person presenting to a health service for help, there is also a need to keep an open mind.

Additionally, health professionals must reflect on the person's age, gender, family background, level of education, past experiences with health services, traumatic personal experiences and reactions (physical and emotional) to stressful situations (Fiani, 2022). How could these factors affect the way the person responds to the assessment process? Some people may feel quite comfortable answering a health professional's questions, while others may not. Some people may feel distressed, in pain, frightened, upset, angry, intimidated, intoxicated with substances, drugs or alcohol or even feeling culturally offended by some assessment questions, while others will accept what is happening without question.

Health professionals are advised to reflect on the many different contextual factors at play before conducting an assessment and determine how they can support the person through the process.

Questions the health professional could ask themselves include the following.

- Is the consumer currently safe and comfortable? Do I feel safe and comfortable? Are others (i.e. family, other staff members) now safe and feeling comfortable?
- What does the consumer want or expect to happen during the assessment?
- Are there factors that may impact how the person engages with me? For example, is the person feeling tired, in pain, nauseous, under the influence of alcohol or substances, distracted or worried?
- How can I use my engagement and communication skills to build collaboration and partnership with the person?
- How can I support the person to feel both physically and emotionally safe?
- How can I use this time to promote hope, respect and Recovery for the consumer and their family?

In addition, the health professional must consider the timing of the questions they ask during an assessment. Adapting approaches to assessment according to context to meet the needs and preferences of the person will improve communication and the quality of the assessment.

Culture can affect an assessment in diverse ways. On the one hand, people from some cultural groups (e.g. refugee populations, Aboriginal and Torres Strait Islander peoples, lesbian, gay, bisexual, transgender or gender diverse, queer, intersex, asexual and other gender non-conforming identities [LGBTQIA+]) have a higher risk of developing mental illness than the general population. On the other hand, symptoms of mental illness may not be recognised or acknowledged in some cultures and, therefore, be difficult to identify or uncover (Cosgrove et al., 2021). A lack of recognition of mental health issues may lead to some people ignoring what they are feeling and postponing seeking help, which can impact health outcomes.

Cultural understandings can also influence how people describe their symptoms, the type of help they seek for mental health problems, their coping styles and the level of support they receive from their family, friends and the community. For example, some cultures may view symptoms of mental illness as 'weakness' or 'shameful', while other cultural groups may view the same symptoms as 'a word from God'. People from some cultures may prefer to talk privately with family members or faith leaders about their experiences; others will seek out medical practitioners, and others again will seek out alternative health solutions.

Migrants and refugees who had little to no access to mental health services in their countries of origin may also be unaware that mental health services are available in Australia. In addition to overcoming language barriers, there is also a need for health professionals to support people from diverse cultures with their mental health literacy, including how they can obtain help when experiencing distress. You can read more about mental illness and culture in the chapter focusing on cultural considerations in mental health.

UPON REFLECTION

Mental illness in LGBTQIA+ populations

Most LGBTQIA+ people live meaningful lives. However, research suggests that LGBTQIA+ people are more likely to experience bullying, harassment, traumatic loss, intimate partner violence, physical and sexual abuse and traumatic forms of societal stigma, bias and rejection than the general population (Waling et al., 2019). LGBTQIA+ people also face discrimination when accessing health care. Such experiences are associated with an increased risk of mental illness, including suicidal ideation.

QUESTIONS

1. What can health professionals do to improve how they assess LGBTQIA+ people who may be experiencing mental health concerns?
2. What can health professionals do to support LGBTQIA+ people to access culturally safe and inclusive health care?

Relationship

Person-centred, recovery-oriented approaches to assessments provide health professionals with an opportunity to engage with and build a relationship with the person who has come to them for help.

The assessment process involves at least two people: the person being assessed and the person undertaking the assessment, with the person's spouse or partner and other health professionals also often involved. Connection with the key people involved is necessary before the assessment can proceed (Geldard et al., 2021).

There are many different ways in which health professionals can connect with consumers. For example, in emergency situations, the engagement will be brief and involve the health professional asking questions that require 'yes' or 'no' answers. When the situation is less pressing, health professionals can take more time to build a relationship, with the quality of their interactions often dependent upon the unconditional positive regard they show the person (Stein-Parbury, 2021).

Unconditional positive regard

The notion of **unconditional positive regard** was originally coined by Carl Rogers (1951, 1961, 1980) and involves showing empathy and support for a person, regardless of what they say or do. The health professional focuses on supporting the person and their health needs rather than expecting the person to conform to a predetermined set of values. Giving a person unconditional positive regard does not mean that any attitude and behaviour is acceptable, but rather that the person with the health problem is treated positively. Demonstrating unconditional positive regard is particularly important when supporting people who have experienced discrimination or stigmatising attitudes in the past, leaving them feeling anxious about how they will be treated in health settings (Geldard et al., 2021).

People who are shown unconditional positive regard are more likely to feel respected and safe, accept themselves and engage in socially constructive behaviour (Bullard, 2020). The outcomes of unconditional positive regard include personal growth and development, and more trusting and effective therapeutic relationships.

Therapeutic relationships

Some health professionals prefer to use the term **therapeutic alliance** when describing the relationship between a health professional and the person seeking assistance because it suggests an active and mutual collaboration between the health professional and consumer as they work together towards a common goal (Horvath, 2018). The term 'therapeutic relationship' is used in this text as it more commonly occurs in various health and para-health settings.

Not all relationships are therapeutic — the **therapeutic relationship** is distinct from other relationships because it enables positive change through therapeutic interactions (Stein-Parbury, 2021). For example, the therapeutic relationship has been shown to positively influence a person's mental health outcomes. Therapeutic relationships support consumers to engage with health interventions, solve problems more effectively and experience improvements in their quality of life (DeAngelis, 2019; Tishby & Wiseman, 2018). Indeed, the opportunities and potential for change achieved through the therapeutic relationship are such that proponents of the biomedical model also promote its centrality in mental health settings (Malhi et al., 2021).

The online therapeutic relationship

The E-Mental Health Strategy for Australia was instituted in 2012 (Department of Health and Ageing, 2012) to promote and guide the use of virtual mental health strategies to enhance the accessibility of services. Progress in this area was rapid during the COVID-19 pandemic when many people were limited in their mental health service options (Australian Institute of Health and Welfare, 2022). Outcomes of the use of online strategies and services to support people with mental illness are promising (Charbonnier et al., 2022)

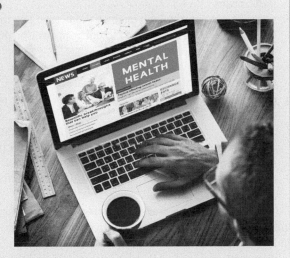

In Australia, e-therapy is offered to children and adolescents, adults and older adults by multiple organisations. These services are listed by Healthdirect (2021), a free Australian health advice web resource funded by the Australian Government. Many private providers of mental health services also deliver personal relationship and family counselling services online.

There are benefits to engaging online with people with mental health problems. For example, people who engage online feel less likely to experience stigma and more comfortable with the relative anonymity of these services (Strand et al., 2020). For some people, using e-mental health services can help them to initially engage with a health professional, leading to face-to-face contact once they have established trust and a positive relationship online. This approach can be especially important for people with a history of trauma who may find it difficult to trust others (Shannon et al., 2021).

The use of e-mental health strategies can also pose challenges for health professionals. For example, some people may find it difficult to connect meaningfully online and prefer face-to-face interactions. There is also a need for organisations or health professionals to develop pathways to follow if a person expresses suicidal ideation online.

A systematic review of studies of the therapeutic alliance in guided internet therapy programs for depression and anxiety found limited evidence supporting the benefits for this mode of service delivery (Pihlaja et al., 2017). In a single study by Tremain et al. (2020), the digital therapeutic alliance was associated with increased engagement and adherence to digital interventions. However, it was also noted that more research is required in this area.

In light of the central nature of the therapeutic relationship in supporting people to achieve the best possible health outcomes, health professionals must reflect on the benefits and challenges of delivering online services, ensuring that they develop the skills required to engage well with people regardless of the setting.

The assessment process allows health professionals to lay the foundations for establishing a therapeutic relationship with the consumer and family. There are various theories and approaches to explain the process, including:

- modelling and role modelling (Erickson, 2006; Erickson et al., 1983, 2005)
- Newman's theory of health as expanding consciousness (Newman, 1995)
- Orem's self-care agency approach (Orem, 1991)
- Peplau's interpersonal relations theory (Peplau, 1952, 1991)
- Roy's adaptation model (Roy, 2009).

Each of these theories or approaches posits its own key factors in building a therapeutic relationship. Other approaches highlight the person's strengths and how they can contribute to the therapeutic relationship, the ecological factors that can influence the therapeutic relationship and the role of culture and social justice (Evans & Hannigan, 2016).

As an introduction, the therapeutic relationship scan be described through the nine concepts posited by Dziopa and Ahern (2009a, 2009b). These concepts are:

1. *understanding and empathy*, which are connected to the notion of unconditional positive regard that helps the person to feel accepted
2. *individuality*, which ensures health professionals approach the person as having unique needs and preferences
3. *providing support*, which enables the person and their family to feel safe and cared for
4. *being there/being available*, including answering questions, providing information and following up on requests in a timely way
5. *demonstrating respect*, which is also connected to **unconditional positive regard** and allows a person to feel physically and emotionally safe
6. *demonstrating clear boundaries* to ensure that the person understands the health professional's role and expectations
7. *demonstrating self-awareness*, including awareness of the health professional's reactions to the person and situation, and managing those reactions appropriately
8. *being 'genuine'*, including open and honest, which helps to build trust with the person
9. *promoting equality*, including a willingness to actively collaborate so that the person receives the best possible health care.

Implementing these nine constructs can be easier said than done. Therapeutic relationships do not occur spontaneously. The following practice suggestions are the first steps health professionals can take to build and maintain strong therapeutic relationships.

- *Introduce yourself.* All relationships, including therapeutic relationships, begin with a respectful introduction. In the busyness of their working day or in urgent situations, some health professionals may forget this simple courtesy when approaching consumers, their families or friends. Your introduction should include your name, role or profession and how you can help them. Also, assure the person that the information they share with you will be treated confidentially.
- *Show kindness.* The simple act of showing kindness in health settings has been linked to increased levels of wellbeing of health professionals and those they are helping (Kaazan, 2020). Maintaining kindness can be challenging in high-stress settings or when faced with aggressive behaviours. Nevertheless, such acts can help to build trust between health professionals, consumers and their families, and will reap the benefits of the therapeutic relationship in the long term.
- *Clarify expectations.* Many people are unsure about what to expect from health professionals. Anxieties can be allayed by opening communication channels and clarifying expectations. For example, some people who seek help from health services are hoping for a 'quick fix' solution (Snell-Rood & Carpenter-

Song, 2018). While there may be cases when such solutions can be provided, mental health concerns usually have complex contributing factors that require help and support over time. This possibility must be explained to the person, with recovery framed as a positive journey and process of change.

- *Empower the person.* Health professionals are in a position of power in health settings. Awareness of this power differential is crucial if health professionals are to build and strengthen trust and collaboration in the therapeutic relationship (Bhattacharya & Priya, 2022). This is possible, even in times of crisis, by:
  - inviting the person's partner or family members to attend the interview
  - asking the person if they would like a drink
  - asking permission to take notes while conducting the assessment
  - providing the person with information that will help them to make decisions about their health needs.
- *Involve partners, family members or friends.* Research suggests that people are happier with their health services when partners, family members or friends are included in the initial interview, assessments, ongoing discussions and interventions (Moen et al., 2021). Health professionals are building better therapeutic alliances with people when they explain the process of assessment and engagement to all involved, invite questions and actively collaborate with the person and their significant others.

LIVED EXPERIENCE

Showing kindness

My Indigenous grandfather grew me up. He died when I was 18. All I can remember is feeling lost and alone, with a grief that felt grey and heavy. I was supposed to start university, but I couldn't. Everything and everyone around me made me feel anxious — I couldn't make decisions, and I couldn't talk to new people or do new things. As time went by, I couldn't leave the house and I couldn't get out of bed.

My mother made me go to a community health centre. When I sat there, I was sure everyone was looking at me. I felt so much shame. When I saw the health professional, I was sure he was laughing at me. He talked down to me and asked me a lot of questions that didn't make sense. He also told me I shouldn't tell anyone I was Aboriginal because I didn't look black enough. I felt even more ashamed and like he was wanting me to betray my grandfather. So I left.

Things didn't get any better. I tried a lot of different health professionals but found it hard to connect with any of them. Then, one day, I talked to someone who was kind to me. She listened to me, accepted my story and didn't judge me. She seemed interested in who I am and how she could support me, without telling me what to do or how to live my life. It was this attitude that helped me on my recovery journey.

Using effective therapeutic communication

Effective communication is critical for establishing, developing and maintaining a functional therapeutic relationship (Fan et al., 2022). Therapeutic communication helps a health professional 'connect' with the person and recognise what is happening to or for them at that moment (Geldard et al., 2021). It allows a health professional to listen to and validate the person's concerns, even when those concerns cannot be immediately resolved (Henderson, 2019). Effective therapeutic communication can also reduce anxiety and feelings of helplessness for the person and encourages people to share essential information, which is essential during the assessment process (O'Toole, 2020). You can read more about effective therapeutic relationships in the chapter that focuses on common reactions in people who are experiencing stress.

The link between health service complaints and poor communication with consumers suggests too many health professionals fail to translate their knowledge about the importance of good communication into practice (Jolly et al., 2020).

Table 2.1 outlines some techniques and strategies that health professionals can use to develop effective skills in therapeutic communication, including those needed to conduct an assessment. The same techniques can also be used for other one-to-one interactions between health professionals and consumers or carers, such as providing health care.

TABLE 2.1   Therapeutic communication

Intervention by the health professional	Rationale and/or strategy
Preparation	
Arranges a quiet, private and safe environment	Promotes confidentiality and minimises interruptions.
Seeks agreement from all involved regarding the agenda, whether formal or informal	Keeps the communication focused.
Discusses a specific timeframe for the interview	Paces the interaction according to the available time. Guards against the person commencing a discussion about very distressing issues just as the time is about to run out.
Non-verbal	
Actively listens	In addition to the verbal, active listening skills required, actively listening involves nodding and leaning forward towards the person.
	Keeps a relaxed, open posture to convey interest.
	Makes eye contact, as appropriate to the person's cultural background.
Looks for non-verbal cues	Observes and reads the body language (including facial expressions) of the person.
	Identifies incongruities between what the person is saying verbally and what their body language is saying — for example, the person says everything is 'fine', but their body language suggests they are depressed.
Uses or tolerates short silences	Enables those at the meeting to reflect on what has been said and what it means.
Maintains appropriate body language and posture	Ensures physical congruence with what is said — for example, if a person verbally expresses great distress, lean towards them to express empathy.
Empathises with or recognises what the other person is feeling	Validates the other person's position.
	Reflects content and feeling, expresses empathy.
	Responds in a way that indicates an understanding of the person's emotions and perspectives, whether stated or not.
Demonstrates a genuine attitude	Demonstrates congruence to the situation — for example, responds with empathy if the person is sharing distressing information.
	Maintains focus on the person and their individual characteristics.
	Is accepting of other person's experiences and points of view.
Verbal	
Actively listens	Verbally summarises the context of the person's story, including keywords that the person uses.
	Verbally acknowledges and affirms the feelings the person is expressing.
	Frequently checks with the person that the health professional understands what the person is saying.
Uses simple language with as little jargon as possible	Regularly checks with the person that they understand what the health professional is asking.
Uses open questions to encourage elaboration; allows the person to direct the interaction	Uses questions such as 'What do you think is happening?' or 'How do you feel about what is happening?'
Clarifies unclear information	Uses sentences, such as 'I'm not sure what you mean. Please tell me some more about what is happening to you.'
Re-states, where appropriate	Uses questions, such as 'So you're saying that you find that difficult?'

Engages with the person's agenda, works to align themselves with the person	Finds out what the person wants and why (e.g. the needs and preferences of the person).
Sets clear boundaries	Clarifies with the person what is acceptable behaviour in the given context.
Knows how to close down the interview appropriately, especially when feeling out of their depth or unsure how to respond	Uses sentences, such as 'I can see this is distressing for you and I think it best that we pause at this time. My colleague, who is more experienced in this area, will talk some more with you about it'.
Summarises	Towards the end of the discussion, goes over the key points and checks whether or not the person needs further information or would like to discuss anything in more detail.
Confronts appropriately	Uses statements, such as 'I do not feel comfortable when you start shouting at me. Also, it doesn't help me understand how to help you. Please tell me about your most pressing issue'.
Problem solves	Uses statements, such as 'I can see this is very distressing for you … I'm wondering what might help or has helped you in similar situations?'
After the interview or discussion	
Uses diagrams where appropriate	Demonstrates flexibility and willingness to illustrate difficult technical concepts or anatomical information if the person has difficulty understanding.
Uses visual aids where appropriate	Demonstrates flexibility and willingness to consider people who prefer diagrams to written information, who have dyslexia or have problems reading, or are from culturally and linguistically diverse backgrounds.
Uses interpreters when required	Understands that interpreters are essential for people for whom English is their second language or who have a hearing disability.
Provides other sources of information (e.g. the internet, self-help organisations and leaflets)	Utilises a variety of sources, including a written record of the key points of the discussion or an audio recording. Leaflets from self-help or community organisations can also be made available, as well as website addresses and anything else that may help the person.
Documents, in detail, what has been discussed	Understands that these can be used as part of the feedback to the rest of the multidisciplinary team.

Source: Adapted from Geldard et al. (2021); Henderson (2019); O'Toole (2020).

Recording

The third step to conducting an assessment — or any clinical interaction — is recording or documenting the findings. Documenting assessment findings facilitates the communication of the information to other health professionals and enables effective planning and continuity of care (Cooper et al., 2021). Clinical documentation is used to audit the quality of health care services delivered and to investigate serious incidents and complaints.

Alongside the legal and ethical requirement for health professionals to record clinical activities, clinical documentation supports patient safety and improved health outcomes (Hay et al., 2020). Before documenting a clinical interaction, however, health professionals must communicate their intentions to the person they are helping and, if appropriate, family members (Treichler et al., 2021). As explained in the chapter that focuses on recovery-oriented health services, ongoing consumer participation in decision making about treatment choices is consistent with the philosophies and principles guiding mental health service delivery in Australia.

Before recording or documenting a health assessment, health professionals are advised to stop a moment to reconsider the following questions.

- What was the primary focus of the assessment?
- What information is missing that could help to improve the person's health outcomes?
- As you document the assessment findings, how can you acknowledge this person as an individual with a history and a social context who is not reducible to a set of symptoms?
- Why is it important to accurately document all the information you have gathered about the person?

- How may this information be used in the days, months or years ahead?

Answers to these questions will enable health professionals to be specific, accurate and comprehensive in their documentation.

Health services across Australia will have different ways of recording clinical information. In general, however, the following is a guide.

- The information must be brief, succinct, legible, and include the date, time, place and people present at the interview.
- The information must be factual. Health professionals must not write judgemental or value-laden statements when referring to the person's physical appearance, behaviour or lifestyle. Remember, consumers can apply to health services to read their records, so do not write information that could be offensive.
- The information must be jargon-free. It is best for health professionals to quote the words of the person they are assessing or describe behaviours rather than to use jargon inaccurately. For example, reporting that 'the person is manic and grandiose' could instead be communicated as 'the person is talking very quickly, very loudly, cannot sit still, and is claiming to be the ruler of the world'.

Finally, clear and factual documentation will allow health professionals to measure the progress of the person's recovery journey over time. Questions that could be answered as part of the ongoing process of documentation include the following.

- Has the person's presentation and mental health status changed? If so, how? Do, or could, the changes affect individual safety or that of others around them?
- Is there improvement in how they are feeling?
- Have family members or others who have known the person — for example, another nurse on duty — noted or recorded recent changes in the person?

Without the relevant records, these questions cannot be answered, and the person's health outcomes could be reduced.

Reporting

Many health professionals make the mistake of presuming that 'someone (else) will do something' once they have documented the findings of an assessment. However, unless health professionals report the findings to colleagues or those responsible for the person's overall care, follow-up may not occur (Agency for Healthcare Research and Quality, 2020). This lack of follow-up can place people, families, community members and health professionals at risk of reduced health outcomes.

Failure to report on or follow up after an assessment can cause consumers and carers to express high levels of frustration. For example, when findings are not reported, other health professionals may presume an assessment has not been conducted, and the consumer is subjected to the same questions all over again. In health settings, such **duplication** is a common source of complaints to health service managers from consumers and family members (Looi et al., 2021).

The power of assessments to make a difference for people is undermined when findings are not reported promptly to relevant health professionals. A lack of reporting means that suitable responses cannot be developed. In contrast, timely reporting enables timely decision making and development of the most appropriate interventions — at the right time, in the right place, by the right people, with the right services delivered at the right level, in a consistent and coordinated way (Cook, 2019).

UPON REFLECTION

The ethics of not reporting

There are many reasons why health professionals don't report clinical information. Reasons for not reporting include being too busy or forgetting; a lack of understanding of the need and necessity to report; presuming others will read the clinical notes; a fear of repercussion; and a culture of non-reporting. Many health professionals are also unaware of the ethical implications of not reporting.

....

QUESTIONS

1. Consider the ethical guidelines of your profession. Where does reporting — or not reporting — fit within these ethical guidelines?

---

2. What impact may non-reporting have on the effectiveness of mental health assessment?

3. How can you, as a health professional, encourage others to report findings of an assessment or other important information related to a consumer, carer or professional practice?

2.3 Assessment tools

LEARNING OBJECTIVE 2.3 Explain the most common mental health assessments.

Assessments are active, collaborative and continuous, conducted each time a health professional has contact with the person they are helping. Assessments can also be informal or formal, as determined by the situation or needs of the person. Informal assessments include observing body language and behaviours or asking questions that seem relevant to an individual at a particular time. Formal assessments employ tools or templates, such as structured formats or checklists, consistent interview plans, validated questionnaires or rating scales that minimise the influence of the health professionals' biases, opinions or value judgements to obtain comprehensive information about the person's experiences, health and wellbeing (Wilson & Giddens, 2020).

The tools, templates, structured formats or checklists used to support a formal assessment have been developed to:
- enable health professionals to gather information in a systematic and structured way
- facilitate the consistency and objectivity of the assessment — for example, different health professionals can conduct the same assessments on a person over time
- support discussions about the most appropriate interventions for the person consumer (Kaplan & Bernstein, 2022).

Two commonly used mental health assessment tools are the mental state examination (MSE) and the suicide risk assessment. These assessment tools are described in the following sections. Mental health assessments should not be confused with **psychometric assessments or screening**, which psychologists commonly use. Psychometric tests evaluate a person's cognitive ability, personality, values, motivations and behaviours in a measured and structured way. Such tests are specific to the field of psychology and comparatively narrow in focus. For example, on the MSE, psychometric tests largely fall into only two domains — behaviour and cognition. Mental health assessments, in contrast, have a broad focus and consider a range of factors.

UPON REFLECTION

Culturally appropriate mental health assessments

Most mental health assessments and psychometric screening tools used in Australia have been developed according to Western scientific traditions (Coelho et al., 2020). Although validated and standardised, they are not necessarily suitable or appropriate for diverse populations who view mental health and illness differently.

Researchers are developing more culturally appropriate assessment tools for some cultural groups. For example, the Kessler Psychological Distress Scale (K10) is a well-known tool used in Australia to assess a person's psychological distress. However, during use in Indigenous Australian populations, it was found that this tool lacked cultural suitability. The tool has since been adapted to be more culturally appropriate (McNamara et al., 2014).

Other cross-cultural mental health assessments in multi-cultural settings have also been developed to enable health professionals to understand the influence of cultural diversity on mental health. Culturally adapted assessment tools include the recovery self-assessment instrument (Ricci et al., 2020) and psychosocial wellbeing (Rasmussen et al., 2014).

QUESTIONS

1. How can health professionals be sure that a mental health assessment is culturally appropriate?

2. What are the benefits and challenges of a culturally-informed approach to mental health assessment?

3. What skills are needed to undertake culturally appropriate mental health assessments?

The comprehensive mental health assessment

When a person first presents with mental health concerns, the health professional must undertake a brief assessment in the first instance to gauge the most appropriate course of action. The focus of the shorter assessment would be to identify:

* the presenting issue or problem (i.e. why they sought help at this time)
* how long the person has had these experiences
* how the person and their daily lives may be affected by their experiences
* the urgency of a follow-up by a mental health specialist.

Health professionals use the information generated by this preliminary assessment to support a referral of the person to specialists, such as the mental health consultation-liaison team, a mental health nurse, psychiatrist or psychologist (Strauss et al., 2021).

Following the preliminary assessment, a health professional conducts a comprehensive mental health assessment. This assessment is much broader in focus and incorporates various aspects of the person's health and wellbeing. The contributing factors for mental health problems are **multifactorial** — that is, mental illness results from many different factors. These factors are summarised in the following sections.

Physical assessment

First and foremost, health professionals must determine if there is a physical cause for the person's current presentation or a physical health condition that has exacerbated the mental illness. Many physical illnesses, such as chronic pain, kidney disease or diabetes, can cause or have been connected to anxiety or depression (Khodarahimi et al., 2021; Sommer et al., 2019); and Alzheimer's disease, Parkinson's disease, brain tumours and even hypoglycaemia have been linked to psychosis (Morgan et al., 2021). Pregnancy provides another example where hormone changes and potential increases in social stressors may impact a person's mental health (McCauley et al., 2019). Ensuring people who present with mental health problems receive a complete physical assessment before a mental health assessment can save misdiagnoses.

A person who is intoxicated or withdrawing from alcohol or drugs may also experience symptoms of mental illness. For this reason, health professionals must wait until the person is no longer intoxicated or withdrawing from alcohol or drugs before assessing them for mental health issues. If the mental health assessment is conducted too soon, it will most likely be inaccurate and may mean that significant risks are not identified and managed. You can read more about the symptoms experienced by a person when withdrawing from substances in the chapter that focuses on substance use disorders.

IN PRACTICE

Physical illness in people with a mental illness

Fiachra, a 38-year-old man, was diagnosed with schizophrenia in his early 20s. At the time of his diagnosis, he experienced paranoia, believing people would hurt him in the street or break into his home to harm his parents.

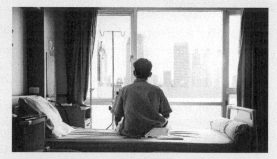

Since that time, Fiachra has taken a range of antipsychotic medications, including but not limited to haloperidol, stelazine, risperidone, quetiapine and olanzapine. Additionally, he has had four mental health hospital in-patient admissions, each for four weeks, throughout his 20s and early 30s. Fiachra has been relatively stable for the past five years, despite having short self-determined breaks of several weeks from the antipsychotic medications.

Health professionals have been concerned recently because of Fiachra's changing physical health. He gained nine kilos in weight in 6 months, has low energy, feels low in mood, has reduced interest in day-to-day activities and complains of a constant need to urinate.

....

QUESTIONS

1. What are Fiachra's current and potential physical health concerns?
2. How could health professionals work with Fiachra to assess and better manage his physical and mental health?
3. What strategies could health professionals have used to help avoid his initial weight gain?

Precipitating factors

Conducting a comprehensive mental health assessment includes asking a consumer or carer to describe the circumstance(s), situation(s) or event(s) that prompted, precipitated or 'triggered' them to seek help from a health professional. Such factors can indicate what is happening in the person's life and how they are coping, and suggest a way forward for the health professional in their assessments. For example, someone who has quite recently experienced or observed a traumatic event may be experiencing symptoms of an acute stress reaction. Another example is the person who experiences hallucinations as a direct result of smoking cannabis. Once such precipitating factors are identified, the health professional can help the person in the short term with appropriate interventions.

Alternatively, a person may have a long history of mental illness and be well aware of stressors, including particular situations or events that trigger an episode of mental illness. In this case, the health professional must note this information in the clinical records.

Biographical history

Obtaining biographical details is a necessary part of a mental health assessment. Such details will include information about different aspects of the person's life, such as:

- early childhood
- education
- relationships to parents, siblings and other family members
- school and work
- experiences or perceptions of experiences as a child and adolescent
- family history of mental health issues
- past and present behaviours related to alcohol and drug use
- past and present functional, occupational and recreational activities
- past and present financial situation
- lifestyle and social situation
- spiritual beliefs
- sexual activities
- onset and course of past mental health issues
- onset and course of current issues of concern.

Every person is a product of their background, as well as their past and present experiences and lifestyles. The ways in which people perceive and manage what is happening to them in the 'here-and-now' will be affected by what has occurred in the past. Knowing and understanding how past events and significant experiences have shaped a person can help them to make positive changes that will generate better outcomes for the future (Trenowth & Moone, 2017).

Collaborative history

A person experiencing symptoms of mental illness may struggle to organise their thoughts due to their distress or symptoms. Collaborative — and corroborative — histories can help clear up confusion about a distressing situation. Obtaining these histories includes talking to partners, family members and friends to obtain a more in-depth understanding of the person and their circumstances. People do not become unwell in a vacuum. Instead, their experience exists within their immediate personal context and larger social and cultural networks. Obtaining information from the partners, families, friends or significant others who are a part of these networks can be crucial to understanding the person's experience and presenting issues.

In an emergency, it is often not possible for health professionals to ask permission from the person before obtaining information from friends and family. Ordinarily, however, health professionals must keep the person informed of whom they intend to speak to. Maintaining clear and transparent communication channels is integral to engaging with the person and building a trusting relationship.

Mental state examination

While some people may refer to the MSE as the mental *status* examination, this term is more commonly used in the United States than in Australia, where the assessment is known as the mental state examination. The MSE is a core component of the comprehensive mental health assessment and focuses on the person's mental state at a particular moment in time. Through observation and an interview, the health professional assesses the person's appearance, behaviour, mood and affect, speech, thought process, thought content, perception, cognition, insight and judgement, as follows.

- *Appearance and behaviours*. A person's appearance (e.g. the grooming, hygiene, hair and condition of the nails); and behaviour (e.g. slow, restless, tremors, inappropriate or concerning behaviour) can reveal much about their inward state. The person's attitude to the situation and those around them can also be telling (e.g. hostile or withdrawn). All of these observable factors are included in this domain of assessment.
- *Mood and affect*. This component of the MSE assesses the subjective and objective perceptions of the person's feelings. 'Mood' is measured and described by the person (e.g. happy, euphoric, sad, fearful, hopeless, helpless, hurt, lonely or worthless). 'Affect', on the other hand, is observed by the health professional (e.g. the expression observed on the person's face or the posture of the person's body). A person's facial expression may be reactive (e.g. their face expresses emotion), restricted (e.g. they are showing no emotion on their face), or incongruent with their stated feelings or to a particular event or situation (e.g. they report feeling sad, but the expression on their face is bright and reactive, or they are laughing inappropriately).
- *Speech*. Different aspects of a person's speech can cast light on their mental state. The rate of the person's speech may be slow, sporadic, monotonous, rapid or pressured, reflecting their thought patterns. The volume of their speech may be soft or loud. The quantity of information provided by the person may be restricted or voluminous. Speech can also be spontaneous or reserved.
- *Thought form*. Thinking is most often expressed verbally, which explains why this domain is closely connected to the domain of 'speech'. Thinking can also be expressed in writing, artwork or other creative activities, so health professionals can potentially use a range of communications when assessing this domain. A good way to understand thought form is to relate it to the thinking process.
  For example, a person's thinking may be hesitant, blocked or vague, and this could be reflected in how they speak. The person may also experience a flight of ideas, that is, ideas that are not sequential or linked, but instead 'fly' from concept to concept with little apparent connection or continuity. Sometimes, the words used by the person may be confusing, or the person may invent new words or use common words in a 'word salad' that no-one but they can understand.
- *Thought content*. The content of a person's thoughts includes the subject matter, meaning or details of their thinking, such as possible delusions and suicidal thoughts, plans or intent. The health professional also needs to assess obsessive or compulsive thoughts.
- *Perception*. People's perceptions include what they see, hear, smell, taste and physically feel. Altered perceptions (where a person may see, hear or smell things that no one else sees, hears or smells) are called hallucinations. Other perceptual disturbances include derealisation (where the person feels that their surroundings are not real), depersonalisation (where the person feels a loss of contact with their reality) or heightened/dulled perception.
- *Sensorium and cognition*. This domain describes a person's level of consciousness (e.g. drowsiness, delirium, clouding of consciousness). The health professional will also assess the person's memory (immediate, recent or remote). This could include providing the person with several words and asking them to recall the words several minutes later to assess short-term memory. Orientation of the person to time, place and person are also relevant, along with the person's concentration level. Health professionals may test this by asking the person to subtract a series of 7s from 100 (i.e. 100, 93, 86, 79, etc.). Finally, the health professional may consider the person's capacity for abstract thinking.
- *Insight and judgement*. This includes examining a person's understanding or awareness of their experiences and how these experiences will affect the way they live.

The framework provided by the MSE enables the health profession to systematically consider each aspect of the person's mental state and their overall mental health.

Process of conducting a mental health assessment

Conducting a mental health assessment involves more than obtaining information from the person with mental health concerns. The assessment process is also used to positively engage consumers and the person's carer, partner or family members, and to facilitate understanding for them and their significant others of what is happening and why.

Some health professionals feel challenged by the idea of conducting a mental health assessment, including how to obtain information from the person with mental health concerns. Table 2.2 provides some of the more common questions or aspects of the mental health assessment, including the MSE, to support health professionals through the assessment process.

TABLE 2.2   Common questions to consider when conducting a mental health assessment

Factors to consider before assessment	Has a physical cause or illness for the person's presentation been ruled out?
	Has drug and/or alcohol intoxication, or withdrawal, been ruled out as a cause?
	Is the person physically well (e.g. not sedated, intoxicated, traumatised, vomiting or in pain) to interview?
	Does the person have a known history of mental illness? If so, is it possible to access a collaborative or corroborative history?
History of presenting issue or event that prompted the assessment at this time	What recent event(s) precipitated or triggered this presentation or made the health professional think an assessment was necessary now?
	Does the person pose an immediate risk (i.e. within the next few minutes or hours) with specific plans to self-harm or perpetrate aggression/violence towards others?
	Allow the person to tell their 'story' and place the experience of their illness or accident in context.
Biographical history	What is the person's personal, family, social and cultural history?
	How is the person placed financially?
	What does the person do for recreation?
	Is the person employed? Are they in a relationship? Is this relationship functional?
Past mental health history	Does the person have a history of self-harm, suicidal ideation or perpetrating aggressive/violent acts towards others? If so, what are the details?
	Does the person have a history of mental illness or mental health concerns? If so, what are the details?
	Does the person have a history of using alcohol or drugs? If so, what kind of alcohol or drugs have they used?
	Has the person required mental health-related hospitalisations in the past? If so, why, when and what was the duration of stay?
	Has the person ever been scheduled under the Mental Health Act? If so, why and when?
	Family history of mental health concerns, mental illness or suicide thoughts/behaviours.
Past and current medical information	Has the person had any past medical concerns, treatments or surgery?
	Is the person currently prescribed medications for medical reasons?
	Any family history of medical concerns?
Appearance and behaviour	Does the person have any distinguishing features?
	How does the person look in terms of body build, posture, gait and obvious marks (e.g. tattoos)?
	Is the person clean-shaven and well-groomed? What are they wearing?
	Is the person dishevelled and unkempt?
	Is there eye contact, unusual body movements, mannerisms or behaviours such as tics or posturing?
	Is the person agitated or restless? Are their movements fast, slow, erratic or other?
	Is the person obviously distressed, markedly anxious or highly aroused?
	Is the person quiet and withdrawn?
	Is the person behaving inappropriately for the situation?
	How attentive and engaged is the person with the assessment process?
	How does the person respond to and interact with the health professional?
	What degree of engagement is there with the health professional?
	Is there any suggestion or does it appear likely that the person may try to leave?
Speech	How much does the person talk? Is it fast or slow, loud or soft, disjointed, vague or lacking meaningful content? Do they respond slowly or quickly? Is the speech 'pressured' (i.e. a rush of words that is difficult to stop)?
	Is the person skipping from one subject to another?

(continued)

TABLE 2.2 *(continued)*

Mood and affect	How does the person describe their mood?
	How does the health professional see the person's mood? What is the expression on their face?
	How do they interact?
	How congruent are these descriptions? The descriptions can be different; for example, the person may say that their mood is 'fine' or 'okay' (subjective), but the health professional may observe in the interview that the person's mood is 'low', 'depressed' or 'elevated' (objective).
Thought form and thought content	Does the person express their thoughts in a confusing, illogical or incoherent manner? Are the person's thoughts racing, or are they very slow? Does their conversation go around in circles and never get to the point? Do ideas tumble out without any link between them? Does the person use words or sentences that don't make sense? Do they use words they have made up?
	What are the themes emerging from the person's thoughts?
	Does the person experience negative, obsessive or unwanted, intrusive thoughts?
	Does the person have delusions? If so, what are they? Health professionals should write down what the person says rather than use psychiatric jargon (such as 'grandiose' or 'paranoid') to describe the person's thoughts. Also explore the details of delusions with questions, such as, 'How certain are you that you are being followed?', 'How certain are you that other people can read your mind?' or 'What do you intend to do to stop the world from ending?'
	Does the person have any unusual beliefs about their experience of mental ill-health or physical health that are not congruent with the information given or the situation?
Perceptions	Does the person hear voices, or strange or unusual sounds? If so, what do the voices say? Are they male or female, or inside or outside of the head? When does the person hear them? Do the voices talk to the person directly? Do they tell the person what to do?
	Does the person see unusual things? Smell unusual odours? Feel things crawling across their skin or inside their body?
	Does the person feel controlled or influenced by external forces?
Judgement/insight	Does the person think they are unwell? Do they think they need to be helped or treated? Are they aware that others think they are unwell?
	What does the person think about their illness, treatment and prognosis?
Cognition	Is the person oriented to time and place? Are they aware of their surroundings? Can the person focus and shift attention appropriately?
	Does the person have the capacity to consent; that is, can the person understand and retain information and then make balanced judgements based on an evaluation of their options?
	What is the person's level of concentration?
	What is the person's ability to make decisions or choices, and think critically or abstractly?
Risk	Is the person at risk of suicide? Self-harm? Abuse? Aggression and/or violence to or from others? Are there particular risks associated with the person's mental state and physical illness (e.g. hopelessness, prompting non-adherence with treatment)?
	Is the person vulnerable or at risk of self-neglect?
	How immediate is the risk?
	What would be the likely impact of any actions if the person were to act upon their ideas?
Collaborative formulation	What is the health professional's understanding of the issues the person has described? Does the consumer and/or carer share this understanding?
	What is the level of risk? Does the consumer and/or carer share this understanding?
	Is immediate action required? If so, does the consumer and/or carer share this understanding?
	Is a referral to the mental health consultation-liaison team advisable? If so, does the consumer and/or carer share this understanding?
	How urgent is the referral? Does the consumer and/or carer understand the urgency?

Mental health assessments and corroborative information

As part of conducting a comprehensive mental health assessment, health professionals are advised to speak to spouses or partners, carers, family members, friends and other professionals who may be supporting the person for corroborative or additional information. Corroborative information can be helpful if there are unanswered questions about the person's descriptions of situations or circumstances. Health professionals will need to obtain consent to obtain this corroborative or additional information to maintain positive engagement with the person. The exception to this would be emergencies or crises.

QUESTIONS

1. What are the possible explanations for differences between the perceptions of the person and their significant others?

2. How could you manage these discrepancies as a health professional?

Risk assessments

Risk assessments conducted in health settings are determined by physical, biological, mental, psychological, social, functional, environmental and other factors that could place a person at risk. In the mental health sector, the most common risk assessments are:
- risk of harm to self, such as self-harm, suicide or self-neglect (e.g. homelessness)
- risk of harm to or from others, such as aggression or violence, or child protection matters.

Central to all risk assessments is identifying the risk factors in a person's life. **Risk factors** increase the likelihood of a person or group of people developing a mental health concern. Risk factors can be weighed against **protective factors**, which reduce the likelihood of a person or group developing a mental health concern.

Risk of harm to self

People can harm themselves in various ways, including self-harming behaviors, such as cutting, burning, head-banging and suicide. People can also harm themselves, intentionally or unintentionally, by using substances, neglecting themselves, not adhering to health treatments, absconding from a hospital or falling (usually for older people).

In light of the focus on suicide prevention in the current national mental health plan (Council of Australian Governments [COAG] Health Council, 2017), health professionals are most likely to conduct a suicide risk assessment in the course of their work. Various suicide risk assessment tools are available, with all of these tools connected to the risk factors for suicide. Suicide risk factors are complex but can be divided into individual, relationship, community and social components, such as those outlined in table 2.3.

TABLE 2.3	Common risk factors for suicide
Individual	Previous suicide attempt
	Mental illness, such as depression or psychosis
	Social isolation
	Criminal problems
	Financial problems
	Impulsive or aggressive tendencies
	Job problems or loss
	Legal problems
	Serious illness
	Substance use disorder

(continued)

TABLE 2.3 *(continued)*

Relationship	Adverse childhood experiences such as child abuse and neglect
	Bullying
	Family history of suicide
	Relationship problems, such as a break-up, violence, or loss
	Sexual violence
Community	Barriers to health care
	Cultural and religious beliefs, such as the belief that suicide is a noble resolution to a personal problem
	Suicide cluster in the community
Societal	Stigma associated with mental illness or help-seeking
	Easy access to lethal means among people at risk (e.g. firearms, medications)
	Unsafe media portrayals of suicide

Source: Centers for Disease Control and Prevention (2021).

Asking a person who may be experiencing challenging circumstances about these aspects of their life will help to determine a person's level of risk for suicide.

On the other hand, a person may also have protective factors to help them cope with challenging situations. These protective factors could include:

- coping and problem-solving skills
- cultural and religious beliefs that discourage suicide
- connections to friends, family and community support
- supportive relationships with care providers
- availability of physical and mental health care
- limited access to lethal means of harm (Centers for Disease Control and Prevention, 2021).

When health professionals conduct a suicide risk assessment, they must determine whether and how the risk factors outweigh the protective factors. An important consideration here is the notions of 'impulsivity' and 'changeability'. If a person is impulsive and known for changing their mind, then they will be at a higher risk of suicide than those who do not act immediately on their impulses. If a person is impulsive and also uses substances, which tend to disinhibit a person, then their risk of harm is higher again. You can read more about the assessment of suicide and self-harm in the chapter that focuses on the person who has self-harmed.

Risk of harm to others and from others

Risk assessments can also be conducted to assess a person's risk of harming others or being harmed by others. Examples of these types of risk assessment could include:

- risk of perpetrating aggression and violence
- risk to children (physical, emotional, sexual)
- level of vulnerability (e.g. risk of being exploited or experiencing elder abuse, risk of homelessness, risk of being unable to self-care).

Health professionals are also at risk of harm from others. These risks are usually occupational, such as the possible risk of harm from a vicious dog during a home visit or the risk of being abused by angry patients.

As with all risk assessments, health professionals are advised to weigh the known risk factors with the protective factors. For example, when determining a person's risk of perpetrating aggression and violence, the most significant risk factor is the person's history of violence or aggression. Contrary to popular belief, people who experience psychosis are not at a higher risk of aggression and violence than others; instead, there is no higher risk factor for future acts of aggression and violence than previous acts of aggression and violence.

Once identified, any risk level must be carefully evaluated, and steps taken to manage the risk. Risk management is always a collaborative venture between the person, their carers or family members and other health professionals.

Mental health assessment of older people

While most older adults experience good mental health, many others are at risk of developing mental or neurological disorders, substance use problems and physical health conditions (WHO, 2017). Some physical health problems can give rise to mental health problems — for example, people with cardiac disease are more likely to have depression than the general population, and those who have depression will have poorer outcomes (National Institute of Health, 2017).

As with all population groups, the assessment of older people must focus on risk factors. Older people experience the same risk factors as younger adults but may have the added risks of:

- cumulative stress issues
- ongoing grief and loss issues
- loss in capacities and a decline in functional ability, including reduced mobility
- chronic pain from physical health problems or disability
- reduced socio-economic status
- isolation, loneliness or psychological distress in older people, for which they may require long-term care (WHO, 2017).

Older adults are vulnerable to elder abuse. This type of abuse includes physical, verbal, psychological, financial and sexual abuse; neglect or abandonment; and loss of dignity and respect. Such experiences, in turn, can lead to mental health issues (Australian Human Rights Commission, 2021).

Older people are also more likely to experience depression, dementia or delirium. There is a need for all health professionals to accurately assess and differentiate between these three quite distinct conditions to ensure appropriate interventions. In particular, delirium is a potentially life-threatening condition often overlooked in health settings; and depression in older people increases the likelihood of suicide. For more information about dementia, delirium and depression, and the similarities and differences among the three conditions, see table 2.4.

TABLE 2.4   **Comparison of main features of dementia, delirium and depression**

Feature	Dementia	Delirium	Depression
Onset	Slow and insidious (months to years)	Acute (hours to days)	Acute or insidious (weeks to months)
Course	Progressive	Fluctuating	May be chronic
Duration	Months to years	Hours to weeks	Months to years
Consciousness	Usually normal	Altered	May be decreased
Attention	Normal except in severe dementia	Impaired	May be decreased
Psychomotor activity	Often normal	Increased or decreased	May be slowed in severe cases
Reversibility	Irreversible	Usually reversible	Usually reversible

Source: Adapted from Dening and Aldridge (2022); Department of Health (2015).

More information about assessing older people who may have depression, delirium or dementia is available in the chapter focusing on older people's mental health.

Outcome assessments

Outcome assessments or measures are used in mental health to monitor a mental health intervention's quality and effectiveness (Kwan & Rickwood, 2015). The process of assessing outcomes is essential to ensure that people receive high-quality services and progress towards recovery. For this reason, alongside assessing the person's physical and mental health, an assessment must include outcome measures from a broad range of perspectives, including those of health professionals, consumers and carers.

One of the best ways a person's outcomes can be determined is by comparing findings of standardised assessments over time. Such comparisons can determine areas of improvement or decline and provide evidence for continuing with a particular intervention, treatment or support (Department of Health, 2015).

Some health departments provide their own mental health assessments or frameworks. For example, in New South Wales, the Mental Health Outcomes and Assessment Tools (MH-OAT) standardise how mental health assessments and reviews are undertaken and documented across the state (NSW Health, 2021). The clinical documentation package includes assessment tools for triage, mental health assessment (including the MSE; substance use; physical examination; family, social and developmental history), review, care planning, discharge planning and also outcomes measures, such as the Health of the Nation Outcomes Scales (HoNOS) and Kessler 10 (K10). Other states, territories, organisations and services across Australia have similar processes to measure the outcomes of the mental health services they provide.

HoNOS and K10

Two assessment tools commonly used across Australia to measure outcomes are Health of the Nation Outcomes Scales (HoNOS) and Kessler-10 (K10).

HoNOS is rated by the health professional. It comprises 12 simple scales measuring behaviour, impairment, symptoms and social functioning and has been validated for use by adults aged between 18 and 64 (AMHOCN, 2022).

Kessler-10 or K10 is a self-report tool — that is, consumer completes the assessment themselves. The K10 measures psychological distress, and the results can be used to identify those needing fur-

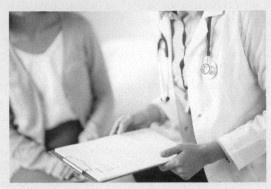

ther assessment for anxiety and depression. The K10 comprises 10–14 questions about how the person has felt over the past four weeks. It takes about 15 minutes to complete (Beyond Blue, 2022).

Both of these assessment tools can be used by health professionals, regardless of specialty area. Findings of these assessments can be readily stored, and comparisons made over time. Many health professionals find it useful to discuss the results of such assessments with the person and their carer or family member.

QUESTIONS

1. What are the potential benefits of discussing their assessment results with the person?

2. What are the potential challenges of discussing their assessment results with the person?

3. How could you overcome the challenges?

2.4 Diagnostic manuals

LEARNING OBJECTIVE 2.4 Outline the place of diagnostic manuals in mental health assessments.

There is a tendency in humans to categorise the world around them. For example, people have assigned categories or types to activities, food, books, music, vehicles and numbers. Categories are also evident in the health context, with classification or diagnostic systems forming an integral part of assessment and treatment.

Health classification systems are developed through international scientific consensus on the research evidence related to disease and disorder and provide a consistent, 'shorthand' language by which people can communicate about symptoms and assessments (WHO, 2022). Health professionals also identify patterns in the signs and symptoms experienced by people, diagnose the problem based on these patterns and recommend health care options.

Systems of health classification are beneficial because they:
- provide a means of consistently classifying health conditions, which is required for the coding of morbidity and mortality (i.e. different types of health conditions and causes of death). This is necessary to help health service managers and governments to determine where resources are best placed
- are a necessary part of the administrative and legal documentation required by health authorities
- enable health professionals to measure the outcomes of the treatments used and, as such, enable examination of standards or quality of care
- can be used to facilitate international conversations about mental illness across differing populations.

Some health professionals regard classification systems as unhelpful because they can reduce personal experience to simplistic diagnostic labels. There are also times when diagnostic labelling can lead to the person being stigmatised; and undermine person-centred care, with a consumer sometimes treated as a group of symptoms or a disease rather than a person with individual needs and preferences ((O'Connor et al., 2022)). Despite such challenges, awareness of the most commonly used classification systems will assist the health professionals when communicating with colleagues and governing bodies, and accessing research evidence to support practice development.

Today, the main diagnostic manuals used in the specialty field of mental health in Western health settings are the *International Statistical Classification of Diseases and Related Health Problems*, 11th Revision (ICD-11) and the *Diagnostic and Statistical Manual of Mental Disorders,* 5th ed. (DSM-5). These diagnostic manuals are by no means the only way of identifying a disease or other health problem. For example, complementary, alternative or Eastern health systems align with their distinctive worldviews. Even so, the ICD-11 and DSM-5 are Australia's most commonly encountered medical classification systems.

ICD-11

The **ICD-11** was endorsed by the WHO as the standard diagnostic tool for epidemiology, health management and the clinical management of people with diseases or other health conditions. The ICD-11 is not specific to psychiatry or mental illness. Rather, it codes all diseases and other health problems; and describes signs and symptoms, abnormal findings and complaints, as well as the social circumstances and external causes of injury and disease. The ICD-11 is used by health systems worldwide to aid decision-making related to reimbursement and resource allocation. This classification system also monitors the incidence and prevalence of diseases and other health problems.

The ICD-11 publication is used to diagnose mental health problems in preference to the DSM-5 in many states and territories across Australia. In addition, the ICD-11 is used extensively by national government organizations, such as the Australian Institute of Health and Welfare. One reason for this preferential use is the status of the ICD-11 as the only classification manual endorsed by the WHO. Also, the ICD-11 sets standards consistent across all diseases and health conditions, not just mental health conditions, on the international stage. Another consideration is that this classification system is available free of charge through the WHO website.

DSM-5

The *Diagnostic and Statistical Manual of Mental Disorders, Fifth Edition, Text Revision* (**DSM-5-TR**) focuses on abnormal psychology, mental disorder or mental illness. It was developed in the United States by the American Psychiatric Association, with critics describing the categorisation as US-centric. There have been five updates since its original publication in 1952, each describing the diagnostic categories of mental health conditions consistent with societal views at the time of development.

A significant feature of the DSM-5 is the 'axis' system used to differentiate symptoms, which includes three separate axes.
1. *Axis I* — all medical conditions, including physical conditions, psychiatric disorders, personality disorders and mental retardation.
2. *Axis II* — psychological or social stress factors affecting the person, including situations that date back to childhood, up to the present day.
3. *Axis III* — person's global functioning or level of disability.

While some commentators have described these three axes as less than optimal, research suggests that their use warrants ongoing utilisation until a better system can be developed (Fowler et al., 2021).

Another useful section of the DSM-5 comprises the self-assessment tools that mental health professionals can use to improve their work.

Why diagnose human distress?

Critics of diagnostic manuals such as the DSM-5 argue that labelling and treating common reactions to human distress can be counterproductive for people, families and communities. For example, when the bar is set too low, there is a risk of pathologising and over-diagnosing normal states of being (Young, 2016). Other critics suggest the DSM-5 serves to colonise the world by prescribing what is acceptable ▶

in the United States as acceptable worldwide, thereby driving the economic interests of multinational pharmaceutical companies (Cosgrove & Krimsky, 2012). Interestingly, however, the DSM-5 does not recommend treatments.

Specific examples of issues identified with the DSM-5 include the state of 'possession' which is acceptable behaviour in some religious communities (Padmanabhan, 2017). In contrast, the DSM-5 identifies possession as a dissociative identity disorder. Transgender populations also have objections to the new diagnosis of 'gender dysphoria' and 'transvestic disorder' (Hsu, 2019). Others have argued that grief trajectories are better tracked in the ICD-11 than in the DSM-5 (Bonanno & Malgaroli, 2020).

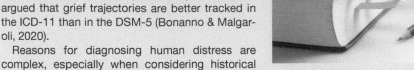

Reasons for diagnosing human distress are complex, especially when considering historical perspectives. For example, 'hysteria' was often diagnosed in women by medical practitioners in the late nineteenth century, but today this state is no longer a recognised illness. Likewise, while homosexuality was once identified as a mental disorder, it is now accepted in Western cultures as one of many expressions of human sexuality. Even the DSM being in its fifth iteration suggests that perceptions of mental illness are fluid.

In the United States, the DSM-5 is used to determine which mental disorders will attract health insurance reimbursement.

In Australia, the ICD-11 codes are used by health services and health professionals to assign funding and resources to particular conditions. Without such diagnostic coding, funding would be more likely to be assigned according to lobbying rather than identified needs. For example, through diagnostic coding, Australian governments have determined the prevalence rates of anxiety, mood and substance use disorders, and channelled funding to support the development of appropriate services.

Health professionals can reduce concerns about trends in diagnosing human distress by ensuring that the assessments they conduct are comprehensive and collaborative, engaging with and supporting the person with mental health concerns, connecting with them personally and building strong and effective therapeutic relationships.

2.5 Young people and mental health assessment

LEARNING OBJECTIVE 2.5 Describe the risk and protective factors for young people with mental health concerns.

About one in seven children and adolescents in Australia report a recent experience of a mental disorder in Australia, with the most common condition attention deficit and hyperactivity disorder, followed by anxiety, depression and conduct disorder (Healthdirect, 2021). The wellbeing of children and adolescents can be substantially impacted by mental ill-health (Australian Institute of Health and Welfare [AIHW], 2022).

This section describes the processes of providing young people with comprehensive, age-appropriate mental health assessments. These assessments are generally undertaken so that **early intervention** strategies can be commenced to manage the diverse stressors they experience in their lives (Theodoisou et al., 2019). Young people in Australia today face many challenges, suggesting the need for all health professionals to support children and adolescents to face these challenges, build resilience and live fulfilling lives.

Young people presenting for assessment

Young people experience the symptoms of mental illness differently from adults. For example, depression can be diagnosed in an adult if the person has been feeling sad, down or miserable for more than two weeks; takes no pleasure in the activities they usually find pleasurable; and has at least three signs and symptoms across the emotional, behavioural, cognitive and physical categories (APA, 2013). Depression experienced by young people, however, is less clear-cut and may include a prolonged sad mood, a loss of interest or withdrawal from normal activities, such as playing or sport; uncharacteristic behaviors, such as stealing or bullying; tiredness, particularly in the afternoons; sleep disturbances; and bed wetting (Headpsace, 2021).

Likewise, young people will react to stress differently than adults, depending on their age and stage of development (see the chapter on the common reactions to stressful situations). Health professionals must understand these differences and respond appropriately.

Another factor to consider when assessing young people for mental health concerns is how they express emotional or behavioural symptoms. For example, a young person who is tired may become agitated, loud, angry and disruptive, and not think of resting or lying down. Such differences can make it difficult for parents and health professionals to gauge what is happening, especially if the young person cannot articulate what they are feeling.

The behavioural and emotional symptoms experienced or expressed by the young person can also be a consequence of life's events or experiences, rather than mental illness. While these behaviours and emotions may not be a mental health concern, they can be an early indicator that mental health concerns may occur later in life (McGorry & Yung, 2021).

Challenging behaviours in young people may be triggered by events or experiences, such as family violence (Mehlhausen-Hassoen & Winstok, 2019), childhood sexual abuse, bullying at school or physical health concerns. While such behaviours require specialist attention, all health professionals must be familiar with the processes involved in assessing a young person, so they can provide the young person and their families with information on what to expect and support them as required.

UPON REFLECTION

Ethical considerations when assessing young people

There are many variations in how mental health problems are assessed and diagnosed in young people globally. These variations may reflect cultural, social, family or educational differences, including different expectations of how children should behave. Another factor is the diagnostic criteria used when assessing children. For example, many specialists avoid diagnosing a young person until they reach a particular age.

Some commentators argue that children and adolescents have a wide range of temperaments and ways of adjusting to their social worlds and that this variation is normal. They suggest that dysfunctional behaviour is subjective and that parents and teachers should be better supported to manage such behaviour in preference to children or adolescents being labelled. Others suggest that if a young person and their family are experiencing challenging behaviours or emotions, and these challenges can be alleviated by a diagnosis and treatment, then why withhold that diagnosis and treatment? This topic remains hotly debated in many contexts.

QUESTIONS

1. What is your view on the ethics of conducting a mental health assessment on a young person to provide a diagnosis? Explain your answer.
2. Who do you think should differentiate between the helpful and unhelpful emotions or behaviours in young people? Parents? Teachers? Counsellors? Social workers? Medical practitioners? Psychologists? The young person? Explain your reasons.

Assessment frameworks for young people

The assessment framework used by mental health professionals when assessing a young person with possible mental health problems is similar to the framework used to assess adults, described earlier in this chapter. The assessment framework includes person-centred and recovery-oriented approaches, practising unconditional positive regard, and developing a therapeutic relationship with the young person. There is a need to explore the presenting problem and biographical history of the young person, and conduct an MSE and risk assessment.

The main differences between the assessment frameworks used for adults and children lie with the adaptations made to meet the needs and preferences of young people and their families. Such adaptations are necessary because young people's mental health and wellbeing are greatly influenced by family members, peer groups and social or community factors, with key family members and significant others included in the assessment process. Other adaptations may include how the assessment is undertaken. For example, if a young person communicates through play or electronic media, health professionals are advised to use play or electronic media to facilitate communication with the young person (Cotter & Bucci, 2021).

As with the assessment of adults experiencing changes in mental health status, there are also various screening tools or questionnaires available for use by mental health professionals to enable comparison of a young person's thoughts, feelings or behaviours to other people of the same age. However, these tools are most often employed by psychologists and enable the diagnosis of a particular disorder rather than an assessment of the young person's mental health. Indeed, the comprehensive mental health assessment has a much broader focus than the psychological screening tools alone, which should never be used as substitutes for a more thorough and personal examination.

Health professionals conducting the assessment must focus on the young person's past and present experiences and explore the young person's stages of development. Such information can be gathered from various sources, including the young person and their parents, other family members, staff at childcare centres, teachers, school counsellors, general practitioners and paediatricians.

Because young people often find it challenging to articulate precisely what is happening to them or how they feel, observation is an integral aspect of the assessment. Mental health professionals identify how the young person relates or reacts to other people and new situations. The young person or their parent(s) may also be asked to keep a record of behaviours over time to help the mental health professional — as well as the young person and/or their parent(s) — to gain a more accurate picture of what is occurring in the home or school environments. While observations help to develop the assessment information further, they should not be used in place of actively engaging with a young person and their parents or family.

Risk and protective factors for children

According to the Victorian Government's Department of Health (2021), risk factors for children and young people in developing a mental health problem include:
- Aboriginality
- alcohol and drug misuse
- disability
- having a parent with a mental illness
- homelessness
- involvement with the youth justice system
- living in out-of-home care
- refugee status
- sexuality and gender issues.

Research studies have also identified the protective factors that guard against a young person developing mental illness. These include:
- secure relationships and a good attachment between the young person and their family, other adults and peers
- positive expectations of self and hopefulness for the future
- a sense of independence and autonomy
- effective therapeutic communication skills
- good problem-solving skills
- well-developed social skills
- the capacity to self-regulate behaviours and emotions
- a warm and supportive environment at home
- a supportive environment in childcare or school
- a sense of security through consistency with firm limits and boundaries
- opportunities for participation in a range of activities (Robinson et al., 2021).

Figure 2.2 provides a guide for the different aspects of the young person's social and emotional life, examined by the mental health professional to obtain this information.

| FIGURE 2.2 | Questions to consider when assessing young people |

When exploring the experiences of young people to identify possible mental health issues, the specialist mental health professional will consider the following areas of interest.

Reasons for presentation
- What has happened, or is happening to lead the young person and/or their family to seek support?
- Is a particular situation or circumstance increasing the young person's distress? If so, what is this situation or condition? How can I help to reduce the person's immediate distress?

Home life
- Are the young person's family and other significant relationships supporting them at this time or are they a source of possible distress?
- Has the young person been placed away from home or lived away from home at any time? If so, where, when, for how long? What is the young person's understanding of the reason for this? What was the young person's reaction to this experience?

School life
- Are there any factors influencing the young person's learning? If so, what are they? Is the young person aware of these factors? How does the young person manage them?
- What is the young person's attitude to school, schoolwork, games, teachers and peers?

Play life
- How does the young person play? What is the content of the play? To what extent is play symbolic? To what extent is the play constructive or destructive?
- Does the young person have a fantasy life? If so, what does it entail? The mental health professional may ask the young person to make three magic wishes or name their three most desired companions on an uninhabited island. The mental health professional may also ask the young person to describe the best thing that could happen to them. Is there a situation or event the young person has imagined that has caused them to feel distressed? The answers to these scenarios can often provide a great deal of information about the young person's inner life.
- Is the young person able to concentrate on their play, or are they easily distracted?

Personal life
- What are the young person's interests? What are their strengths?
- Does the young person experience any particular worries or relationship difficulties? Does the young person have someone they can trust and feel emotionally attached to?
- What is the young person's self-image? Has this changed over time or recently? Self-image is sometimes determined by what the young person says or does, the fantasy ideas or goals expressed and the young person's estimation of what others think of them.

Sleep
- What are the patterns of sleeping of the young person? How long does it take the person to sleep? What are their evening habits that may impact the quality and quantity of sleep?
- Does the young person experience nightmares? If so, what is the content of these nightmares?
- Does the young person sleepwalk or sleep-talk?

Behaviours
- Are there signs of premature sexual interest or activity?
- Is the young person distressed, anxious or depressed? Does the young person have self-harm or suicidal thoughts or behaviours?
- Is the young person feeling anxious, vulnerable or powerless?
- Is there evidence that the young person is using alcohol and other drugs?
- Is there evidence that the young person has other challenging behaviours — for example, acting out, aggression or violence or self-destructive or reckless behaviours?
- Is there evidence of changing eating habits or eating concerns/disorder?

Stages of development
- When does the young person reach each of the developmental stages?

Physical examinations are a crucial aspect of the mental health assessment of a young person. This is because there may be an underlying physical or biological reason for the young person's experiences. Health professionals must consider the many causes of physical symptoms, such as headaches and pain. At the same time, a physical examination can also identify abuse, neglect or maltreatment, which are risk factors for mental illness. All health professionals must assess for the signs of abuse, neglect or maltreatment when undertaking the physical assessment. When undertaking a comprehensive mental health assessment of a young person, the health professional must also consider the following physical factors, which may signify the young person's abuse, neglect or maltreatment:
- failure to thrive
- weight and height
- signs of head injuries, a torn lip or unexplained dental injury
- bilateral black eyes with a history of single blow or fall
- traumatic hair loss

- retinal haemorrhage
- skin injuries
- bruises or burns in the shape of an object or an immersion injury
- bite marks
- bruises of various colours (in various stages of healing)
- injuries to soft-tissue areas that are normally protected (thighs, groin, stomach or upper arms)
- injuries of the gastrointestinal or genitourinary tract
- bone injuries, for example, unexplained or unusual fractures (Royal Children's Hospital Melbourne, 2021).

2.6 Communicating with young people

LEARNING OBJECTIVE 2.6 Highlight the importance of age-appropriate communication when assessing young people.

Positive engagement with any person, young or old, involves the health professional establishing, developing, and maintaining a connection with the person they are helping. Early and constructive engagement helps the young person with mental health concerns to feel supported, receive the care they need and prevent the progression or recurrence of mental illness (Stavely et al., 2018). Such benefits suggest why health professionals need to develop the skills to connect with or relate to young people experiencing mental health concerns. A critical skill is the use of age-appropriate communication.

For example, the methods of communicating with very young children are quite different to those used when communicating with children in their middle childhood and different again to teenagers and young adults. All health professionals are encouraged to familiarise themselves with the developmental stages of young people to gain an awareness of differences in how they express themselves. Specifically, it may be necessary to observe very young children as they play, or communicate with them through their play, rather than asking them questions they do not understand or for which they lack the vocabulary to answer.

Indeed, and as with young people who experience physical illness, young people with mental health problems will often find it challenging to describe what they are experiencing. Such situations suggest the importance of health professionals engaging with them to access their perspectives, understand what is happening to them and work towards meeting their needs. Consequently, all health professionals must consider how best to connect and communicate with the young person.

Figure 2.3 provides some strategies to assist health professionals in connecting with and communicating with young people. As with all strategies, following these suggestions will not guarantee engagement; however, with practice and reflection, health professionals will develop the skills required to support them in their work, including helping young people with mental health concerns.

FIGURE 2.3 Communication strategies and young people

- Arrange a time and place that fits in with their world, rather than expecting the young person to feel comfortable with attending unfamiliar interview rooms or clinical environments.
- Communicate with the young person on their terms, such as using sandboxes, doll houses, crayons, clay or online environments. Be creative!
- Listen more than you speak. While this principle must guide how health professionals work with all people, young and old, it is crucial when supporting children and adolescents. If the health professional does most of the talking, the young person may feel irritated, intimidated or overwhelmed, and they may decide that it is easier to simply agree with the health professional, rather than share what they are thinking.
- Respect the young person and their views. Don't speak 'down' or condescendingly to the young person, or tease them about how they look, dress or speak. The best therapeutic relationships are authentic; young people will be able to sense if a health professional is not genuine or not interested. Young people will not share their feelings or private thoughts with someone they do not trust.
- Take time to be with the young person and hear about their experiences. Mental health assessment is a continuous process. Take time to think about how new information changes your overall impression of the person's situation. Continually review safety assessment and management plans.
- Don't make presumptions. Some health professionals will presume that because they experienced a particular emotion, thought or behaviour as a child or because their own children experienced these

emotions, thoughts or behaviours, other young people will have similar experiences. There is no 'one-size-fits-all' with children; they are individuals with their own way of dealing with their experiences.
- Avoid telling the young person what they should or shouldn't be thinking or feeling, or how they should be behaving. While the young person may (or may not) listen politely, it is unlikely that they will follow the directions given to them by someone they hardly know.
- Don't assume that the parent's or family's story about the young person's thoughts, feelings or behaviours is the same as the young person's. Health professionals must always ensure that they give the young person the time, space and privacy to tell their own stories.

Source: Adapted from Butterfly (2021); Macmillan et al., (2022); Rickwood (2021); Stavely et al., (2018).

The need to avoid 'labelling' young people

The health professional must take time and care before suggesting a diagnosis or 'label' for the young person experiencing mental health concerns. A mental health diagnosis carries stigma (see the chapter on mental health care in Australia), and this stigma can add to the young person's distress.

A young person's emotions and behaviours are expressed along a continuum or spectrum, with differences resulting from personal preference, cultural and religious differences, education and their parent's expectations. Variations will also arise from the diverse diagnostic systems used in different countries. For example, the diagnostic criteria for some mental health disorders in the DSM-5 differ from those in the ICD-11. These many factors suggest that deciding what is 'normal' for young people will always involve a degree of subjectivity.

While it is essential to provide young people with a rigorous and comprehensive mental health assessment, it is not necessary to use the findings of this assessment to develop a diagnosis. Instead, the focus of the assessment for the health professional is to find ways to support the young person, helping them to manage their emotions, thoughts or behaviours as they move through life. This support will include exploring the young person's risk and protective factors, educating them and their families and working with them to build on their strengths (McGorry & Yung, 2021).

UPON REFLECTION

Children of parents with a mental illness

Over a million Australian children have at least one parent with a mental illness (Emerging Minds, 2021). Children whose parents have a mental illness have an increased risk of developing mental health issues. The national government funded the Children of Parents with a Mental Illness (COPMI) initiative to support these children with resources and additional help.

When assessing children whose parents have a mental illness, additional risk factors include:
- low socioe-conomic status
- parent unemployment
- stressful life events
- challenging family constellations.

Parents with mental illness could also be assessed for:
- current circumstances and safety of the child or children
- capacity to provide physical and emotional care
- the parent's access to appropriate supports and services, and/or willingness to access support if needed
- the direct effect of the parent's mental illness, on the child or children
- the availability of alternative care and support for the child or children (RANZCP, 2016).

To ensure that children whose parents have a mental illness receive the support they need, they should be referred to school counselling services and, where appropriate, community groups.

....

QUESTIONS

1. Reflect on the risk factors for children of parents with a mental illness. What steps could you take to ensure the safety of the child?

2. Reflect on the situation of parents with a mental illness who also have children. What steps could you take to ensure that the person receives the best possible health care?

SUMMARY

This chapter provided an overview of mental health assessment, including biopsychosocial assessment frameworks and person-centred and recovery-oriented approaches. The most common mental health assessments were discussed, together with diagnostic frameworks. The final sections of the chapter focused on the mental health assessment of young people, including their risk and protective factors, and the importance of age-appropriate communication.

KEY TERMS

assessment A comprehensive evaluation of the health needs and preferences of a person.

biomedical model The Western, scientific approach to treating illness or disease. The causes of illness are viewed as biological. The health professional's role is to make a diagnosis, prescribe treatment interventions and achieve measurable outcomes.

biopsychosocial approach An approach to health care provision that addresses the full range of a person's health needs and preferences.

DSM-5 (TR) The *Diagnostic and Statistical Manual of Mental Disorders, Fifth edition, Text Revision*, published by the American Psychiatric Association; its focus is psychiatry or abnormal psychology.

duplication Similar or identical health services provided to or imposed on people with no added benefit for the consumer and reduced efficiency for the health organisation.

early intervention Strategies that target individuals who are displaying the early signs and symptoms of a health issue.

empathy A human quality demonstrated by a person that shows they are able to identify with the thoughts, feelings or experiences of another person.

ICD-11 The *International Statistical Classification of Diseases and Related Health Problems* manual, 11th revision, developed by the World Health Organization. The ICD-11 encompasses all diseases and related health problems and is not specific to psychiatry or mental illness.

mental health assessment A comprehensive assessment of a person's social, emotional, relational, behavioural, cognitive and functional wellbeing.

mental state examination (MSE) A systematic and structured way of observing and describing a person's current levels of mental health.

multifactorial The term used to describe a state that involves, depends or is controlled by a number of elements or factors.

person-centred care An approach to health care that involves the health professionals being responsive to the individual differences, needs and preferences of the person receiving the care.

personhood The state or condition of being a person; defined by one's individuality and aspects such as family background, culture, ethnicity, systems of beliefs, occupational and recreational activities and sexuality.

protective factors Factors that decrease the likelihood that an individual or group of people will develop a condition or illness; they are measured in terms of consequence and likelihood.

psychometric assessment An assessment that focuses on the educational and psychological measurement of knowledge, abilities, attitudes and personality traits.

risk factors Factors that increase the likelihood that an individual or group of people will develop a condition or illness; they are measured in terms of consequence and likelihood.

suicide risk assessment The formal process by which a health professional gauges or estimates a person's short-term, medium-term and long-term risk for suicide.

therapeutic alliance The mutual and active collaboration between a health professional and consumer to bring about change and healing.

therapeutic communication The communication techniques utilised by a health professional to engage with a person, build and maintain a relationship and enable the person to achieve personal change.

therapeutic relationship The relationship between the health professional and person that enables change in or for the person.

unconditional positive regard The positive and accepting attitude that is demonstrated by the health professional towards the person they are helping, regardless of who that person is or what they say or do.

REVIEW QUESTIONS

1 What is the difference between self-reflection and practice reflection?
2 How are person-centred approaches different to recovery-oriented approaches to assessment?
3 What are the benefits of using a 'biopsychosocial' framework?
4 Why is it important to record and report an assessment after completing it?
5 What differentiates a therapeutic relationship from other types of relationships?
6 Why is it necessary to undertake a physical assessment of a person who is experiencing mental illness?
7 What are the benefits of supporting families, including children, of people experiencing mental health concerns/mental illness?
8 What is the difference between 'mood' and 'affect'?
9 What are the main domains of the mental state examination (MSE)?
10 What are five risk factors for suicide?
11 Differentiate between depression, delirium and dementia
12 What are the main challenges for the health professional assessing a young person with mental health concerns?

DISCUSSION AND DEBATE

1 How can a health professional ensure a person experiencing mental health changes remains the central focus of their care?
2 What strategies can you use to maintain your own positive wellbeing?
3 What are the benefits and challenges of reflective professional or clinical supervision?
4 Why is it essential to combine person-centred and recovery-oriented approaches to mental health assessment?
5 Why are assessments a continuous process?
6 What strategies can health professionals use to communicate assessment and risk information within their team?
7 Which aspects of the comprehensive mental health assessment do you think are the most important? Justify your answer.
8 What steps can health professionals take to develop the acumen to work effectively with young people?

PROJECT ACTIVITY

MENTAL HEALTH ASSESSMENTS IN EMERGENCY SITUATIONS

The role of first responders in supporting the mental health of people in distress is under-recognised. For example, first responders (including paramedics, emergency nurses and medical practitioners) are often required to make complex safety decisions. These may involve maintaining safety to one's self and others. A person may have escalating aggressive behaviours, may present with acute psychosis or mania, may be under the influence of substances, may be experiencing distressing panic attacks or express suicidal thoughts or behaviours.

1 How can health professionals ensure that accurate risk assessment and management strategies are implemented while maintaining positive relationships with consumers and their families?
2 Which skills are helpful for health professionals when engaging with people experiencing acute distress and high-risk situations?
3 How can facilitating hope be a positive strategy for people experiencing acute distress? What strategies can health professionals use to build hope for people experiencing acute distress?

WEBSITES

1 The Black Dog Institute provides an online Psychological Toolkit, where health professionals can access various mental health and psychological assessment tools to utilise during their work. These practice resources can assist health professionals in managing mental health conditions in their clinical work: www.blackdoginstitute.org.au.

2 Children of Parents with a Mental Illness (COPMI) and Emerging Minds are national initiatives that develop information for parents, their family and friends, and health professionals to support young people. The website provides a range of resources to assist professionals and organisations working with children and/or parents/families with the skills to identify, assess and support children at risk of mental health conditions. www.copmi.net.au.

3 The National Institute of Mental Health in the United States provides information and resources that aim to transform understanding of the assessment and treatment of mental illness. This information includes a wide range of sources, toolkits, pathways and screening tools for mental health assessment. www.nimh.nih.gov.

4 GROW is a national organisation that provides a peer-supported program for growth and personal development to people with a mental illness and those people experiencing difficulty in coping with life's challenges: www.grow.org.au.

5 The National Institute for Health and Care Excellence (NICE), located in the United Kingdom, provide comprehensive resources on health-related topics, including mental health assessments. Use the search bar to access the information you need: www.nice.org.uk.

6 Headspace, the National Youth Mental Health Foundation, provides a range of resources on its website related to young people, assessment, early intervention, resilience and how to support parents and carers: www.headspace.org.au.

7 The Mental Illness Fellowship of Australia (MIFA) is a non-government, not-for-profit, grassroots, self-help, support and advocacy organisation dedicated to helping people with serious mental illnesses, their families and friends. Serious mental illness includes schizophrenia, bipolar disorder, major depression, obsessive-compulsive disorders and anxiety disorder: www.mifa.org.au.

REFERENCES

Agency for Healthcare Research and Quality. (2020). *Follow up with patients: Tool #6: Health Literacy Universal precautions toolkit* (2nd ed.). www.ahrq.gov/health-literacy/improve/precautions/tool6.html#

American Psychiatric Association. (2013). *Diagnostic and statistical manual of mental disorders* (5th ed.). APA.

Australian Human Rights Commission. (2021). Elder abuse. *Australian Government*. www.humanrights.gov.au/elderabuse

Australian Institute of Health and Welfare (AIHW). (2022). *Australia's children*. Australian Government. www.aihw.gov.au/reports/children-youth/australias-children/contents/health/children-mental-illness

Australian Institute of Health and Welfare (AIHW). (2022). *Mental health services in Australia. Australian Government.* www.aihw.gov.au/reports/mental-health-services/mental-health-services-in-australia/report-contents/mental-health-impact-of-covid-19

Australian Mental Health Outcomes and Classification Network (AMHOCN). (2022). *Health of the National Outcomes Scales (HoNOS)*. www.amhocn.org/publications/health-nation-outcome-scales-honos

Beyond Blue. (2022). *Anxiety and depression checklist (K10)*. www.beyondblue.org.au/the-facts/anxiety-and-depression-checklist-k10

Bhattacharya, P., & Priya, K. (2022). Stakeholders facilitating hope and empowerment amidst social suffering: A qualitative documentary analysis exploring lives of homeless women with mental illness. *International Journal of Social Psychiatry, 68*(4), 908–918. https://doi.org/10.1177/00207640211011186

Bolton, D., & Gillet, G. (2019). The biopsychosocial model 40 years on. In D. Bolton & G. Gillet (Eds.), *The biopsychosocial model of health and disease: New philosophical and scientific developments* (pp. 1–43). Springer.

Bonanno, G., & Malgaroli, M. (2020). Trajectories of grief: Comparing symptoms from the DSM-5 and ICD-11 diagnoses. *Depression & Anxiety, 37*(1), 17–25. https://doi.org/10.1002/da.22902

Bor, R., Eriksen, C., Oakes, M., & Scragg, P. (2017). *Pilot mental health assessment and support: A practitioner's guide*. Routledge.

Briggs, H., Clarke, S., & Rees, N. (2021). *Mental health assessment and triage in an ambulance clinical contact centre. Journal of Paramedic Practice*. www.paramedicpractice.com/features/article/mental-health-assessment-and-triage-in-an-ambulance-clinical-contact-centre

Burns, A., Dannecker, E., & Austin, M. (2019). Revisiting the biological perspective in the use of biopsychosocial assessments in social work. *Journal of Human Behavior in the Social Environment, 29*(2), 77–194. https://doi.org/10.1080/10911359.2018.1500505

Butterfly, L. (2021). What makes a good youth mental health service? In A. Yung, J. Cotter, & P. McGorry (Eds.), *Youth Mental Health: Approaches to emerging mental ill-health in young people* (pp. 100–105). Routledge.

Centers for Disease Control and Prevention. (2021). *Risk and protective factors*. US Department of Health and Human Services. www.cdc.gov/suicide/factors/index.html

Charbonnier, E., Trémolière, B., Baussard, L., Goncalves, A., Lespiau, F., Philippe, A., & Le Vigouroux, S. (2022). Effects of an online self-help intervention on university students' mental health during COVID-19: A non-randomized controlled pilot study. *Computers in Human Behavior Reports, 5*, 100175. https://doi.org/10.1016/j.chbr.2022.100175

Coelho, J., Ribeiro, A., Sampaio, F., Sequeira, C., Lleixà Fortuño, M., & Roldán Merino, J. (2020). Cultural adaptation and psychometric properties assessment of the NOC Outcome "Cognition" in a sample of Portuguese adults with mental illness. *International Journal of Nursing Knowledge, 31*(3), 180–187. https://doi.org/10.1111/2047-3095.12268

Coffey, M., Hannigan, B., Meudell, A., Jones, M., Hunt, J., & Fitzsimmons, D. (2019). Quality of life, recovery and decision-making: A mixed methods study of mental health recovery in social care. *Social Psychiatry & Psychiatric Epidemiology, 54*(6), 715–723. https://doi.org/10.1007/s00127-018-1635-6

Cook, A. (2019). Taking a holistic approach to acute mental health crisis. *Journal of Paramedic Practice, 11*(10), 426–432. https://doi.org/10.12968/jpar.2019.11.10.426

Cooper, A., Brown, J., Eccles, S., Cooper, N., & Albrecht, M. (2021). Is nursing and midwifery clinical documentation a burden? An empirical study of perception versus reality. *Journal of Clinical Nursing, 30*(11–12), 1645–1652. https://doi.org/10.1111/jocn.15718

Cosgrove, L., Morrill, Z., Karter, J., Valdes, E., & Cheng, C. (2021). The cultural politics of mental illness: Toward a rights-based approach to global mental health. *Community Mental Health Journal, 57*(1), 3–9. https://doi.org/10.1007/s10597-020-00720-6

Cotter, J., & Bucci, S. (2021). E-mental health for young people. In A. Yung, J. Cotter, & P. McGorry (Eds.), *Youth mental health: Approaches to emerging mental ill-health in young people* (pp. 125–138). Routledge.

Council of Australian Governments (COAG) Health Council. (2017). *Fifth National mental health and suicide prevention plan. Australian Government.* www.mentalhealthcommission.gov.au/getmedia/0209d27b-1873-4245-b6e5-49e770084b81/Fifth-National-Mental-Health-and-Suicide-Prevention-Plan.pdf

Cummin, N., & Schuller, B. (2020). Five crucial challenges in digital health. *Frontiers in Digital Health, 2,* 536203. https://doi.org/10.3389/fdgth.2020.536203

Davies, S., Sriskandarajah, S., Staneva, A., Boulton, H., Roberts, C., Shaw, S., & Silverio, S. (2022). Factors influencing 'burn-out' in newly qualified counsellors and psychotherapists: A cross-cultural, critical review of the literature. *Counselling & Psychotherapy Research, 22*(1), 64–73. https://doi.org/10.1002/capr.12485

DeAngelis, T. (2019). Better relationships with patients lead to better outcomes. *Monitor on Psychology, 50*(10), 38. www.apa.org/monitor/2019/11/ce-corner-relationships

Delderfield, R., & Bolton, G. (2018). *Reflective practice: Writing and professional development.* (5th ed.). SAGE Publications Ltd.

Dening, K., & Aldridge, Z. (2022). The three Ds: Dementia, delirium and depression. *Journal of Community Nursing, 35*(6), 59–64. [DOI not evident]

Department of Health (2015a). *Differential diagnosis — depression, delirium and dementia.* Victoria State Government. www.health.vic.gov.au/patient-care/differential-diagnosis-depression-delirium-and-dementia

Department of Health. (2015b). *Measuring outcomes in mental health services. Victoria State Government.* www.health.vic.gov.au/practice-and-service-quality/measuring-outcomes-in-mental-health-services

Department of Health. (2021). *Risk factors for children and young people. Victoria State Government.* www.health.vic.gov.au/mental-health-services/risk-factors-for-children-and-young-people

Department of Health and Ageing. (2012). *E-Mental health strategy. Australian Government.* www.mqhealth.org.au/__data/assets/pdf_file/0011/1010630/emstrat.pdf

Driscoll, J., Stacey, G., Harrison Dening, K., Boyd, C., & Shaw, T. (2019). Enhancing the quality of clinical supervision in nursing practice. *Nursing Standard, 34*(5), 43–50. https://doi.org/10.7748/ns.2019.e11228

Dziopa, F., & Ahern, K. (2009a). Three different ways mental health nurses develop quality therapeutic relationships. *Issues in Mental Health Nursing, 30,* 14–22. https://doi.org/10.1080/01612840802500691

Dziopa, F., & Ahern, K. (2009b). What makes a quality therapeutic relationship in psychiatric/mental health nursing: A review of the research literature. *The Internet Journal of Advanced Nursing Practice, 10*(1), 18. https://doi.org/10.5580/1060

Emerging Minds. (2021). *COPMI: About COPMI. Children of Parents with a Mental Illness Initiative.* www.copmi.net.au/about-copmi-2

Engel, G. (1977). The need for a new medical model: A challenge for biomedicine. *Science, 196,* 129–136. https://doi.org/10.1126/science.847460

Engel, G. (2012). The need for a new medical model: A challenge for biomedicine. *Psychodynamic Psychiatry, 40*(3), 377–396. https://doi.org/10.1521/pdps.2012.40.3.377

Erickson, H (Ed.). (2006). *Modeling and role-modeling: A view from the client's world.* Unicorns Unlimited.

Erickson, H., Tomlin, E., & Swain, M. (1983, 2005). (8th Printing) *Modeling and role-modeling: A theory and paradigm for nursing.* Prentice Hall/EST Company.

Evans, N., & Hannigan, B. (2016). *Therapeutic skills for mental health nurses.* Open University Press.

Fan, C., Hazlett, J., & Taylor, R. (2022). Perceiving therapeutic communication: Client–therapist discrepancies. *American Journal of Occupational Therapy, 76*(3), 1–6. https://doi.org/10.5014/ajot.2022.047670

Fiani, T. (2022). Practical functional assessment and behavioral treatment of challenging behavior for clinically based outpatient Services: A consecutive case series evaluation. *Education & Treatment of Children, 45*(2), 211–230. https://doi.org/10.1007/s43494-022-00071-9

Fowler, J., Carlson, M., Orme, W., Allen, J., Oldham, J., Madan, A., & Frueh, B. (2021). Diagnostic accuracy of DSM-5 borderline personality disorder criteria: Toward an optimized criteria set. *Journal of Affective Disorders, 279,* 203–207. https://doi.org/10.1016/j.jad.2020.09.138

Geldard, D., Geldard, K., & Foo, R. (2021). *Basic personal counselling: A training manual for counsellors* (9th ed.). Cengage Australia.

Gibbs, G. (1988). *Learning by doing: A guide to teaching and learning methods.* Oxford Polytechnic.

Hay, P., Wilton, K., Barker, J., Mortley, J., & Cumerlato, M. (2020). *The importance of clinical documentation improvement for Australian hospitals.HIM-Interchange, 49*(1), 69–73. https://doi.org/10.1177/1833358319854185. www.himaa.org.au/files/himinterchange/2020/Volume10Issue1/4-Hay.pdf

Headspace. (2021). *What is depression? .* www.headspace.org.au/explore-topics/for-young-people/depression/

Healthdirect. (2021). *Kids and mental health. Canberra, Australian Government.* www.healthdirect.gov.au/kids-mental-health

Healthdirect. (2021). *Online therapy (eTherapy). Canberra, Australian Government.* www.healthdirect.gov.au/etherapy

Henderson, A. (2019). *Communication for health care practice.* Oxford University Press.

Horvath, A. (2018). Conclusions: The tapestry of the therapeutic relationship and recommendations for clinicians and researchers. In O. Tishby & H. Wiseman (Eds.), *Developing the therapeutic relationship: Integrating case studies, research, and practice* (pp. 15–28). American Psychological Association.

Hsu, S. (2019). Fanon and the new paraphilias: Towards a trans of color critique of the DSM-V. *Journal of Medical Humanities*, *40*(1), 53–68. https://doi.org/10.1007/s10912-018-9531-3

Jarva, E., Oikarinen, A. , Andersson, J., Tuomikoski, A., Kääriäinen, M., Meriläinen, M., & Mikkonen, K. (2022). Healthcare professionals' perceptions of digital health competence: A qualitative descriptive study. *Nursing Open*, *9*(20), 1379–1393. https://doi.org/10.1002/nop2.1184

Johns, C. (2022). *Becoming a reflective practitioner* (6th ed.). Wiley Blackwell.

Jolly, J., Bowie, P., Dawson, L., Heslington, L., & Dinwoodie, M. (2020). Evaluation of a simulation-based risk management and communication masterclass to reduce the risk of complaints, medicolegal and dentolegal claims. *BMJ Simulation & Technology Enhanced Learning*, *6*(2), 69–75. https://doi.org/10.1136/bmjstel-2018-000392

Kaazan, P. (2020). Going viral with kindness. *Internal Medicine Journal*, *50*(6), 773–773. https://doi.org/10.1111/imj.14868

Kaplan, R., & Bernstein, K. (2022). *Psychiatric mental health assessment and diagnosis of adults for advanced practice mental health nurses*. Routledge, Taylor & Francis.

Khodarahimi, S., Veiskarami, H., Mazraeh, N., Sheikhi, S., & Rahimian Bougar, M. (2021). Mental health, social support, and death anxiety in patients with chronic kidney failure. *Journal of Nervous & Mental Disease*, *209*(11), 809–813. https://doi.org/10.1097/NMD.0000000000001386

Kwan, B., & Rickwood, D. (2015). A systematic review of mental health outcome measures for young people aged 12 to 25 years. *BMC Psychiatry*, *15*, 279. https://doi.org/10.1186/s12888-015-0664-x

Lewis, P., & Foley, D. (2020). *Health assessment in nursing* (3rd ed.). Wolters Kluwer.

Lonergan, A., Timmins, D., & Donohue, G. (2021). Mental health nurse experiences of delivering care to severely depressed adults receiving electroconvulsive therapy. *Psychiatric & Mental Health Nursing*, *28*(3), 309–316. https://doi.org/10.1111/jpm.12692

Looi, J., Allison, S., Bastiampillai, T., & Kisely, S. (2021). Headspace, an Australian youth mental health network: Lessons for Canadian Mental Healthcare. *Journal of the Canadian Academy of Child & Adolescent Psychiatry*, *30*(2), 116–122. www.pubmed.ncbi.nlm.nih.gov/33953763/

Ma, Y., Xiang, Q., Yan, C., Liao, H., & Wang, J. (2021). Relationship between chronic diseases and depression: the mediating effect of pain. *BMC Psychiatry*, *21*, 436. https://doi.org/10.1186/s12888-021-03428-3

Macmillan, I., Mahony, L., & Tindall, R. (2022). *How can GPs help young people engage with treatment for mental health issues? NPS MedicineWise*. www.nps.org.au/news/how-can-gps-help-young-people-engage-with-treatment-for-mental-health-issues

Malhi, G., Bell, E., Basset, D., Boyce, P., Bryant, R., Hazell, P., Hopwood, M., Lyndon, B., Mulder, R., Porter, R., Singh, A., & Murray, G. (2021). The 2020 royal Australian and New Zealand clinical practice guidelines for mood disorders. *Australian and New Zealand Journal of Psychiatry*, *55*(1), 1–111. www.ranzcp.org/files/resources/college_statements/clinician/cpg/mood-disorders-cpg-2020.aspx

McCauley, M., Brown, A., Ofosu, B., & Nynke Van Den, B. (2019). 'I just wish it becomes part of routine care': Healthcare providers' knowledge, attitudes and perceptions of screening for maternal mental health during and after pregnancy: A qualitative study. *BMC Psychology*, *19*(279), 1–8. https://doi.org/10.1186/s12888-019-2261-x

McCormack, B., McCance, T., Bulley, C., Brown, D., McMillan, A., & Martin, S. (2020). *Fundamentals of person-centred healthcare practice*. Wiley Blackwell.

McGorry, P., & Yung, A. (2021). Transition to adulthood. In A. Yung, J. Cotter, & P. McGorry (Eds.), *Youth mental health: Approaches to emerging mental ill-health in young people* (pp. 3–12). Routledge.

McKay, K., Ariss, J., & Rudnick, A. (2021). RAISe-ing awareness: Person-centred care in coercive mental health care environments—A scoping review and framework development. *Journal of Psychiatric & Mental Health Nursing*, *28*(2), 251–260. https://doi.org/10.1111/jpm.12671

McNamara, B., Banks, E., Gubhaju, L., Williamson, A., Joshy, G., Raphael, B., & Eades, S. (2014). Measuring psychological distress in older Aboriginal and Torres Strait Islanders Australians: A comparison of the K-10 and K-5. *Australian and New Zealand Journal of Public Health*, *38*(6), 567–573. https://doi.org/10.1111/1753-6405.12271

Mehlhausen-Hassoen, D., & Winstok, Z. (2019). The association between family violence in childhood and mental health in adulthood as mediated by the experience of childhood. *Child Indicators Research*, *12*, 1697–1716. https://doi.org/10.1007/s12187-018-9605-9

Mirea, D., Martin-Key, N., Barton-Owen, G., Olmert, T., Cooper, J., Han, S., Farrag, L., Bell, E., Friend, L., Eljasz, P., Cowell, D., Tomasik, J., & Bahn, S. (2021). Impact of a web-based psychiatric assessment on the mental health and well-being of individuals presenting with depressive symptoms: Longitudinal observational study. *JMIR Mental Health*, *8*(2), e23813. https://doi.org/10.2196/23813

Moen, Ø., Skundberg-Kletthagen, H., Lundquist, L., Gonzalez, M., & Schröder, A. (2021). The Relationships between Health Professionals' Perceived Quality of Care, family involvement and sense of coherence in community mental health services. *Issues in Mental Health Nursing*, *42*(6), 581–590. https://doi.org/10.1080/01612840.2020.1820119

Mollica, R., & Fricchione, G. (2021). Mental and physical exhaustion of health-care practitioners. *The Lancet*, *398*(10318), 2243–2244. https://doi.org/10.1016/S0140-6736(21)02663-5

Morgan, V., Waterreus, A., Ambrosi, A., Badcock, J., Cox, K., Watts, G., Shymko, G., Velayudhan, A., Dragovic, M., & Jablensky, A. (2021). Mental health recovery and physical health outcomes in psychotic illness: Longitudinal data from the Western Australian survey of high impact psychosis catchments. *Australian & New Zealand Journal of Psychiatry*, *55*(7), 711–728. https://doi.org/10.1177/0004867420954268

Nathan, R., & Lewis, E. (2021). Assessment of coexisting psychosis and substance misuse: Complexities, challenges and causality. *Advances in Psychiatric Treatment*, *27*(1), 38–48. https://doi.org/10.1192/bja.2020.45

National Institute of Health. (2017). *Heart disease and depression: A two-way relationship*. National Heart, Lung, and Blood Institute. www.nhlbi.nih.gov/news/2017/heart-disease-and-depression-two-way-relationship

Newman, M. (1995). Recognizing a pattern of expanding consciousness in persons with cancer. In M. A. Newman (Ed.), *A developing discipline: Selected works of Margaret Newman*. NLN, Jones and Bartlett.

NSW Health. (2021). *Mental health outcomes and assessment tool (MH-OAT)*. www.health.nsw.gov.au/mentalhealth/professionals/Pages/mhoat.aspx

O'Connor, C., Brassil, M., O'Sullivan, S., Seery, C., & Nearchou, F. (2022). How does diagnostic labelling affect social responses to people with mental illness? A systematic review of experimental studies using vignette-based designs. *Journal of Mental Health, 31*(1), 115–130. https://doi.org/10.1080/09638237.2021.1922653

O'Toole, G. (2020). *Communication: Core interpersonal skills for healthcare practitioners* (4th ed.). Elsevier.

Orem, D. E. (1991). *Nursing: Concepts of practice* (4th ed.). Mosby-Year Book Inc.

Padmanabhan, D. (2017). From distress to disease: A critique of the medicalisation of possession in DSM-5. *Anthropology & Medicine, 24*(3), 261–275. https://doi.org/10.1080/13648470.2017.1389168

Palmer, C., Richardson, D., Rayner, J., Drake, M., & Cotterill, N. (2022). Professional perspectives on impacts, benefits and disadvantages of changes made to community continence services during the COVID-19 pandemic: Findings from the EPICCC-19 national survey. *BMC Health Services Research, 22*(1), 1–12. https://doi.org/10.1186/s12913-022-08163-3

Peplau, H. (1952, 1991). *Interpersonal relations in nursing*. MacMillan.

Pihlaja, S., Stenberg, J., Joutsenniemi, K., Mehik, H., Ritola, V., & Joffe, G. (2017). Therapeutic alliance in guided internet therapy programs for depression and anxiety disorders – A systematic review. *Internet interventions, 11*, 1–10. https://doi.org/10.1016/j.invent.2017.11.005

Rasmussen, A., Ventevogel, P., Sancilio, A., Eggerman, M., & Panter-Brick, C. (2014). Comparing the validity of the self reporting questionnaire and the Afghan symptom checklist: Dysphoria, aggression, and gender in transcultural assessment of mental health. *BMC Psychiatry, 14*, 206. https://doi.org/10.1186/1471-244X-14-206

Raudenská, J., Steinerová, V., Javůrková, A., Urits, I., Kaye, A., Viswanath, O., & Varrassi, G. (2020). Occupational burnout syndrome and post-traumatic stress among healthcare professionals during the novel coronavirus disease 2019 (COVID-19) pandemic. *Best Practice Research in Clinical, 34*(3), 553–560. https://doi.org/10.1016/j.bpa.2020.07.008

Ricci, E., Leal, E., La-Rotta, E., Onocko-Campo, R., & O'Connell, M. (2020). Cross-cultural adaptation of the recovery self-assessment instrument (RSA–R) person in recovery version to Brazilian Portuguese (Pt/Br). *Journal of Public Mental Health, 19*(4), 333–347. https://doi.org/10.1108/JPMH-02-2020-0008

Rickwood, D. (2021). Help-seeking in young people. In A. Yung, J. Cotter, & P. McGorry (Eds.). *Youth mental health: Approaches to emerging mental ill-health in young people* (pp. 35–52). Routledge.

Rietkerk, W., Uittenbroek, R., Gerritsen, D., Slaets, J., Zuidema, S., & Wynia, K. (2021). Goal planning in person-centred care supports older adults receiving case management to attain their health-related goals. *Disability & Rehabilitation, 43*(12), 1682–1691. https://doi.org/10.1080/09638288.2019.1672813

Robinson, J., Cox, G., Hetrick, S., & Byrne, S. (2021). Youth suicide: Predictors, predictors and prevention. In A. Yung, J. Cotter, & P. McGorry (Eds.), *Youth Mental Health: Approaches to emerging mental ill-health in young people* (pp. 195–223). Routledge.

Rogers, C. (1951). *Client-centered therapy: Its current practice, implications and theory*. Houghton Mifflin.

Rogers, C. (1961). *On becoming a person: A therapist's view of psychotherapy*. Houghton Mifflin.

Rogers, C. (1980). *A way of being: The founder of the human potential movement looks back on a distinguished career*. Houghton Mifflin.

Roy, C. (2009). *The Roy adaptation model* (3rd ed.). Prentice Hall Health.

Royal Australian and New Zealand College of Psychiatrists (RANZCP). (2016). *Children of parents with mental illness: Position Statement 56*. www.ranzcp.org/news-policy/policy-and-advocacy/position-statements/children-of-parents-with-mental-illness

Royal Children's Hospital Melbourne. (2021). *Child abuse*. VIC Health. www.rch.org.au/clinicalguide/guideline_index/Child_Abuse_Guideline

Shannon, P., Vinson, G., Horn, T., & Lennon, E. (2021). Defining effective care coordination for mental health referrals of refugee populations in the United States. *Ethnicity & Health, 26*(5), 737–755. https://doi.org/10.1080/13557858.2018.1547369

Snell-Rood, C., & Carpenter-Song, E. (2018). Depression in a depressed area: Deservingness, mental illness, and treatment in the contemporary rural U.S. *Social Science & Medicine, 219*, 78–86. https://doi.org/10.1016/j.socscimed.2018.10.012

Snowdon, D., Leggat, S., Harding, K., Boyd, J., Scroggie, G., & Taylor, N. (2020). The association between effectiveness of clinical supervision of allied health professionals and improvement in patient function in an inpatient rehabilitation setting. *Disability & Rehabilitation, 42*(8), 1173–1182. https://doi.org/10.1080/09638288.2018.1518493

Sommer, J. L., Blaney, C., & El-Gabalawy, R. (2019). A population-based examination if suicidality in comorbid generalized anxiety disorder and chronic pain. *Journal of Affective Disorders, 257*, 562–567. https://doi.org/10.1016/j.jad.2019.07.016

Standsfield, J., & Shah, N. (2021). Mental health recovery and transformation: Lessons for action. *International Journal for Health Promotion and Education, 59*(3), 131–134. https://doi.org/10.1080/14635240.2021.1905967

Stavely, H., Redlich, C., & Peipers, A. (2018). *Engaging young people and their families in youth mental health: Strategies and tips for mental health workers*. Orygen. www.orygen.org.au/About/Service-Development/Youth-Enhanced-Services-National-Programs/Primary-Health-Network-resources/ENGAGING-YOUNG-PEOPLE-AND-THEIR-FAMILIES-IN-YOUTH/orygen-Engaging-young-people-and-their-families-in.aspx?ext=

Stein-Parbury, J. (2021). *Patient and person: Interpersonal skills in nursing* (7th ed.). Elsevier.

Strand, M., Eng, L., & Gammon, D. (2020). Combining online and offline peer support groups in community mental health care settings: A qualitative study of service users' experiences. *International Journal of Mental Health Systems, 14*, 39. https://doi.org/10.1186/s13033-020-00370-x

Strauss, P., Lin, A., Winter, S., Waters, Z., Watson, V., Wright Toussaint, D., & Cook, A. (2021). Options and realities for trans and gender diverse young people receiving care in Australia's mental health system: Findings from Trans Pathways. *Australian & New Zealand Journal of Psychiatry, 55*(4), 391–399. https://doi.org/10.1177/0004867420972766

Theodoisou, L., Knightsmith, P., Lavis, P., & Bailey, S. (2019). *Children and young people's mental health: Early intervention, ongoing support and flexible evidence-based care*. Pavillion Publishing.

Tishby, O., & Wiseman, H. (2018). Conclusions: The tapestry of the therapeutic relationship and recommendations for clinicians and researchers. In O. Tishby & H. Wiseman (Eds.), *Developing the therapeutic relationship: Integrating case studies, research, and practice* (pp. 341–348). American Psychological Association.

Treichler, E., Evans, E., & Spaulding, W. (2021). Ideal and real treatment planning processes for people with serious mental illness in public mental health care. *Psychological Services, 18*(1), 93–103. https://doi.org/10.1037/ser0000361

Tremain, H., McEnery, C., Fletcher, K., & Murray, G. (2020). The therapeutic alliance in digital mental health interventions for serious mental illnesses: Narrative review. *JMIR Mental Health, 7*(8), e17204. https://doi.org/10.2196/17204

Trenowth, S., & Moone, N. (2017). Chapter 1: Overview of assessment in mental health care. In S. Trenowth & N. Moone (Eds.), *Psychosocial assessment in mental health*. Sage.

van Weeghel, J., Boertien, D., van Zelst, C, & Hasson-Ohayon, I. (2019). Conceptualizations, assessments, and implications of personal Recovery in mental illness: A scoping review of systematic reviews and meta-analyses. *Psychiatric Rehabilitation Journal, 42*(2), 189–181. https://doi.org/10.1037/prj0000356

Waling, A., Lim, G., Dhalla, S., Lyons, A., & Bourne, A. (2019). *Understanding LGBTI+ Lives in Crisis. Australian Research Centre in Sex, Health and Society*. La Trobe University & Lifeline Australia. Monograph 112 www.lifeline.org.au/media/usdp3jhq/understanding-lgbti-lives-in-crisis-2019.pdf

Watts, L. (2019). Reflective practice, reflexivity, and critical reflection in social work education in Australia. *Australian Social Work, 72*(1), 8–20. https://doi.org/10.1080/0312407X.2018.1521856

Wilson, S., & Giddens, J. (2020). *Health assessment for nursing practice* (7th ed.). Elsevier.

Wong, Y., & Vinsky, J. (2021). Beyond implicit bias: Embodied cognition, mindfulness, and critical reflective practice in social work. *Australian Social Work, 74*(2), 186–197. https://doi.org/10.1080/0312407X.2020.1850816

World Health Organization (WHO). (1948). *Constitution of the World Health Organization*. WHO. www.who.int/about/governance/constitution

World Health Organization (WHO). (2017). *Mental health of older adults*. WHO. www.who.int/news-room/fact-sheets/detail/mental-health-of-older-adults

World Health Organization (WHO). (2022). *Classifications and terminologies*. WHO. www.who.int/standards/classifications

Young, G. (2016). *Unifying causality and psychology: Being, brain and behaviour*. Springer.

ACKNOWLEDGEMENTS

Photo: © Monkey Business Images / Shutterstock.com

Photo: © RossHelen / Shutterstock.com

Photo: © Monkey Business Images / Shutterstock.com

Photo: © Rawpixel.com / Shutterstock.com

Photo: © namtipStudio / Shutterstock.com

Photo: © Pressmaster / Shutterstock.com

Photo: © ktasimar / Shutterstock.com

Figure 2.1: © University of Edinburgh, (2020). *Gibb's Reflective Cycle*. Retrieved 15 July 2022 from www.ed.ac.uk/reflection/reflectors-toolkit/reflecting-on-experience/gibbs-reflective-cycle.

Table 2.3: © Centers for Disease Control and Prevention. (2021). *Risk and Protective Factors*. US Department of Health and Human Services. Retrieved 12 July 2022 from www.cdc.gov/suicide/factors/index.html. Public Domain.

Table 2.4: © Adapted from Dening, K & Aldridge, Z. (2022). The three Ds: Dementia, delirium and depression. *Journal of Community Nursing, 35* (6), 59–64 and State of Victoria Department of Health, www.health.vic.gov.au/patient-care/differential-diagnosis-depression-delirium-and-dementia.

CHAPTER 3

The legal and ethical context of mental health care

LEARNING OBJECTIVES

This chapter will:

3.1 identify the key legal, ethical and professional principles guiding the provision of mental health care

3.2 describe the challenges for health professionals when making ethical decisions

3.3 discuss the concepts of consent, capacity and competence

3.4 explain the importance of advance care agreements or directives in the field of mental health

3.5 discuss the concept of duty of care

3.6 outline the use and application of mental health legislation across Australia

3.7 provide an introduction to the interface between legal and mental health systems known as forensic mental health.

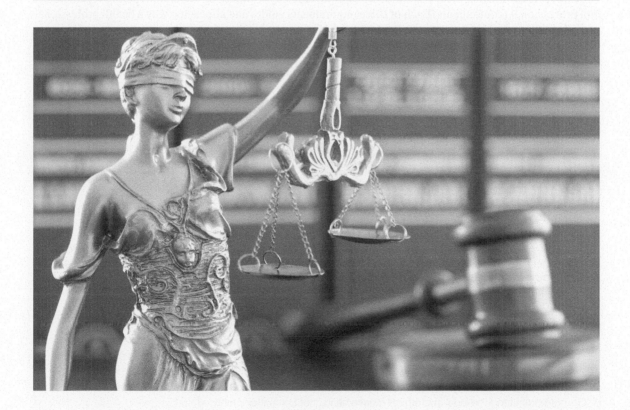

Introduction

The legal and ethical principles that underpin the provision of mental health care in Australia may seem complex to those who practise in non-mental health settings. For example, some health professionals may wonder about the capacity or competence of a person with a mental illness to give informed consent for a medical procedure; health professionals may also be uncertain about their duty of care to the person with a mental illness in particular situations, others may feel that they lack knowledge of the requirements of the mental health legislation relevant to their state or territory.

This chapter identifies the key legal, ethical and professional issues for health professionals who provide care to people with a mental illness wherever they are geographically situated, for example, in acute inpatient care, non-mental health hospital or community settings. It includes a discussion of the concepts of capacity, competence, consent and duty of care. An outline is also provided of the importance of advance care agreements or directives for people with a mental illness, and the development of forensic care. The chapter concludes by explaining the mental health legislation that is in place in states and territories across Australia and how this legislation generally relates to health professionals working in a variety of contexts.

The discussion and examples provided in the chapter are broad in focus. This is because each of the states and territories have different laws. Even so, it is anticipated that this broad focus will enable health professionals to consider how best to integrate the major principles into their everyday practice, regardless of their location or place of work. The broad focus will also serve as a means by which health professionals can increase their overall awareness of the legal and ethical frameworks within which they work and effectively meet the requirements of these frameworks.

3.1 The legal and ethical context

LEARNING OBJECTIVE 3.1 Identify the key legal, ethical and professional principles guiding the provision of mental health care.

A health professional's practice is informed and governed by a variety of factors, including legal, ethical and professional requirements. Each of these requirements guides and affects the way a health professional provides care to those in need. In the field of mental health, the legal, ethical and professional requirements are quite complex. One reason for this is that each state and territory in Australia has enacted its own distinct mental health legislation to consistently guide the way in which people with a mental illness receive treatment and care. Some of the specifics are discussed in the last section of this chapter.

This section outlines the legal, ethical and professional principles that guide the provision of health care to people with mental health problems, no matter where they are located geographically, or in what type of health setting they occupy. The outline also includes a brief discussion of the major issues that may arise from applying these principles in practice.

UPON REFLECTION

'But I'm not a lawyer!'

Many health professionals are reluctant to learn about the legal and ethical requirements that frame the way they practise. The complexities of this area of health service delivery are such that they would prefer to leave these issues to the lawyers. However, given the political climate of the day, social media usage and the knowledge the community has regarding mental health, human rights and appropriate health care, it is vital that we understand the legal and ethical boundaries that underpin our practice in order to minimise compromising the care we provide, as well as uphold our professional standing.

....

QUESTIONS

1. What are the potential consequences for the health professional who does not understand the legal and ethical requirements that frame their practice?
2. What are the potential consequences for the consumer and/or carers when the health professional does not understand the legal and ethical requirements that frame their practice?
3. What are the potential consequences for the health service provider and governments when the health professional does not understand the legal and ethical requirements that frame their practice?
4. What are your thoughts regarding the use of social media to highlight potential ethical and legal breaches perpetrated by first responders and health care professionals?

Legal requirements

Australia's legal system was inherited from the British legal system and comprises common law and statute law. The terms '**statute law**' and '**common law**' will be used throughout this chapter, so it is important to clarify their meaning. Statute law refers to laws that are also known as the 'laws of the land'; for example, the *Aboriginal and Torres Strait Islander Peoples Recognition Act 2013*. These laws are passed by an Act of Parliament, whether state, territory or Commonwealth. The relevance of the proposed law and the way it will be enacted in the community is debated in parliament to ensure it reflects the will of the people. Common law refers to the principles that guide the interpretation of the law based on decisions made by judges in individual cases. Table 3.1 outlines some of the characteristics of each of these types of laws.

TABLE 3.1   **Characteristics of statute law and common law**

Statute law	Common law
A law made by parliament (state, territory or Commonwealth). Its relevance and enactment is openly debated in parliament prior to becoming law. The law is written down and can be consulted and referred to by others. Statute laws take precedence over all other laws.	Also referred to as case law or judge-made law. These are common law principles based on the decisions made by judges in individual cases. The 'Bolam principle' provides an example of case law informing health care practice: the case of *Bolam v Friern Hospital Management Committee* (1957) produced a definition of what is reasonable in terms of the standard of competence expected of health professionals when carrying out their duties.
Statute law is applicable as long as it remains on the statute — the only way for legislation to cease to be law is for it to be repealed.	They may be based on interpretations of statute law (but not necessarily so), or decisions made by a court.
Examples of Commonwealth statute laws relevant to health care include the *Privacy Amendment Act 2004*, the *Freedom of Information Act 1982* and the *Work Health and Safety (Transitional and Consequential Provisions) Act 2011*.	A further example of common law principles applied to health care is the concept of a 'duty of care'. It has long been established in common law that health professionals and health service providers owe their consumer a duty of care (Aboriginal and Torres Strait Islander [ATSI] Health Practice Board of Australia, 2014).

In the health context in Australia, an important statute law is the *Health Practitioner Regulation National Law Act 2009*. This law has given rise to nationwide registration and accreditation standards for health professionals as part of the National Registration and Accreditation Scheme for Health Professionals, which commenced on 1 July 2010. For 15 specific health professional groups across Australia, this law means one national registration fee, one set of registration and general professional standards and one registration process, rather than the previous inconsistent state and territory-based registration processes. The Australian Health Practitioner Regulation Agency (AHPRA) supports this law and currently regulates more than 800 000 health practitioners across the country (AHPRA, 2021).

Other statute laws that inform how health professionals practise in Australia include privacy Acts, health record Acts and freedom of information Acts. Table 3.2 provides an outline of these and other laws that are particularly relevant for health professionals who care for a person with a mental illness. For example, mental health legislation that has been enacted in each of the states and territories guides the health care and treatment that is provided to people with a mental illness, and guards against human rights abuses. This legislation is discussed in more detail later in the chapter. Also important are the privacy laws that are in place in all states and territories. These laws are discussed in the section 'Confidentiality and privacy'.

TABLE 3.2   **Examples of statute laws applicable when caring for people with mental health problems**

Statute	Comments
Mental Health Acts (various)	Allows for care, treatment and control of people experiencing mental illness or disorder in either a voluntary or involuntary capacity (Mental Health Coordinating Council, 2015). Health professionals need to be aware of the common sections of the Act in the state or territory in which they are practising.

(continued)

TABLE 3.2 *(continued)*

Statute	Comments
Health Records Acts (various), and the *Privacy Act 1988* (in particular National Privacy Principle 6)	Allows individuals to access personal information, including health-related information, unless providing access to the information would pose a serious threat to the life or health of the individual (National Privacy Principle 6.1[b]).
Human Rights Acts or Charters (various)	Enshrined in law are the following civil and political rights (ACT Parliamentary Counsel, 2017). • The right to life • The prohibition of torture and inhumane and degrading treatment • The right to liberty and freedom of movement • The right to privacy and reputation • Freedom of expression, including thought, conscience, religion and belief • The prohibition of discrimination • The right to humane treatment when deprived of liberty
Freedom of Information Act 1982 (FOI Act)	Gives the right to access written information from public bodies (including health care providers). Members of the public may request information relating to health services policies (e.g. local policy on the prescribing and administration of medication). It needs to be noted that access to information may be denied in situations where it is considered that disclosure of sensitive information might be detrimental to the applicant's physical or mental health, or wellbeing (FOI Act s. 41).
Guardianship and Management of Property Acts or Guardianship and Administration Acts (various)	Set out the legal terms under which it is possible to make decisions — including those relating to health care — for people who are not able to make decisions for themselves.

Ethical requirements

All health professionals are required by their professional bodies to practise in a lawful and ethical manner (e.g. Australian Association of Social Workers (Draft), 2022; International Council of Nurses, 2021; Paramedicine Board of Australia, 2018). The primary ethical requirement of all health professionals is to respect the:

• right of the individual to make decisions about their care (i.e. autonomy, freedom and self-determination)
• need to avoid inflicting harm (non-maleficence)
• need to do good (beneficence)
• need to treat people fairly and with respect (justice and fairness) (Beauchamp & Childress, 1994; Kurpad, 2018).

These ethical principles are particularly important when caring for people with a mental illness in contemporary Australian society. This is because of the way people with a mental illness have historically been treated in Australia.

As noted in the chapter on mental health care in Australia, it is only since the 1980s that people with mental health issues have been assured the same rights as other citizens, including the right to make their own decisions about their own care, and to be treated fairly and with respect. Consequently, many people with a mental illness may be fearful or suspicious of health professionals and their potential to disempower them. Effective health professionals have learnt from the past and work hard to inspire hope in the future of all those for whom they care.

The ethical frameworks provided by the professional bodies also uphold the need to avoid paternalism, whereby health professionals assume they always know what is best for the consumer. While the health professional's motivation may be informed by the desire to do good, this must always be balanced with an individual's right to autonomy. It is the role of the health professional to respect this right and to be aware that notions of 'doing good' are often open to subjective interpretations. On the other hand, consideration should also be given to the consequences and risks of such a decision when the offer of treatment is declined or consumers make choices that sit uncomfortably with the health professional (Woolford et al., 2020).

This ethical tension is sometimes referred to as the **dignity of risk** principle (Lifeplan, 2022). The issues involved, then, are complex and best dealt with by using an approach that involves active dialogue between all members of the multidisciplinary team and the individual concerned.

Secondary ethical requirements are also important considerations for health professionals, and include the principles of truthfulness, equity and equality, respect and dignity, sanctity and quality of life, and privacy and confidentiality. In the course of their work, health professionals interact with a range of people with diverse views, family backgrounds, cultures, aspirations, expectations and behaviours. When caring for a person with a mental illness, the principles of equity and equality, respect and dignity, and privacy and confidentiality have particular relevance for health professionals. Reasons for this include the need to counter the stigma that is attached to people with a mental illness in Australia today. For example, the personal values that a health professional holds in relation to mental health and illness must be set aside in the workplace and secondary ethical principles must be upheld. The way in which this can be achieved by health professionals is considered in the chapters that look at common reactions to stressful situations, and people displaying challenging behaviours.

Confidentiality and privacy

Confidentiality is both an ethical and legal principle that prohibits disclosure of privileged information without the person's informed consent. This includes information about a person's mental health status. There may be times, however, when such disclosure is necessary.

For example, if the person temporarily lacks capacity and there is no appointed guardian, then the wishes of family members, carers or significant others need to be taken into account when reaching decisions about treatment and ongoing care. However, the eventual outcome is the responsibility of the health professional, based on their assessment of what is in the person's best interests and the preferences of the person (if known).

The legal context regarding capacity and consent is fairly clear, although the issue of whether a person with a permanent incapacity is absolutely unable to give consent has been challenged in the United Kingdom (Selinger, 2009). This has led to calls to ensure that decisions regarding capacity are derived not only from the legal definitions, but also from factors such as personal wellbeing, personhood, previously stated wishes (e.g. an advance care directive), beliefs and preferences.

When caring for people with a mental illness, there are a number of issues around confidentiality and privacy that the health professional may not ordinarily encounter. One of these issues relates to the notions of stigma, as previously noted. For example, many consumers and carers will be sensitive about their clinical record and how the information about their mental health issue is being documented. There can also be issues for partners or carers, who may be anxious about what is happening to their family member and react by pressing the health professional for details or information. This situation can become quite complex as health professionals work to balance the provision of information to partners or carers to assist them in their supportive roles, with the consumer's right to confidentiality and privacy. Some jurisdictions have legislation supportive of care relationship principles (e.g. *Carers Recognition Act 2021*) which may guide health professional practice and service delivery policy. It is further recommended that health professionals discuss such issues as they evolve with the consumers, carers and other members of the multidisciplinary team.

My Health Record

In 2020, on an average day across the country, there were 430 000 general practitioner appointments, 830 000 Pharmaceutical Benefits Scheme (PBS) and Repatriation Pharmaceutical Benefits Scheme (RPBS) medication prescriptions filled and 32 000 hospitalisations (Australian Institute of Health and Welfare [AIHW] 2020). Additionally, during 2020–21 there were almost 5.2 million ambulance service responses (Productivity Commission, 2022). All these contacts generate significant information regarding a person's health and the treatment they receive from various health

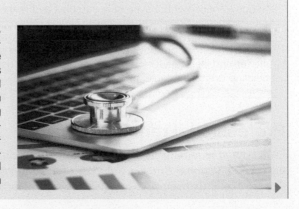

professionals. This information is not usually stored in the same place and is not always easy to access in a timely manner.

In a measure to address this issue, the Australian Department of Health developed the My Health Record (previously known as the Personally Controlled Electronic Health Record System), which commenced in Australia in July 2012. The My Health Record is a secure electronic document that contains a summary of a person's past and current health status. This initiative has evolved from an original voluntary 'opt-in' program, to the current 'opt-out' program. During a 2016 review, the federal government considered the uptake of this program to be slow, with less than 1 million Australians electing to have a My Health Record. There was then an intensive national government campaign to inform the public of the benefits of the My Health Record strategy. Between July 2018 and January 2019, Australians were given the option to opt out of the program, with the consequence being that those members of the public who did not opt out would automatically have a My Health Record developed for them. At the conclusion of the opt-out period, 2.5 million people had formally opted out and 23 million people became recipients of a My Health Record (Australian Digital Health Agency, 2019). This figure means 90.1 per cent of eligible Australians have a My Health Record. If an individual opted out and changes their mind, they can register for a My Health Record online, over the phone, by mail or in some Department of Human Services centres where Medicare services are available.

A person's My Health Record can be updated in three ways: by authorised health professionals, by Medicare and by consumers themselves for example, parents can enter information regarding their child's immunisation status. Health care organisations need to register to enable authorised staff in their facilities to access and update the My Health Records of consumers. Once an agency has My Health Record authorisation, approved health professionals from that particular health agency may upload information such as discharge summaries, diagnostic test results, referrals and specialist letters. Medicare is able to submit information relating to:

- all Medicare Benefits Schedule (MBS) appointments and Department of Veterans' Affairs (DVA) occasions of service where a Medicare claim is made
- all medication claim details under the PBS or the RPBS
- immunisations and organ donor preferences if this information is recorded with the approved governmental agencies.

Personal details, allergies, current medication and advance care agreement templates can all be accessed and amended by the individual person within the My Health Record document.

The advantages of such a system include:

- quick and efficient sharing between health professionals
- health professionals not being solely reliant on consumers' memories for past treatments and procedures
- increased treatment time through decreased medical record retrieval time
- faster access to relevant medical information, especially after hours
- the ability to temporarily access health information in medical emergencies where consumers are unable to give information themselves (e.g. where they are experiencing trauma, unconsciousness or delirium)
- a mobile app for parents to monitor their child's immunisation history
- the option for members of the public to cancel their My Health Record at any time.

However, there are a number of system limitations, for example, the information in the My Health Record may not be accurate, current or complete; the owner of the My Health Record cannot remove or modify a clinical comment made by a health professional; consumers are able to restrict specific information to health professionals via advanced controls settings if they choose; and the My Health Record is certainly not a replacement for the numerous electronic or paper medical record depositories that currently exist. Additionally, despite active governmental processes and policies, there have been concerns raised about the minimum technological and security requirements that are needed to maintain the privacy of such highly personal information.

Given that health care facilities and selected health professionals need to be registered for this system, the governance of the system is complex and is therefore legislatively supported at the federal level by the *Personally Controlled Electronic Health Records Act 2012* and the *Personally Controlled Electronic Health Records Regulation 2012*. For further information about My Health Record, access the website www.myhealthrecord.gov.au, where a large number of fact sheets, frequently asked questions, consumer stories and interactive modules are available for consumers and health professionals. A My Health Record helpline is also available: phone 1300 901 001.

Professional requirements

Professional requirements are identified for the mental health workforce in general. These are outlined in the revised *National Practice Standards for the Mental Health Workforce*, which consists of 13 standards that are explicitly planned to augment the specific practice standards for the nursing, occupational therapy, psychiatry, psychology and social work professions (Victorian Government Department of Health, 2013). There are also a number of discipline-specific requirements to guide the way in which a health professional practises, outlined in documents such as the *Code of Conduct for Nurses* (Nursing and Midwifery Board of Australia [NMBA] 2018), the *Australian Psychological Society Code of Ethics* (Australian Psychological Society, 2007) and *Practice Standards for Mental Health Social Workers* (Australian Association of Social Workers (Draft), 2022). These documents require health professionals to act in the best interests of the health consumer at all times. Although these documents are not legally binding, failure to act within the guidelines constitutes a breach of the Code, which could be used to demonstrate a failure to follow approved practice and may potentially lead to civil action or professional registration consequences (AHPRA, 2020).

3.2 Challenges for health professionals

LEARNING OBJECTIVE 3.2 Describe the challenges for health professionals when making ethical decisions.

The nature of mental illness, the presentation of acute distress and the impact of behavioural disturbance can present specific challenges to health professionals within clinical settings. For example, not everyone presenting for assessment or treatment will behave as the health professional expects them to; that is, they may not be cooperative, compliant or adherent, or uncomplaining or grateful. This is the natural consequence of numerous factors that influence the way in which people respond to the experience of being injured or unwell and in need of assistance (including feelings of pain, discomfort, acute fear, stress and anxiety) sometimes leading to difficult or challenging behaviour. (See the chapters that look at common reactions to stressful situations, and people displaying challenging behaviours.)

On occasion, such challenging behaviour may manifest as the consumer declining treatment or refusing to accept well-intentioned advice or requests from health professionals. Other examples include occasions when the consumer may lack the capacity to make decisions. Challenging behaviours can also be exhibited by people with marked cognitive impairment or substance abuse issues, someone with an acute exacerbation of a mental illness, or a person who is profoundly depressed and expresses a wish to be allowed to die.

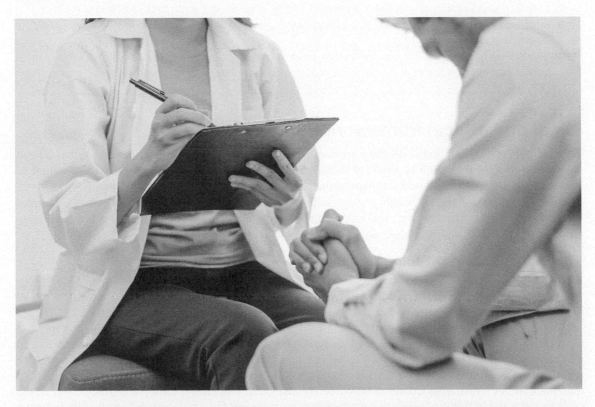

In these circumstances, it is necessary for the health professional to abide by the ethical framework that informs their practice. This will include utilising approaches such as unconditional positive regard (see the chapter on common reactions to stressful situations). It is also important to demonstrate an attitude of respect, acceptance, dignity and equity. Further, the health professional would be wise to consider how they can best uphold and/or protect the human rights of a person in all situations (see the chapter that focuses on people displaying challenging behaviours).

'To tell or not to tell?'

Phillip and Antonio, both aged 27 years, are a same-sex married couple. Within their friendship group, they have lost three friends in the past two years to suicide, which they both found difficult to come to terms with. Following some psychological treatment for workplace stress and thoughts of self-harm, Antonio has been diagnosed with a major depressive disorder. You and your colleagues have provided Antonio with comprehensive information regarding treatment options for his depressive disorder, but Antonio is very distressed by the diagnosis, as his friends were all diagnosed with depression prior to their deaths. Additionally,

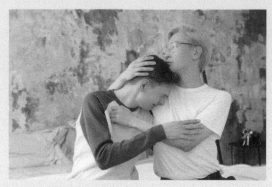

at the best of times, Phillip tends to exaggerate and catastrophise any minor life event and to protect Phillip from further psychological anguish, Antonio informs you that under no circumstances are you to disclose this information to his partner.

Many health professionals struggle with knowing what information they can legally share with the carers and family of people they provide care to. Some health professionals disclose all information related to the consumer, while others have a position that they share nothing unless the consumer has signed a release of information form.

QUESTIONS

1. What risk factors contribute to poor health outcomes in the gay male population?

2. If this scenario was related to a same-sex female couple, what would the risk factor profile look like?

3. What legal and ethical rights do carers and those with a genuine interest in the consumers wellbeing have in such circumstances?

4. What are some strategies that may be helpful to health professionals in achieving a communication balance between consumers and others who have a genuine interest in the consumers' wellbeing?

Legal and ethical frameworks

This section provides an outline of the important legal and ethical frameworks or principles that inform the way in which health care is provided in Australia. Topics covered include the individual's right to autonomy, informed consent and the harm principle. Ethical theories and decision making will also be discussed. It is important for health professionals to understand how these frameworks and principles shape their practice. This, in turn, will enable them to comply with the requirements of law and, in so doing, provide ethical and equitable care to consumers with a mental illness.

The individual's right to autonomy

As noted in the chapter on mental health care in Australia, current health practices have seen a shift away from the conventional model of health care in which the patient is treated as the passive recipient, to one in which the consumer has changing health-related characteristics, is an active and involved co-contributor who participates in the planning, feedback and delivery of preferred health services for themselves, and works with the multidisciplinary team towards a common goal (McIntyre et al., 2021). Consumer-centred models and person-focused approaches to care have given rise to health professionals focusing more upon collaboration and partnerships with consumers and their significant others to achieve better health outcomes for all (Australian Commission on Safety and Quality in Health Care [ACSQHC], 2017). One such model is the 'triangle of care' model where the consumer, professional staff and an identified support person are all equal partners (Mind Australia & Helping Minds, 2016). However, ensuring the meaningful involvement of consumers, carers, partners and family in making treatment decisions requires health professionals to employ a sound ethically-driven perspective.

One of the fundamental principles framing the sound ethically-driven perspectives is the recognition of the individual's right to autonomy. While this may seem straightforward, respecting the individual's right to exercise their free will may, in reality, present major dilemmas for health professionals who are caring for a person with a mental illness.

For example, a health professional might wish to prevent a person with a mental illness, who is also experiencing suicidal ideation, from leaving a clinical setting. Suicide and suicidal ideation are a major concern for all health professionals (see the chapter on caring for a person who has self-harmed). The incidence of suicide among people with serious mental health conditions is at least seven times higher than for the general population (SANE Australia, 2021). Despite this, the individual's right to autonomy means they are free to come and go as they please, regardless of whether they have a mental illness. This creates a dilemma for health professionals seeking to provide care to a person considered to be at risk. Action taken by the health professional can sometimes be perceived as denying the individual's right to free will. To resolve this dilemma, the health professional must be able to demonstrate that the individual's risk of self-harm is significant enough to warrant limiting autonomy.

Informed consent

Australia's health care system is based on a doctrine of **informed consent**. This means that an individual has the right to choose to accept or reject recommended medical care. For such decisions to be considered legally and ethically sound, they must be informed and voluntary, undertaken before the procedure, specific to the procedure in question, and the individual (inclusive of supportive substitute decision makers) must be competent to make decisions about interventions and consequences that affect them (Victorian Department of Health & Human Services, 2019).

It is important to demonstrate an individual's capacity to understand their situation, which directly affects their responses. In assessing a person's capacity to make a decision, the Communities and Justice Department of the NSW Government offers the advice in the figure 3.1.

FIGURE 3.1	Assessing capacity in health

Legal test

This is what you are looking for when you are assessing whether a person has the capacity to make medical or dental decisions: Capacity = Understanding the nature + Effect of the actual treatment being proposed at the time the consent is required.

Checklist

- Does the person understand the nature and effect at the time that the medical or dental decision is required, not hours or days before or after it is made?
- Does the person know the 'nature' of the treatment? That means, do they understand broadly and in simple language.
  - What the medical or dental treatment is?
  - What the procedure involves?
  - Why it is proposed?
  - That there are other options? (If choosing between options, the person must understand what each option is, what it involves, the effect of each option, and the risks and benefits.)
  - What it means if they don't have the treatment?
- Does the person understand the 'effect' of the treatment? Are they aware, in simple terms, of the main benefits and risks of the treatment? Does the person have the ability to indicate whether they want the treatment? Can they communicate any decision made, with assistance if necessary?
- Has the person made the decision freely and voluntarily?
  Also consider that a person has a right to refuse treatment. What most people would decide to do in the situation is irrelevant. Consider the following.
- Is refusal of treatment consistent with the person's views and values?
- Is this behaviour usual for the person?
- Has all the relevant information been given to the person in a way they can understand?

▸

Additionally, the Office of the Public Advocate has a medical decision-making flowchart available to guide and assist processes in relation to decision-making capacity. The website also provides links for this tool to be utilised via a smartphone app (Office of the Public Advocate, 2022). More information is available here: www.publicadvocate.vic.gov.au/medical-treatment/patient-consent/patient-capacity-to-consent.

All adults, including those with a mental health problem, are to be presumed to have capacity until the contrary is proved and significantly, where capacity is contested, the burden of proof lies with the person asserting the incapacity (End of Life Directions for Aged Care [ELDAC], 2022)

This means that the health professional must be very sure of the way they assess incapacity before presuming a person is unable to consent to a procedure. It is important to note that the vast majority of people with a mental illness are able to give informed consent in the health context. Significantly, this includes the person who has been detained under the Mental Health Act. Generally, health professionals should not make presumptions about a person's capacity, especially when these presumptions may be based upon preconceived ideas. Rather, assessment of capacity needs to be undertaken by a health professional who has specialised knowledge and experience in this area of assessment, or has undertaken specific training related to clinical and legal capacity assessment requirements.

The 'harm principle'

Intervention in a situation where an individual chooses to leave a hospital setting without treatment, and against medical advice, is based on the utilitarian ethical philosophy espoused by John Stuart Mill (1963), known as the **harm principle**. Adhering to the harm principle means that a degree of intervention that limits a person's autonomy may be justified in certain situations. The same principle is followed when the Australian government enacts legislation that limits individual autonomy in order to reduce the likelihood of harm to the individual and/or others. Examples of such interventionist policies — or, depending on the point of view, paternalistic legislation — aimed at minimising harm include the legal requirement to wear seatbelts in cars and the ban on smoking in public places. However, a health professional who limits the autonomy of a consumer without first obtaining consent, where such consent is required, may be liable to accusations of battery and assault and/or negligence (Cheluvappa & Selvendran, 2020; Queensland Judgments, 2018).

The harm principle raises interesting issues for those who self-harm. For example, the incidence of self-harm by people post hospital discharge was explored in the Commonwealth Senate enquiry into suicide prevention (Commonwealth of Australia, 2010). The recommendations of the inquiry include establishing protocols for the follow-up support of people who are discharged from hospital following an admission for self-harm behaviours. Additionally, the Northern Territory Government has made a commitment to also provide services to those people who have been assessed as being at risk of self-harm, and those who have been treated following a self-harm episode but not admitted to hospital (Select Committee on Youth Suicides in the NT, 2012). Such protocols may go some way to reducing the burden on health professionals to ensure the safety of individuals with mental health issues who have left the hospital setting.

Concern has also been raised about individuals who attend a hospital emergency department with a mental health presentation and prematurely leave the hospital either prior to the assessment being completed or without receiving treatment or care (Duggan et al., 2020). One reason for this concern relates to the way people with mental health issues are triaged (Coroners Court of Victoria, 2021). Another reason is the negative perceptions exhibited by some health professionals towards individuals who have self-harmed (see the chapter on caring for a person who has self-harmed). It is important that health professionals are aware of their own values in relation to mental health and ill-health, self-harming, suicide and so on, and do not allow these values to compromise the way they provide health care to people in need (see the chapter on common reactions to stressful situations). It is also important that health professionals are aware of the legal and ethical issues involved and, when unsure, refer such situations to the multidisciplinary team for consideration.

Ethical theories

Appendant to the aforementioned ethical principles are the ethical theories relevant to the provision of mental health care. Ethical theories are based on ethical principles and each person uses their life experiences, personal values system and cultural perspectives to determine the theory to which they align their choices and behaviours. This is especially so when the person faces an ethical dilemma.

Ethical egoism is a term used to describe when the person making the treatment decision decides what is right and advantageous for them even though the decision may not necessarily be advantageous for others. How others view the outcome of the decision is irrelevant, even when the decision is not obviously supported by family, carers and significant others (ELDAC, 2022). However, there are occasions when the health professional must make a clinical decision and this is when ethical theories can be helpful.

Ethical theories and principles that are useful in assisting decision making when faced with an ethical dilemma include virtue ethical theory, deontological ethical theory, consequentialism or utilitarianism ethical theory, casuist ethical theory and rights-based theory. Deontological and consequentialism are two of the most important ethical theories and their principles are frequently used when caring for a person with a mental illness.

In short, the principles of deontological ethical theory are that choices and actions are either morally right or morally wrong, and that every individual has a moral obligatory duty to undertake those actions that are morally right. This is illustrated in figure 3.2. For example, a consumer following a deontological philosophy who is prescribed medication while detained under mental health legislation would always take the medication even if they did not believe that they needed the treatment. This consumer would adhere to the prescribed treatment because there is a legal directive to do so and the person believes in being a good law-abiding citizen and will follow the law at all costs.

FIGURE 3.2 Deontological versus consequential ethics

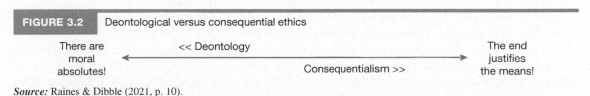

Source: Raines & Dibble (2021, p. 10).

Conversely, consequentialism ethical theory proposes that the decision to do something is determined by the anticipated outcome, which usually translates to the greatest benefit to the greatest number of people. All options may be considered, and the option for the best outcome is then selected, irrespective of the rightness of the procedures required to obtain the outcome. People subscribing to consequentialism believe that any action taken is acceptable if the best outcome is achieved.

Ethical decision making

Ethical decision making by health professionals does not occur in a vacuum, but is informed by a complex interplay of professional judgement, ethical principles and legal requirements. Reconciling all these factors within the health care setting can be challenging, especially when providing care to people with a mental illness. Health professionals are best to seek the appropriate level of advice, support and supervision to enable them to participate in decision making that is based on sound ethical principles. It is also important that health professionals practise adequate self-care, keep up-to-date in their learning and achieve acceptable levels of competence to ensure the decisions made are translated into sound ethical practice.

The process of ethical decision making is supported by a number of professional bodies. For example, the Nursing and Midwifery Board of Australia [NMBA] (2020) has developed a national decision-making framework to assist nurses and midwives to make calculated and informed decisions regarding their clinical work. This framework can be effectively utilised by all health professionals, across the multidisciplinary team in the course of their work, and is further supported by an illustrative flowchart (NMBA, 2020). A further example is the *Decision Making Framework for NSW Health Aboriginal Health Practitioners* (New South Wales Ministry of Health, 2018).

In addition to utilising decision-making frameworks, there is a need for health professionals to reflect upon the way in which they enter into a social contract with their clients, other health professionals and the wider community (Magill & Prybil, 2020). This social contract demands that health professionals utilise a particular set of clinical skills and demonstrate appropriate ethical, legal and social behaviours (Nimita & Carol, 2014). Such behaviours include those that are viewed as acceptable by the societies and cultures within which the health professional is located, and uphold the basic values of those societies or cultures. Indeed, there is an implicit expectation that health professionals in Australia will support the moral, ethical and legal principles of the socio-cultural context in which they live. In so doing, their work will serve to maintain the fundamental social fabric of the Australian community and thus improve population health outcomes (see the chapter on culturally appropriate mental health care).

This section described the most important legal and ethical principles in the provision of health care in Australia today, and applied these principles to situations that involve people with a mental illness. In the next section, notions of capacity and competence are described. Understanding these notions is important for health professionals who encounter people with mental health problems. This is because the perceptions of capacity or competence can significantly affect the type of care and treatment the consumer receives.

3.3 Capacity and competence

LEARNING OBJECTIVE 3.3 Discuss the concepts of consent, capacity and competence.

An understanding of the concepts of **capacity** and **competence** is vital to ensuring the consumer's autonomy and right to self-determination are respected. Under common law in Australia, all adults have the right to refuse any treatment that is offered to them, as long as it can be demonstrated that they possess the (legal) capacity to make this decision, which may include supported decision-making processes. This legal right remains, even if the expected outcome could be detrimental to the person concerned (Queensland Government, 2018). In these situations, people who refuse treatment may pose a significant challenge to the practice of the health professional, particularly if the person's wishes differ from those of the multidisciplinary team, partners, carers, family members or significant others.

Prior to discussing the concepts of capacity and consent, the **doctrine of necessity** needs to be considered. This doctrine, or principle, is paternalistic in nature. Even so, it allows for the provision of care to a person, with or without their consent, where it is considered necessary to save the person's life, and prevent serious damage or impairment to the person's health (Chandler et al., 2016). In the field of mental health, an example of the adoption of this principle occurred in an ACT Supreme Court case that was heard in August 2009. Chief Justice Higgins made a legal judgement that the rights of an elderly man with a history of paranoid schizophrenia who was starving himself would not be violated if medical practitioners intervened to save his life (*Australian Capital Territory v JT* [2009] ACTSC 105). Conversely, there is now documented international instances when the doctrine of necessity intervention in acute medical/psychiatric situations, even when death is anticipated, has not occurred (Nowland et al., 2019). This scenario, sometimes referred to as 'suicide by advance directive' occurs when a person presents to the emergency department, for example, following an episode of self-harm and either (i) remains competent but does not consent to emergency care, or (ii) presents with an advanced agreement/living will clearly stating that medical intervention is not to be attended. This phenomenon is increasing in Australia; the advance care directives and attempted suicides guidelines produced by the Victorian Department of Health & Human Services (2017) provides further advice on this issue.

These examples demonstrate that health professionals will sometimes be placed in situations where necessity requires them to act against the specific wishes of a person; or when conversely, they are prevented from delivering life-saving treatment and care due to a pre-determined legal position. When providing care to people with a mental illness, such situations will often be made based on the level of competence or capacity of the person requiring treatment. Determining competence and capacity, however, is no easy task. This is discussed in the following section.

Principles of capacity and competence

As mentioned previously, in order to determine if an individual is able to give their informed consent to a treatment option, it is important to demonstrate their capacity and competence to make such decisions. It is therefore necessary to understand the meaning of the terms 'capacity' and 'competence' as applied to the health care setting. These principles enable health professionals to determine whether a person has given valid consent for a particular treatment or investigation to be carried out.

In Australia, a person is considered to have the capacity to make decisions about their health care and/or treatment unless it can be demonstrated otherwise (e.g. they have an impairment or disturbance of mental functioning that affects their capacity to make a particular decision). This is the first principle of defining competence. The second principle is that the level of competence required is proportional to the seriousness of the medical decision. This is sometimes referred to as 'requisite competence'. For example, a greater level of competence is required for contemplating whether to consent to a total hysterectomy than choosing between oral and intravenous antibiotic therapy (Sorrentino, 2014). The final principle is that the determination of competency is only specific to one particular decision and time frame. This is important to remember as consumers who are receiving involuntary care and treatment may still be competent to consent to other medical care (Office of the Public Advocate, 2019). Moreover, people with a mental health impairment who are considered to have the capacity to make a particular decision have the same rights to make unwise or risky decisions as those without such an impairment.

At the same time, the issue of informed consent is complicated because the individual's capacity to make an informed decision may be compromised by their mental illness. It is therefore important that an assessment is made of the person's capacity to give their informed consent (Queensland Health, 2017). Consideration also needs to be given to the 'levels' or 'degrees' of capacity and incapacity.

For example, incapacity may be permanent, temporary or partial. Someone who is intoxicated after drinking a large amount of alcohol may temporarily lack capacity, as could someone who has recently had a general anaesthetic. Other causes of incapacity — temporary, partial or permanent — include:
- being under the influence of alcohol or other drugs, including prescribed and non-prescribed medication and prohibited substances
- dementia
- pain
- mental illness or mental dysfunction including psychosis, depression, hypomania and some anxiety states
- intellectual disability
- brain injury
- hypoxia (Queensland Ambulance Service, 2019).
  Further conditions identified include:
- delirium
- progressive neurological disease
- communication disability
- emotional shock
- fatigue
- panic and fear
- illness itself
- overwhelm
- information overload (Bester et al., 2016).
  Incapacity is a key factor to consider when determining the ability of a person to make a reasonable or competent decision regarding their health care.

As already mentioned, an adult is assumed to have competence unless it can be proved otherwise. Varkey (2021) describes the domains underpinning determinations in relation to whether a person has capacity and is competent to consent to a certain treatment or make a particular treatment decision. The clinical tests for competency must demonstrate that the person:
- must be competent to understand and decide
- receives a full disclosure
- comprehends the disclosure
- acts voluntarily
- consents to the proposed action (Varkey, 2021).
  In the main, people with mental health problems are able to meet each of these criteria. As already noted, they are therefore presumed by the health professional to have competence until it is demonstrated otherwise.

Incapacity

In Australia there is no single definition for **incapacity**. Instead, legal definitions of incapacity are based on a range of common laws with varying statute definitions. For example, in South Australia, mental incapacity is defined in the *Guardianship and Administration Act 1993* (s. 3.1, p. 7) as:

> the inability of a person to look after their health, safety or welfare, or to manage their affairs as a result of any damage, illness, disorder, imperfect or delayed development, impairment or deterioration of the brain or mind (i.e. brain damage or neurological disease), or any physical illness or condition that renders the person unable to communicate their intentions or wishes in any manner whatsoever.

Others have suggested that a person may not have the capacity to make decisions about certain aspects of their lives but retain the capacity to make decisions about other matters (Office of the Public Advocate, 2019). For example, a person may not be capable of making decisions about their financial affairs or major medical treatment, but still have capacity to make decisions about basic health care and general lifestyle issues, such as who they would like information given to or where they want to live. Notions of capacity and incapacity, then, are very complex.

The notion of incapacity is also enshrined in statute law; for example, various state and territory guardianship Acts. As with common law, the provisions of these Acts assume that a person, including the person with a mental illness, has the capacity to make their own decisions unless it can be proved otherwise. These Acts contain specific provision for the administration of treatment to an adult who is unable to give consent.

UPON REFLECTION

Convenience and consent

It is curious that, generally speaking, when a consumer agrees with the recommendations of the treating team, the competence question is not raised or challenged. However, at certain times, when a consumer does not agree to a treatment proposal, their ability to consent may be further scrutinised.

....

QUESTIONS

1. What are your organisation's processes and procedures regarding the consenting process?
2. What role can the multidisciplinary team play in assisting with consent issues?
3. What systems and supports are in place for people who require assistance to understand information, prior to consenting?
4. What additional tools could you use with Indigenous peoples or those from a culturally or linguistically diverse background?

Different types of consent

The concept of consent is derived from the ethical principle of autonomy. As noted, consent to a proposed treatment, intervention or medical procedure needs to be informed. It also needs to be given voluntarily and the individual must demonstrate capacity to provide, understand and communicate their consent (New South Wales Health Care Complaints Commission, 2014).

In practice, there are three distinct types of consent.

1. *Implied consent* — indicated by conduct or action; for example, by proffering an arm when a pathology technician explains that they would like to obtain a blood sample
2. *Verbal consent* — when an individual is directly asked if they are agreeable to information being recorded, accessed or shared, and the response is provided verbally
3. *Written consent* — when consent is agreed to on a signed paper consent form (ACT Health, 2018).

Although all three forms of consent are equally valid in practice, written and verbal consent need to be obtained for all potentially serious investigations or interventions, for example, surgical procedures and general anaesthesia. In summary, for consent to be valid, it must be:

- based on an informed decision, that is, full information needs to be provided to the person regarding risks, benefits and alternatives
- given freely and without duress

- given by someone who is competent to make the decision (or the legal representative of the person)
- specific and cover only the proposed intervention or procedure (ACSQHC, 2020).

Awareness of these different types of consent is especially important when providing care to a person with a mental illness. For example, a health professional may interpret a particular gesture or behaviour as implied consent, when, in reality, the consumer is exhibiting a sign of mental illness or a medication side effect. This can create problems as the consumer may then react against the health professional's presumption of consent.

Treatment decisions made by a third party

In Australia there is no consistent nationally recognised process whereby another person (including the individual's relatives, carer or significant other) can consent to something on behalf of another adult (ACSQHC, 2020). In situations involving minors, it is important to check the relevant state or territory legislation governing both privacy issues and consent to health care and treatment for younger age groups, particularly for 14–16-year-olds (Australian Law Reform Commission, 2010a). However, in a medical emergency and where there is no written directive to the contrary, health professionals are not required to obtain consent before starting the minimum treatment required to preserve life.

Power of attorney

In the majority of states and territories it is now possible for an individual to appoint another person to make treatment decisions on their behalf; for example, by appointing someone to act in the role of 'enduring power of attorney (medical treatment)'. This allows the person appointed (the 'attorney') to make medical decisions (in consultation with health professionals and other relevant people) when the signatory is no longer capable of making such decisions for themselves. Anyone can be appointed to act in this role. The attorney is not permitted to refuse reasonable medical procedures for the relief of pain, suffering and discomfort or the reasonable provision of food and water, although they can refuse other forms of treatment if expressly authorised to do so (Austin Health, 2021).

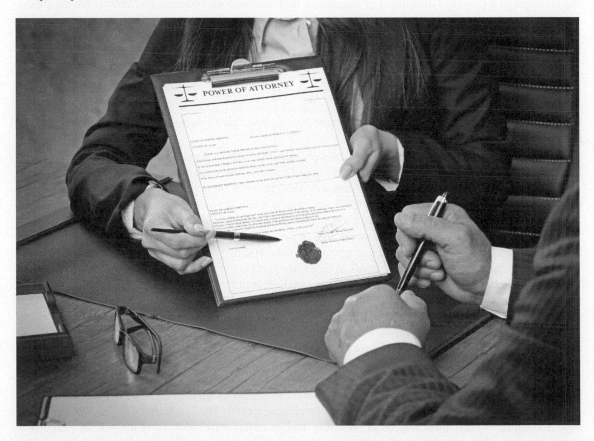

There are four main types of power of attorney; each state and territory has slightly different types, each with varying uses and powers.

1. *General power of attorney* can be used when an individual is unable to manage their affairs or sign documents because they are overseas or in hospital.
2. *Enduring power of attorney* comes into effect when individuals are no longer able to look after themselves. A general power of attorney would not continue to be effective if the person loses their mental capacity, but an enduring power of attorney would. In some states and territories there may be some crossover with enduring guardianship.
3. *Medical power of attorney* is known by the names 'enduring power of attorney' (Australian Capital Territory, South Australia and Queensland), 'medical treatment decision maker' (Victoria), 'enduring guardianship' (New South Wales, Western Australia and Tasmania) and 'advance personal plan' (Northern Territory). The person appointed to take on any one of these roles is able to make life and death decisions about the individual concerned, including whether the individual should continue on life support equipment.
4. *Enduring guardianship* becomes important when an individual is no longer able to make certain lifestyle decisions, such as where and with whom to live, what health care to receive, and daily issues such as diet and dress. An enduring guardian can consent (or refuse to consent) only to treatments that are provided to promote or maintain the health and wellbeing of the person for whom they have been appointed to act. They can make decisions regarding:
   - medical and dental treatment that will promote the individual's health and wellbeing
   - access, that is, who the individual will see
   - restrictive practices function (to protect the individual from self-harm)
   - how the individual will receive treatment; for example, whether the individual needs to be registered with a particular doctor.

An appointed enduring guardian cannot provide a lawful consent to euthanasia. In some states and territories the individual may need to appoint an enduring guardian rather than an enduring power of attorney.

It is important that all health professionals have some understanding of the processes related to the appointment of a power of attorney. For example, consumers with an enduring and serious mental illness may have someone acting in the role of attorney to oversee their finances or to determine what kind of health care they will receive. Health professionals are responsible for checking such arrangements are in place and with whom, and for ensuring that the correct processes are followed.

3.4 Advance care agreements

LEARNING OBJECTIVE 3.4 Explain the importance of advance care agreements or directives in the field of mental health.

Advance care agreements have become increasingly important across Australia. These documents are also known in some states and territories as advance care directives, advance health care directives or advance health directives. Advance care agreements are a written record of an individual's wishes about serious and sensitive health care issues, such as their views on invasive medical procedures and appropriate treatments. In the field of mental health, an advance care agreement or directive is written by a consumer when they have the capacity to make decisions about the type of mental health treatment that they wish to be provided when they are acutely unwell or unable to give informed consent.

An advance care agreement or directive can be written, only if the individual concerned has the capacity to do so. It can be changed or updated as often as required until the individual no longer has the capacity to change it. These documents can also include directions about life-sustaining treatment. For example, a person with multiple, long-term and/or painful life-limiting conditions may request in their advance care directive that in the event of a medical crisis they are not to be resuscitated. It is essential that family, carers and/or significant others are aware of such requests well in advance of a medical crisis to ensure they understand and support the wishes of the person making the directive.

Excluding the commencement of a medical emergency, it is important for health professionals to clarify whether a person has an advance care directive before initiating treatment. The existence of an advance care directive needs to be recorded in the person's clinical record. The instructions of this document are legally binding in most jurisdictions in Australia, and, if advance care directives are not legislated in a particular state, they may be valid under common law (Advance Care Planning Australia, 2018). The directives in an advance care agreement must be respected and considered by health professionals and the multidisciplinary team who are making the treatment decisions.

Legal issues

From a legal hierarchy perspective, Australian mental health Acts override advance care directives, but recognise the importance of these documents within the legislation (Mental Health Coordinating Council, 2015). The Australian Government (2021) have published the *National framework for advance care planning documents* to provide ethical considerations and principle-based information regarding the current position, and expectations of advance care directives, particularly for policy makers, regulators and health administrators. This document is not intended for the general public.

As already noted, the use of advance care directives has gathered momentum in Australia, notwithstanding the very limited Australian case law supporting the legality of advance care directives. Figure 3.3 explains the history behind advance care directives (referred to in this example as advance statements) becoming legislated and describes why theses advance care directives are particularly important for consumers of mental health services and their carers, who are seeking to empower themselves and feel strongly about their right to self-determine.

FIGURE 3.3 Improving recovery journeys

Mental health consumers have pushed for formal recognition of Advance Statements for many years. In 2014 Victoria became the first state to legally recognise Advance Statements.

The Mental Health Legal Centre (MHLC) maintains a strong position that each consumer knows best about the lived experience of their 'illness' and that decisions made by others on their behalf will never adequately substitute for the decisions people make for themselves about their own lives. Self-determination is crucial to anybody's ongoing wellbeing.

Advance Statements help consumers to have a greater say in how they are treated when receiving compulsory treatment. This includes information about what treatments have been effective in the past and those that have been less effective or have had unwelcome side effects. It can also include views on receiving Electro Convulsive Treatment.

An Advance Statement can be made at any time and must meet some basic formal requirements. It needs to be in writing, signed and dated by the person making the statement and witnessed by an authorised witness. The authorised witness must confirm that the person making it understands what an Advance Statement is and the consequences of making one.

Advance Statements are recognised under Victoria's Mental Health legislation (*Mental Health Act 2014*) and must be considered by treating teams when they are making decisions about treatment and also by the Mental Health Tribunal when deciding whether to make an order for compulsory treatment.

Sometimes treating teams will not follow your Advance Statement, if they do not offer the treatment requested or do not think it will work. If this happens consumers can ask for written reasons, these reasons must be given within 10 days.

While it is only treatment preferences that must be considered under the Mental Health Act, consumers often also record other personal information that they want their treating team to know. This might include things like information about family and home life, needing access to art supplies or music while in hospital or what will happen to pets.

The MHLC website also offers an application 'Your Treatment Your Voice', which provides guidance for individuals in developing the initial steps of an Advance Statement.

Source: Mental Health Legal Centre Inc. (n.d.).

Information required to make an informed decision

To make an informed health care decision, the individual must demonstrate that they understand in broad terms the:
- nature of the proposed intervention
- purpose of the proposed intervention
- risks and benefits of the proposed intervention
- possible risks and consequences associated with not carrying out the proposed intervention
- possible risks and benefits of alternative interventions.

For consent to be valid it must be given voluntarily and the person must be in possession of all the relevant information pertinent to the intervention being proposed. Consent is not necessarily valid just because the person has signed a consent form. It is up to the health professional to demonstrate that they have provided the information required for informed decision making.

There are some professional codes that provide direction for this type of circumstance. For example, the Paramedicine Board of Australia *Code of conduct* (2018) guides paramedics' practice in relation to consent and refusal to treatment, stating:

> Informed consent is a person's voluntary decision about healthcare that is made with knowledge and understanding of the benefits and risks involved, and informing patients or clients of the nature of and need for all aspects of their clinical care, including examination and investigations, and giving them adequate opportunity to question or refuse intervention and treatment, and when working with a patient or client whose capacity to give consent is or may be impaired or limited, obtaining the consent of people with legal authority to act on behalf of the patient or client and attempting to obtain the consent of the patient or client as far as practically possible (Paramedicine Board of Australia, 2018).

This statement also reinforces the importance of advance care directives or agreements. A significant role of the health professional, then, is to promote the use of these agreements to consumers and carers. If the preferences of the consumer or carer are clearly articulated and made available to health professionals, then informed decisions are more likely to be made.

3.5 Duty of care

LEARNING OBJECTIVE 3.5 Discuss the concept of duty of care.

Health professionals owe the consumer a duty of care and need to ensure that the consumer does not come to any unnecessary harm as a result of negligence or omission (ATSI Health Practice Board of Australia, 2014). Duty of care is established through common law (see *Masson v State of Queensland* [2018] QSC 162) and is applicable to all health care settings and individual professionals. Exercising a duty of care means that an individual health professional must take responsibility for ensuring that they are competent to meet the care needs of the people they help or care for.

It is important to note that duty of care extends to police and paramedics. In the case of *The Australian Capital Territory v Crowley* and *Commonwealth of Australia and Pitkethly* [2012] ACTCA 52, Mr Crowley was a 32-year-old man who had been reported to police as disturbing the neighbourhood and threatening individuals with a sword and a kendo stick during an apparent psychotic episode. Two police officers attempted to subdue Mr Crowley by using verbal de-escalation strategies, capsicum spray and then a police baton — none of which were effective in reducing his aggression. Mr Crowley continued to threaten and assault police, and was subsequently shot in the neck by one of the officers. The gunshot injury resulted in Mr Crowley sustaining a spinal injury and quadriplegia. Some months later, Mr Crowley sued both the Federal Government (Australian Federal Police) and ACT Health for negligence and breach of duty of care. Initially Mr Crowley's claim was upheld and he was awarded $8 million compensation. However, on appeal the decision was overturned with a finding of no negligence and no liability towards either the police or health service (Australian Government Solicitor, 2012).

Health services and other institutions responsible for the organisation and provision of health care also have a corporate duty of care and need to ensure that there are adequately trained staff and facilities to meet the person's needs. A review of these responsibilities is routinely undertaken by agencies such as the Australian Commission on Safety and Quality in Health Care during the health service accreditation processes.

At times, the health professional's duty of care may appear to be in conflict with a consumer's right to autonomy and self-determination. For example, it can be difficult to reconcile the wishes of an individual client to refuse treatment (autonomy) with the professional and legal obligation to provide care. In essence, health professionals need to demonstrate that their actions are:

- reasonable
- in the person's best interests
- undertaken with the person's informed consent.

An exception to this would be when the person fails the test of capacity. In such cases, the health professional's duty of care will form the basis of subsequent actions.

A prime example of this would be the presentation of a mental health consumer who is exhibiting aggressive or destructive behaviour that seems to be out of control, in the community or in an emergency department. The consumer is unable to give consent and is refusing treatment. To protect the consumer, community members and also the health professionals from physical harm, a decision is made by the medical officers, nursing staff or (in some states and territories) the paramedics, to rapidly tranquilise the consumer. In light of the overall context, this decision is deemed to be reasonable and in the consumer's best interests, even though it is undertaken without their consent and is contrary to the consumer's right to autonomy and self-determination. The decision is also consistent with the doctrine of necessity, the harm principle and notions of duty of care.

Practical issues to consider

As the phenomenon of advance care agreements prohibiting life-sustaining treatment becomes more evident in Australia, the potential impact of moral distress related to a preventable death on health professionals must be addressed and managed. Moral distress develops given the ethical conflict between the choice of allowing a person to die that could be saved versus actively providing life-saving treatment against the person's explicit wishes. These situations illustrate the delicate balance of beneficence and autonomy in practice.

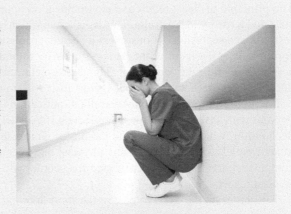

QUESTIONS

1. What legal strategies can you adopt in order to prepare yourself/your team and your organisation for such presentations?
2. What ethical strategies can you adopt in order to prepare yourself/your team and your organisation for such presentations?
3. What professional strategies can you adopt in order to prepare yourself/your team and your organisation for such presentations?
4. What personal qualities, resources or strategies can you call upon to assist and guide you with this matter?
5. How can your health service further mitigate potential personal, professional and organisational risks in these situations?

Reasonable and unreasonable

An important principle in deciding whether to act contrary to a person's expressed wishes concerns the issue of 'reasonableness'; that is, to what extent the health professional can directly intervene in a particular situation or with a particular client. For example, if a person is admitted to hospital following a deliberate overdose of medication, it would be reasonable to ask the person whether they had any substances on them that they could use to harm themselves during their admission in hospital. Such a request is reasonable because of the risks associated with overdose and the likelihood of someone repeating their actions (see the chapter on caring for a person who has self-harmed), even when they are in hospital.

To ask the question of the person demonstrates accountability to the health professional's duty of care and may be considered a reasonable action, illustrating the health professional's commitment to the safety of the consumer. However, despite being aware of the potential risk of repeated self-harm, it would be unreasonable in this situation to search the person and their belongings without the person's permission, as the degree of force associated with this action would be disproportionate to the degree of risk posed (see the following section on restraint).

The principle of acting in a way that is contrary to a person's expressed wishes (or in the absence of knowing whether the person would wish the treatment to proceed) is connected to the health professional's duty of care. Common law provides the legal framework by which health professionals can:
- detain someone against their will
- give urgent treatment in an emergency situation to someone who lacks capacity to give consent.

In practice, common law allows an individual to apprehend or restrain a person if there are reasonable grounds to believe that person poses a significant danger to themselves or others and would continue to do so if allowed to leave a safe environment or to continue to engage in risk-taking behaviours. The degree of physical intervention, such as physical restraint, needs to be enough to bring the emergency situation to an end, but must not be excessive. Any restraint that involves disproportionate force, or which continues after the immediate crisis is over, cannot be justified. Additionally, the person carrying out the restraining action may be legally compromised if they continue to maintain force that is considered unnecessary or excessive.

Least restrictive environment

The principle of 'least restrictive environment' is upheld by the mental health legislation enacted in each state and territory in Australia. This legislation, which is described in the next section, also guides the use of restraint and seclusion of consumers by health professionals. The fundamental issue is that a complete and appropriate assessment of the person's capacity to make a decision must be undertaken prior to initiating action to restrain the individual. This assessment, and any other information that is used to inform the decision to restrain an individual against their will, must be documented.

It is important to note that Australia's ratification of the United Nations Convention on the Rights of Persons with Disabilities came into effect on 16 August 2008. Australia subsequently lodged an interpretive declaration, which states that the nation recognises that anyone with a disability must be respected and treated equally in regard to their physical and mental integrity and that the Convention permits safe compulsory treatment and assistance for people with disabilities, where the treatment is necessary and is a last resort.

This suggests the need to ensure the most appropriate actions are taken and that health professionals act in the consumer's best interests by examining all relevant factors and events that have led to the presenting situation. This will include issues such as the person's previously expressed wishes, the views of family, carers and/or significant others, and an evaluation of the risks and benefits of intervening versus not intervening (Kurpad, 2018). A framework for reflecting in practice is suggested in table 3.3 as a means of planning actions in situations that may be challenging or complex (Harrison & Hart, 2006).

TABLE 3.3 **Framework for responding to challenging situations**

Consider	Rationale
Personal safety. Does the person present an immediate risk to self or others?	If refusing the proposed intervention is likely to have life-threatening consequences for the person or others, intervention is justified under common law. If failing to act is subsequently proved to have been negligent, the health professional will be in breach of their duty of care.
Does the health professional possess all the relevant information about the situation?	It is important to obtain as much collateral history and supporting information as possible. Sources of information include: • the person's family/carer or significant other • background to the current presentation • current social or interpersonal difficulties/problems • effects of alcohol or illicit drugs on the person's mental state • effects of shock, sedation or medication on the person's ability to communicate • the person's previously expressed wishes regarding the situation (e.g. have they prepared an advance care directive regarding treatment in this situation?).
The health professional's knowledge and skills base. Does the health professional consider themselves confident to respond to this situation?	Health professionals and/or their colleagues must have adequate training and access to clinical supervision. • Health professionals must have adequate knowledge, training and experience to be able to assess capacity competence. • Ensure the health service has up-to-date policies and clinical guidelines in place for the management of such situations. – Do the health professionals know how to access specialist help? – Are they aware of their role in assessing capacity? – What support and advice, such as additional staff, access to on-site security personnel, can they expect to receive? (See the chapter on caring for a person who has self-harmed for additional information.)

What alternatives are available to the health professional in this situation?	If the situation is not life threatening, it is likely that a number of planned alternatives to direct physical intervention could be adopted. Are there other staff in the health service to whom the health professional can refer for assistance? Queensland Health, Clinical Excellence Division (2017, p. 20) suggests: • deferring the health care until such time as the patient is able to make a decision, if the clinical condition allows • repeating the assessment on a number of occasions at times when the patient appears best able to understand and retain the information • involving those people whom the patient considers might help them reach a decision • seeking the views of those who personally know the patient well, on the patient's ability to decide and best ways of communicating with the patient • using different communication methods • recording any decisions made at times when the patient has capacity • considering any previous views expressed directly to the clinical team or documented in the clinical records by the patient when they had capacity, including through a valid advance health directive • seeking advice from suitably experienced specialist medical practitioners.
Is the health professional familiar with the mental health legislation of the state or territory in which they are working?	Mental health legislation across Australia only allows for treatment of a mental illness, not a physical illness or treatment of the physical consequences of a mental illness. Given the differences in the federated Acts, there are general core elements that health professionals need to address when considering the use of initiating a course of treatment under their local Act. These elements will be similar to the following. • The person has a mental illness or mental dysfunction. • The person is declining treatment. • The person cannot be treated in a less restrictive environment. • The person is at risk of harm to either self or others. • The person is likely to deteriorate within a short period of time if they are not treated.
The consequences of not acting	The health professional must be able to defend and justify their actions if challenged (Morrison-Valfre, 2017; Queensland Judgments, 2018). It is therefore important to ensure that the rationale for the chosen course of action is clearly described and documented in the person's clinical records. Details of conversations with partners, families, carers, significant others and colleagues also need to be recorded.

UPON REFLECTION

Least restrictive environment principle

Despite the intentions of health professionals to uphold least restrictive principles in practice, there are times when the physical environment restricts choice and freedom of movement. These limitations are often deliberately designed for safety and may include swipe only access doors into and within health facilities, locked fire exits only activated during a code and general area access restrictions for consumers and or visitors.

QUESTIONS

1. From a legal perspective, is a locked environment warranted in a health care setting?
2. From an ethical perspective, is it appropriate to admit voluntary consumers into a locked psychiatric or aged care setting?
3. From an autonomy perspective, is the consumer being treated in the most respectful, least restrictive manner for a hospital admission?
4. Using a least restrictive environment lens, what other environmental implications are there in your particular work setting that impact freedom of movement? What practices could you adopt to mitigate these identified constraints in order to uphold least restrictive principles as much as possible?

3.6 State and territory mental health legislation

LEARNING OBJECTIVE 3.6 Outline the use and application of mental health legislation across Australia.

In Australia, each state and territory has enacted its own mental health legislation, commonly called a 'Mental Health Act' (MHA). The names of these MHAs are provided in table 3.4. While these MHAs have a number of differences, all are based upon principles ensuring the right of people with a mental illness to autonomy, freedom and self-determination, and the provision of least restrictive health care.

TABLE 3.4   **Australian state and territory Mental Health Acts**

State/territory	Mental Health Act
Australian Capital Territory	*Mental Health Act 2015* *Mental Health (Secure Facilities) Act 2016*
New South Wales	*Mental Health Act 2007* *Mental Health Amendment (Statutory Review) Act 2014*
Northern Territory	*Mental Health and Related Services Act 1998*
Queensland	*Mental Health Act 2016*
South Australia	*Mental Health Act 2009*
Tasmania	*Mental Health Act 2013*
Victoria	*Mental Health Act 2014*
Western Australia	*Mental Health Act 2014*

The majority of state and territory MHAs have been significantly revised within the past decade with the inclusion of Recovery principles and, significantly, a noticeable swing towards supported decision-making models rather than traditional guardianship-type models (Parker, 2016). In many jurisdictions it is now a mandated requirement that a person's cognitive capacity and decision-making abilities are to be assessed and/or determined prior to involuntary care provisions being initiated (e.g. see ACT, NSW, QLD and VIC MHAs). However, there is limited legal justification for short-term involuntary detention of a person in the event of an ambiguous decision-making assessment, with some authors proposing that this practice is discriminatory against those with a mental health diagnosis (Szmukler, 2020). The increasing focus on supportive and collaborative practices that further enhance individual decision making in relation to treatment and care decisions, is further supported by the principles of treatment in the least restrictive environment. The many human right principles mentioned are further supported by The Convention of the Rights of Persons with Disabilities (CRPD), and Byrne, White and McDonald (2018) have developed an audit tool to assist mental health law makers to ensure the legislation is CRPD compliant.

The essential function of each of these MHAs is to protect individual people and the community as a whole. The following interventions may be included and explicitly prescribed in the mental health legislation enacted in the particular state or territory in which the health professional is working:

- mental health assessment orders
- forensic mental health orders
- involuntary mental health treatment orders and breach requirements
- restriction orders
- community care orders
- the Mental Health Tribunal membership, function and role
- electroconvulsive therapy and psychosurgery
- referrals by courts
- the provision of official visitors
- private mental health facilities
- the rights of consumers and carers, and the responsibilities of the health professionals
- seclusion and restraint guidelines.

All Australian state and territory MHAs allow for an individual to be detained against their will, sometimes for long periods of time, usually on the basis of what medical practitioners consider that an individual might do, rather than on what they have already done. Ethically, this is a clear case of beneficence overriding autonomy. For example, a person may be detained when they articulate thoughts of harming themselves and/or others, but have not actually attempted to harm the identified person. The MHA is designed exclusively for the treatment of mental illness and mental dysfunction, not physical illness or the physical consequences of a mental illness.

The Mental Health Act in action

The State of Victoria conducted a Royal Commission into Victoria's Mental Health System with the goal of gathering feedback and lived experience voices to develop recommendations that would underpin the overhauling and improvement of state mental health services. The Royal Commission delivered their final report in 2021, culminating in 65 recommendations across several key areas, including improvement in treatment frameworks and systems, delivery of mental health and wellbeing services, and workforce capacity and retention.

One young person who shared their story at the Commission hearings was Erika Williams, who feels she would have taken her life if health care professionals had not instigated involuntary care to ensure she stayed in hospital, and in treatment.

Erika reported that during previous admissions for mental health treatment, she had absconded a number of times from the health facility, always with the intent to immediately take her life. Erika further stated that for her, the involuntary use of the Mental Health Act during her hospital admission prevented an early discharge occurring, which ultimately kept her safe.

She further stated that there were times she felt she could be admitted in a voluntary capacity, but that her treating psychiatrist would sometimes utilise involuntary mental health care provisions when he feared for her safety and wanted to delay a premature discharge.

Erika also commented that while involuntary mental health care is often considered as a negative intervention due to the infringement and limitation of basic human rights during the admission, she clearly believes that if she had not been admitted under these conditions, she would have ended her life.

Source: Adapted from Bennett (2019) and State of Victoria (2021).

Sectioning and scheduling

Each MHA is divided into several parts, sections or schedules, from which comes the term 'sectioning' or 'scheduling'. Being sectioned or scheduled means an individual has been compulsorily admitted to a hospital for assessment or to receive treatment for a mental disorder. This includes disorders such as schizophrenia, bipolar disorder, depression, anxiety, eating disorders and obsessive-compulsive disorders. There are a number of conditions that must be met before someone can be compulsorily admitted to hospital. For example, under section 5 of the Victorian MHA, a person can be compulsorily admitted only if all of the following are met (Fizroy Legal Service, 2021).

- The person has a mental illness.
- Because the person has a mental illness, the person requires immediate treatment to prevent serious:
  - deterioration in the person's mental or physical health, or
  - harm to the person or to another person.
- If the person is subject to a temporary treatment order, immediate treatment will be provided.
- There are no less restrictive means reasonably available to enable the person to receive the immediate treatment.

It also needs to be noted that not all sections of the MHAs are relevant to an acute care facility setting, although a number of sections are seen in this setting with some frequency. MHAs are also used to treat people in the community.

The application of the MHA can be a complex and time-consuming process, particularly for health professionals who do not have to deal with this legislation on a regular basis. Table 3.5 provides a brief example of the continuum of involuntary care pathway that is generally followed by mental health legislation across Australia. The Royal Australian and New Zealand College of Psychiatrists (RANZCP) have a national comparison of mental health acts available for review on their website.

Despite the complexities, it is important for health professionals to remember that failure to ensure the MHA is interpreted accurately or to ensure that people are detained only as specified in the legislation, could result in the person being detained unlawfully. Interpretation of an MHA is generally undertaken by health professionals, including medical practitioners, psychologists, registered nurses, social workers and paramedics. Lawyers and the police also have an important role. This interpretation is supported by a number of legal instruments, protocols and procedures that provide 'checks and balances' to guard against misinterpretation. The protocols and procedures also provide detailed guidance for health professionals to support them in their work of caring for the person with a mental illness.

TABLE 3.5 Example of the continuum of involuntary care pathway provided under Australian state and territory Mental Health Acts

Duration of detention	Reason	Comments*
4 hours	Detention of a person who a police officer, a paramedic or appointed health professional suspects has a mental illness or mental dysfunction that requires urgent treatment	This short detention is a mechanism under the Act to allow the person to be transported to a scheduled or gazetted facility for further assessment. The person detained must be taken to a 'place of safety'**, usually a police station or a hospital.
72 hours	Detention of a person who requires a further assessment period in hospital	This is the section most likely to be used within an acute care facility and this detention can only be attended and authorised by a medical officer. Treatment without consent (except any that needs to be given as a life-saving measure) cannot be given while the person is subject to the MHA.
Up to a further 7 days	Assessment	The treating team makes an application to the Mental Health Tribunal for a further detention period. This is generally used if the person has no recent history of admission under the Act, or where the diagnosis is unclear, or the response to treatment is slow and risk issues remain. This detention period is approved/declined by the Mental Health Tribunal (or equivalent). The person has the right of appeal to the Mental Health Tribunal.
Up to 28 days	Assessment and treatment	The diagnosis remains unclear and progress is slow. This detention period is approved/declined following an application to the Mental Health Tribunal (or equivalent). The person has the right of appeal to the Mental Health Tribunal (or equivalent).
Up to 6 months	Treatment	The clinical progress is slow and risk issues may still be present. This detention period is approved/declined following an application to the Mental Health Tribunal (or equivalent). The person has the right of appeal to the Supreme Court. People subject to this section are likely to be receiving treatment under the Act in a community or rehabilitation setting.

* Formal documentation accompanies all sections.

** Gazetted facility is not defined in law, but is a matter for local determination. The relevant health services, police force and local government must all agree as to where the local place of safety is. The place of safety should not routinely be the local police station or 'watch house', but rather an appropriate health care setting.

If the MHA is applied inappropriately, the consumer may have a case against the individual health professional or health organisation involved for unlawful detention (false imprisonment) or breach of human rights (Morrison-Valfre, 2017, p. 27). False imprisonment is an intentional tort — the intentional unjustified, nonconsensual detention or confinement of a person within fixed boundaries for any length of time. Restraint may be physical, chemical or emotional (e.g. intimidation or threat) (Mosby, 2017, p. 674). A high-profile example of false imprisonment is the case of Cornelia Rau, who disappeared from the psychiatric unit of a Sydney hospital in March 2004 and, when subsequently stopped by police in Far North Queensland, identified herself as a German tourist who had overstayed her visa. Initially detained as an 'unlawful non-citizen', Ms Rau spent six months in a Queensland prison alongside convicted criminals before being transferred to the Baxter immigration detention centre. It was not until February 2005 that Ms Rau's true identity became known. Ms Rau has since received a large compensation payment.

A second high-profile and extremely controversial false imprisonment claim is that lodged by asylum seekers in search of refuge in Australia, but who were held in the Papua New Guinea Manus Island Detention Centre between 2012 and 2014. In April 2016, the Papua New Guinea Supreme Court ruled that the offshore detention of Australian asylum seekers on Manus Island was illegal (Lewis, 2016).

Upon this ruling, it was assumed that, from a legal perspective, it followed that the Australian government and associated service providers were also acting unlawfully. The Australian law firm Slater and Gordon, acting as lawyers representing the asylum seekers, then lodged a class action claim in the Supreme Court of Victoria seeking compensation for physical and psychological injuries that are directly attributable to the living conditions of asylum seekers while detained in the centre. However, the Australian government maintained a position of denial in relation to the alleged false imprisonment and mistreatment of those initiating the claim. Nevertheless, rather than going through a trial process, in July 2017 the government settled the class action by agreeing to pay compensation of $70 million (plus costs) to the 1905 plaintiffs (Koziol, 2017).

Further to false imprisonment issues, the following list highlights some known problems that have occurred during the application of the previous *Mental Health Act 2000* (Qld), particularly in a non-mental health setting.

- *Incorrect reason for detention.* The MHA only allows for detention and treatment relating to a mental illness; for example, citing the need to give physical treatment for non-emergency medical problems is not allowed, nor is detaining a person who is considered a public nuisance.
- *Forcing physical treatment on a non-consenting person.* Treatment can only be given against a person's expressed wish in certain circumstances.
- *Failing to ensure that the relevant MHA documentation has been accepted by the necessary governing bodies.* If this does not take place within the time frame stipulated in the Act, the health professional may be fined, have penalty points recorded against their name, or be jailed in extreme breaches.
- *Failing to provide the person and their nearest relative with written and verbal information regarding their rights.* Under the MHA, people have certain rights; for example, to speak with an advocate and access legal representation. It is therefore essential that these rights are explained in easy-to-understand language.

IN PRACTICE

What to do?

During the initial phase of the COVID-19 pandemic, most states and territories enacted Emergency Public Health Directives, which essentially restricted free movement of all community members. This was generally termed 'lockdown'. Some occupational groups and a limited number of personal activities were excluded from these rules. Consequences for breaching these rules differed across jurisdictions; however, national police intervention was common with arrests, fines and jail terms reported for extreme quarantine breaches. There were occasions when people with a mental health illness refused to comply with the Emergency Public Health Directives, including the donning of a mask in public areas. This created a quandary for police, who were required to maintain social control throughout this period.

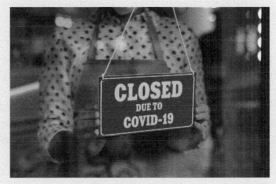

QUESTIONS

1. From an ethical perspective, is it appropriate for known mental health consumers to be admitted against their will for the purposes of upholding an Emergency Public Health Directive?
2. What are the legal and professional ramifications for health professionals who may be involved in scenarios like this?
3. What are the actual and perceived risks for the community if people continually flaunt Emergency Public Health Directives?
4. Does the immunisation status of the individual change the degree of risk for the community?
5. In what creative ways could police, ambulance and mental health services work together to better address this issue, without undermining the rights of any particular group?

The appropriate application of mental health legislation requires considerable experience. Even so, health professionals who follow the core principles that underwrite all mental health legislation across

Australia are well on the way to providing care that is both legal and ethical. These core principles include upholding the person's human rights within the limitations of the legislation, ensuring the care they receive is delivered in the least restrictive manner as possible, and providing evidenced-based care and treatment that is appropriate for that person as an individual.

3.7 Forensic mental health care

LEARNING OBJECTIVE 3.7 Provide an introduction to the interface between legal and mental health systems known as forensic mental health.

The Preamble of the National Statement of Principles for Forensic Mental Health (Australian Health Ministers' Advisory Council, 2006) states:

> Forensic mental health is a specialised field within mental health. In terms of service planning and development, forensic mental health has been neglected and reform has lagged behind mainstream mental health services.
>
> There is a high occurrence of mental illness amongst inmates in correctional settings. Often mental illness is present in association with other disabilities such as substance abuse and intellectual disability.
>
> Offenders with a mental disorder are a highly stigmatised and marginalised group in our community. There are a number of particularly vulnerable populations within this group, including juveniles, Aboriginal and Torres Strait Islander peoples and people from culturally and linguistically diverse backgrounds. The marginalisation is increased by sensationalised media representations that often give misleading accounts of forensic mental health issues.
>
> These Principles have been developed in the context of, and are underpinned by, international and national policy frameworks including: the United Nations Principles on the Protection of People with a Mental Illness, the International Covenant on Civil and Political Rights, the Australian Health Ministers' Mental Health Statement of Rights and Responsibilities, the National Mental Health Strategy, the National Standards for Mental Health Services and the Royal Commission into Aboriginal Deaths in Custody.
>
> The National Mental Health Strategy acknowledges that forensic populations are a group requiring access to the same range of services as the wider community. The Second National Mental Health Plan identified forensic populations as one of the target groups for which the following reforms are essential: improved service access, better service responses, further development and evaluation of appropriate service models.

In Australia, in general terms, a forensic consumer is considered to be a person who has committed a crime and been found not guilty by reason of mental illness or impairment, or unfit to be tried due to a mental illness or mental disorder (Royal Australian & New Zealand College of Psychiatrists, 2016). In 1993, the Australian Human Rights Commission (AHRC) reported that 'mentally ill people detained by the criminal justice system are frequently denied the health care and human rights protections to which they are entitled' (Human Rights and Equal Opportunity Commission, 1993). Unfortunately (from a health care perspective), more than 25 years later, ill-health of male and female Australian prisoners continues to be at higher levels than reported in the general population (AIHW, 2019).

Nationally, under the various crimes or mental health Acts where forensic provisions or procedures apply, there continues to be inconsistent detention or forensic orders that may be enacted. There is furthermore a national lack of uniformity regarding the treatment, care, detention and release processes of forensic patients (O'Donahoo & Simmonds, 2016). However, there has still been significant national progress since forensic mental health care was included in the second National Mental Health Plan (Department of Health and Family Services, 1998) and the National Statement of Principles for Forensic Mental Health 2006 (Australian Health Ministers' Advisory Council, 2006). One such advancement has been the National Statement of Principles Relating to Persons Unfit to Plead or Found Not Guilty by Reason of Cognitive or Mental Health Impairment (Australian Government, 2019).

The Statement goes some way to addressing that a nationally consistent expectation of culturally appropriate services are provided to all people in forensic settings across the country. Additionally, the 2006 National Statement of Principles is scheduled for review in order to consider important changes to the Forensic landscape including increasing recognition of Indigenous cultures, inclusion of Lived Experience perspective, adoption of International Agreements (including the United Nations Nelson Mandela Rules), enhanced alignment with the delivery of contemporary mental health services and the impact of the National Disability Insurance Scheme in a forensic setting (Victorian Institute of Forensic Mental Health, 2022).

In most Australian jurisdictions, forensic mental health care may now be provided in a number of locations including courts, police custody centres, prisons, secure hospitals and community settings (Victorian Institute of Forensic Mental Health, 2019), and the human rights of people detained under forensic orders has begun to be addressed within the recent amendments to the various state and territory MHAs. For example, in NSW, the Mental Health Review Tribunal has the power and authority to decide:

- where a forensic patient should be detained
- whether the patient can have any leave from the hospital (i.e. go outside of the hospital)
- if a patient is ready to be released into the community with conditions
- if a patient is ready to be unconditionally released (so that they are completely free to resume their life in the community without conditions) (New South Wales Mental Health Review Tribunal, 2019).

SUMMARY

This chapter summarises the relevant ethical, legal and professional requirements of health professionals in relation to the care of people with mental health issues. Particular emphasis is placed on the need for health professionals to develop clarity regarding the relevant legal frameworks that inform their practice. To assist with this process, the difference between statute and common law is explained. A number of statute laws pertinent to the delivery of mental health care are identified. The impact of common law from the perspectives of duty of care and assault and battery are also discussed.

This is followed by a description of the domains of capacity, competence and informed consent; the harm principle; ethical egoism; and the doctrine of necessity. In particular, it is suggested that an understanding of capacity, informed consent and duty of care is vital if health professionals are to provide care that is legally and professionally accountable and defensible in a court of law. Consumer autonomy and informed decision-making options for people receiving care for a mental illness are also discussed, including advance care directives or agreements.

The chapter also outlines the mental health legislation prescribing the legal requirements that must be met by health professionals when involuntary detention is authorised. The chapter then identifies the need for all health professionals to meet the legal requirements of the state, territory or jurisdiction in which they work, and the need for all health professionals to have a sound ethical framework that guides their relationships and the care they provide to the consumer, their partner, carer, family or significant others.

The chapter concludes by providing a definition and an historical overview of forensic mental health care in Australia, and issues related to the provision of care for this population.

KEY TERMS

capacity A legal term that is used as a basis to determine that a person has understood the information provided to them, and that the person has made a decision based on their ability to process this information, including the benefits and risks involved.

common law Principles based on the decisions made by judges in individual cases.

competence When a person can speak, understand and comprehend the language used to communicate information to members of a community; satisfactory processing of this information allows a person to perform tasks and duties to an expected level within the community.

dignity of risk The concept of supporting the right of a person to take reasonable risks is essential for dignity and that the impeding of this right can stifle personal growth, self-esteem and the overall quality of life.

doctrine of necessity Allows health professionals to provide non-consenting care to a person in order to save the person's life, to prevent serious deterioration of the person's health and to minimise ongoing significant pain or distress.

ethical decision making Process of making a decision based on personal moral, ethical and legal positions, that needs to be made between two or more often unfavourable alternatives, in any given circumstance.

ethical egoism An ethical theory proposing that people are entitled to make choices and decisions based on their own self-interest, over and above the interest of others.

harm principle The principle that a person has the right to complete freedom of choices and actions, regardless of what the greater community believes, on the proviso that their actions do not directly harm, infringe or violate the same freedom of choice of others.

incapacity The inability of a person to look after their health, safety or welfare or to manage their affairs due to a cognitive deficit that impairs their decision-making abilities.

informed consent When a person agrees to a recommended course of treatment, a medical or surgical procedure, or participation in a clinical trial, following thorough explanation of the proposed treatment, including actual and potential risks involved, which the person has been able to understand.

statute law A law made by parliament (Commonwealth, state or territory); the relevance and enactment of this law is openly debated in the parliament prior to becoming law.

REVIEW QUESTIONS

1 Identify six relevant statute laws from your state or territory that directly impact on your practice.
2 What are the four primary ethical principles that all health care providers are required to practise?
3 What must a person be able to demonstrate for a health professional to determine that the person has the capacity to consent?
4 What additional consent procedures exist for young people aged 14–18 years?
5 List the advantages and disadvantages of the My Health Record. How would you explain this system to a person unaware of its existence?
6 There are three types of consent. What are they?
7 Consequentialism and deontology are just two of many ethical theories. Define these two theories.
8 Define 'duty of care'.
9 Under which circumstances would an advanced care directive not be followed?
10 What are the legal requirements for involuntary detention in your state or territory?
11 What does the term 'less restrictive environment' mean?
12 What is the definition of 'forensic consumer'?

DISCUSSION AND DEBATE

1 Suicide attempts and treatment refusals using an advance care directive have been identified by Australian governments as a growing concern. What are the legal and ethical considerations of such an act for the person, the health care professional, the organisation, the legal system, the family? What are the actual duty of care principles and the potential assault and battery ramifications?
2 Discuss what you think are the main issues related to notions of 'capacity' and 'incapacity' in the mental health context.
3 How does dignity of risk fit with Recovery principles? How can health care professionals reconcile beneficence in this situation?
4 Access the mental health legislation (Mental Health Act) in your state or territory.
   (a) What are the requirements for detaining someone against their will under your Mental Health Act?
   (b) Who has the authority to do this?
   (c) Who needs to be informed when detention is activated under the Act? How do you inform the relevant body or people? Is there a time frame stipulated to do this?
   (d) What information do you need to give to the consumer and their family?
5 Consider the following statement.

   Legislation directs, guides and impacts on the practice of health professionals. Much of the work in a clinical care setting is governed by Commonwealth and state or territory legislation. This legislation is particularly significant for health care practitioners who are working in a clinical setting.

   (a) What legislation is applicable on a daily basis for health care practitioners in a clinical setting?
   (b) How does that legislation impact on your day-to-day work? How can health care practitioners ensure they are performing their role in accordance with the relevant legislation?
6 Describe a potential 'duty of care versus individual rights' (dignity of risk) conflict or ethical dilemma that may arise in your particular workplace. Discuss the scenario from the personal values, professional standards and ethical principle perspectives. How might you manage this situation?
7 A 17-year-old woman gives birth. Is the woman able to consent to medical treatment for herself? As a mother and parent, is the woman able to consent to medical treatment for her child? Discuss.
8 Given the importance of the National Statement of Principles for Forensic Mental Health advocating for baseline health care for people who are incarcerated, and acknowledging that comorbid rates of physical conditions is higher amongst detained populations than community members, who is responsible for providing physical health care in a forensic setting, the judicial system or the primary health system? Discuss.

PROJECT ACTIVITY

Capacity and competence are key factors when determining the cognitive ability of a person to make a decision regarding their health care. A person is capable of making decisions about their own health care for mental illnesses or disorders, if they understand when a decision about their health care needs to be made, the facts involved with the decision, the choices they have available to them and the consequences of each possible choice. If they can make their decision with the discussed criteria taken into consideration, and they are able to communicate their choice (in whatever way is possible for them), then they are deemed competent enough to make decisions about their own health care.

1 What factors must a health professional consider when assessing capacity and competence?
2 What tools or information may be of assistance to help determine the decision-making capacity of a consumer?
3 How does the complexity of the proposed health care intervention affect your determination of whether a person is competent to consent or not?
4 What roles do the consumer and carer play in the assessment of the consumer's capacity and competence?
5 What are the options available to health professionals when a capacity assessment is inconclusive or there are differing opinions?
6 For those identified as requiring additional support during the consent process, what surrogate and supported decision-making tools and processes can be offered to them?

WEBSITES

1 The Australian Association of Social Workers is the professional representative body of social workers in Australia, with over 16 000 members nationwide. The Association is an incorporated company, guided by a constitution and nationally managed by a board of directors, elected from and by the membership: www.aasw.asn.au.
2 The Australian Health Practitioner Regulation Agency is the organisation responsible for the implementation of the National Registration and Accreditation Scheme across Australia: www.ahpra.gov.au.
3 The Australian Commission on Safety and Quality in Health Care (ACSQHC) is proactive in developing and strengthening a health system that is better informed, supported and organised to deliver safe and high-quality care. To achieve this the Commission works in partnership with many stakeholders including government, states and territories, the public and private health sector, those with lived experience, clinical experts and carers: www.safetyandquality.gov.au.
4 The Australian Psychological Society is committed to advancing psychology as a discipline and profession. It spreads the message that psychologists make a difference to people's lives, through improving scientific knowledge and community wellbeing: www.psychology.org.au.
5 Forensicare (Victorian Institute of Forensic Mental Health) is Victoria's leading clinical provider of forensic mental health care, and provides services across a range of settings including police custody centres, courts and prison, mental health services, secure hospitals and within the community: www.forensicare.vic.gov.au.
6 The Paramedicine Board of Australia began registration processes for paramedics in December 2018, meaning that paramedicine has now become a nationally regulated profession under the *Health Practitioner Regulation National Law Act 2009* and the titles 'paramedic' and 'paramedicine' are now protected by law: www.paramedicineboard.gov.au.
7 Advance Care Planning Australia provides information regarding the documentation of future preferences for health care. Additional information is available for health professionals including underpinning laws and ethical considerations of advance care planning. www.advancecareplanning.org.au.

REFERENCES

Aboriginal and Torres Strait Islander Health Practice Board of Australia. (2014). *Code of conduct for registered health practitioners.* www.atsihealthpracticeboard.gov.au/Codes-Guidelines/Code-of-conduct.aspx

ACT Health. (2018). *Consent.* ACT Government. www.health.act.gov.au/research/research-ethics-and-governance/consent

ACT Parliamentary Counsel. (2017). *Human Rights Act 2004 (ACT).* www.legislation.act.gov.au/a/2004-5

ACT Legislative Assembly. (2021). *Carers Recognition Bill (ACT).* www.parliament.act.gov.au/__data/assets/pdf_file/0007/17940 67/Carers-Recognition-Bill-2021.pdf

Advance Care Planning Australia. (2018). *Advance care planning and the law.* www.advancecareplanning.org.au/for-health-and-care-workers/legal-requirements

Australian Association of Social Workers (Draft). (2022). *AASW Practice Standards.* www.aasw.asn.au/practitioner-resources/practice-standards

Austin Health. (2021). *Advanced care planning Australia: Advance care planning laws in the Australian Capital Territory.* www.advancecareplanning.org.au/law-and-ethics/state-and-territory-laws/advance-care-planning-laws-in-act

Australian Commission on Safety and Quality in Health Care. (2020). *Fact sheets for Clinicians.* www.safetyandquality.gov.au/sites/default/files/2020-09/sq20-030_-_fact_sheet_-_informed_consent_-_nsqhs-8.9a.pdf

Australian Commission on Safety and Quality in Health Care. (2017). *National safety and quality health service standards* (2nd ed.). ACSQHC.

Australian Digital Health Agency. (2019). *9 out of 10 Australians have a My Health Record.* www.myhealthrecord.gov.au/news-and-media/australians-to-have-my-health-record

Australian Government. (2019). *National statement of principles relating to persons unfit to plead or found not guilty by reason of cognitive or mental health impairment.* Attorney General Department. www.ag.gov.au/rights-and-protections/publications/national-statement-principles-relating-persons-unfit-plead-or-found-not-guilty-reason-cognitive-or-mental-health-impairment

Australian Government. (2021). National framework for advance care planning documents Department of Health. www.health.gov.au/sites/default/files/documents/2021/06/national-framework-for-advance-care-planning-documents.pdf

Australian, Government Solicitor. (2012). *ACT Court of Appeal confirms police responsibilities for prevention of crime are critical to determining whether a duty of care is owed.* Express Law No. 178 www.ags.gov.au/publications/express-law/el178

Australian Health Ministers' Advisory Council Mental Health Standing Committee. (2006). *National statement of principles for forensic mental health.* Australian Government Department of Health and Ageing.

Australian Health Practitioner Regulation Agency. (2021). *How we manage concerns: Possible Outcomes.* www.ahpra.gov.au/Notifications/How-we-manage-concerns/Possible-outcomes.aspx

Australian Health Practitioner Regulation Agency. (2021). *What we do.* www.ahpra.gov.au/About-Ahpra/What-We-Do.aspx

Australian Institute of Health and Welfare. (2019). *The health of Australia's prisoners 2018,* cat. no. PHE 246. Canberra: AIHW.

Australian Institute of Health and Welfare. (2020). *Australia's health 2020: Media Release Canberra.* AIHW. www.aihw.gov.au/news-media/media-releases/2020/july/national-report-card-examines-covid-19-and-other-h

Australian Law Reform Commission. (2010a). *Capacity and health information.* www.alrc.gov.au/publication/for-your-information-australian-privacy-law-and-practice-alrc-report-108/68-decision-making-by-and-for-individuals-under-the-age-of-18/capacity-and-health-information

Australian Psychological Society. (2007). *Code of ethics.* Flinders Lave: Victoria.

Beauchamp, T., & Childress, J. (1994). *Principles of biomedical ethics* (4th ed.). Oxford University Press.

Bennett, J. (2019). Mental health care 'diminished dramatically' by bed shortages, Royal Commission told. *ABC News online.* www.abc.net.au/news/2019-07-10/patients-falling-through-gaps-mental-health-royal-commission/11295670

Bester, J., Crisite, M., & Kodish, E. (2016). The limits of informed consent for an overwhelmed patient: Clinicians' role in protecting patients and preventing overwhelm. *AMA Journal of Ethics, 18*(9), 869–886.

Byrne, M., White, B., & McDonald, F. (2018). A new tool to assess compliance of mental health laws with the Convention on the Rights of Persons with Disabilities. *International Journal of Law and Psychiatry, 58,* 122–142.

Chandler, K., White, B., & Wilmott, L. (2016). The doctrine of necessity and the detention and restraint of people with intellectual impairment: Is there any justification? *Psychiatry, Psychology and Law, 23*(3), 361–387.

Cheluvappa, R., & Selvendran, S. (2020). Medical negligence - Key cases and application of legislation. *Annals of Medicine and Surgery, 57,* 205–211. https://doi.org/10.1016/j.amsu.2020.07.017

Clinical. (2010). *Technical and Ethical Principal Committee of the Australian Health Ministers' Advisory Council. A national framework for advanced care directives: Consultation draft.* Consumers Health Forum of Australia.

Commonwealth of Australia. (2010). *Commonwealth response to the hidden toll: Suicide in Australia, report of the senate community affairs reference committee.* Attorney-General's Department, Commonwealth of Australia.

Coroners Court of Victoria. (2021). *Finding into death without inquest of Christopher Douglas Ritson.* State of Victoria. www.coronerscourt.vic.gov.au/sites/default/files/2021-05/ChristopherDouglasRitson_156020.pdf

Department of Health and Family Services. (1998). *Second national mental health plan.* Commonwealth of Australia.

Department of Health WA. (2016). *WA health consent to treatment policy 2016.* Government of Western Australia.

Duggan, M., Harris, B., Chislett, W. K., & Calder, R. (2020). *Nowhere else to go: Why Australia's health system results in people with mental illness getting 'stuck' in emergency departments. Mitchell Institute Commissioned report 2020.* Victoria University.

End of Life Directions for Aged Care. (2022). *Factsheet: Capacity and consent to medical treatment.* www.eldac.com.au.

Fitzroy Legal Service. (2021). *The Law Handbook. Your practical guide to the law in Victoria. Compulsory mental health treatments and patients.* Fitzroy Legal Service. www.fls.org.au/law-handbook/disability-mental-illness-and-the-law/mental-illness/compulsory-mental-health-treatment-and-patients

Harrison, A., & Hart, C. (2006). *Mental health care for nurses: Applying mental health skills in the general hospital.* Blackwell Publishing.

Human Rights and Equal Opportunity Commission. (1993). *Report of the national inquiry into the human rights of people with mental illness*. Australian Human Rights Commission.

International Council of Nurses. (2021). *The ICN code of ethics for nurses*. ICN. www.icn.ch/system/files/2021-10/ICN_Code-of-Ethics_EN_Web_0.pdf

Koziol, M. (2017). Court approves $70 million compensation payout to Manus Island detainees *The Sydney Morning Herald*. www.smh.com.au/politics/federal/court-approves-70-million-compensation-payout-to-manus-island-detainees-20170906-gybpjy.html

Kurpad, S. (2018). Ethics in psychosocial interventions. *Indian Journal of Psychiatry*, *60*(4), S571–S574.

Lewis, R. (2016). PNG court rules detention of asylum seekers on Manus Island is illegal. *The Australian*. www.theaustralian.com.au/national-affairs/png-court-rules-detention-of-asylum-seekers-on-manus-island-is-illegal/news-story/2241b33cc1de8c05f8d92d92d5eea151

Lifeplan. (2022). *Dignity of risk and duty of care: A balancing act?* www.lifeplan.org.au/news/dignity-of-risk-duty-of-care-balance.

Magill, G., & Prybil, L. (2020). *Governance ethics in healthcare organizations*. Routledge.

McIntyre, E., Oorschot, T., Steel, A., Leach, M. J., Adams, J., & Harnett, J. (2021). Conventional and complementary health care use and out-of-pocket expenses among Australians with a self-reported mental health diagnosis: A cross-sectional survey. *BMC Health Services Research*, *21*(1), 1266. https://doi.org/10.1186/s12913-021-07162-0

Mental Health Coordinating Council. (2015). (4th ed.). MHCC.

Mental Health Legal Centre. (n.d). *Advance statements: Improving recovery journeys*. www.mhlc.org.au/advance-statements

Mill, J. (1963). *Collected works of John Stuart Mill*. University of Toronto Press.

Mind Australia and Helping Minds. (2016). *A practical guide for working with carers of people with a mental illness*. In *Mind Australia, Helping Minds, Private Mental Health Consumer Carer Network (Australia), Mental Health Carers Arafmi Australia and Mental Health Australia*.

Morrison-Valfre, M. (2017). *Foundations of mental health care* (6th ed.). Elsevier.

Mosby. (2017). *Mosby's medical dictionary* (10th ed.). Elsevier.

New South Wales Mental Health Review Tribunal. (2019). *Forensic patients*. www.mhrt.nsw.gov.au/forensic-patients.

New South Wales Ministry of Health. (2018). *Decision making framework for NSW health Aboriginal health practitioners. Workforce planning & development (WPD)*. NSW Ministry of Health.

Nimita, L., & Carol, I. B. (2014). The modern social contract between the patient, the healthcare provider, and digital medicine. *Journal of Socialomics*, *3*, 105

Nowland, R., Steeg, S., Quinlivan, L. M., Cooper, J., Huxtable, R., Hawton, K., Gunnell, D., Allen, N., Mackway-Jones, K., & Kapur, N. (2019). Management of patients with an advance decision and suicidal behaviour: A systematic review. *British Medical Journal Open*, *9*(5), e023978.

Nursing and Midwifery Board of Australia. (2018). *Code of conduct for nurses in Australia*. Professional Standards. www.nursingmidwiferyboard.gov.au/Codes-Guidelines-Statements/Professional-standards.aspx

Nursing and Midwifery Board of Australia. (2020). *Nursing practice decision flowchart. www.nursingmidwiferyboard.gov.au/Codes-Guidelines-Statements/Frameworks.aspx*.

Nursing and Midwifery Board of Australia. (2020). *A national framework for the development of decision making tools for nursing and midwifery practice*. www.nursingmidwiferyboard.gov.au

O'Donahoo, J., & Simmonds, J. G. (2016). Forensic patients and forensic mental health in victoria: Legal context, clinical pathways, and practice challenges. *Australian Social Work*, *69*(2), 169–180.

Office of the Public Advocate. (2022). *Patient capacity to consent*. www.publicadvocate.vic.gov.au/medical-treatment/patient-consent/patient-capacity-to-consent

Office of the Public Advocate. (2019). *About mental capacity*. www.opa.sa.gov.au/page/view_by_id/21.

Paramedicine Board of Australia. (2018). *Code of conduct for paramedics*. Paramedicine Board of Australia. www.paramedicineboard.gov.au/professional-standards/codes-guidelines-and-policies.aspx.

Parker, M. (2016). Getting the balance right: Conceptual considerations concerning legal capacity and supported decision-making. *Journal of Bioethical Inquiry, 13*, 381–393 https://doi.org/10.1007/s11673-016-9727-z

Productivity Commission. (2022). Report on Government Services 2022 Part E, section 11: Ambulance Services. www.pc.gov.au/research/ongoing/report-on-government-services/2022/health/ambulance-services

Queensland Ambulance Service. (2019). *Digital clinical practice manual, version 2019*. The State of Queensland. www.ambulance.qld.gov.au/clinical.html.

Queensland Government. (2018). *Potential healthcare choices. Refusing treatment*. www.qld.gov.au/health/support/end-of-life/advance-care-planning/choices.

Queensland Health, Clinical Excellence Division. (2017). *Guide to informed decision-making in health care* (2nd ed.). State of Queensland.

Queensland Judgments. (2018). *Masson v State of Queensland* QSC Queensland Supreme Court. www.queenslandjudgments.com.au/case/id/310290.

Raines, J. C., & Dibble, N. T. (2021). *Ethical decision-making in school mental health* (2nd ed.). Oxford University Press. https://doi.org/10.55521/10-019-112

Royal Australian & New Zealand College of Psychiatrists. (2016). *Principles for the treatment of persons found unfit to stand trial. Position statement 90*. RANZCP.

SANE Australia. (2021). *Fact sheets and guides: Suicidal behaviour*. www.sane.org/information-and-resources/facts-and-guides/suicidal-behaviour

Select Committee on Youth Suicides in the NT. (2012). *Gone too soon: A report into youth suicide in the Northern Territory*. Northern Territory Government.

Selinger, C. P. (2009). The right to consent: Is it absolute? *British Journal of Medical Practitioners*, *2*(2), 50–54.

Sorrentino, R. (2014). Performing capacity evaluations: What's expected from your consult? *Current Psychiatry*, *13*(1), 41–44

State of Victoria. (2021). Royal Commission into Victoria's Mental Health System, Final Report, Volume 1: A new approach to mental health and wellbeing in Victoria, Parl Paper No. 202, Session 2018–21 (document 2 of 6). www.finalreport.rcvmhs.vic.gov.au/fact-sheets ISBN 978-1-925789-66-9 (pdf/online/MS word

Szmukler, G. (2020). Involuntary detention and treatment: Are we edging toward a "Paradigm Shift"? *Schizophrenia Bulletin*, *46*(2), 231–235. https://doi.org/10.1093/schbul/sbz115

Varkey, B. (2021). Principles of clinical ethics and their application to practice. *Medical Principles and Practice*, *30*, 17–28.

Victorian Department of Health & Human Services. (2019). *Informed consent. Recovery and supported decision making*. State of Victoria.

Victorian Department of Health & Human Services. (2017). *Advance care directives and attempted suicides*. State of Victoria. www2.health.vic.gov.au/about/publications/policiesandguidelines/advance-care-directives-and-attempted-suicides

Victorian Government Department of Health. (2013). *National practice standards for the mental health workforce*. State of Victoria.

Victorian Institute of Forensic Mental Health. (2019). *Our services*. www.forensicare.vic.gov.au/our-services/community-forensic-mental-health-services.

Victorian Institute of Forensic Mental Health. (2022). *National principles for forensic mental health*. www.forensicare.vic.gov.au/national-principles/

Woolford, M. H., de Lacy-Vawdon, C., Bugeja, L., Weller, C., & Ibrahim, J. E. (2020). Applying dignity of risk principles to improve quality of life for vulnerable persons. *International Journal of Geriatric Psychiatry*, *35*(1), 122–130. https://doi.org/10.1002/gps.5228

ACKNOWLEDGEMENTS

Photo: © izzet ugutmen / Shutterstock.com

Photo: © smolaw / Shutterstock.com

Photo: © Pormezz / Shutterstock.com

Photo: © Vasyl Nagernyak / Shutterstock.com

Photo: © Africa Studio / Shutterstock.com

Photo: © Syda Productions / Adobe Stock

Photo: © New Africa / Shutterstock.com

Figure 3.1: © Section 5.2: Assessing capacity in health, NSW Government: Communities & Justice, 2005. Licensed under CC BY 4.0.

Figure 3.2: © Raines, J. C. & Dibble, N. T. (2021). *Ethical decision-making in school mental health* (2nd ed.). Oxford University Press.

Figure 3.3: © Mental Health Legal Centre (n.d.) *Advance statements: Improving recovery journeys*. Retrieved December 11, 2019 from www.mhlc.org.au/our-programs/advance-statements www.mhlc.org.au/advance-statements.

Extract 3A: © *Guardianship and Administration Act 1993*, South Australian Legislation. Licensed under CC BY 4.0.

Extract 3B: © Paramedicine Board of Australia (2018) *Code of conduct for paramedics*. Canberra: Paramedicine Board of Australia. Retrieved November 5, 2019 from www.paramedicineboard.gov.au/professional-standards/codes-guidelines-and-policies.aspx

Extract 3C: © National Statement of Principles for Forensic Mental Health, 2006. Australian Institute of Health and Welfare. Licensed under CC BY 4.0.

Culturally appropriate mental health care

LEARNING OBJECTIVES

This chapter will:

4.1 define the concepts of 'culture' and 'subculture'

4.2 consider the cultural constructions of mental health and illness

4.3 discuss the mental health and wellbeing of Aboriginal and Torres Strait Islander peoples

4.4 describe the major mental health issues for people from rural and remote cultures

4.5 outline the main concerns that affect the mental health of migrants and refugees

4.6 consider the mental health needs of lesbian, gay, bisexual, transgender, queer, intersex and asexual people

4.7 explain the importance of providing culturally appropriate care to all people with mental health issues.

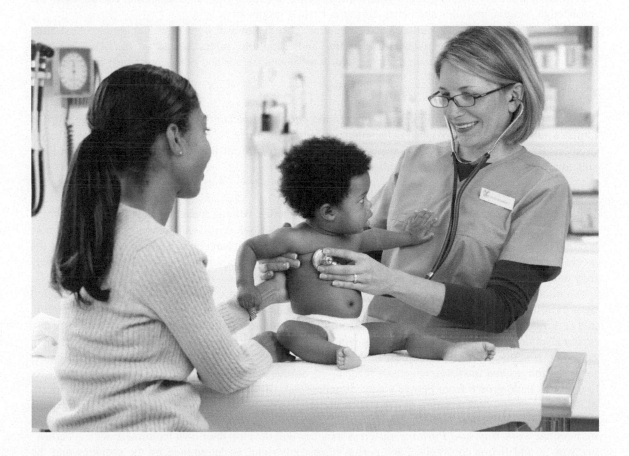

Introduction

All health professionals will interact with people from different cultures during their work. Australia is one of the most multicultural nations in the world (Minas, 2018). Population groups include the traditional custodians of Australia, the Aboriginal and Torres Strait Islander peoples, and immigrants and refugees — past and present — from Africa, America, Asia, Britain, Europe, India, the Middle East and other regions. Australia also has many different subcultural groups based on age, context, education, employment, gender, sexuality and religion. Each of these cultural and subcultural groups has distinct characteristics, preferences and needs for their mental health and wellbeing.

This chapter introduces cultural diversity in the context of mental health and illness. The chapter examines the notions of 'culture' and 'subculture', then outlines the major issues for health professionals when providing mental health care to Aboriginal and Torres Strait Islander, rural and remote, migrant and refugee, and LGBTQIA+ peoples. A broad approach to supporting diverse people is recommended, including acknowledging the diversity between and within cultural groups. The chapter also outlines how health professionals can effectively negotiate cultural differences through acceptance, respect and a commitment to listen to people from culturally and linguistically diverse backgrounds. Finally, the chapter concludes by emphasising the importance of engaging with social and cultural networks when caring for people who live with mental illness.

4.1 The pervasive nature of culture and subculture

LEARNING OBJECTIVE 4.1 Define the concepts of 'culture' and 'subculture'.

Until the 1970s and the development of cultural studies as an intellectual movement (Hall, 1980), the meaning of 'culture' was relatively narrow. A person could enjoy 'culture' by going to the opera, ballet or an art exhibition. Alternatively, nations or ethnic groups often promote a way of life or 'culture' that was quite distinct from other groups. Today, the meaning of culture is much broader and encompasses the knowledge, beliefs, attitudes and behaviours of particular groups of people.

In this section, the terms 'culture' and 'subculture' are defined in light of contemporary Australian society. Consideration is also given to how cultures and subcultures affect the interactions between health professionals and consumers, their carers or family members, friends and other community members.

Culture and subculture

The Australian culture is difficult to define. Some people associate Australia with Bondi Beach, the Outback, and kangaroos or koalas. Others think of 'a fair go', the ANZAC tradition, the outdoor lifestyle or sport. But where does that leave the Aboriginal and Torres Strait Islander peoples, multiculturalism, subcultural minority groups and **globalisation**?

Definitions of 'culture' and 'subculture'

Culture has been defined as the accepted patterns of knowledge, beliefs, attitudes and behaviours by which a group of people live; the shared history, traditions, values, attitudes, goals and practices that characterise a group (Wesch, 2018; Williams, 1963). A person's cultural background helps them to make sense of the world because it shapes and guides every aspect of their life (including their professional life), the way they understand health and ill-health, and how they view and relate to others.

A culture is not the same as a **society**. Human societies comprise large groups of people connected by proximity, politics, the economy, social status, social networks or some other shared interest (Barkan, 2017). While this description has many similarities to the notion of culture, people who make up a society do not always share the same cultural mores. For example, Australian society has one national government but comprises many different cultures. In the same way, the capital cities in Australia have quite distinct local economies and interests, which are made up of various cultural minorities.

Cultures have grown from people's need to make sense of their world through shared understandings of 'the way things are' (Bhugra et al., 2021). These shared understandings give rise to cultural groups defined by distinct beliefs, values, and ways of life or seeing the world. As Erikson (1966, p. 10) wrote in his seminal work *Wayward Puritans*, different societies will develop their own 'cultural space . . . "ethos" or "way"', and live accordingly. Each person's sense of 'right' is determined by the societies and the culture(s) to which they belong; this sense of right or most appropriate way of doing things encourages a person's adherence to the established social order. To exemplify, if a person desires to be accepted as part of the group, they are less likely to behave in a way other people in the group view as 'wrong' or 'just not the way we do things around here'. This dynamic provides one reason why cultural influences are powerful, able to shape — even control — a group's thoughts, feelings and behaviours.

Another aspect of culture is a **subculture**, which describes the culture of smaller discrete groups of people located within larger cultural groups. These groups share a subset of common attitudes, values, goals and practices (Bhugra & Bhui, 2018). A person who has grown up in Western Sydney will have a different view of the world and of what it is to be Australian than a person raised in Melbourne's Toorak or much further afield in Cairns, Launceston or Kalgoorlie. These differences are the result of geographic and socio-economic factors. Again, an Australian who is a Christian will have a different understanding of the world than an Australian who is a Muslim; an Australian who has lived most of their life in the twentieth century will see things differently than an Australian who has lived most of their life in the twenty-first century. In short, more than 25 million people live in Australia, each of whom will be connected to, shaped by and interpret the world according to the larger Australian culture. At the same time, each person will also be influenced by the various subcultures and groups to which they belong.

The influence of culture on health professionals

Cultural and subcultural influences affect the health professional in many ways. First, the cultural background of a health professional forms an integral part of how they work. Health professionals' cultural backgrounds are a filter through which they observe, act, react to and interact with others, suggesting why health professionals must develop an awareness of how their cultural background influences their work.

Second, cultural influences will shape how other people relate to the health professional. A person's cultural background affects their reactions to challenging situations, and how they communicate or disclose information and complete tasks. Likewise, a person's understanding of health and illness will influence their perceptions and interactions with health professionals and the health system. For instance, a person with a positive view of health professionals may be more open-minded about receiving health interventions. A person's culture and subculture will also affect how they understand mental health and illness, including the symptoms they experience and their recovery journey.

UPON REFLECTION

'Normal' and 'abnormal'

In some cultures or subcultures, it is 'normal' for people to self-flagellate to express negative feelings about themselves. However, other cultures or subcultures view this type of behaviour as 'abnormal', with self-harming indicating a mental health problem.

Another, more common example is the 'drinking culture' that characterises mainstream Australian society, with a widespread acceptance of people regularly drinking alcohol to excess and behaving in a disinhibited manner. Health professionals who understand the risks of this behaviour will view such behaviours as unhealthy.

QUESTIONS

1. Identify some of the behaviours that are viewed as 'normal' by the cultural, subcultural or religious group to which you belong but viewed as 'abnormal' by other cultural, subcultural or religious groups.
2. Identify some of the behaviours of other cultural, subcultural or religious groups that you perceive as 'abnormal', 'different' or 'odd'.
3. What behaviours or 'ways of being' are universal or accepted by all groups as 'just the way things are'?

4.2 Cultural constructions of mental illness

LEARNING OBJECTIVE 4.2 Consider the cultural constructions of mental health and illness.

Over the years, the various ways cultural groups understand or perceive mental illness have been given considerable attention in the academic literature (Bhugra & Bhui, 2018). For example, seminal philosophers Goffman (1961) and Foucault (1961) were among the first to associate 'madness' with notions of social exclusion, social control, disempowerment and 'other'. Levine and Levine (1970) went on to discuss the arbitrary construction of mental illness in Western societies, noting that during conservative times the causes of mental illness tended to be framed according to an individual's internal make-up; while in times of social and political reform, causes of mental illness were more likely to be related to the influence of cultural environments. Social or cultural understandings of mental illness are not fixed but change according to the circumstances of the time and location.

More recently, it has been argued that people with mental health issues will look to those around them and the attitudes, values, goals and practices of the communities to which they belong for explanations for their distress (Bhugra et al., 2021). These explanations will differ in contemporary Australian society, with its diverse cultural histories, practices, spiritual beliefs and lifestyles. A variety of cultural myths abound and include the following.

- People with mental illness are dangerous and more violent than other people.
- Mental illness is a punishment for something bad the person or their parents have done.
- People with a mental illness are more likely to be victims of violence.
- Schizophrenia is a spiritual problem — a demon possesses the person.
- Schizophrenia is the mother's fault, caused by her poor style of relating.
- People will never recover from a mental illness — once they have it, they will always have it.
- People who belong to some cultural groups are more likely to become mentally ill than people from other cultural groups.

As explained in the chapter on mental health care in Australia, such views are baseless. Moreover, they have the potential to stigmatise or cause distress to people with the lived experience of mental illness. For this reason, it is right to question their validity.

Indeed, health professionals must take the time to think critically about how cultural issues may impact the person with mental ill-health, their family and community. For example, the research evidence does not support the view that people with a mental illness are dangerous or more violent than others (Saleh, 2020). Unrealistic representations in movies are often based on cultural perceptions rather than facts. Health professionals must differentiate between fact and fiction, between research evidence and cultural myth, while at the same time respecting the beliefs of others and dealing with cultural differences proficiently. Ways of achieving cultural proficiency are discussed in later sections of this chapter.

Alternative views on mental health care

The vast majority of health professionals in Australia have been educated according to Western biomedical values. As noted in the chapter on mental health care in Australia, this model is characterised by diagnostic labelling and linear modes of treatment that are prescribed according to a particular set of symptoms. In the mental health sector, such interventions aim to modify thoughts and behaviours to be consistent with dominant cultural **norms** (Thompson, 2018). Alternative or 'other' approaches to health care tend to be given token consideration by health professionals (Dudgeon & Bray, 2018).

However, exploring the value of cultures or subcultures can open health professionals' minds to other views and ways of being. For example, some people firmly believe that the DSM-5 is a tool developed by powerful capitalistic and hegemonic influences in the United States (Padmanabhan, 2017). Consequently, common reactions to stressful situations, such as grief reactions to death, may be pathologised. Moreover, they argue, health professionals and multinational pharmaceutical companies can benefit from these approaches through an increase in business and profits from prescribing medication or psychotherapy for these so-called conditions.

While this point of view may or may not have some basis, it differs from Australia's dominant understandings of mental health and illness . In a multicultural landscape, health professionals must be aware of and open to ideas of difference. Even the American Psychiatric Association (APA, 2013), the creators of the DSM-5, urge health professionals to consider cultural norms before making a diagnosis. Those who do not consider cultural differences risk pathologising culturally-based variations in behaviour, belief or experiences.

The remainder of the chapter describes the main issues for people from various cultures who live in Australia today and experience symptoms of mental illness. The information is provided in three sections: Indigenous Australian cultures, rural and remote cultures, and other diverse cultures. Although introductory, the information enables health professionals to understand how a person's cultural background influences their perceptions of 'normal' and the effect of these influences on health service provision.

Biomedicine and the Western culture

Biomedical approaches to health care are generally framed by mainstream 'Western' culture. Alternative therapies tend to be aligned with 'Eastern' cultures, such as Chinese medicine, Ayurvedic medicine, Shamanic healing and yoga.

Interestingly, over the past decade or so, many mental health professionals, including medical practitioners who work within the biomedical model of health care, have begun to advocate for approaches that include mindfulness to help people manage their anxiety. Mindfulness is derived from Eastern approaches to help treat anxiety and depression.

QUESTIONS

1. How open are you to alternative approaches to health care?
2. To what degree are your perceptions of alternative approaches to health care shaped by your cultural background?
3. How do your cultural biases influence how you support people in need of health care?

4.3 Mental health and Indigenous Australian cultures

LEARNING OBJECTIVE 4.3 Discuss the mental health and wellbeing of Aboriginal and Torres Strait Islander peoples.

There are around 810 000 Indigenous Australians, comprising 3.2 per cent of the national population (Australian Bureau of Statistics [ABS], 2022). The life expectancy for Indigenous Australians is approximately 8.2 years less than estimates for non-Indigenous Australians (Hendrie, 2018), with the leading causes of death for Indigenous Australians being circulatory diseases (23 per cent) and cancer (23 per cent), with infant mortality still higher than non-Indigenous Australians (Australian Institute of Health and Welfare [AIHW], 2021a). The **burden of disease** was approximately 3.5 times higher in Indigenous Australians than non-Indigenous Australians in 2018, result of living with illness rather than from premature death (AIHW, 2022b). Also of concern is the rate of suicide. In 2020:

- suicide accounted for 5.5 per cent of all deaths of Aboriginal and Torres Strait Islander peoples while the comparable proportion for non-Indigenous Australians was 1.9 per cent
- one-quarter (25 per cent) of all deaths by suicide in Indigenous Australians were female, which was greater than in non-Indigenous populations (23 per cent females) (AIHW, 2021e).

This section focuses on the mental health and wellbeing of Aboriginal and Torres Strait Islander peoples. First, the diversity of Indigenous Australian cultures across Australia is considered, together with the trauma many Aboriginal and Torres Strait Islander peoples have experienced since colonisation, leading to psychological and other distress in many Indigenous Australian communities. Second, the section explains why there is a need for all health professionals to understand the significant issues experienced by Indigenous Australians and work together to redress the inequities involved.

What is meant by 'indigenous'?

The United Nations has reserved the right of indigenous peoples to define who and what is 'indigenous' and to maintain and develop their own distinct identities, characteristics and cultures (Department of Economic and Social Affairs, n.d.). This right to self-define is necessary as it is only through self-definition that indigenous peoples can self-determine. Likewise, it is only through self-determination that indigenous peoples can shape their futures. With an estimated 5000 distinct cultures arising out of the 300–350 million indigenous peoples currently living across 72 countries globally, reaching some understanding of what it means to be indigenous is a complex task (International Working Group on Indigenous Affairs, 2001).

Indigenous peoples are diverse groups of people with similarly diverse backgrounds who share various traditions related to religious or spiritual practices, language, lifestyle and family systems or community beliefs, together with close ties with the environment, ancestral lands or Country (Australian Institute of Aboriginal and Torres Strait Island Studies, 2018). Figure 4.1 details common characteristics across the cultural, political, spiritual, ecological and social spectrums.

Similarities between the many and diverse indigenous cultures worldwide include:

- distinct traditions concerning spiritual practices, languages, lifestyles, family systems and beliefs, together with a desire to preserve these traditions for future generations
- close ties or long traditions with the environment, land, Country or ancestral sites. In some communities, this may relate to notions of managing and protecting the environment and ancestral or sacred sites. In other, now urbanised communities, these ties may be more spiritually metaphorical
- strong family and community connections
- a sense of shared collectivity with indigenous peoples and cultures worldwide, including common ways of knowing the world around them
- a history of repression by the dominant cultures, resulting in current disparities in standards of living and health status
- a shared view of the importance of self-determining to enable political, social and economic equity
- a whole-of-life view of health and wellbeing.

Source: Adapted from Australian Institute of Aboriginal and Torres Strait Island Studies (2018); Cultural Survival (2018); Department of Health and Aged Care (2022a); Secretariat of the Permanent Forum on Indigenous Issues (2009).

In Australia, the term Indigenous Australian is commonly used to describe the Aboriginal and Torres Strait Islander peoples — the traditional custodians of Australia. Some groups, however, have challenged using the term Indigenous Australian because it does not acknowledge the many differences between the Aboriginal and Torres Strait Islander cultures. For example, before British settlement, there were many hundreds of languages and social groups in Australia; today, while less than 200 remain, each group has its own distinct way of understanding the world. Using the plural 'peoples' is one way of acknowledging this diversity (Taylor & Guerin, 2019).

Indigenous Australians in urban areas

According to the Australian Institute of Health and Welfare (2022), 38 per cent of Indigenous Australians live in the capital cities, 44 per cent live in inner and outer regional areas and 17 per cent live in remote and very remote areas. Overall, approximately 80 per cent of Indigenous Australians live in areas designated as 'urban' (ABS, 2017). Consequently, Indigenous cultures and communities across Australia are often described as urbanised.

The urbanisation of Indigenous Australians has given rise to substantial change to their socio-cultural practices. Urbanisation has meant that many of the traditional structures and beliefs that were part of traditional Indigenous cultures and communities before colonisation have been broken down or have disappeared. This situation has given rise to some Indigenous peoples feeling they have lost many of their traditions and direction.

Another significant influence on the Indigenous Australian cultures has been the inter- and intra-generational influences of the Stolen Generations. It has been argued that the forced removal of Indigenous children from their parents up until the 1970s played a pivotal role in the breakdown or disappearance of family structures in many Indigenous Australian communities (Yu, 2019). Children who were removed from their parents and placed in residential or other facilities located in urban areas had no parenting or family role model(s) as they were not a part of the communities that are integral to Indigenous cultures. When those who were removed became adults and began to produce families of their own, they struggled to know how to raise their children or what it meant to be part of an Indigenous family, community or culture (Krakouer et al., 2018). Such difficulties have added to the lack of cohesion and breakdown of traditional structures and cultures caused by colonisation and urbanisation.

Indeed, many urbanised Indigenous Australians feel a lack of connection to the land or Country of their elders, past and present (Busija et al., 2018). While notions of Country can be spiritual or metaphorical for many Indigenous Australians, this lack of a lived experience of connection can distress those who feel weighed down by the expectations placed on them by people from other cultures. For example, there is a tendency among non-Indigenous peoples to stereotype Indigenous populations and presume their lifestyles should be more traditional. Consequently, Indigenous Australians living in urban areas may feel they lack legitimacy.

The urbanisation of Indigenous Australian cultures has given rise to several challenges, including those related Indigenous peoples' and communities' health and wellbeing (Porter et al., 2018). These challenges are described in the following sections.

The Indigenous view of health

Generally speaking, Indigenous peoples share a **whole-of-life view of health**. Notions of 'health' are understood by Indigenous peoples as a state of wellbeing achieved by balancing the mind, body, emotions, spirit, culture and environment (Fisher et al., 2019). For Aboriginal and Torres Strait Islander peoples, when this balance is upset in one person, the entire community suffers.

The whole-of-life view of health shared by Indigenous peoples can be linked to Western notions of the social determinants of health (Butler et al., 2019). The World Health Organization (WHO) (n.d.) defines the **social determinants of health** as the conditions in which people are born, develop, live, work and grow old. The social determinants of health are factors that determine the health status of all people and include income and its distribution, education, unemployment and job security, employment and working conditions, early childhood development, nutrition, housing, social exclusion, social safety networks, health services, gender, race and disability (AIHW, 2022c). The social determinants of health are also shaped by the general distribution of wealth, power and resources at global, national and local levels (Vallesi et al., 2018). The whole-of-life view of health maintains that good health relies on access to the resources that support quality of life and equal opportunity (AIHW, 2022d).

Of concern, then, is that:

- at least 25 per cent of Indigenous Australians aged 15 years of age and over live in overcrowded housing (AIHW, 2019)
- secondary school retention rates for Indigenous Australians in Years 7/8 to Year 12 are 61 per cent, compared to 86 per cent for non-Indigenous Australians (AIHW, 2021b)
- on average, Indigenous Australians earn half the gross adjusted household income of non-Indigenous Australians (AIHW, 2021c)
- almost one-quarter of Indigenous Australians have used an illicit substance in the last 12 months, which is 1.4 times higher than non-Indigenous Australians (AIHW, 2022a).
- Indigenous Australians have a shorter life expectancy than non-Indigenous Australians (AIHW & NIAA, 2020a).

When compared with non-Indigenous Australians, Indigenous Australians are also:

- 2.7 times as likely to smoke
- 2.7 times as likely to experience high or very high levels of psychological distress
- 1.7 times as likely to have a disability or restrictive long-term health condition (AIHW, 2018a).

Other consequences of the social disadvantage of Indigenous Australians include the high level of emotional distress and other mental health issues they experience (Doyle et al., 2017). There is a pressing need, then, for all health professionals to acknowledge that Indigenous Australians have a socially constructed view of mental health and illness, and recognise the importance of taking culturally informed approaches to delivering health care (Hensel et al., 2019).

International and national directives

International conventions and national policy directives frame and inform health care delivery to Aboriginal and Torres Strait Islander peoples. These policy directives drive the design, goals and provision of equitable and accessible, culturally respectful health services for Indigenous Australians. They also influence the work and education of health professionals and the outcomes of their practices.

In 1986, the WHO's *Ottawa Charter for Health Promotion* (1986) presented an action plan to enable 'health for all' by 2000. This action plan addressed the social determinants of health, such as peace, shelter, education, food, income, a stable ecosystem, sustainable resources, social justice and equity. The WHO's *Jakarta Declaration* (1997), built on the *Ottawa Charter,* identified the urgency for further investment in health, especially for disadvantaged groups such as women, children and older people, together with indigenous peoples, the poor and other marginalised populations. Since then, initiatives such as the WHO Mental Health Gap Action Programme have supported the scaling up of services for mental health, neurological and substance abuse disorders in low- to moderate-income peoples, including those who belong to indigenous cultures (WHO, 2020). These charters, declarations and programs have been the impetus behind various initiatives worldwide to improve indigenous peoples' mental health and wellbeing (see Abbott et al., 2018; Michaelson et al., 2018).

In Australia, the principles of these declarations are evident in the various national mental health plans the Australian government developed over the last decades. The more recent of these plans place particular emphasis on Indigenous communities; and include prioritising the development of community-controlled services to improve the mental health and wellbeing of Aboriginal and Torres Strait Islander peoples, together with fostering partnerships between sectors, thereby encouraging community services and organisations to work together (Fisher et al., 2019).

There are varied examples of such partnerships already in action. For instance, a locally designed community pilot study was developed to determine the effectiveness of culturally appropriate, community-driven, intensive child-centred play therapy programs in a remote Aboriginal community for children who have experienced adversity (Wicks et al., 2018). It was found that the difficulties and emotional problems experienced by the children, as reported by parents and teachers, diminished over time. This project also highlights what can be achieved when a local or community-specific approach is taken, with health care developed according to the socio-cultural, economic, political and ideological needs rather than biomedical factors alone. Moreover, the outcomes of this project demonstrate the effectiveness of empowering communities to improve their health through self-determination (McPhail-Bell et al., 2018; Mulder et al., 2022).

The mental health and wellbeing of Indigenous Australians

Because Indigenous cultures in Australia share a whole-of-life view of health, the mental health and wellbeing of Indigenous Australians cannot be considered in isolation from their physical wellbeing. Even so, differentiating between the two can be helpful for health professionals who belong to non-Indigenous cultures and seek to understand the issues faced by Indigenous Australians today.

As already explained, the mental health of Indigenous Australians incorporates more than the individual's level of functioning. Notions of mental health and wellbeing are linked to the people's connections with the land, spirituality, ancestry, family and community. For Indigenous Australians, mental health and wellbeing encompass a broad range of problems that can result from unresolved grief and loss, trauma and abuse, domestic violence, removal from family, substance misuse, family breakdown, cultural dislocation, racism and discrimination, and social disadvantage (Joseph 2019; Temple et al., 2019). In short, when Indigenous Australians feel connected to their Country, culture, spirituality and community, they see themselves as socially and emotionally healthy.

Five broad discourses influence the mental health and wellbeing of indigenous peoples worldwide:
1. culture and spirituality
2. strong extended family and community relationships
3. historical, social and economic factors
4. fear, shame and stigma
5. an overwhelming sense of loss (Fogarty et al., 2018).

The first of the discourses — culture and spirituality — includes the notions of storytelling, ceremonies, ancestors, sacred sites, tribal areas and identity (Butler et al., 2019). If an indigenous community feels culturally and spiritually 'in balance', that community is more likely to feel socially and emotionally well. Alternatively, if a community feels culturally and spiritually out of balance, then that community will feel socially and emotionally unwell (Fay, 2018).

This state of imbalance expresses itself in many ways. Health professionals from Western cultures may diagnose an Indigenous Australian with clinical depression, but members of their community will recognise the mood or behaviour as a cultural condition known as 'longing', 'crying' or 'being sick for Country' (Martin et al., 2019). In the same way, some behaviours of an Indigenous Australian may be viewed as innapropriate by people who do not belong to or understand the person's culture. However, this behaviour may be due to the person or community being unable to achieve cultural resolution to an incident, often because of constraints exercised by the surrounding, dominant non-Indigenous culture (Schultz & Cairney, 2017). A person's thoughts, feelings and behaviours must be interpreted from within their own cultural framework or view of the world (Blignault & Kaur, 2019). Likewise, Indigenous Australians' mental health and wellbeing must be measured according to their cultural and spiritual understandings.

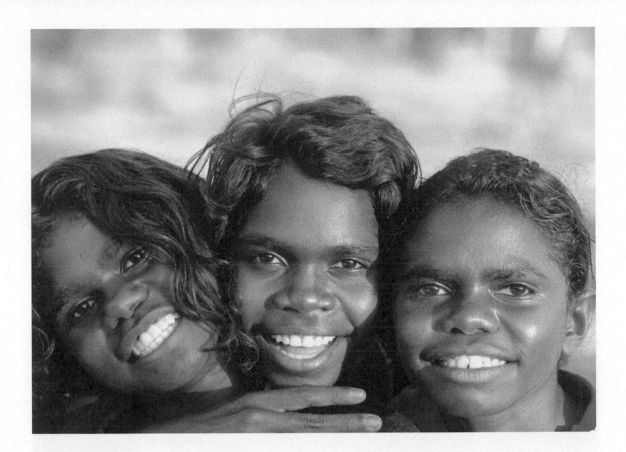

Mental illness as a 'punishment'

In some Indigenous Australian cultures, illness may be viewed as punishment for breaking cultural laws. For instance, if a male visits a sacred woman's site, the cultural group may expect him to become unwell. Similarly, some Indigenous Australian communities may view mental illness as a manifestation of spirituality. A person may see or hear people who passed, which may be viewed as a spiritual gift rather than a grief reaction. Indigenous communities can also feel vicarious, collective grief. If a child is stillborn in a community, the entire community will feel unwell.

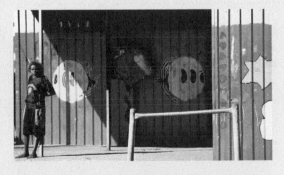

This collective approach also provides opportunities, with some organisations partnering with Indigenous Australian communities to build social and emotional wellbeing. For example, the Healthier Futures Initiative brings Captain Starlight to remote Aboriginal and Torres Strait Islander community health clinics to provide a positive distraction for kids through song, dance, games and storytelling and boost community engagement in the health care system. You can read more about this initiative at: www.starlight.org.au/about-us/what-we-do/healthier-futures-initiative.

QUESTIONS

1. What does 'collective grief' look like?

2. How can health professionals assess individuals for 'collective grief'?

3. What can you do, as a health professional, to support those experiencing 'collective grief'?

The remaining four framing discourses (strong family and community relationships; historical, social and economic factors; fear, shame and **stigma**; and an overwhelming sense of loss) also provide fertile ground for exploring aspects of Indigenous Australians' mental health and wellbeing. For example links have been identified between the lower levels of wellbeing of Indigenous Australians and the breakdown in family and community ties due to colonisation and urbanisation (Doyle et al., 2017). To reiterate, reasons for this breakdown include the injustices and **discrimination** that Indigenous Australians have experienced since colonisation, such as genocide, where whole families and communities were wiped out; the seizure of their land without recompense; and the Stolen Generations.

The 1997 report of the National Inquiry into the Separation of Aboriginal and Torres Strait Islander Children from their Families titled *Bringing Them Home*, acknowledged that Indigenous Australian children had been forcibly separated from their families and communities by governments and missionaries from the first days of European settlement (Australian Human Rights Commission, 1997). Events in Australia since colonisation have led to experiences of intergenerational trauma, grief and loss, a degraded sense of belonging and low self-esteem. These events have significantly affected the mental health and wellbeing of Aboriginal and Torres Strait Islander peoples (Ringland, 2019), leading to an erosion of contemporary Indigenous Australians' general health and wellbeing (Strobel, 2019).

On 13 February 2008, the Australian Government passed a motion of *Apology to Australia's Indigenous Peoples*, on behalf of the Australian people. The Prime Minster of the time apologised to all Australian Aboriginal and Torres Strait Islander peoples for their profound grief and suffering since colonisation. Many perceived the apology as a turning point in the relationship between the Indigenous Australians and non-Indigenous Australians, and for the mental health and wellbeing of Indigenous Australians (Passi, 2018).

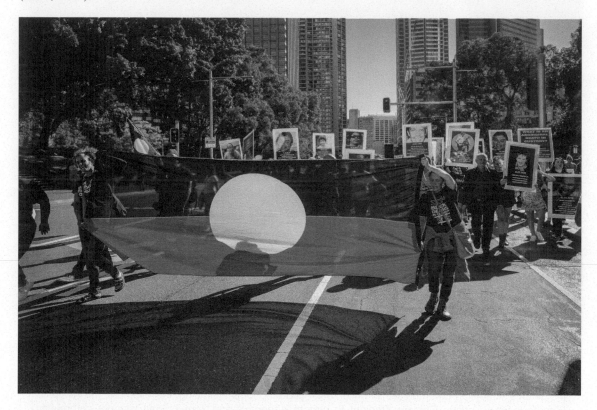

While some gains have been made in addressing the effects of colonisation on the mental health and wellbeing of Indigenous Australians, many issues remain. Anxiety/depression and suicide are two of the top four leading causes of illness in Indigenous males; and anxiety/depression is the top cause of illness for Indigenous females (Titov et al., 2019). In addition, Indigenous Australians are more often exposed to activities that impact their mental health and wellbeing, such as smoking, poor nutrition, alcohol misuse, overcrowded living conditions and domestic violence (Butler et al., 2019). These statistics highlight just some of the challenges facing Indigenous Australian communities, health professionals, health services and governments.

Also of concern is the racism that continues in many parts of Australia. Examples include:
- Indigenous Australians and cultures are often represented as the subjects of documentary programs or news items that suggest an intractable problem that won't go away (McCallum & Waller, 2017)
- Indigenous Australians are framed as tourist novelties to be observed or exploited (Calma et al., 2017)

- the Indigenous 'problem' is often portrayed as 'distant', belonging to remote outposts like 'up north', the 'Top End' or 'Outback', and well away from — even irrelevant to — the Indigenous Australians who live in urban locations (Dudgeon et al., 2018).

Although the publicly promoted attitudes towards people who belong to Indigenous cultures have been sanitised of the overt racism of the past, there is no doubt that Indigenous Australians continue to be positioned as 'other' in Australian society (Markwick et al., 2019). One consequence is that Indigenous Australians affected by symptoms of mental illness are doubly stigmatised — labelled and marginalised for exhibiting symptoms of mental illness, and likewise labelled and marginalised for belonging to a minority racial group (Coates et al., 2019). Indigenous Australians are, therefore, less likely to disclose symptoms of mental illness, leading to a reduced likelihood of early intervention strategies being implemented promptly (Stanley et al., 2019). The potential consequences of this **double stigma** are serious.

The chapter that focuses on mental health care in Australia explains that stigma is the perception that a person or group of people is less worthy than another person or group of people. When stigma is acted upon, and a person is treated differently because they have a mental illness or other condition, that person is experiencing discrimination. Discrimination is illegal under the Commonwealth *Disability Discrimination Act 1992* (DDA). Health professionals are required to practise according to this legislation.

Although the law can partly control overt behaviour, it is far more challenging to change the attitudes of individuals and societies. The urgent need for ongoing intervention in this area continues to be addressed in Australia's evolving National Mental Health Strategy, which supports the achievement of better health outcomes for Indigenous Australians by acknowledging the:
- unique contribution of Australia's Indigenous heritage and cultures to the broader society and culture
- right of Indigenous Australians to status, culture, self-determination and land
- absolute necessity of upholding these rights.

Significantly, the focus of both the DDA and the National Mental Health Strategy is social and cultural, rather than biomedical. The key to improving the mental health and wellbeing of Indigenous Australians, then, lies not with diagnosis and treatment, but with inclusion and upholding the human rights of Indigenous Australians across the nation, including their right to self-determination (Australian Human Rights Commission, 2017).

For this reason, all health professionals can assist with closing the gap in the levels of health between Indigenous Australians and the non-Indigenous population. The first step is mutual resolve. Another, more practical step for health professionals is to ensure that they ask those who attend a health service if they identify as Indigenous and if so, offer them the support of an Aboriginal health worker. Unfortunately, some health professionals may presume a person who doesn't 'look' Indigenous in appearance could not possibly belong to an Indigenous culture. All health professionals must understand that indigeneity does not depend on a person's appearance, but rather on their place in an Indigenous Australian community. For this reason, health professionals must give each person the choice to speak with an Aboriginal and Torres Strait Islander mental health worker, regardless of their appearance.

Finally, health professionals can support improving health outcomes for Indigenous Australians by providing culturally appropriate information to individuals, families and communities (McGough et al., 2018). This information must include suggestions to the person and their family about their health care options. Such options include participating in health promotion and illness prevention activities aimed at Indigenous communities across the nation, culturally appropriate interventions for the grief, loss and trauma experienced by Indigenous Australians, and contributing to community-driven and culturally appropriate research and evaluation to empower indigenous communities to self-determine (Department of Health, 2019).

Issues to consider when supporting the mental health and wellbeing of Indigenous Australians

This section outlines some of the major issues that face health professionals when delivering health care (including mental health care) to Indigenous Australians, and the steps health professionals can take to address these issues. Topics considered are the mobility of many Indigenous Australians, the under-representation of Indigenous Australian health professionals in the health workforce and the general lack of understanding in the mainstream health workforce about the roles of Aboriginal and Torres Strait Islander health workers.

Under-representation of Aboriginal and Torres Strait Islander health workers

An Aboriginal and Torres Strait Islander health workforce is integral to the Australian health care system (Mbuzi et al., 2018). The development of an Indigenous Australian health workforce has occurred over the past twenty years, with the latest National Aboriginal and Torres Strait Islander Health Workforce Strategic Framework and Implementation Plan published in 2022. This framework and plan recognise the need for quality Aboriginal and Torres Strait Islander health workers in the primary, secondary and tertiary health care sectors (Department of Health and Aged Care, 2022a). The strategy also emphasises the importance of supporting and appropriately utilising 'Aboriginal and Torres Strait Islander mental health workers', a broad term that refers to Aboriginal and Torres Strait Islander peoples working in wide-ranging roles in both government and community-controlled organisations, with varied qualifications, skill sets and criteria (RANZCP, 2016).

There are several reasons why it is necessary to develop a quality Aboriginal and Torres Strait Islander mental health workforce. First, the under-representation of Aboriginal and Torres Strait Islander mental health workers can be linked to the lower health status of Indigenous Australians more generally (AIHW & NIAA, 2020b).

Despite the diversity in Indigenous cultures across the nation, Indigenous Australians share enough in common to know the most appropriate ways of supporting other Indigenous Australians. Second, Indigenous Australians must be at the table to support the development, planning and provision of culturally appropriate health services and thereby self-determine (Hefler et al., 2018).

It is necessary, then, for governments and employing organisations to work to address the under-representation of Indigenous Australians in the health workforce. Likewise, Indigenous peoples must be empowered to bring their cultural knowledge(s), skills, experiences and general expertise into the mental health sector. Finally, there is a need to understand the role of Aboriginal and Torres Strait Islander mental health workers. This role is explained in the next section.

Lack of understanding of roles

Today there is no single educational pathway to becoming an Aboriginal and Torres Strait Islander mental health worker; nor is there a single condition of employment or way of interacting with Aboriginal and Torres Strait Islander mental health workers (Department of Health and Aged Care, 2022a). The roles of Aboriginal and Torres Strait Islander mental health workers are many and varied. In addition, the model within which Aboriginal and Torres Strait Islander mental health workers practise does not necessarily fit Western-oriented mental health service delivery models. Consequently, there is some general misunderstanding about what Aboriginal and Torres Strait Islander mental health workers actually do (Wright et al., 2019).

What is certain, however, is that Indigenous Australian-specific roles are proving to be effective (Harfield et al., 2018). For this reason, all health professionals must support and advocate for Aboriginal and Torres Strait Islander mental health workers and be aware of the nature of the work, especially those in the mental health sector.

Indigenous Australian mental health professionals are most often employed from within their own community(ies) and work to support the community as a whole rather than as specialists who provide therapy to individual consumers with psychiatric diagnoses (Wright et al., 2019). The different roles undertaken by Aboriginal and Torres Strait Islander mental health workers may include a:
- clinical function, often as the first point of contact for an Indigenous Australian with the health service, particularly in rural or remote areas
- liaison function, working with the primary non-Indigenous health professional to mediate cultural issues
- health promotion and education function in their communities
- community care, management, policy development or program planning function.

Perhaps most important is that health professionals ascertain the availability of Aboriginal and Torres Strait Islander mental health workers in their area and how this person may be contacted. Although Aboriginal and Torres Strait Islander mental health workers are currently under-represented, they are nevertheless there to be utilised wherever possible.

A mobile population

The relative mobility of Indigenous Australians presents challenges to health professionals and services (Shand et al., 2019). It is challenging to provide continuity of care for any person, Indigenous or non-Indigenous, who frequently relocates. Also, the vagaries of the Australian health system (which comprises eight states and territories, each with its own clinical records and health-related legislation) present hurdles for the transfer of information and communication between health professionals and services, and for individuals who must negotiate the different systems (Best & Fredericks, 2018). Moreover, for some Indigenous Australians, moving from town to town or from state to state, can give rise to feelings of disconnection from the communities in which they live. Their own Country or mob is in another place, so they may feel dislocated.

For this reason, health professionals must ensure they follow up on the care being delivered to an Indigenous Australian. For example, if the person does not attend an appointment for some time, the following questions could be asked: Has that person moved on? Has the person been supported to enter their health information into the national My Health Record database? Have their clinical records been forwarded to the appropriate services? Does the health professional need to speak personally to health professionals who are now supporting the person? By following up, health professionals are enabling the person to achieve the best possible health outcome.

'How would you like us to help you?'

Empowerment is a somewhat abstract concept. It is a means by which people develop a capacity to influence the world around them. Empowering other people, however, is not without its challenges. First and foremost, where does the health professional start?

A crucial first step involves listening to the person and their preferred family member or community representative, providing culturally appropriate information, and allowing the person and their family or community members to make their own decisions (Butler et al., 2019). The role of storytelling for many Indigenous Australians and communities is of particular importance.

IN PRACTICE

Listening with big ears

Aunty Kerrie Alaylee Doyle, a Winninninni woman from Darkinjung Country, is a Professor of Indigenous Health and an Indigenous Australian health professional. She has many stories to tell to those who will listen — just as she listens to many of the stories that are told to her.

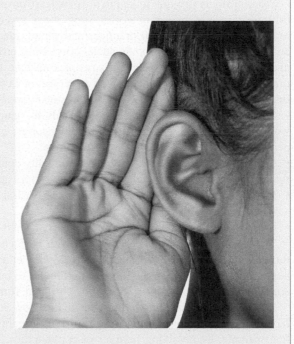

> I go out and I listen with 'big ears'. It's only with 'big ears' and not 'hard ears' that I can hear what the mob are saying.

> If you listen hard enough, you hear the mob groaning. Some of them, they are often told that change is coming and things are going to get better. But when they talk together about their health, they talk about freedom. They talk about being able to live life without the government and police and tourists staring, and of being able to go into a shop without security officers checking up on them, and of being able to find a job that's more than just menial and of being able to do their 'business'. But there's no freedom for some of them now; there's only sadness.

> Some of them, they've taken to using drugs and alcohol. They know it makes them sick, but they do it anyway and then they're locked up by the police. They need help — not jail — but they don't tell anyone that they're sick because they know if they do they'll be moved away, off Country. They know it brings shame and the mob will groan even more. Listen hard enough, you'll hear it.

> One time, I was looking after this one young lad. He was in prison for break and enter. I was the first Aboriginal counsellor he had seen. His records said he was non-compliant and he wouldn't take his

▶

medication and he wouldn't cooperate. I sat with him for a long while and we didn't say anything. Then I asked him where his mob was from. He started to cry. He said he didn't know his Country. He was adopted when he was a baby but he was not athletic and his adoptive father had bashed him because he had wanted a boxer. That lad, he grew up in a good white place in the city but he never felt he fitted in, he never felt accepted by his white family or by the local Aboriginal kids or by anyone. So he grew up angry and alone with no-one to talk to and no-one who wanted to listen. Then they told him he was depressed and put him on medication.

I reckon if those health workers who had been looking after him, if they'd been listening to what he was saying, things would have been better for him. My mob have a saying, we say, you listen with 'big ears', not hard ears that are waiting for us to make a mistake or ears that think they know better, but 'big ears' that listen to your story. I reckon if those doctors and nurses had been listening with big ears, I reckon things might have been different for him.

QUESTIONS

1. What do you see as the difference between 'big ears' and 'hard ears'?

2. What do you find it easier to do — talk or listen? Why?

3. What practical strategies could you adopt to help you to, firstly, listen with 'big ears' and, secondly, suggest therapeutic strategies to Indigenous Australians?

Listening

Storytelling is central to many indigenous cultures and a significant component of the Indigenous understanding of mental health and wellbeing worldwide (Wendt, 2017). Indigenous peoples use stories to construct, represent and develop their communities, community identity and their view of themselves (Fernando & Bennett, 2019).

Storytelling is strongly linked to the **oral traditions** of Indigenous peoples. As already noted, these oral traditions include the use of stories, song, dance and craft-making; and giving instructions and directions to pass on specific cultural practices and values, language and laws, histories and family relationships, and beliefs (Friskie, 2020). As such, storytelling provides an ideal medium by which the major issues and preoccupations of indigenous peoples may be understood and approached. Indeed, through their oral traditions, the heart and soul of an indigenous community (the emotions, activities, motivations and insights) may be best observed and understood (Coombes et al., 2018).

Storytelling enables health professionals to gauge an Indigenous Australian's mental health and wellbeing (McBride et al., 2021). A person's stories, which can include cultural stories, community stories, personal stories and anecdotes, will tell of the:

- strength of the person's family and community connections
- impact of historical, social and economic factors upon communities and their wellbeing
- fear, shame and stigma many Indigenous Austraians feel when it comes to their mental health and wellbeing
- the overwhelming burden of loss they carry (Lewis et al., 2017).

The health professional can connect with Indigenous Australians and their families or communities through the stories of their communities (Molloy et al., 2019b). Once this connection has been made, the health professional will have more opportunities to build a genuine and trusting alliance with Indigenous Australians, in collaboration with Aboriginal and Torres Strait Islander mental health workers.

Provideing mental health care to Indigenous Australians will also involve the steps shown in figure 4.2, which provides some suggestions for health professionals who support Indigenous Australians. For example, by involving families or communities, listening carefully to what is being communicated, providing information, and showing a willingness to be flexible to meet the needs of the person, the health professional will be well placed to support the process of making a difference for the mental health and wellbeing of Indigenous Australians (Fogarty et al., 2018).

When providing mental health care for an Indigenous Australian:

☐ involve their preferred family and/or community members in discussions about their mental health and wellbeing and ask them what they think is happening

☐ listen carefully to what the person and family may be trying to tell you; that is, listen to their stories as they will contain valuable information about the health and wellbeing of the person

☐ involve their preferred family or community members in discussions about possible care or treatment

☐ contact an Aboriginal and Torres Strait Islander mental health worker for advice and support

☐ offer relevant, culturally appropriate information to the family; assess their understanding of the information and offer alternative sources of information if needed

☐ if in a hospital, be flexible about the timing and number of visitors, and enable the person to adhere to their cultural practices and keep personal belongings nearby. Remember, many Indigenous Australians fear hospitals after experiencing relatives and friends dying in hospital. Fear can sometimes make a person react in ways that seem inappropriate

☐ be aware that many people from Indigenous Australian cultures feel shame if they or their relative experiences symptoms of mental illness. Discuss the issues and reassure all those involved.

UPON REFLECTION

Indigenous Australians and emergencies

Emergency situations present particular challenges for health professionals when helping Indigenous Australians. Involving family or community members in discussions about the situation at hand or urgent treatment options can be difficult. Even so, there will be times when health professionals are required to support an Indigenous Australian experiencing a health emergency. This support must be culturally appropriate.

QUESTIONS

1. What steps can you take to ensure that the health care you provide to Indigenous Australians during an emergency is culturally appropriate?

2. What other strategies could be used to ensure the health care you provide to Indigenous Australians during an emergency is culturally appropriate?

This section focused on how to provide **culturally appropriate care** to Indigenous Australians.

The following section discusses the mental health of people who live in rural and remote areas of Australia, including Indigenous and non-Indigenous peoples. The section discusses the main issues faced by people who live in rural and remote locations, how these issues impact the mental health of geographically isolated populations, and the services available to support people who live in rural and remote areas in Australia.

4.4 Mental health and rural and remote cultures

LEARNING OBJECTIVE 4.4 Describe the major mental health issues for people from rural and remote cultures.

Australia has been described as one of the most urbanised nations in the world, with less than 28 per cent of the population living in rural and remote areas (AIHW, 2022e). This level of urbanisation raises many questions, particularly for those living in farming communities, mining towns, coastal villages and regional centres across the nation. For example, how relevant are rural and remote issues to most Australians? How are rural and remote cultures different from mainstream Australian culture? What role do health professionals play in supporting the mental health of rural and remote populations?

Many of the answers to these questions are connected to notions of equity. Access and equity are two foundation stones of public health care (including mental health service delivery) in Australia. An essential part of the health professional's role is to advocate for services and practices that support access and equity for all people, including those who live in rural and remote locations (Baum et al., 2019).

What is a 'rural' or 'remote' culture in Australia?

In the past, Australian rural and remote populations were defined by bush iconographies, such as unique fauna and flora, desert or bushland, and a harsh climate; isolation and long distances; agricultural or mining land-use; and populations that were slow-paced, conservative, lacking sophistication, stoical, but also self-reliant, resilient, independent and strongly community-minded (Driscoll et al., 2017). Today, with advancements in transport and communication networks, and the effects of globalisation, there have been profound changes in how 'rural' and 'remote' are experienced or understood (Lebaron, 2018). Indeed, some commentators now argue that the boundaries differentiating notions of rural, urban, state, national and international are blurred (Brown et al., 2019).

The Department of Health and Aged Care (2022b) provides some direction for health professionals by classifing rural, remote and metropolitan areas according to population (including density) and distance to urban centres containing a population of 10 000 persons or more. Also significant are socio-cultural characteristics, the number of community resources and the economic characteristics of a region (Malatzky & Glenister, 2019).

Another consideration is the notion of the **rural–urban continuum**, which measures how particular communities conform to varying levels of ruralism and urbanism (Cohen et al., 2018). Different rural and remote locations and communities (from coastal rural to inland rural and remote areas; from farmers and miners to the people living in small towns and regional centres that service these industries) all exhibit unique cultural characteristics (see figure 4.3). The rural–urban continuum acknowledges the diversity, complexity and evolving nature of rural populations and cultures (van Spijker et al., 2019). Health professionals must understand the inherent diversity of rural populations and cultures.

| FIGURE 4.3 | The rural–urban continuum |

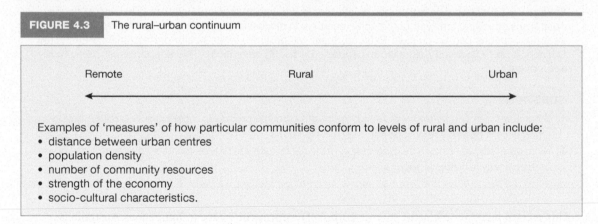

Although most health professionals do not work in rural and remote locations, the dearth of services and health resources in these places means that people from rural and remote locations will often travel to the city to access health care. Another consideration is the increasing number of 'fly-in fly-out' health professionals now servicing rural and remote locations. Health professionals aware of the issues for rural and remote Australians will be better equipped to deliver the most effective treatment and care.

Major issues for people living in rural and remote areas

There are many benefits to living in rural and remote areas. Life in rural towns is associated with higher levels of resilience and satisfaction with safety and community connections, when compared to the experiences of those living in cities (Hine et al., 2018). These benefits suggest why many older people are now choosing to move to rural areas for a 'tree change' or 'sea change' on retirement (Henderson et al., 2018).

On the other hand, rural and remote locations have also been linked to discourses of disadvantage. These discourses include geographic isolation from metropolitan centres and services; shrinking and dispersed populations and social networks; and structural disadvantage, including poor roads and technology (Cheers, 2019).

Moreover, when compared to metropolitan Australia, rural and remote populations are associated with a long list of negative indicators, including lower socio-economic indices, lower education levels, higher unemployment rates, higher morbidity and mortality rates in almost all of the health categories, higher rates of hospitalisation, fewer health care services and lower utilisation of these services, fewer health professionals, and issues around the location or distribution of these health professionals (Fennell et al., 2018). In short, rural and remote populations have many social issues that impact their levels of health, including mental health.

Mental health issues for people living in rural and remote areas

Research suggests that the prevalence of mental health conditions in rural and remote Australia is equivalent to levels in major cities (National Rural Health Alliance, 2017). The one exception has been the higher rates of suicide in rural and remote areas, which are proportionally higher than in major cities (AIHW, 2021f).

Despite the general equivalence in mental health status, rural and remote Australians face many more barriers when seeking support for mental health problems than people who live in metropolitan areas (Fennell et al., 2018). One reason for this is the difficulty in effectively accessing treatment. As already noted, there are proportionately fewer health professionals practising in rural and remote areas and issues with the location and distribution of these health professionals (Smith et al., 2019). This situation means that while the prevalence of mental health conditions in rural and remote Australia is equivalent to levels in the major cities, there are fewer services.

Another challenge is that rural and remote Australians are less likely to seek out mental health care than their city counterparts (National Rural Health Alliance, 2017). Reasons for this include:

- lack of anonymity in small communities
- less availability and accessibility of services
- cost of travel and accommodation when accessing services in the larger centres
- cultural understandings of mental illness that discourage people from disclosing mental health problems
- greater visibility of mental health issues in small communities
- the stigma associated with the use of mental health services.

This situation raises questions about the disclosure rates to health professionals by rural and remote people with symptoms of mental illness. It also raises questions about the statistical equivalence between those with mental health issues who live in rural and metropolitan locations. For example, the lack of anonymity in rural areas and the limited services remain the greatest barriers to diagnosing and treating mental illness (Fennell et al., 2018). Such issues suggest yet another hurdle to overcome when supporting rural and remote people with mental health concerns: stigma.

Attitudes and values

The stigma attached to mental health issues in rural areas has been well documented in the research literature (Handley et al., 2018). People in smaller rural communities may fear the stigma that is sometimes associated with mental illness, with individuals more visible and confidentiality less assured (Dwyer et al., 2021). One explanation for such attitudes may relate to the value placed by rural and remote Australians on maintaining performance or productivity, despite adversity (National Rural Health Alliance, 2017). This view is consistent with the culture of independence, self-reliance and stoicism, and notions of 'getting over it and getting on with it' that have been associated with many rural and remote communities (Handley et al., 2018). People from rural and remote cultures tend to privilege physical 'strength' and frown upon emotional 'weakness'. While stoicism provides one way of dealing with hardship, in the long term, it may also discourage people from seeking help when they are in need.

Health professionals must be aware of this stoical cultural mindset and ask rural and remote Australians questions about these potential issues, so they can assist the person and their family members as needed. In addition, health professionals must assure the person from a rural or remote location, especially if they live in a small community, that their answers to questions about their health (including their mental health) will be treated confidentially. The experience of stigma in a small community can be devastating to a person and lead to reductions in their mental health outcomes.

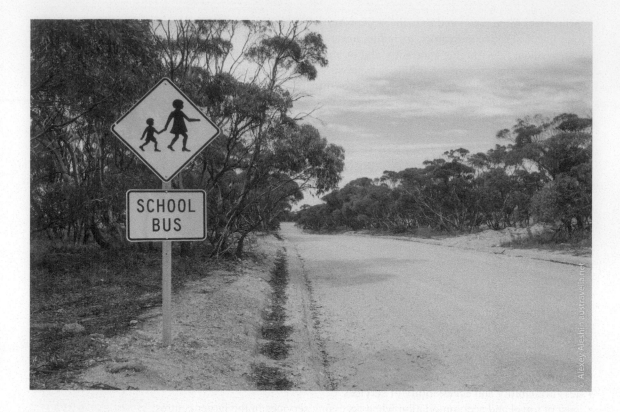

Considering the challenges

According to the AIHW (2022e), people who live in remote or very remote parts of Australia are more likely to report:

- not having a general practitioner nearby as being a barrier to visiting a general practitioner for health care
- not having a specialist medical practitioner nearby as being a barrier to receiving specialist assistance
- having visited an emergency department in the past 12 months because no general practitioner was available when they needed one.

QUESTIONS

1. What would be the health outcome for people with mental health problems who are unable to access a general practitioner?
2. What is the role of nursing, paramedicine and allied health professionals in these situations?
3. How can patients be best informed about the services offered by nursing, paramedicine and allied health professionals?

Ongoing loss

As noted in the seminal texts of Ward (1958) and White (1981), rural and remote populations have traditionally held a significant position in Australian society and the national identity or psyche. In the past, images such as the Outback, pioneers and bushmen have proudly represented what it means to be Australian. However, with the increasing urbanisation, notions of 'rural' and 'remote' have lost their status in Australian society. Indeed, some argue that rurality is irrelevant to most Australians, leaving many rural and remote communities feeling marginalised and experiencing a sense of loss (National Rural Health Alliance, 2017).

Compounding the effects of this loss are the ongoing issues of droughts, cyclones, floods, fires and plagues, increasingly faced by rural, regional and remote Australians (Ellis & Albrecht, 2017). In addition to natural disasters are the other hardships often associated with rural areas, including lower education levels, higher unemployment rates, and higher morbidity and mortality rates than those living in cities (Cheers 2019). The stresses and hardships experienced by rural and remote populations on an ongoing basis are therefore profound.

Experiences involving ongoing or protracted loss can substantially impact the mental health of a person or group of people. For example, links have been identified between feelings of alienation or detachment, marginalisation, loss of meaning, and levels of depression and suicide (Life in Mind, 2023). Regional, rural and remote populations experience many of these feelings, suggesting one reason suicide rates are higher in these locations. Other ongoing mental health and associated problems associated with rural and remote populations include the use of alcohol and other drugs, and the culture of violence (AIHW, 2022e). All of these factors have the potential to impact the health outcomes of rural and remote Australians.

Helping rural communities through natural disasters

Ongoing natural disasters in Australia affect people in all locations, particularly those who live in regional, rural and remote locations, experiencing the results of drought, flood or fire. Such experiences give rise to high stress and anxiety for all involved. According to the Department of Home Affairs (2022), people in rural townships and communities who recently experienced devastating floods that destroyed their homes, property and farmlands reported that, during the emergency itself, all of those involved worked well together. In contrast, for the protracted clean-up phase, the long-term effects were:

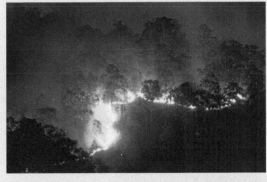

- financial hardship for households and businesses (e.g. small and large businesses, including but not limited to farmers)
- family and relationship problems (e.g. arguments due to the levels of long-term stress they were experiencing, lack of communication, physical conflict, relationship breakdown)
- job pressure and overwork, as people commenced the process of cleaning up while still trying to maintain their regular employment
- people (particularly those who are young) moving away due to fear of the flood reoccurring and/or inability to rebuild and/or lack of income
- environmental problems such as unsanitary water supplies, loss of vegetation and animals, soil erosion and increased risk of bushfires
- lack of community services, including health care, education, housing and employment organisations
- higher incidence of physical and mental health problems among community members, as well as suicide attempts
- loss of social networks and a breakdown in community spirit (Healthdirect, 2018).

Health professionals helped community members manage the stress of the flood, in both the short term and long term, by:

- encouraging people to seek help from a crisis support service (e.g. 13 11 14, www.lifeline.org.au)
- ensuring people, including children and adolescents, had the opportunity to talk about what had happened or was currently happening to them
- talking to community members about how they are managing the situation and the different options for help that are available
- informing people and communities of the support and other services offered by the Australian government and relevant state governments for those affected by natural disasters and/or helping people to explore available financial help
- teaching people how to manage their stress
- supporting people to be positive and proactive
- encouraging people to seek and accept help from others
- raising awareness about the need for people to seek help if they have thought of harming themselves (Department of Home Affairs, 2022).

Health professionals must stay abreast of the support and other services that people who experience natural disasters can access so they can help and advise people and communities accordingly.

Source: Department of Home Affairs (2022); Healthdirect (2018).

Systemic issues

Rural or remote Australians also face several systemic issues when seeking help for mental health concerns. As already suggested, rural and remote populations receive less treatment for mental health issues than their city counterparts (AIHW, 2022e). In addition, the mental health resources available are more fragmented and limited than those received by the general health sector (Malatzky & Glenister, 2019). Such issues present challenges for governments, health services, health professionals and consumers.

One reason for these inequities is the current trend for governments across Australia, at both national and state levels, to centralise the administration of services. An outcome of this centralisation is a reduced capacity for smaller communities to be involved in shaping how local services are delivered. The plans and decisions affecting the lives of rural or remote people are often made by distant agents who have little understanding of local issues, local culture and local know-how. People in rural and remote areas are further disempowered and marginalised because they are given little or no involvement in how services are developed or implemented.

Another inhibiting factor is the **one-size-fits-all** or **universalist approach** that often characterises how governments plan and develop health services across Australia, including mental health services. 'Standardisation' is a common catch-cry of health managers and policymakers alike, arguably to assist with managing risks and promoting equity (Mollah et al., 2018). However, this approach presumes that all populations have the same needs and that these needs will be met in the same way. As a result, there is the potential to overlook the many cultural, social, geographical and other differences evident within and between different localities, populations and cultures.

Mental health service delivery cannot be uniform when considering the multifaceted nature of rural and remote Australia. Instead, addressing mental health issues for those living in rural and remote Australia requires an approach that considers the diversity of the populations and meets the potential needs of each locality (Molloy et al., 2019a). For this reason, health treatment and care is best understood in terms of local or community specificity. Health services must be flexible and allow communities to develop their own solutions. Likewise, health professionals must be flexible and allow individuals from rural and remote areas to develop their own answers.

Last, but not least, there is a systemic shortage of suitably qualified health professionals in rural and remote Australia (AIHW, 2022e). The issues generated by this shortage cannot be overstated. Without a health workforce, people cannot be treated or cared for in their own communities (Jackson et al., 2019). Travelling long distances to consult with health professionals or for admission to a hospital gives rise to multiple issues. These issues include higher costs to access health services and feelings of dislocation for the person with the health issue, who is isolated from the support of family and friends. Indeed, the lack of health professionals willing or able to deliver health care in regional, rural and remote locations is an issue for governments across Australia, requiring innovative approaches to delivering health care in these locations.

Addressing the issues in rural and remote areas

Identifying and implementing ways to reduce health inequities and closing the **gap in health service provision** to people in rural and remote regions is receiving increasing attention. For example, governments and health service organisations are focussed on addressing the absence or lack of services in rural and remote areas, as demonstrated by the many innovative projects, programs and initiatives that have now been implemented by the federal, state and territory governments to address the various issues involved (Bryant et al., 2018).

Several approaches are now being used to attract health professionals to live and work in rural and remote locations, including lifestyle and financial incentives (Gwynne & Lincoln, 2017). In addition, mobile health teams, telehealth and video-conferencing services and online resources have been developed to support health professionals, communities, families and individuals located in rural and remote Australia (Bryant et al., 2018). Another key initiative is the community development work being undertaken in some locations to assist rural and remote Australians to support themselves, with projects taking on a 'capacity building' focus (Moran et al., 2019). This approach is fundamental to rural and remote communities, enabling them to withstand the natural disasters that are an increasingly common part of the Australian way of life (Ellis & Albrecht, 2017).

Figure 4.4 lists various programs and projects currently in progress to support people in rural and remote areas. Although by no means exhaustive, this list provides an introduction for health professionals to develop an awareness of the available resources. In turn, the information can be used to support people from rural and remote areas who may be experiencing symptoms of mental illness.

FIGURE 4.4   Rural and remote programs and initiatives

Programs and initiatives supporting rural and remote populations

- Digital health services, which allow people to access help from a mental health professional by phone or online without leaving their homes.
- Online resources, including health promotion, illness prevention, education and other resources for consumers and health professionals.
- Mental health first aid (MHFA) programs, developed specifically for rural, remote and Indigenous populations, aim to improve rural and remote mental health literacy and overcome stigma.
- National Rural Health Alliance, which is Australia's peak non-government organisation for rural and remote health. This organisation aims to enable better health and wellbeing in rural and remote Australia and provides a range of resources on its website to support this vision.
- The University Departments of Rural Health (UDRH) program. This program encourages students of medicine, nursing and other health professions to pursue a career in rural practice by providing clinical opportunities. UDRH programs also support rural health professionals with various resources.
- Scholarship and incentives for tertiary and vocational education and training programs in rural and remote areas.

Digital mental health initiatives

Digital health or eHealth involves using phone or internet connections to provide health services, such as mental health information and services, electronic prescribing and electronic health records, including the national 'My Health Record'. In Australia, eHealth services are supported by the Australian Digital Health Agency (www.digitalhealth.gov.au), which provides information, guidance and initiatives to support the development of digital health services. During the COVID-19 pandemic, digital health services grew exponentially, supported by additional Medicare items. The Australian government (2022c) describes digital initiatives as transformational in addressing the health inequities within and between rural and remote communities.

Benefits for service users of digital or eHealth services include:
- decreased travel time
- time/cost saving
- increased access to services
- reduced anxiety related to access and health issues
- reduced disruption when accessing health services (e.g. travel time, overnight accommodation)
- improved recovery times (LeBlanc et al., 2020).

Despite these benefits, however, barriers remain for rural and remote service users and the health professionals who provide these services. These barriers include:
- lack of suitable internet connection, especially in rural and remote Australia
- consumers being aware of or unable to access telehealth services
- lack of clinicians providing telehealth services

- lack of resourcing of consumers (e.g. many people do not own a computer or do not have the internet in their home)
- lack of education or skills of consumers to use telehealth or problem-solve technological issues
- digital technologies do not always meet the needs of people or health professionals (e.g. some people prefer face-to-face contact, and some physical examinations cannot be conducted using home-based telehealth technologies)
- limited training of health professionals in the use of equipment (St Clair & Murtagh, 2019).

Such challenges also suggest the need for additional investment into telecommunications infrastructure and public education about digital health services.

Digital mental health services

Digital mental health services include telephone (calls or texts) and online services (via desktops and mobile devices) to support people with mental health concerns (Department of Health and Aged Care, 2021). In Australia, digital mental health services include:
- crisis support (e.g. Blue Knot Foundation Helpline, Kids Helpline, Lifeline, MensLine Australia, QLife)
- counselling and other treatment options (e.g. automated self-help programs, multiple online counselling providers, webchat, peer support forums, headspace, consultations with a psychiatrist and e-prescribing)
- mental health promotion and education (e.g. Beyond Blue, Emerging Minds, Black Dog Institue, HealthInfoNet)
- recovery support (e.g. Healthdirect, Mental Health Carers, Mind Australia)
- support for health professionals (e.g. Health to Health).

These services support not only rural and remote populations but also people located in metropolitan Australia who cannot or prefer not to leave their homes to access mental health services. However, measuring the effectiveness of these services, particularly for rural and remote Australians, remains a work in progress (Renfrew et al., 2021).

'Fly-in fly-out'

'Fly-in fly-out' (FIFO) workers are people who live in metropolitan or urban locations, travel by aircraft to a rural or remote location to work, stay in that location for an intensive period of work (e.g. 1–4 weeks), and then travel home again. Some workers also drive-in and drive-out (DIDO) of these locations. FIFO and DIDO workers are common in rural and remote Australia, particularly in the mining sector (Cottrell et al., 2021). However, while FIFO workers have been heralded as a solution to the problems of providing skilled labour to undertake the available work in rural and remote locations, several risks have been identified for the health (including mental health) of these workers; together with the communities into which they fly-in and fly-out and drive-in and drive-out (Adams et al., 2019).

For the FIFO workers, such issues include those related to the work pressures involved in meeting productivity demands, extended rosters, social isolation (especially affecting those living away from their families), poor help-seeking behaviours and limited access to support services (Atkins & Lay, 2018). For the communities into which these workers fly-in and fly-out, issues include the perceptions that these outsiders are taking their jobs and do not contribute meaningfully to the local communities where they reside for such a short time (Sutherland et al., 2017).

These issues raise questions for governments at all levels and the organisations delivering health care in these locations. For example, how can accessible, equitable and effective health care be provided in remote locations to people who live there for such short periods? How can health professionals best support the communities where FIFO workers are travelling?

FIFO health professionals

FIFO health professionals fly into rural and remote Australia to deliver health services in various specialties, including mental health (Sutherland et al., 2017). The FIFO health professionals include medical practitioners, such as specialists and consultants, nurses, paramedics and allied health professionals.

From the point of view of the rural and remote communities, the benefits of utilising FIFO health professionals include reduced financial costs for those who would otherwise need to access health care in the cities or regional centres. Using FIFO health professionals can also reduce feelings of dislocation in rural people. To exemplify, FIFO consultant psychiatrists fly into rural locations to support GPs treating a person with a mental illness in the local hospital rather than transferring the person to a larger facility some distance away (Carey et al., 2018).

From the point of view of the health professional, the FIFO option allows them to continue to live in their own home in the city, while simultaneously delivering a much-needed service to people in rural and remote areas (Cottrell et al., 2021). Some health professionals being paid financial incentives to fly into a rural or remote location, stay for several days of intense work, and then fly out again to relax for a relatively long period of work-free time.

There are also issues with the FIFO approach to providing health care. FIFO health professionals are not part of the communities they visit and, consequently, lack understanding of the community's major preoccupations, ways of being and culture. The lack of involvement of the FIFO health professionals in the community also undermines public health approaches to building resilience and capacity of communities — that is, helping the community to help itself. Instead, FIFO health professionals tend to be associated with the city — an expert from the outside who arrives to deliver health care, with little commitment to the people or place. Additionally, the large financial incentives paid to FIFO health professionals can create resentment in the local population.

Of course, the FIFO approach is just one way forward. Governments and health service providers across Australia will continue to explore ways to address the issues related to providing health care (including mental health care) to rural and remote Australians. Meanwhile, health professionals can support the progress by maintaining awareness of the issues involved, and ensuring they take a culturally appropriate approach to helping all people with mental health problems, regardless of their background. The need to take such an approach is discussed in the next section, which focuses on helping people from culturally or linguistically diverse backgrounds who are experiencing symptoms of mental illness.

UPON REFLECTION

Isolation, loneliness and mental health

Many Australians in metropolitan and rural locations experienced social isolation during the COVID-19 pandemic. Social isolation, which involves having minimal contact with others, is different from loneliness, a subjective state of negative feelings about having a lower level of social contact than desired (AIHW, 2021d). Some people (e.g. introverts) enjoy having fewer social contacts and opportunities to take a break from people, while others (e.g. extroverts) find social isolation stressful.

According to the National Rural Health Alliance (2017), the physical isolation experienced by many rural and remote Australians can negatively affect their physical and mental health. During the COVID-19 pandemic, many people who were required to socially isolate, reported increased feelings of loneliness, stress, anxiety and depression and, for some, suicidal ideation (AIHW, 2021d).

The negative impact of social isolation and loneliness can be reduced by:
- membership in communities or sporting organisations
- volunteering to help others
- paid and volunteer carers and companions
- companion animals
- developing stronger community connections (including online community connections) (AIHW, 2021d).

QUESTIONS

1. How comfortable do you feel with isolation?
2. When have you felt the most isolated or lonely?
3. What steps can you take, as a health professional, to support people who feel unable to manage isolation or loneliness?

4.5 Mental health and multiculturalism

LEARNING OBJECTIVE 4.5 Outline the main concerns that affect the mental health of migrants and refugees.

Australia is one of the world's most culturally diverse nations (Bharadwaj, 2018). It is populated by over 25 million people, with almost half reporting having at least one parent born overseas and some 30 per cent stating they were born in another country (ABS, 2021). In total, Australians have identified more than 200 different countries of origin, with the United Kingdom, New Zealand, China and India predominating. This diversity suggests the need for health professionals to be familiar with the issues encountered when providing health care to **culturally and linguistically diverse (CALD)** populations.

Multiculturalism has added to the richness of Australia's social fabric; however, it has also given rise to several challenges, including how best to deliver health care to people with CALD backgrounds (AIHW, 2018). This section examines notions of multiculturalism in the context of mental health and illness. Rather than focusing on the details of Australia's many cultures and subcultures, a broad perspective is taken, emphasising the importance of mutual respect for and accepting the differences involved. Also highlighted is the need for collaboration between health professionals, the person and their family members or community to find the most culturally appropriate ways of delivering high-quality mental health services.

The language of multiculturalism

There are a large number of terms and acronyms that are used in the multicultural context in contemporary Australia. These terms include 'acculturation', 'assimilation', 'asylum seekers', 'culturally and linguistically diverse' or 'CALD', 'ethnicity', 'integration', 'migrant', 'nationality', 'non-English-speaking background', 'race', 'refugee' and 'transcultural'. When the concepts of 'cultural safety', 'cultural awareness', 'cultural knowledge', 'cultural competence' and 'cultural proficiency' are also taken into account, it is understandable that many health professionals struggle to negotiate this minefield of terminology.

Health professionals often use the term 'culturally and linguistically diverse' or CALD to describe the cultural differences between groups of people, including how diverse people communicate and dress, their social traditions, food, social structures, art and religion. Another term commonly used in the health sector is **transcultural** (Wolf et al., 2019). This word describes an approach to health care that requires the health professional to extend or move through more than one culture to focus on each person's health needs and the care required (Khawaja et al., 2021).

Transcultural approaches were first developed by nursing professionals, in particular Madeleine Leininger (1988), who realised that people from different cultural backgrounds had different expectations of health care. These differences often led to inequities in health care as the dominant culture imposed its ways of being and doing onto minority groups with a different culture (Parfitt, 2018). As a consequence, the health outcomes of these minority groups were compromised.

Leininger decided that health professionals required a theoretical framework to deliver culturally appropriate care. She described transcultural health care as:

> a formal area of study and practice focused on comparative holistic cultural care, health, and the illness patterns of people with respect to differences and similarities in their cultural values, beliefs, and life ways with the goal to provide culturally congruent, competent, and compassionate care (Leininger, 1997).

Today, transcultural health professionals form an integral part of the health system in Australia. Transcultural practices are person-centred and seek to meet the specific needs of the person and their family (Khawaja et al., 2021).

State and territory governments across Australia have now developed transcultural mental health resource centres (e.g. Queensland Transcultural Mental Health Centre, 2019; Transcultural Mental Health Centre, 2019). Resources are freely available online, and include leadership in and support for clinical consultation and assessment; transcultural (mental) health promotion, prevention and early intervention; publication and resource development; and education and training. Web addresses related to transcultural approaches are provided at the end of this chapter.

Another descriptor often used in the multicultural context is 'non-English-speaking background'. All cultures have their own language(s) or dialect(s). In Australia, the dominant language is Australian English. People for whom English is not a first language may be referred to as having a 'non-English-speaking background'. In the health context, this often means that an interpreter is required to assist with communication (Yick & Daines, 2019). Interpreters are discussed in more detail later in this chapter. At this point, it is necessary to explain that people for whom English is a first language do not always share the same culture as mainstream Australians. For example, although more than 73 per cent of people in Australia speak English at home, their cultural background may be Canadian, English, Irish, Scottish, Welsh or from another country that belongs to the Commonwealth (including many African countries) (World Population Review, n.d.). Likewise, there are cultural differences between Australia and the United States; health care is universally available to all Australian residents or citizens at minimal cost, whereas the provision of health care in the United States is different. Any such differences, including the alternative perspectives these differences produce, must be considered by the health professional when helping a person.

Refugees and migrants

The WHO (2019) identifies that there are currently an estimated 1 billion migrants worldwide, including 258 million international migrants and 763 million internal migrants. This situation equates to one in seven of the world's population. WHO (2019) also estimates that 68 million internal and international migrants have been forcibly displaced. Refugees and migrants have a right to good health — but often lack access to health services and financial protection.

Today, people may come to Australia as either a **refugee** or a **migrant**. Health professionals need to understand the differences between these two diverse groups of people so they can appropriately assess their different health needs.

Refugees have been forced to leave their home countries (Amnesty International, 2022). This situation is often the result of well-founded fears of being persecuted for their race, religion, nationality or membership in a particular social group or political perspective. Consequently, some refugees may be relieved to arrive in their new country and will settle in relatively quickly. Others, however, may struggle to settle in due to racist attitudes towards them, their past experiences or mental health issues.

People who resettle in Australia on humanitarian grounds experience a lower health status than other refugees and migrants (Dowling et al., 2019). Also, many refugees who have witnessed or experienced torture or significant trauma before arriving in Australia — or even after arriving in detention centres — will be affected by their experiences (Nickerson et al., 2019). Issues that may develop as a result of trauma can include depression, anxiety and **post-traumatic stress disorder (PTSD)** (Shen et al., 2018).

While many refugees seek help from health professionals to manage their symptoms, others may be less willing to seek support. This unwillingness could be due to a lack of knowledge about the kind of help available (Parajuli & Horey, 2019). A lack of willingness to seek support can also be due to cultural differences (Samuel et al., 2018). For this reason, mental health screening or assessment must be conducted on people who have arrived in Australia as refugees. It is also important that refugees are informed of the various health services that are available for them to access across Australia.

UPON REFLECTION

Health services for refugees and asylum seekers

As noted by Shawyer and colleagues (2017), refugees and asylum seekers often have a low health status and complex health needs, due to limited access to health care in their countries of origin. Once in Australia, refugees and asylum seekers can experience access issues due to language and cultural differences. To further complicate their situation, they may also be traumatised from their experiences before arriving in Australia and distressed by the resettlement process.

....

QUESTIONS

1. Access to health care is a fundamental human right. What can we do to ensure that refugees are supported to access health care?
2. Some refugees will not be familiar with the mental health services available in Australia. What can we do to ensure that refugees understand the different services available?
3. Some refugees will not be familiar with the signs and symptoms or diagnoses of conditions such as PTSD. What can we do to ensure refugees receive the help they need?

In contrast to refugees, migrants have chosen to leave their country of origin and move to Australia (Amnesty International 2022). For this reason, many migrants will be happy about their move and settle into their new home with few difficulties. Some migrants, however, may feel homesick and geographically and linguistically isolated (Silove et al., 2017), leading to family members holding on to the traditions of their old country and being reluctant to become a part of the broader Australian culture. While this may provide some reassurance for these families, it can also impact their children. For example, the parents may refuse to allow their children to participate in regular school activities, which leads to marginalisation and a reduced sense of belonging or 'fitting in' for these children (Valibhoy et al., 2017). Other problems for migrants can result when they return to visit their country of origin and find that things have moved on or changed. When this occurs, the person can experience a reduced sense of belonging to their old country, leading to further unhappiness, loneliness and depression (Jetten et al., 2018). Despite initial hopes, then, a move to another country for some people can give rise to profound disappointment.

The different experiences of refugees and migrants suggest the need for health professionals to seek out information from the person with a CALD background, rather than make assumptions. Different approaches are needed to help diverse people, according to their backgrounds and experiences. To provide the most effective care (including mental health care), health professionals need to familiarise themselves with the backgrounds and cultures of the people they help (Wamwayi et al., 2019).

People in detention

Incarceration under Australia's system of manda-tory immigration detention, all non-citizens without a valid visa must be detained. This detention can be onshore or offshore.

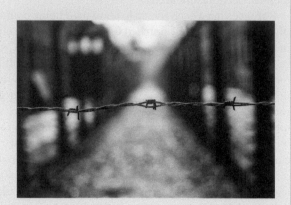

According to the Refugee Council of Australia (2020), Australia's offshore detention policy has given rise to mental illness in refugees caused by:
- uncertainty about their future
- their lack of independence and loss of control
- the monotony of life in detention
- concern about family members still living in dan-ger overseas
- the impacts of past torture and trauma
- witnessing the negative impacts of detention on other people in detention.

A national campaign in 2018 against mandatory offshore detention led to the transfer of all children held in offshore detention centres to mainland Australia. The years spent on Nauru by the children and adolescents had a devastating effect on their mental health (Vasefi, 2019). Diagnoses included ongoing depression, anxiety and stress-related disorders, with many of these children experiencing difficulty sleeping, fatigue, feelings of worthlessness and hopelessness, difficulties with memory and concentration, and recurring thoughts of suicide. The restrictive nature of the onshore community detention also delayed their road to recovery, as the children could not participate in regular community or educational activities.

According to the Australian Child and Adolescent Trauma, Loss and Grief Network (n.d.) at the Australian National University, refugee children and families can take many years to recover from their experiences before arrival to Australia, during detention and once they have been resettled.

Key factors for supporting refugees, in particular children and adolescents, to achieve recovery and, ultimately, wellbeing include:
- supporting them to rebuild a sense of safety and security
- exploring ways to develop social groups and interpersonal attachments
- helping them to develop plans and goals for the future
- encouraging them to maintain a sense of cultural identity
- enabling them to find a safe way to talk about their traumatic experiences (Tomasi et al., 2022).

It would be impossible for a health professional to possess enough knowledge of every culture to provide culture-specific care to all the people they encounter. However, health professionals can develop the understanding required to familiarise themselves with the major **cultural discourses** that frame the worldview of different cultures. By doing this, health professionals will be better equipped to understand the main differences between the cultures and adapt their practices accordingly.

The discourses of individualism and collectivism, which inform all cultures to some degree, are discussed in the next section. Cultural constructions of gender roles and how these may impact the role of health professionals are also considered. Finally, the outcomes of stigma on people with mental health problems who also have a CALD background are discussed.

Individualism and collectivism

As noted earlier, cultural norms and influences are often invisible or taken for granted, understood as 'fact', 'reality' or 'just the way things are'. To illustrate, many health professionals unquestioningly accept the 'obvious' value placed by Australian health services on the person through individualised care or treatment plans. **Individualism**, however, is a very Western construct or belief system and stands in contrast to the notions of **collectivism**, which frame other systems of belief (Cendales & Ortiz, 2019; Triandis, 2018).

Generally, individualistic cultures, including the dominant culture in Australia, have the following characteristics in common.

- The 'self' is the most important consideration.
- Priority is given to personal or individual goals.
- Identity is defined in terms of personal or individual attributes or achievements.
- The individual is encouraged to stand out, be unique, and express themselves.
- Self-reliance and independence are admired.
- Rules are made to ensure individuals' independence and freedoms, and to promote individual rights and choice. However, adherence or conforming to these rules can be arbitrary or 'individualised', as people are encouraged to make their own way.
- Notions of 'in-groups' and 'out-groups' are less distinct than in collectivist cultures.
- Individualists are more likely than collectivists to pre-judge people based on their personal attributes (Hogan, 2019).

Examples of countries in which individualism is prominent include Australia, Canada, France, Italy, New Zealand, the United Kingdom and the United States.

Generally, collectivistic cultures have the following characteristics in common.

- The 'group', 'collective' or community is the most important consideration.
- Priority is given to the group's goals.
- Personal identity is defined in terms of the group's attributes or achievements.
- Everyone is encouraged to conform and do what is best for the group.
- Everyone is discouraged from openly expressing opinions or beliefs that may contravene the beliefs of the group.
- Group, family or rights for the common good are seen as more important than the rights of individuals.
- Rules are made to promote group stability and order. Adherence or conforming to these rules is essential.
- Clear distinctions are made between 'in-groups' and 'out-groups'.
- Working with others and cooperating is the norm. Refusal to cooperate and a desire to be independent or to stand are viewed as shameful. All in the group rely upon each other for support.
- Collectivists are more likely than individualists to pre-judge people based on group identity. As such, the whole group will try to protect a member, and the group itself, from outside influences (Gao et al., 2019; Triandis, 2018).

Examples of countries in which collectivism is prominent include Argentina, Brazil, China, Egypt, Greece, India, Japan, Korea, Mexico, Portugal, Taiwan and Vietnam. In addition, many indigenous cultures are framed by the discourse of collectivism.

The invisible nature of these two worldviews gives rise to many issues when offering a health service. Health professionals born and raised as part of the dominant Australian culture, which is individualistic in orientation, may make assumptions about how health care 'should' be delivered based on their cultural values. Consequently, health professionals may not be able to understand why the person they are trying to help is not interested in, for example, exploring notions of self-esteem or self-actualisation. The health professional may even perceive this person's lack of interest as 'insightless', 'uncooperative' or 'non-compliant'. However, the person from a collectivist culture who enters the Australian health system may find themselves separated from the family or the community group to which they belong and through which they find meaning (Tseris, 2019). For this reason, when they are expected to make decisions about themselves as individuals — a concept that is foreign to their system of values — they feel stressed or become anxious or depressed (Wood et al., 2019).

Understanding the notions of individualism and collectivism is necessary to accept the fundamental differences between some cultures. Health professionals who are aware of these differences will be better able to adapt their practices to engage the person from a different culture and develop health care that is more appropriate to the particular needs of the person.

Gender roles

Another crucial aspect of culture that will influence how health care is delivered to CALD populations is the role of gender (Perales & Todd, 2018). Every culture has its own particular understandings, values, traditions and rules (spoken and unspoken) about the role of males and females, be they adults, teenagers, children or infants (Kiely et al., 2019). Contemporary Western-oriented cultures have been significantly influenced by the feminist, gender, anti-discrimination and human rights movements, to name a few (Coleman, 2018). Some cultures, however, have a different view of gender roles, marriage, relationships, and the place of children, from the dominant Australian culture. These differences may challenge health professionals and raise questions about their role in the decision making of people with CALD backgrounds.

Supporting people who have culturally and linguistically diverse backgrounds

The national Department of Health and Aged Care has developed Head to Health, which provides resources for health professionals who support people with diverse cultures (Department of Health and Aged Care, 2020). These resources include information for carers of people from CALD cultures who may be experiencing mental health problems.

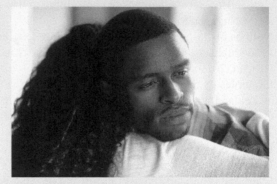

The Department of Health (n.d.) has also provided information on mental health services for people with CALD backgrounds, available on the Department's website. The Department notes that people with culturally diverse backgrounds have low access to mental health care and support in the broader community. Barriers to accessing mental health care and support are cultural, structural and service-related.

Take, for instance, Owusu, who had recently arrived in Australia with his family from Ghana. The cultural barriers he faced upon his arrival included:

- language barriers. Even though Owusu spoke English, he found that many of the slang words used by Australians were unfamiliar, and the accents were sometimes difficult to understand
- not being accustomed to speaking to strangers about the difficulties faced by his family
- not feeling comfortable with his wife and daughters seeking help when he was not present
- feeling fearful of the authorities, including the child services, social services, immigration and the police, due to his previous experiences in his home country
- feeling resentful that his qualifications, achieved in Ghana were not recognised in Australia
- afraid to seek out mental health support due to the high levels of stigma in the community about mental health problems.

The structural barriers he encountered included:

- lack of knowledge or understanding of the kinds of services available and how these services could help his family
- uncertainty about where to go or how to access the services.

The service-related barriers that held him back included:

- fear that he might be judged or stereotyped by health professionals
- confusion about the model of health care used in Australia
- uncertainty about whether the health care would suit him and his family and/or if health professionals would listen to their distinct needs.

As a result, he and his wife tried to manage without seeking help, leading to his family missing out on receiving the care they needed.

QUESTIONS

1. As a health professional, what practical steps can you take to help people with CALD backgrounds open up?
2. As a health professional, what can you do to help break down the structural and cultural barriers for people from CALD backgrounds?
3. As a health professional, what can you do to help break down the service-related barriers for people from CALD backgrounds?

Unless a practice contravenes Australian law or a person with a culturally diverse background asks for assistance to deal with problems they are experiencing with aspects of their culture, it is not the role of the health professional to interfere with cultural behaviours or situations with which they personally disagree.

Rather, the focus of the health professional must remain on the person's health. Health professionals who feel confused by culturally influenced behaviours are strongly encouraged to seek the advice of the manager or another health professional who has specialised in this area.

Finally, it is also vital that health professionals recognise that different cultures have different rules about appropriate male–female interactions, regardless of the context. If unsure, the health professional may ask the person with a culturally diverse background or their family members the following questions.

- Is it culturally appropriate for the health professional of one gender to speak to a person of the other gender in this situation?
- Is there a need for a cultural mediator or worker to assist before the interview proceeds?
- Is privacy being protected?
- Are cultural expectations being respected?

Answering these questions enables the health professional to deliver culturally appropriate health care.

Cultural diversity, stigma and mental illness

As discussed in the chapter on mental health care in Australia, people with mental health problems are often stigmatised. The stigma attached to mental illness in diverse societies and cultures worldwide, including Australia (Kirmayer et al., 2018). Reasons for this are cultural, historical, religious, social and political (Mirza et al., 2019). The consequences of stigma for people with mental illness are always negative.

The main stigma-related issues for CALD communities in Australia in relation to mental illness include:

- limited understanding of the concepts of mental health and illness
- cultural perceptions that any kind of disability is shameful, particularly a disability related to mental illness
- a consequent reluctance to seek assistance for mental health issues (Gopalkrishnan, 2018; Coates et al., 2019).

Of course, it is unhelpful to generalise. Different cultures will have different perceptions or understandings of mental health and illness, resulting in different levels of stigma. Nevertheless, many cultural barriers exist for people with culturally diverse backgrounds who seek help or support for mental health problems (Poon & Lee, 2019). It is the responsibility of the health professional to be aware of these barriers, and reach out to people with culturally diverse backgrounds.

Breaking down negative attitudes is always challenging. Even so, health professionals can lead the way by providing culturally appropriate information, role-modelling acceptance, and developing clear communication channels (Loganathan & Varghese, 2019). The final section of this chapter provides some practical suggestions on how this can be achieved.

UPON REFLECTION

Mental health and multicultural considerations?

Uche is a 34-year-old male from Nigeria who lives with his parents in an Australian capital city. Uche presents to the health professional with anxiety and depression.

The health professional engaged with Uche and found out he had a girlfriend he could not take home as his parents would disapprove. Uche doesn't like being lectured by his parents about who he can and can't see. He wants to be with his girlfriend and spend more time with her before they get married. On the other hand, he also knows that he needs to go for religious counselling before he can get married and, in line with tradition, take his girlfriend for a medical checkup to ensure she isn't pregnant. The problem is that Uche knows she is pregnant, and he is the father. The medical tests will be positive, which means his parents won't let him get married because marrying a pregnant woman is taboo in his culture.

Uche says that this is why he feels anxious and depressed.

....

QUESTIONS

1. How would you support Uche in this situation?

2. How would you support Uche's girlfriend?

3. How will the health professionals manage confidentiality issues if Uche's parents approach them for information?

4.6 Supporting people who are members of subcultures or minority groups

LEARNING OBJECTIVE 4.6 Consider the mental health needs of lesbian, gay, bisexual, transgender, queer, intersex and asexual people.

Approximately 3.5 per cent of Australians describe themselves as a minority sexual identity of the population (Wilson et al., 2020). The introduction of marriage equality laws in Australia in 2017 raised awareness of many issues experienced by lesbian, gay and bisexual people. Likewise, an increased presence in the electronic media of trans, queer or questioning, intersex and asexual people has increased awareness of alternative ways of being (Goldberg et al., 2018). Even so, **lesbian, gay, bisexual, trans, queer or questioning, intersex, asexual and other gender non-conforming identities (LGBTQIA+)**, or other people who belong to communities that support the LGBTQIA+ cause, face many barriers and hurdles, particularly in relation to their mental health and wellbeing (Hughes, 2018). This section examines the challenges experienced by LGBTQIA+ people in the context of their mental health and wellbeing. Questions addressed include: Is there an LGBTQIA+ subculture in Australia, and if so, does this subculture support the health and wellbeing of LGBTQIA+ people? And how does it do so? What are the primary risk factors for LGBTQIA+ people, and members of other minority groups, for developing a mental health problem? What are the main mental health problems experienced by LGBTQIA+ people?

Definitions of LGBTQIA+ people

While the acronym 'LGBTQIA+' tends to be viewed as a single category; it actually comprises various people with diverse lifestyles, needs and preferences (Pennay et al., 2018). LGBTQIA+ people have different but overlapping demographics, histories, and experiences (Hughes, 2018). Moreover, the plus sign at the end of LGBTQIA+ can include people who support the LGBTQIA+, also called 'allies', who likewise have diverse backgrounds.

The common factor that connects LGBTQIA+ people is the notion of 'difference' in terms of their sexuality and/or gender and/or physical sexual characteristics. While the dominant perspective in almost all cultures is that people are either male/female and heterosexual; LGBTQIA+ people have the lived experience of a different view of the world. This difference is not homogenous, however. Therefore, LGBTQIA+ people should be approached through a multifaceted lens.

Some health professionals confuse the various terms LGBTQIA+ people use to describe themselves. Table 4.1 provides a list of the terms and descriptions. Using these terms appropriately can help LGBTQIA+ people to feel more understood and accepted.

TABLE 4.1 Common terms used by LGBTQIA+ groups

Term	Description
Agender	People who do not identify as any gender at all.
Ally	People who actively support LGBTQIA+ people.
Asexual	People who do not feel sexual attraction or a desire for partnered sexuality. Asexuality is not to be mistaken for celibacy, which is about choice more than sexual orientation.
Bisexual	Either male or female, with a primary sexual and affectional orientation towards people of either gender.
Demisexual	People who require an emotional bond to form a sexual attraction.
Gay	A primary sexual and affectional orientation towards people of the same gender.
Genderfluid	People who use gender identity as self-expression and not something that is static.
Genderqueer	People who do not conform to binary gender identities.
Greysexual	Refers to the 'grey area' between asexuality and sexuality.
Intersex	Umbrella term that describes people who are born with indeterminate physical sexual characteristics. Note, not all intersex people have undergone medical transition.

Lesbian	Female with a primary sexual and affectional orientation towards people of the same gender.
Non-binary	People who do not conform to binary gender identities.
Pansexual	People with a desire for all genders and sexes.
Polyamorous	People who are open to multiple consensual romantic or sexual relationships at one time.
Queer	People who overtly celebrate that they do not fit into traditional binary or heterosexual norms.
Questioning	People in the process of exploring the expression or orientation of their gender identity.
Omnisexual	People with a desire for all genders and sexes.
Sapiosexual	People attracted to intelligence, regardless of a person's gender identity.
Trans	An umbrella term that describes a range of experiences or identities for people whose gender identity or expression of that identity differs from the dominant expectations of their assigned sex at birth. Note, not all trans people undergo a medical transition (hormones or surgery).
Two-spirit	A term used by Native Americans to describe a third gender.

Source: Adapted from Human Rights Campaign (n.d.); LGBTQIA Resource Centre (2019).

LGBTQIA+ culture

Many people who identify as LGBTQIA+ describe aspects of their way of life as a 'subculture' of the larger Australian culture, with the LGBTQIA+ culture boasting its own norms, lifestyles or ways of being. This culture includes upholding lifestyles that are different or 'alternative' to the dominant heteronormative culture, which marginalises different or alternative ways of being or doing (McDermott et al., 2018).

In some countries, the LGBTQIA+ culture is widely accepted, and includes a good understanding of the LGBTQIA+ social movement, support for works of art by LGBTQIA+ people, and the celebration of significant figures in the LGBTQIA+ community, alongside attendance of LGBTQIA+ events. For this text, the LGBTQIA+ culture is defined by the patterns of knowledge, beliefs, attitudes and behaviours by which LGBTQIA+ people live, including their shared history, values, attitudes, goals and practices. This culture — or way of being or doing — helps LGBTQIA+ people make sense of the world, guides how they view themselves and others, and connects them to one another. The LGBTQIA+ culture is an important means by which LGBTQIA+ people feel they are not alone and have a place in society.

The LGBTQIA+ culture and its place in Australian society continues to be 'other' — that is, an alternative culture — with members often reporting they feel and are marginalised or ostracised. Despite growing acceptance of difference, the heteronormative influences that characterise mainstream culture in Australia continue to exercise considerable influence that can leave many LGBTQIA+ people feeling like outcasts (Kilicaslan & Petrakis, 2019). The consequences of this on the mental health of LGBTQIA+ people are considerable.

Risk factors for the mental health of LGBTQIA+ people

The LGBTQIA+ population is not a homogenous group, with the different subcultures and individual experiences within the population group giving rise to various risk factors. However, some commonalities exist concerning the mental illness and wellbeing of LGBTQIA+ people. These risk factors are similar to those experienced by minority groups everywhere and include prejudice, aversion, hatred or fear. Other risk factors are more specific to the individual's or group's experiences. For example, the wellbeing of many intersex people is affected if they have undergone challenging or unwanted medical (including pharmacological) or surgical interventions.

Another example is the transphobia experienced by transsexual or transgender people. In particular, young people who experience transphobia are at a higher risk of experiencing anxiety, depression, self-harm, suicidal ideation and substance abuse.

LGBTQIA+ people who live in regional or rural communities are also at risk, as they are more likely to feel isolated and be discriminated against, leading to higher levels of self-harm and suicidal ideation.

Social isolation is another risk factor and takes many forms, including rejection by family, friends and acquaintances, and leads to low self-esteem, anxiety, depression, substance abuse and suicide attempts.

As with all people who belong to other minority cultures, these risk factors can be linked to systemic issues related to access, equity and discrimination (Pienaar et al., 2018). For many health professionals, overcoming such systemic issues may seem outside their sphere of influence. Even so, change begins at the individual level — health professionals can make a difference by advocating for LGBTQIA+ people in need and ensuring their practice supports access, equity and equality of all people, regardless of sexual preference, gender orientation or physical characteristics (Cronin et al., 2021).

LIVED EXPERIENCE

The 'questioning' male

My earliest memories are of me wishing — at times desperately — that I had been born a girl. In my family, the differences between boys and girls were made very clear and there was a lot of pressure for me to line up with the 'shoulds' of being a boy. I remember my parents being angry if I even looked sideways at things or activities traditionally marked as 'female', like playing with dolls or dressing up or wearing jewellery or make-up. So I worked hard to be the son they wanted — I craved love and acceptance. Being part of the family — belonging — was important to me.

As time went by, though, I began to carry around a lot of confusion and distress, including the feeling that life wasn't fair and the world was against me. I began to fight with my parents — wanting them to love and accept me but also trying to drive them away for what they were doing to me. This confused me because I couldn't work out what they were doing to me that was so bad, but I constantly felt torn apart. Before I knew it, I was being treated for 'behavioural issues' at school.

And all the while, I was hiding 'girl things' in my bedroom — things I stole from my cousins or friend's sisters but never my own sister as I was terrified she would find them and tell my parents. Pink things, fluffy things, jewellery and makeup — things that, for some reason, made me feel euphorically happy, and at the same time, guilty and shameful. I hid them in places that no one would ever look and get them out late at night and explore and fantasise — I was a female and I loved the feeling . . . and hated myself.

My feelings of self-loathing became worse as I hit puberty — the more my body became like a man's, the more I wanted to punish that body. So I threw myself into contact sports and soon became known as a 'mad man' who lined up for anyone or anything that would get in the line of fire. Bruises and beatings felt good, like badges of honour.

Then I discovered alcohol, drugs and self-harming. I'd wipe myself out: bang my head, cut my thighs . . . feel the pain . . . take a bizarre joy in watching the dark red blood seeping out across my hated body. Once the initial relief passed me by, I'd hate myself all the more.

Except one day I got careless — drunk, stoned, cutting up and careless. My sister found me after I'd been cutting up. I still remember her screams, my mother's crying, my father's anger, the ambulance sirens. And suddenly I was in hospital, then locked away in a 'looney bin'. I was consumed by guilt at my parent's shame. I decided I wanted — needed — to die and began to make plans.

It was while I was in hospital that I met someone — another teenager, a girl who also hated her body, a girl who wanted to be a boy, a girl who wasn't scared to tell people about it. I was drawn to this person and it didn't take long to figure out why. They talked to me, I talked to them, like I'd never talked to anyone before in my whole life. I felt I could be myself. The relief was like something I'd never experienced before. They gave me the courage to tell the nurses and doctors. But I refused to tell my parents. I'm not ready — I'm not sure I'll ever be ready. I can't let them down. I need my family — I need to belong. Meanwhile, anti-depressants and sharing my secret with the counsellor are helping.

Mental health issues faced by LGBTQIA+ people

In light of the detrimental experiences of the vast majority of LGBTQIA+ people concerning social and cultural acceptance, together with experiences of social exclusion, social control, disempowerment and stigma, it can be no surprise that many of them experience low levels of mental health and wellbeing (Jacobs & Morris, 2016). For example, when compared to the general population, LGBTQIA+ people are more likely to attempt suicide in their lifetime (Hill et al., 2022). Specifically:

- young LGBTQIA+ people aged 16–27 are five times more likely to attempt suicide
- trans people aged 14–25 are 15 times more likely
- intersex people aged 16 and over are nearly six times more likely, particularly those who experience abuse and harassment
- LGBTQIA+ young people are nearly four times as likely to engage in self-harm than heterosexual young people (LGBTIQ+ Health Australia, 2021).

Compared to the general population, LGBTQIA+ people are also more likely to experience mental health problems (Perales 2019). LGBTQIA+ people are two and a half times more likely to be diagnosed and treated for mental illness than the general population (LGBTIQ+ Health Australia, 2021). Depression and anxiety are a particular concern, with LGBTQIA+ people aged 16 or over are three times more likely to experience depression and more than twice as likely to be diagnosed with anxiety than the general population (Wilson & Cariola, 2020). Of particular concern are the rates of suicide and self-harm in LGBTQIA+ people (LGBTIQ+ Health Australia, 2021).

In light of these worrying statistics, it is vital that health professionals understand the issues involved and how best they can support LGBTQIA+ people. Strategies and approaches are outlined in the next section of the chapter.

UPON REFLECTION

What are your biases?

Health professionals will have their own personal, social and cultural biases about LGBTQIA+ people, some positive, some not so positive. Health professionals must be aware of these biases and how they can affect the health care they deliver to people who lead alternative lifestyles. Through self-awareness, health professionals can put their biases aside and respond professionally to all people seeking help for a health concern, regardless of their lifestyles.

QUESTIONS

1. What is your personal, social or cultural view of lesbian, gay or bisexual people? Of trans people? Of queer or questioning people?
2. What are your thoughts on intersex people? In your opinion, do they need to choose one or the other gender to be part of our society?
3. How could your biases affect how you help people with different sexualities or diverse genders?

4.7 Towards providing culturally appropriate mental health care

LEARNING OBJECTIVE 4.7 Explain the importance of providing culturally appropriate care to all people with mental health issues.

As part of their duty of care, health professionals are expected to negotiate the many cultural differences of the people they are helping. This expectation places a responsibility on health professionals to seek the information and education they need to support and develop their practice and deliver culturally appropriate care.

There is some debate about the processes involved in providing culturally appropriate mental health care to people from diverse backgrounds. Some commentators have suggested that teaching cultural awareness or knowledge may work to generate an unhelpful 'us' versus 'them' dichotomy or reinforce views of 'otherness' (Kewley et al., 2018). For this reason, a broad, respectful and accepting approach is required to enable health professionals to become culturally proficient (Power et al., 2018).

Cultural proficiency

Cultural proficiency in providing mental health care occurs when the health professional recognises that a person has a culturally diverse background and ensures that the person's culture, language, customs, attitudes, beliefs and preferred ways of being or doing are accepted and respected (Currie, 2022). Cultural proficiency builds on notions of **cultural safety**, which originated in New Zealand in the 1990s.

Cultural safety involves providing an environment in which people are safe; where there is no challenge to, or denial of, their identity; and where their needs are met (Dawson et al., 2022). A culturally safe health environment will involve respect, shared meaning, shared knowledge, and effective engagement with culturally diverse peoples learning together.

Cultural proficiency goes further than cultural safety and includes five broad principles for the health professional:

1. acquisition of a broad understanding of how different cultures may view health, mental health and illness
2. demonstration of respect for and acceptance of the different cultures

3. a focus on the person together with their families and/or communities to enable genuine interpersonal or therapeutic engagement
4. delivery of ongoing mental health education and the provision of culturally appropriate information to people with culturally diverse backgrounds
5. commitment to lifelong learning and development in this significant area of health care provision (The Center for Culturally Proficient Educational Practice, 2019).

Proficiency is when health professionals have achieved competence in this area of practice, with added awareness that the learning process is lifelong and requires constant ongoing reflection and development of practice.

To achieve cultural proficiency in mental health care delivery, the health professional will move through several stages of practice. These include cultural awareness, cultural knowledge, cultural sensitivity and cultural competence (Mullins & Khawaja, 2018).

Cultural awareness begins with health professionals examining their values-base and beliefs. As discussed at the beginning of this chapter, those who identify with the dominant Australian culture may presume that the values of that culture are 'common sense' or 'just the way things are', rather than cultural constructions or assumptions that influence the way they understand notions of health and illness (Hultsjö et al., 2019). Health professionals who are aware of the impact of their own culture on the way they understand the world are more likely to be accepting of, and respectful towards those with different values and beliefs.

Cultural knowledge can be derived from many sources, including anthropology, sociology, cultural studies, psychology, biology, nursing, medicine and the arts. Acquiring cultural knowledge includes understanding the values, beliefs and nuances of a particular culture's perception of health (including mental health); and understanding the societal and organisational structures and accepted practices of each culture (Stodart & Kai, 2018). This knowledge can assist health professionals in adapting approaches to meet the needs of the person from that culture (Andrade, 2019). Although it is helpful to know the details of different cultural practices and beliefs, the health professional cannot have enough knowledge of all the different cultures that comprise the multicultural mix in Australia. The acquisition of cultural knowledge, then, is an ongoing process.

Cultural sensitivity entails the development of appropriate interpersonal or therapeutic alliances with people from different cultures. Health professionals are encouraged to examine themselves to identify how they view the cultural differences of people in their care (Dur et al., 2022). Questions they may ask themselves would include whether others have an equally legitimate way of life and understanding of the world as the health professional. Reflecting on the answers to such questions will enable the health professional to develop cultural sensitivity (Göl & Özüm, 2019).

Cultural competence is achieved when health professionals demonstrate sensitivity to cultural, race, gender, sexual orientation, social class and economic issues in their practice (Kaphle et al., 2022). Cultural competence involves the skills, awareness, encounters, desire and knowledge required to deliver culturally appropriate care and is achieved by health professionals when awareness, knowledge and sensitivity are integrated into their practice (de Peralta et al., 2019).

Finally, and as already noted, cultural proficiency follows the achievement of cultural competence. A health professional becomes culturally proficient when they have achieved cultural awareness, cultural knowledge, cultural sensitivity, and cultural competence, and continues to work on maintaining and building on this state of being on a lifelong basis. Cultural proficiency is not static, but an ongoing process in which health professionals are actively involved.

Health professionals are strongly encouraged to learn more about these various terms and how they apply in practice. This learning can be achieved by attending training courses on providing culturally appropriate care (Geerlings et al., 2018), which are now required of health professionals by governments and health services across Australia. There is also a list of useful websites at the end of this chapter.

Culturally appropriate approaches to treating mental illness

The approaches to providing mental health care and treatment to people with culturally diverse backgrounds are as multifaceted as the many different cultures the health professional will encounter (Poon & Lee, 2019). The health professional with no cultural awareness may inadvertently discourage the person with a culturally diverse background from seeking help for a mental health issue. This situation could lead to poorer outcomes for the person (Kaphle et al., 2022).

While acknowledging that CALD populations are in no way homogeneous and that each person or group will have different issues and needs, there are several simple but effective steps a health professional may take to assist people with mental health issues, regardless of their background. These approaches include, but are not limited to:

- demonstrating acceptance and respect, regardless of personal bias
- listening to the person and responding constructively to their expressed needs and preferences
- ensuring the involvement of a suitable interpreter when required
- providing culturally and linguistically appropriate information and education to the person, their families and the groups/communities to which they belong
- focusing on the personal interactions and the therapeutic alliance or relationship (Muir-Cochrane et al., 2018).

By taking these steps, health professionals will facilitate communication with the people they are helping, which, in turn, will optimise health outcomes.

Ensuring the availability of interpreters

Many health professionals may be uncertain if a person requires an interpreter. It may seem as if a culturally diverse person understands what is happening to them because, for example, the person smiles and nods when questioned. However, the person may only be demonstrating politeness or deference to the health professionals, as is appropriate to that culture. Health professionals must never take the understanding of others — including Indigenous Australians, for whom English may be a second language — for granted.

There is a need for health professionals to contact an interpreter for a person with a culturally diverse background who also has a mental health issue when the:

- person or family member requests an interpreter
- person prefers to speak, or is more fluent in, a language other than English
- health professional assesses the person as having difficulty communicating in spoken English
- health professional finds they are repeating themselves in more straightforward terms to help the person to understand (Yick & Daines, 2019).

If the health professional is in doubt, it is better to obtain the services of an interpreter than to leave it and hope the person with a culturally diverse background understands (Mollah et al., 2018).

Sometimes a suitable interpreter may not be available. There is a general lack of interpreters across Australia (Tomasi et al., 2022). The health professional also needs to be aware that many countries have multiple dialects. For instance, there are 18 major languages in India and over 1600 regional dialects. Additionally, health professionals must remember that some interpreters may not be well informed on mental health issues, giving rise to additional challenges in the communication process. Specifically, a lack of understanding of the relevant medical terms could lead to the relaying of inappropriate or incorrect information by interpreters to health professionals, or vice versa, which may result in misdiagnosis or inappropriate treatment. For this reason, the health professional must check for understanding with the person's family or community member, on an ongoing basis.

For people with culturally diverse backgrounds who are located in rural and remote areas or where no suitable interpreter is available, interpreters are now available by telephone or video linkup, and health professionals are encouraged to seek the most appropriate interpreter available.

IN PRACTICE

When is an interpreter needed?

Mrs Zhang is a 58-year-old Chinese woman who lives in Canberra with her daughter Min, son-in-law Eric and 6-year-old granddaughter Lina. Mrs Zhang speaks no English, while Min and Eric speak English fluently.

Min and Eric work long hours as they are saving to purchase a house. Mrs Zhang spends her time caring for Lina, and cooking, cleaning and washing for the family.

Mrs Zhang stayed in Australia on a temporary parent visa after her granddaughter was born. This visa required her to return to China periodically. More recently, Min and Eric had managed to secure permanent residency for Mrs Zhang.

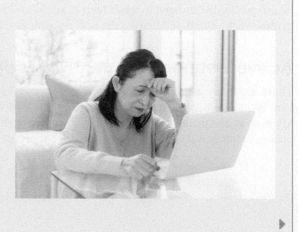

At first, Mrs Zhang felt happy that she was no longer required to travel home so often. As time went by, however, Mrs Zhang found that she missed seeing her extended family and community. She also felt increasingly isolated and excluded in Australia, especially once Lina started school. Lina was now practising speaking English with her parents, and Mrs Zhang could not understand the conversations.

Moreover, Mrs Zhang could not understand the Australian way of doing things. She watched the news each evening and, although she couldn't understand what was being said, she saw some shocking things happening on the screen. It seemed to her that people could do whatever they liked and there was no respect. Mrs Zhang began to feel anxious about her and her family's safety, especially after Min and Eric told her about some recent murders of women in Melbourne. Mrs Zhang decided she didn't want to go outside in case bad men were nearby, and she told Lina that she, too, should avoid going outdoors.

As time passed, Lina began to take on some of her grandmother's anxieties. She cried if her parents tried to take her to the park or on an outing over the weekend. Mrs Zhang would cry too and beg Min and Eric to stay at home where they would be safe. She even started to talk to them about the whole family going home to China.

Min was increasingly worried about her mother, who seemed anxious about everything and sometimes quite depressed. Min was also concerned that Lina might soon refuse to go to school. Min decided it was time to seek medical assistance for Mrs Zhang and Lina.

QUESTIONS

1. Mrs Zhang speaks no English, but her daughter speaks fluent English. Will there be a need for health professionals to obtain an interpreter for Mrs Zhang, or can they rely on the help of Lin to translate? Provide a rationale for your answer.

2. Lina speaks limited English, but her mother speaks fluent English. Is there a need for health professionals to obtain the services of an interpreter for Lina, or can they rely on the help of Lin to translate? Provide a rationale for your answer.

Information and education

The lack of culturally and linguistically appropriate information on mental health issues presents barriers to people with culturally diverse backgrounds, often preventing them from accessing services and achieving satisfactory health outcomes (Baker et al., 2019). People cannot consider the options available within the community without adequate information and knowledge. Information and knowledge are key factors in challenging stigma, empowering people and enabling participation (Fish & Fakoussa, 2018). Further, a lack of knowledge and understanding can generate anxiety, fear and feelings of disempowerment.

Several excellent websites provide resources and information about mental health issues for CALD populations, and a selection of these are provided at the end of this chapter. It is recommended that health professionals download information from relevant websites and offer this information in paper format to people with culturally diverse backgrounds, who may be unable or unwilling to access the internet.

Although ethnicity can impact a person's ability to seek information, support, and access the necessary services, there will also be times when the system fails to deal appropriately with difference or diversity (Moleiro et al., 2018). As noted in the section on rural and remote cultures, the Australian health system tends to take a 'one-size-fits-all' approach to providing treatment and care. For this reason, individual health professionals need to adapt their practice to accommodate the needs of the person with a culturally diverse background, facilitating the best possible outcomes for all concerned.

Actively supporting culturally appropriate services

There are many actions a health professional can take to ensure that culturally appropriate mental health care is made available to a person with a culturally diverse background. Some of these actions may relate to ensuring the health service can support diversity (Kaphle et al., 2022). Figure 4.5 lists the steps health professionals can take to make a difference for people with culturally diverse backgrounds.

Health professional checklist for culturally diverse consumers

☐ Is quality information available to consumers in various forms and languages?

☐ Are professional interpreters available?

☐ Do you provide interpreter services? Is there an interpreter sign in the reception area that people can use to identify their preferred language?

☐ Are there posters, pictures and other promotional materials in the office that reflect the diversity of the service's consumers?

☐ Have all staff and workers received accredited training in providing culturally appropriate health care?

☐ Have interpreters been provided with basic information and training about working with mental health consumers?

☐ Do your organisation's mission statement, policies and procedures incorporate principles and practices that promote diversity and cultural competency?

☐ Do evaluation mechanisms include assessing the number of consumers from diverse backgrounds against ethnic population distribution in the local area?

☐ Does the service work collaboratively with local ethnic-specific services to draw on their expertise?

☐ Does the service provide training to diverse consumers to support and work with other diverse consumers?

☐ Is the service aware of local ethnic-specific support groups? Does it refer to these services where appropriate?

Perhaps most important is the quality of the interactions a health professional has with the person and their family. To deliver culturally appropriate care, the health professional must build and maintain accepting, respectful and genuine therapeutic relationships (Nickerson et al., 2019). Ways to enable such partnerships or alliances are discussed in the chapter focusing on assessment in the mental health context. For people with culturally diverse backgrounds, this will also include the health professional:

- acknowledging cultural and subcultural influences and differences
- taking the necessary time to actively listen to the person and their family to identify how these cultural and subcultural influences may affect the provision of mental health care and mental health outcomes
- taking the necessary time to develop trust, always accepting and respecting differences
- ensuring support workers are engaged (e.g. interpreters, transcultural health professionals, Aboriginal and Torres Strait Islander mental health workers and members of the transgender community)
- providing as much information as possible to all concerned and discussing what this information may mean for them
- being flexible.

The alliance or relationship between a health professional and the person and their family needs to be mutual and therapeutic; the relationship with the health professional makes the most difference and supports the recovery process. In turn, this alliance will allow the health professional to raise issues such as the mental health and ill-health of the person and how they can most effectively address any needs (de Peralta et al., 2019).

UPON REFLECTION

Is your practice culturally appropriate?

Many health professionals assume that they are delivering culturally appropriate care. However, few consider just how cultural appropriateness is measured.

QUESTIONS

1. What three steps can you take to gauge your cultural competence or proficiency?

2. What can you do to improve your cultural competence or proficiency in the future?

3. What can you do to support colleagues to improve their cultural competence or proficiency in the future?

Working with families and communities

Working with families, communities, and individuals is integral to supporting the health and wellbeing of people with diverse cultural backgrounds. A collaborative and inclusive approach is integral to the recovery journey for people with mental illness, regardless of cultural background.

The principles of consumer-centred approaches to health care are described in the chapter on mental health care in Australia. The approaches can be expanded to include families, social networks (where possible) and communities, particularly for people from collectivist cultures. At the same time, a more inclusive approach is helpful for all people, with research on the concept of social capital indicating that socially embedded people are less vulnerable (Villalonga-Olives et al., 2022), particularly if they experince symptoms of mental illness. Family, friends or communities can offer the kind of support that a health professional cannot provide — specifically, unlike the social network, health professionals are not always available outside of business hours. Working with the family, friends and communities — including the leaders or elders of these communities — is an essential means by which health professionals can assist individuals.

The main principle underpinning social network or community strategies is that people with mental health problems are most often closely involved with their friends, families and/or communities, so it makes sense for the friends, family, or community members to be part of the solution. Sustainable outcomes are only achievable when the social network is supportive. The aim of social network or community strategies, then, is to design a more aligned plan to the realities of the world in which the mental health problems live.

Family Group Conferencing

One social network strategy used for people with mental illness from diverse cultures is Family Group Conferencing (FGC), a decision-making model originally established in the 1980s in New Zealand. This model is based on Māori traditions and values, such as involving the extended family in caring for children experiencing problems and their parents.

In the FGC vocabulary, people are not perceived as 'clients' or 'consumers', but rather as citizens experiencing problems who can be encouraged to develop a plan with the assistance of their social network (Meijer et al., 2019). An independent coordinator is assigned to the conference and, in collaboration with the person with a mental illness, invites the extended network (including family, friends and community members) to a meeting at a time and location convenient to each participant. The coordinator needs to be especially capable of encouraging the participation of attendees and ultimately ensuring a plan that is acceptable to and supported by all involved is formed (Schout, 2022). The FCG is family-driven, to address the person's aims as part of a social network and supported by that social network.

THE BIG PICTURE

Community-based education

Community-based education is crucial to improving the levels of mental health literacy in communities. Mental health literacy refers to the knowledge and beliefs of people about mental health and illness. Good mental health literacy can help people to recognise, manage and prevent mental health problems. Mental health literacy is often associated with a person's level of education and social support, the size of the person's social circle, and how individuals rate their health.

To support higher levels of mental health in people with culturally diverse backgrounds, health professionals can work with community leaders,

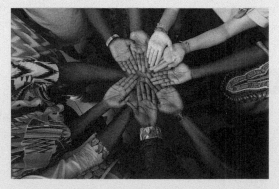

elders or groups to improve the mental health literacy of particular population groups and, in the process decrease stigma (Castillo et al., 2019). This health promotion strategy empowers culturally and linguistically diverse groups to proactively address the mental health issues experienced by community members through community-based education.

For example, the South Sudanese Community Association in Victoria received funding through the Victorian state government's Department of Health and Human Service to assist young people in the western suburbs of Melbourne. The program aims to build relationships and improve the capacity of

---

young people of the Victorian South Sudanese community who are at risk when interacting with the justice system. Activities include addressing behaviours, like substance misuse, that can lead to aggression and violence and roaming the streets. The program also raises awareness of unresolved grief, depression and suicidal feelings in Sudanese youth. Such community programs demonstrate how issues can be addressed when community members join together to address identified issues. Read more about this program at www.premier.vic.gov.au/targeted-support-risk-south-sudanese-youth.

SUMMARY

Australia is one of the most urbanised and multicultural nations in the world. People who belong to Indigenous Australian, rural and remote, CALD, LGBTQIA+ or other minority cultures have a lower health status than those who belong to the dominant Western-oriented culture. Health professionals are responsible for delivering culturally appropriate care, including providing services that are equitable and accessible.

This chapter provided some direction to health professionals to negotiate the complexities of cultural and subcultural diversity in the mental health context. Cultural constructions of mental health and illness were considered, particularly how these constructions influence the work of the health professional. The chapter discussed the mental health and wellbeing of Aboriginal and Torres strait Ilsnader peoples and the approaches health professionals can take to collaborate with Indigenous communities. The main mental health issues for people from rural and remote cultures in Australia were also examined, together with the role of rural and remote cultures in shaping and informing their mental health outcomes. Next, the chapter outlined the most significant aspects of providing mental health care to people with culturally diverse backgrounds and explained the importance of providing culturally appropriate care to all people with mental health issues. A focus was the primacy of the interpersonal or therapeutic relationship between the health professional and the person or community with whom they are working. The chapter concluded by emphasising the importance of families, social networks and communities in supporting the recovery of diverse people with mental health concerns.

KEY TERMS

burden of disease The overall impact of disease or injury on a society, including that which is beyond the immediate cost of treatment. The term incorporates individual, societal and economic costs.

collectivism A set of beliefs that upholds the group or collective/community as more important than the individual; this includes prioritising the goals or 'greater good' and identity of the group over those of the individual.

cultural awareness The state of awareness reached by a person who examines or reflects upon their own value-base and socio-politico-cultural beliefs in relation to the beliefs and value bases of different cultures.

cultural competence A level of practice achieved when health professionals integrate cultural awareness, knowledge and sensitivity into their practice.

cultural discourses Coherent bodies of statements or distinct frameworks that represent, maintain or develop 'reality' as understood by a particular culture.

cultural knowledge Understanding of the details of a particular culture, including the structures and accepted practices of that culture.

cultural proficiency A stage of practice that follows on from cultural competence. It is achieved by health professionals when they become advanced practitioners and lifelong learners in culturally appropriate health care.

cultural safety A state of being, practice or environment that is safe for people from all cultures. Cultural safety is about shared respect, shared meaning, shared knowledge and experience, learning together with dignity, and truly listening.

cultural sensitivity Being receptive and responsive to cultural differences as a means of developing appropriate interpersonal or therapeutic relationships with people.

culturally and linguistically diverse (CALD) A broad concept that refers to the wide range of cultural groups that make up a population or community and differ according to ethnicity, language, race, religion, social traditions and other factors.

culturally appropriate care The care that is provided to a person by a health professional that is consistent with the cultural values of the person who is unwell.

culture The accepted patterns of knowledge, beliefs, attitudes and behaviours by which a group of people live.

digital health Health services that allow people to access help from a health professional by phone or online without leaving their homes. Also known as eHealth services.

discrimination The unfair treatment of a person or group of people based on categories such as gender, age, class, relationship, ethnicity, culture, religion, health issue or disability.

double stigma The stigma experienced by those who have two or more 'labels' that are viewed negatively by a society; for example, a mental illness and racial minority, or a mental illness and unemployed status.

empowerment The process through which people become more able to influence the individuals and organisations that affect their lives.

gap in health service provision The descriptor often used by health professionals and health services to refer to the absence or lack of services in a particular location or area of health.

globalisation The process by which the world's nations, economies and cultures are becoming increasingly interdependent, a result of technological advancement and improved telecommunications infrastructures, transportation and business networks.

individualism A set of beliefs or an ideology where the 'self' is the most important consideration. This includes giving priority to one's own goals and one's own self-definition or actualisation over that of the group.

lesbian, gay, bisexual, transgender, queer or questioning, intersex and asexual and other gender non-conforming identities (LGBTQIA+) A minority group, nationally and internationally, whose sexuality and/or gender lies outside of the dominant heterosexual orientation or binary gender norm. The plus sign also refers to those not included in the LGBTQIA acronym, including allies.

migrant A person who moves from one place, region or country to another at their own volition.

norms The beliefs and values held by a social or cultural group about how members of that group should behave.

one-size-fits-all or **universalist approach** An approach or intervention that does not consider diversity or difference; rather, it demands that a standardised approach or intervention meet the needs of all people.

oral traditions The use of storytelling, song, dance or instructions to pass on specific cultural practices and values and beliefs.

post-traumatic stress disorder (PTSD) A diagnosed mental health condition characterised by the development of a long-lasting anxiety reaction following a traumatic or catastrophic event.

refugee A person who leaves the country of their nationality due to a well-founded fear that they will be persecuted for reasons of race, religion, nationality or membership of a particular social or political group.

rural–urban continuum A measurement of the way particular communities conform to levels of ruralism and urbanism.

social determinants of health The social factors that determine the health status of all people, including (but not limited to) early childhood development, disability, education, employment, gender, health services, housing, income, nutrition, social exclusion, social safety networks and race.

society A large group of people connected by proximity, politics, the economy, social status, social networks or some other shared interest.

stigma An attribute, behaviour or reputation that is perceived, constructed and/or represented by a group of people, society or culture negatively.

subculture The culture of smaller discrete groups of people, located within larger cultural groups, who share a subset of common attitudes, values, goals and practices.

transcultural A combining of the elements of, or extending through, more than one culture.

whole-of-life view of health An understanding of health as a state of wellbeing achieved through the balancing of mind, body, emotions, spirit, culture and the environment. The whole-of-life view of life is similar to the 'holistic' approach to health.

World Health Organization (WHO) An agency of the United Nations that is an overarching authority on international public health and coordinates international public health initiatives. WHO's headquarters are in Geneva, Switzerland.

REVIEW QUESTIONS

1 Define 'culture' and 'subculture'. How can a person's culture affect their view of mental health and illness?

2 What are three common myths about mental illness that many people erroneously believe?

3 Name five broad discourses that frame or inform the understanding of mental health and wellbeing of Indigenous Australians.
4 What are the social determinants of mental health for Aboriginal and Torres Strait Islander peoples?
5 How has urbanisation affected the Indigenous Australians?
6 Name and explain at least six common social determinants of health.
7 What are two issues for people living in rural areas who need to access mental health services?
8 Differentiate between the terms 'multicultural', 'transcultural' and 'culturally and linguistically diverse'.
9 What are the main mental health issues for refugees? What are the main mental health issues for migrants?
10 How can health professionals best support the mental health of people who belong to minority groups, such as lesbian, gay, bisexual, transgender, queer, intersex and asexual people?
11 Outline the differences between 'cultural safety', 'cultural awareness', 'cultural knowledge', 'cultural competence' and 'cultural proficiency'.
12 What can health professionals do to facilitate providing culturally appropriate mental health care to a person with a culturally diverse background?

DISCUSSION AND DEBATE

1 There are many examples to demonstrate the social and cultural construction of mental illness. For instance, before the 1970s, homosexuality was viewed as a mental illness or, in some societies, a criminal offence; but in Australia today same-sex couples are legally permitted to marry. Likewise, post-traumatic stress disorder (PTSD) only became an official psychiatric diagnosis in the 1980s after the Vietnam War to explain the effects of combat on some veterans. Identify other examples of how mental illness has changed with time or according to cultural norms. How do cultural constructions affect how health professionals help a person with a mental health problem?
2 Discuss the myths that many people believe about mental illness. Compare these myths to the representations of people with mental illness in the mass media, including in movies. How do these representations of people with mental illness influence the cultural myths? What more can be done to deconstruct cultural myths?
3 The Australian Human Rights Commission is advocating for recognising Aboriginal and Torres Strait Islander people in the Australian Constitution. What connection is there between recognising Aboriginal and Torres Strait Islander peoples in the Australian Constitution and improving health outcomes?
4 What are the main benefits and challenges facing Aboriginal and Torres Strait Islander health workers and Aboriginal and Torres Strait Islander mental health workers? What more can be done to support thesel health workers to 'close the gap' in the health status of Indigenous Australians?
5 Many rural and remote populations are known for their resilience. What factors have contributed to this resilience? What can health professionals learn from the resilience of rural and remote populations? What steps can people who live in metropolitan Australia take to develop the same resilience as those who live in rural locations?
6 What are the benefits and challenges for emergency services personnel who live and work in rural and remote Australia? What can be done to support emergency services personnel in rural and remote Australia to overcome the challenges of their work?
7 Consider the many barriers faced by migrant and refugee populations in Australia. Also consider the impact of these barriers on the mental health of the migrants and refugees. Discuss the barriers and their impact, considering how they can be overcome by migrant or refugee people.
8 Consider the notions of 'one-size-fits-all' in the context of health service delivery in a multicultural society. When can standardisation be considered a good thing? How can health professionals ensure that a high standard of equitable health services is maintained while also allowing for diversity?

PROJECT ACTIVITY

People with mental health issues will look to those around them and the attitudes, values, goals and practices of the communities to which they belong to explain their distress (Bhugra et al., 2021). This sociocultural construction of mental health and illness can impact how health professionals provide support.

Approach at least four people from different cultures or subcultures and talk to them about how their cultural group perceives mental health and illness. These different cultural groups could include:

- migrant or refugee cultures
- Aboriginal and Torres Strait Islander peoples
- diverse professional groups (e.g. allied health, emergency services personnel, nurses, public servants)
- older people
- young people.

Questions to ask these people could include the following questions.

- How do you and/or your cultural group perceive 'mental illness'?
- How have these perceptions changed over time?
- How do these perceptions influence how you and/or your cultural group interact with people with mental illness?

In light of these conversations, reflect on the following questions, and write answers in your practice reflection journal to the following questions.

- As I was growing up, how did I perceive people with mental illness? What factors influenced these perceptions?
- How have my perceptions of mental illness changed over time? What factors have influenced my current perceptions?
- How do my past and present perceptions of mental illness compare to those of the people I interviewed?
- What struck me most about my conversations about mental illness with people from diverse cultures? Why?
- What did I learn from my conversations? How could this learning change my professional practice?

WEBSITES

1 The Australian Indigenous Health *InfoNet* is an innovative internet resource that aims to inform practice and policy in Indigenous Australian health by making research and other knowledge readily accessible. Health*InfoNet* aims to contribute to 'closing the gap' in health between Indigenous and other Australians: www.healthinfonet.ecu.edu.au.

2 The National Rural Health Alliance (the Alliance) comprises 45 national organisations committed to improving the health and wellbeing of the 7 million people in rural and remote Australia. The diverse membership of the Alliance includes representation from the Aboriginal and Torres Strait Islander health sector, health professional organisations, health service providers, health educators and students: www.ruralhealth.org.au.

3 The Australian Refugee Association (ARRA) believes in the desire and capacity of refugees to be part of Australia's culture and economic life. The ARRA provides advice, assistance, advocacy and practical support with settlement services, migration services, employment services, public education, policy and advocacy: www.australianrefugee.org.

4 Embrace Multicultural Mental Health is run by Mental Health Australia and provides a national focus on mental health and suicide prevention for people from CALD backgrounds. https://embracementalhealth.org.au.

5 LGBTIQ+ Health Australia is the peak health organisation in Australia, supporting and advising individuals and groups that provide health-related programs, services and research focused on lesbian, gay, bisexual, transgender, intersex, queer and other sexuality, gender and bodily diverse people and communities: www.lgbtiqhealth.org.au.

7 Mental Health Australia is the peak, national non-government organisation representing and promoting the interests of the Australian mental health sector. Consumer and carer participation in all levels of decision making is fundamental for the improvement of mental health services and crucial to improving the lives of people with a mental illness: www.mhaustralia.org/about-us.

REFERENCES

Abbott, P., Lloyd, J., Joshi, C., Malera-Bandjalan, K., Baldry, E., McEntyre, E., & Harris, M. (2018). Do programs for Aboriginal and Torres Strait Islander people leaving prison meet their health and social support needs? *Australian Journal of Rural Health*, 26(1), 6–13. https://doi.org/10.1111/ajr.12396

Adams, M., Lazarsfeld-Jensen, A., & Francis, K. (2019). The implications of isolation for remote industrial health workers. *Rural and Remote Health*, 19(2), 5001. https://doi.org/10.22605/RRH5001

American Psychiatric Association. (2013). *Diagnostic and statistical manual of mental disorders* (5th ed.). https://doi.org/10.1176/appi.books.9780890425787

Amnesty International. (2022). *Refugees, asylum-seekers and migrants.* www.amnesty.org/en/what-we-do/refugees-asylum-seekers-and-migrants

Andrade, J. (2019). Determining the associations between dietetic-related activities and undergraduate dietetic students' general cultural knowledge, attitudes, and beliefs. *Nutrients, 11*(6), 1202. https://doi.org/10.3390/nu11061202

Australian Bureau of Statistics. (2021). *30% of Australia's population born overseas.* Canberra, Australian Government. www.abs.gov.au/media-centre/media-releases/30-australias-population-born-overseas

Australian Bureau of Statistics. (2017). *Census of population and housing: Reflecting Australia – stories from the Census, 2016.* ABS. (cat. no. 2071.0)

Australian Bureau of Statistics. (2022). *Census of population and housing – Counts of Aboriginal and Torres Strait Islander Australians.* Australian Government. www.abs.gov.au/statistics/people/aboriginal-and-torres-strait-islander-peoples/census-population-and-housing-counts-aboriginal-and-torres-strait-islander-australians/latest-release

Australian Child and Adolescent Trauma, Loss and Grief Network. (n.d.). *Refugees and asylum seekers: Supporting recovery from trauma.* Australian National University. https://tgn.anu.edu.au/wp-content/uploads/2014/10/Refugees-and-asylum-seekers-Supporting-recovery-from-trauma_0.pdf

Australian Human Rights Commission. (2017). *Aboriginal and Torres Strait Islander social justice.* AHRC. www.humanrights.gov.au/our-work/aboriginal-and-torres-strait-islander-social-justice

Australian Human Rights Commission. (1997). *Bringing them home: Report of the national inquiry into the separation of Aboriginal and Torres Strait Islander children from their families.* www.humanrights.gov.au/publications/bringing-them-home-report-1997

Australian Institute of Aboriginal and Torres Strait Island Studies. (2018). *Indigenous Australians: Aboriginal and Torres Strait Island people.* AIATSIS. www.aiatsis.gov.au/explore/indigenous-australians-aboriginal-and-torres-strait-islander-people

Australian Institute of Health and Welfare. (2022a). *Alcohol, tobacco and other drugs in Australia.* AIHW. www.aihw.gov.au/reports/alcohol/alcohol-tobacco-other-drugs-australia/contents/priority-populations/aboriginal-and-torres-strait-islander-people

Australian Institute of Health and Welfare. (2022b). *Australian burden of disease study: Impact and causes of illness and death in Aboriginal and Torres Strait Islander people 2018.* AIHW. www.aihw.gov.au/reports/burden-of-disease/illness-death-indigenous-2018/summary

Australian Institute of Health and Welfare (AIHW). (2022c). *Determinants of health for Indigenous Australians.* Canberra, Australian government. www.aihw.gov.au/reports/australias-health/social-determinants-and-indigenous-health

Australian Institute of Health and Welfare (AIHW). (2022d). *Profile of Indigenous Australians.* Canberra, Australian government. www.aihw.gov.au/reports/australias-health/profile-of-indigenous-australians

Australian Institute of Health and Welfare (AIHW). (2022e). *Rural and remote health.* Canberra, Australian government. www.aihw.gov.au/reports/rural-remote-australians/rural-and-remote-health

Australian Institute of Health and Welfare. (2021a). *1.23 Leading causes of mortality.* AIHW. www.indigenoushpf.gov.au/measures/1-23-leading-causes-mortality

Australian Institute of Health and Welfare. (2021b). *2.05 Education outcomes for young people.* AIHW. www.indigenoushpf.gov.au/measures/2-05-education-outcomes-young-people

Australian Institute of Health and Welfare. (2021c). *Indigenous income and finance.* AIHW. www.aihw.gov.au/reports/australias-welfare/indigenous-income-and-finance

Australian Institute of Health and Welfare. (2021d). *Social isolation and loneliness.* AIWH. www.aihw.gov.au/reports/australias-welfare/social-isolation-and-loneliness-covid-pandemic

Australian Institute of Health and Welfare. (2021e). *Suicide & self-harm monitoring: Deaths by suicide amongst Indigenous Australians.* AIWH www.aihw.gov.au/suicide-self-harm-monitoring/data/populations-age-groups/suicide-indigenous-australians

Australian Institute of Health and Welfare. (2021f). *Suicide & self-harm monitoring: Deaths by suicide by remoteness.* AIHW. www.aihw.gov.au/suicide-self-harm-monitoring/data/geography/suicide-by-remoteness-areas

Australian Institute of Health and Welfare. (2019). *Indigenous housing.* AIHW. www.aihw.gov.au/reports/australias-welfare/indigenous-housing

Australian Institute of Health and Welfare. (2018). *Australia's health 2018: In brief: 5.5 Lesbian, gay, bisexual, transgender and intersex people. AIHW.* www.aihw.gov.au/reports/australias-health/australias-health-2018

Australian Institute of Health and Welfare (AIHW) & National Indigenous Australians Agency (NIAA). (2020a). *1.19 Life expectancy at birth. Canberra, Australian government.* www.indigenoushpf.gov.au/measures/1-19-life-expectancy-birth

Australian Institute of Health and Welfare (AIHW) & National Indigenous Australians Agency (NIAA). (2020b). *3.12 Aboriginal and Torres Strait Islander people in the health workforce. Canberra, Australian government.* www.indigenoushpf.gov.au/measures/3-12-atsi-people-health-workforce

Atkins, M., & Lay, B. (2018). Association between K10 psychological distress score, Epworth sleepiness scores and physical health in fly in–fly out mine workers. *Internal Medicine Journal, 48*, 24–24. https://doi.org/10.1111/imj.13829

Baker, J., Raman, S., Kohlhoff, J., George, A., Kaplun, C., Dadich, A., Best, C., Arora, A., Zwi, K., Schmied, V., & Eapen, V. (2019). Optimising refugee children's health/wellbeing in preparation for primary and secondary school: A qualitative inquiry. *BMC Public, 19*, 812. https://doi.org/10.1186/s12889-019-7183-5

Barkan, S. (2017). *Health, illness and society: An introduction to medical sociology.* Rowman & Littlefield.

Baum, F., Graycar, A., Delany-Crowe, T., de Leeuw, E., Bacchi, C., Popay, J., & Harris, E. (2019). Understanding Australian policies on public health using social and political science theories: Reflections from an Academy of the Social Sciences in Australia workshop. *Health Promotion International, 34*(4), 833–846. https://doi.org/10.1093/heapro/day014

Best, O., & Fredericks, B. (2018). *Yatdjuligin: Aboriginal and Torres Strait Islander nursing and midwifery care.* Cambridge University Press.

Bharadwaj, J. (2018). *You made the right move, "Australia is one of the world's most inclusive country".* SBS Hindi. www.sbs. com.au/language/english/audio/you-made-the-right-move-australia-is-one-of-the-world-s-most-inclusive-country

Bhugra, D., & Bhui, K (Eds.). (2018). *Textbook of cultural psychiatry.* Cambridge University Press.

Bhugra, D., Watson, C., & Ventriglio, A. (2021). Migration, cultural capital and acculturation. *International Review of Psychiatry, 33*(1–2), 126–131. https://doi.org/10.1080/09540261.2020.1733786

Blignault, I., & Kaur, A. (2019). Integration of traditional and western treatment approaches in mental health care in Pacific Island Countries. *Australasian Psychiatry.* https://doi.org/10.1177/1039856219859273

Brown, L., Jones, G., & Bond, M. (2019). E-health: Psychosocial challenges for South Australian rural mental health consumers. *Rural and Remote Health, 19*(3), 1–10. www.rrh.org.au/journal/article/5103

Bryant, L., Garnham, B., Tedmanson, D., & Diamandi, S. (2018). Tele-social work and mental health in rural and remote communities in Australia. *International Social Work, 61*(1), 143–155. https://doi.org/10.1177/0020872815606794

Busija, L., Cinelli, R., Toombs, M., Easton, C., Hampton, R., Holdsworth, K., & McCabe, M. (2018). The role of elders in the wellbeing of a contemporary Australian Indigenous community. *The Gerontologist, 60*(3), 513–524. https://doi.org/10.1093/geront/gny140

Butler, T., Anderson, K., Garvey, G., Cunningham, J., Ratcliffe, J., Tong, A., Whop, L., Cass, A., Dickson, M., & Howard, K. (2019). Aboriginal and Torres Strait Islander people's domains of wellbeing: A comprehensive literature review. *Social Science & Medicine, 233*, 138–157. https://doi.org/10.1016/j.socscimed.2019.06.004

Calma, T., Dudgeon, P., & Bray, A. (2017). Aboriginal and Torres Strait Islander social and emotional wellbeing and mental health. *Australian Psychologist, 52*(4), 255–260.

Castillo, E., Ijadi-Maghsoodi, R., Shadravan, S., Moore, E., Mensah, M., Docherty, M., Nunez, M. G. A., Barcelo, N., Goodsmith, N., Halpin, L. E., Morton, I., Mango, J., Montero, A. E., Koushkaki, S. R., Bromley, E., Chung, B., Jones, F., Gabrielian, S., Gelberg, L., & Wells, K. B. (2019). Community interventions to promote mental health and social equity. *Current Psychiatry Reports, 21*(5), 35. https://doi.org/10.1111/ap.12299

Carey, T., Sirett, D., Wakerman, J., Russell, D., & Humphreys, J. (2018). What principles should guide visiting primary health care services in rural and remote communities? Lessons from a systematic review. *Australian Journal of Rural Health, 26*(3), 146–156. https://doi.org/10.1111/ajr.12425

Cendales, B., & Ortiz, V. (2019). Cultural values and the job demands-control model of stress: A moderation analysis. *International Journal of Stress Management, 26*(3), 223–237. https://doi.org/10.1037/str0000105

The Center for Culturally Proficient Educational Practice. (2019). *The guiding principles.* www.ccpep.org/home/what-is-cultural-proficiency/guiding-principles

Cheers, B. (2019). *Welfare bushed: Social care in rural Australia.* Routledge.

Coates, D., Saleeba, C., & Howe, D. (2019). Mental health attitudes and beliefs in a community sample on the Central Coast in Australia: Barriers to help seeking. *Community Mental Health Journal, 55*(3), 476–486. https://doi.org/10.1007/s10597-018-0270-8

Cohen, S., Cook, S., Sando, T., & Sabik, N. (2018). What aspects of rural life contribute to rural-urban health disparities in older adults? Evidence from a national survey. *Journal of Rural Health, 34*(3), 293–230. https://doi.org/10.1111/jrh.12287

Coleman, P. (2018). Cultural differences in general and psychiatric nurses: A critical analysis using social identity theory. *Aporia, 10*(2), 17–27. https://doi.org/10.18192/aporia.v10i2.4122

Cottrell, M., Judd, P., Comans, T., Easton, P., & Chang, A. (2021). Comparing fly-in fly-out and telehealth models for delivering advanced-practice physiotherapy services in regional Queensland: An audit of outcomes and costs. *Journal of Telemedicine and Telecare, 27*(1), 32–38. https://doi.org/10.1177/1357633x19858036

Coombes, J., Lukaszyk, C., Keay, L., Ivers, R., Sherrington, C., Tiedemann, A., & Moore, R. (2018). First Nation Elders' perspectives on healthy ageing in NSW, Australia. *Australian and New Zealand Journal of Public Health, 42*(4), 361–364. https://doi.org/10.1111/1753-6405.12796

Cronin, T., Pepping, C., Halford, W., & Lyons, A. (2021). Mental health help-seeking and barriers to service access among lesbian, gay, and bisexual Australians. *Australian Psychologist, 56*(1), 46–60. https://doi.org/10.1080/00050067.2021.1890981

Cultural Survival. (2018). *The issues.* www.culturalsurvival.org/issues

Currie, G. (2022). Yindyamarra Winhanganha: A conduit to indigenous cultural proficiency. *Journal of Nuclear Medicine Technology, 50*(1), 66–72. https://doi.org/10.2967/jnmt.121.262436

Dawson, J., Laccos-Barrett, K., Hammond, C., & Rumbold, A. (2022). Reflexive practice as an approach to improve healthcare delivery for indigenous peoples: A systematic critical synthesis and exploration of the cultural safety education literature. *International Journal of Environmental Research and Public Health, 19*(11), 6691. https://doi.org/10.3390/ijerph19116691

de Peralta, A., Gillispie, M., Mobley, C., & Gibson, L. (2019). It's all about trust and respect: Cultural competence and cultural humility in mobile health clinic services for underserved minority populations. *Journal of Health Care for the Poor & Underserved, 30*(3), 1103–1118. https://doi.org/10.1353/hpu.2019.0076

Department of Economic and Social Affairs. (n.d.). *Indigenous peoples at the UN.* www.un.org/development/desa/indigenouspeoples/about-us.html

Department of Health. (2019). *Primary Health Networks (PHN) primary mental health care guidance — Aboriginal and Torres Strait Islander Mental Health Services.* Australian Government. www.health.gov.au/sites/default/files/documents/2021/04/primary-health-networks-phn-primary-mental-health-care-guidance-aboriginal-and-torres-strait-islander-mental-health-services-primary-health-networks-phn-primary-mental-health-care-guidance-aboriginal-and-torres-strait-isla.pdf

Department of Health and Aged Care. (2022a). *National Aboriginal and Torres Strait Islander health workforce strategic framework and implementation plan 2021–2031.* Australian Government. www.health.gov.au/resources/publications/national-aboriginal-and-torres-strait-islander-health-workforce-strategic-framework-and-implementation-plan-2021-2031

Department of Health and Aged Care. (2022b). *Rural, remote and metropolitan area.* Australian Government. www.health.gov.au/health-topics/rural-health-workforce/classifications/rrma

Department of Health and Aged Care. (2022c). *Telehealth.* Australian Government. www.health.gov.au/health-topics/health-technologies-and-digital-health/about/telehealth

Department of Health and Aged Care. (2021). *Digital mental health services.* Australian Government. www.health.gov.au/initiativ es-and-programs/digital-mental-health-services

Department of Health and Aged Care. (n.d.). *Mental health services for people of culturally and linguistically diverse (CALD) backgrounds.* www.health.gov.au/resources/publications/mental-health-services-for-people-of-culturally-and-linguistically-dive rse-cald-backgrounds

Department of Health and Aged Care. (2020). *Head to health.* Australian Government. www.headtohealth.gov.au

Department of Home Affairs. (2022). *Disaster assist.* Australian Government. www.disasterassist.gov.au

Dowling, A., Enticott, J., Kunin, M., & Russell, G. (2019). The association of migration experiences on the self-rated health status among adult humanitarian refugees to Australia: An analysis of a longitudinal cohort study. *International Journal for Equity in Health, 18*(1). https://doi.org/10.1186/s12939-019-1033-z

Doyle, K., Hungerford, C., & Cleary, M. (2017). Study of intra-racial exclusion within Australian Indigenous communities using eco-maps. *International Journal of Mental Health Nursing, 26*(2), 129–141. https://doi.org/10.1111/inm.12259

Driscoll, C., Darian-Smith, K., & Nichols, D. (2017). *Cultural sustainability in rural communities: Rethinking Australian Country Towns.* Routledge.

Dudgeon, P., & Bray, A. (2018). Indigenous healing practices in Australia. *Women & Therapy, 41*(1–2), 97–113. https://doi.org/10.1080/02703149.2017.1324191

Dudgeon, P., Darwin, L., Hirvonen, T., Boe, M., Johnson, R., Cox, R., Gregory, L., McKenna, R., McKenna, V., Smith, D., Turner, J., Von Helle, S., & Garrett, L. (2018). We are not the problem, we are part of the solution: Indigenous Lived Experience Project Report. *Centre of Best Practice in Aboriginal and Torres Strait Islander Suicide Prevention and Black Dog Institute.* www.black doginstitute.org.au/wp-content/uploads/2020/04/lived-experience-report-final-nov-2018.pdf

Dur, Ş., Göl, İ., & Erkin, Ö. (2022). The effects of nursing students' conscientious intelligence on their cultural sensitivity levels. *Perspectives in Psychiatric Care, 58*(2), 795–803. https://doi.org/10.1111/ppc.12852

Dwyer, A., de Almeida Neto, A., Estival, D., Li, W., Lam-Cassettari, C., & Antoniou, M. (2021). Suitability of text-based communications for the delivery of psychological therapeutic services to rural and remote communities: Scoping review. *JMIR Mental Health, 8*(2), e19478. https://doi.org/10.2196/19478

Ellis, N., & Albrecht, G. (2017). Climate change threats to family farmers' sense of place and mental wellbeing: A case study from the Western Australian Wheatbelt. *Social Science & Medicine, 175,* 161–168. https://doi.org/10.1016/j.socscimed.2017.01.009

Erikson, K. (1966). *Wayward puritans: A study in the sociology of deviance.* Wiley.

Fay, J. (2018). Decolonising mental health services one prejudice at a time: Psychological, sociological, ecological, and cultural considerations. *Settler Colonial Studies, 8*(1), 47–59. https://doi.org/10.1080/2201473X.2016.1199828

Fennell, K., Hull, M., Jones, M., & Dollman, J. (2018). A comparison of barriers to accessing services for mental and physical health conditions in a sample of rural Australian adults. *Rural and Remote Health, 18*(1), 1–12. https://doi.org/10.22605/RRH4155

Fernando, T., & Bennett, B. (2019). Creating a culturally safe space when teaching Aboriginal content in social work: A scoping review. *Australian Social Work, 72*(1), 47–61. https://doi.org/10.1080/0312407X.2018.1518467

Fish, M., & Fakoussa, O. (2018). Towards culturally inclusive mental health: Learning from focus groups with those with refugee and asylum seeker status in Plymouth. *International Journal of Migration, Health& Social Care, 14*(4), 361–376. https://doi.org/10.1108/IJMHSC-12-2017-0050

Fisher, M., Battams, S., McDermott, D., Baum, F., & MacDougall, C. (2019). How the social determinants of Indigenous health became policy reality for Australia's National Aboriginal and Torres Strait Islander Health Plan. *Journal of Social Policy, 48*(1), 169–189. https://doi.org/10.1017/S0047279418000338

Fogarty, W., Lovell, M., Langenberg, J., & Heron, M. (2018). *Deficit discourse and strengths-based approaches: Changing the narrative of Aboriginal and Torres Strait islander health and wellbeing.* Lowitja Institute. www.lowitja.org.au/page/services/res ources/Cultural-and-social-determinants/racism/deficit-discourse-strengths-based

Foucault, M. (1961). *The history of madness.* [trans.] J. Khalfa & J. Murphy. Routledge. 2006

Friskie, S. (2020). The healing power of storytelling: Finding identity through narrative. *The Arbutus Reviews, 11*(1), 19–27. https://doi.org/10.18357/tar111202019324

Gao, S., Corrigan, P., Qin, S., & Nieweglowski, K. (2019). Comparing Chinese and European American mental health decision making. *Journal of Mental Health, 28*(2), 141–147. https://doi.org/10.1080/09638237.2017.1417543

Geerlings, L., Thompson, C., Bouma, R., & Hawkins, R. (2018). Cultural competence in clinical psychology training: A qualitative investigation of student and academic experiences. *Australian Psychologist, 53*(2), 161–170. https://doi.org/10.1111/ap.12291

Goffman, E. (1961). *Asylums.* Anchor.

Göl, İ., & Erkin, Ö. (2019). Association between cultural intelligence and cultural sensitivity in nursing students: A cross-sectional descriptive study. *Collegian, 26*(4), 485–491. https://doi.org/10.1016/j.colegn.2018.12.007

Goldberg, L., Rosenburg, N., & Watson, J. (2018). Rendering LGBTQ+ visible in nursing: Embodying the philosophy of caring science. *Journal of Holistic Nursing, 36*(3), 262–271. https://doi.org/10.1177/0898010117715141

Gopalkrishnan, N. (2018). Cultural diversity and mental health: Considerations for policy and practice. *Frontiers in Public Health, 6,* 179. https://doi.org/10.3389/fpubh.2018.00179

Gwynne, K., & Lincoln, M. (2017). Developing the rural health workforce to improve Australian Aboriginal and Torres Strait Islander health outcomes: A systematic review. *Australian Health Review, 41*(2), 234–238. https://doi.org/10.1071/AH15241

Hall, S. (1980). *Culture, media, language: working papers in cultural studies, 1972–1979.* Hutchinson Centre for Contemporary Cultural Studies University of Birmingham.

Handley, T., Lewin, T., Perkins, D., & Kelly, B. (2018). Self-recognition of mental health problems in a rural Australian sample. *Australian Journal of Rural Health, 26*(3), 173–180. https://doi.org/10.1111/ajr.12406

Harfield, S., Davy, C., McArthur, A., Munn, Z., Brown, A., & Brown, N. (2018). Characteristics of Indigenous primary health care service delivery models: A systematic scoping review. Globalization *and Health, 14*(1), 12. https://doi.org/10.1186/s12992-018-0332-2

Healthdirect. (2018). *Natural disasters*. www.healthdirect.gov.au/natural-disasters

Hefler, M., Kerrigan, V., Henryks, J., Freeman, B., & Thomas, D. (2018). Social media and health information sharing among Australian Indigenous people. *Health Promotion International, 34*(4), 706–715. https://doi.org/10.1093/heapro/day018

Henderson, J., Dawson, S., Fuller, J., O'Kane, D., Gerace, A., Oster, C., & Cochrane, E. (2018). Regional responses to the challenge of delivering integrated care to older people with mental health problems in rural Australia. *Aging & Mental Health, 22*(8), 1031–1037. https://doi.org/10.1080/13607863.2017.1320702

Hendrie, D. (2018). *Major life expectancy gap among Aboriginal and Torres Strait Islander people. NewsGP, Royal Australian College of General Practitioners*. www1.racgp.org.au/newsgp/clinical/life-expectancy-gap-between-remote-and-urban-abori

Hensel, J., Ellard, K., Koltek, M., Wilson, G., & Sareen, J. (2019). Digital Health solutions for Indigenous mental well-being. *Current Psychiatry Reports, 21*(8), 68. https://doi.org/10.1007/s11920-019-1056-6

Hill, A., Lyons, A., Power, J., Amos, N., Ferlatte, O., Jones, J., Carman, M., & Bourne, A. (2022). Suicidal ideation and suicide attempts among lesbian, gay, bisexual, pansexual, queer, and asexual youth: Differential impacts of sexual orientation, verbal, physical, or sexual harassment or assault, conversion practices, family or household religiosity, and school experience. *LGBT Health, 9*(5), 313–324. https://doi.org/10.1089/lgbt.2021.0270

Hine, R., Maybery, D., & Goodyear, M. (2018). Challenges of connectedness in personal recovery for rural mothers with mental illness. *International Journal of Mental Health Nursing, 27*(2), 672–682. https://doi.org/10.1111/inm.12353

Hogan, M. (2019). *Collectivism and individualism: It's not either/or, it's both. Psychology Today*. www.psychologytoday.com/au/blog/in-one-lifespan/201906/collectivism-and-individualism

Hughes, M. (2018). Health and well being of lesbian, gay, bisexual, transgender and intersex people aged 50 years and over. *Australian Health Review, 42*(2), 146–151. https://doi.org/10.1071/AH16200

Hultsjö, S., Bachrach-Lindström, M., Safipour, J., & Hadziabdic, E. (2019). 'Cultural awareness requires more than theoretical education' — Nursing students' experiences. *Nurse Education in Practice, 39*, 73–79. https://doi.org/10.1016/j.nepr.2019.07.009

Human Rights Campaign. (n.d.). *Resources: Glossary of terms*. www.hrc.org/resources/glossary-of-terms

International Working Group on Indigenous Affairs. (2001). *Indigenous Peoples and the United Nations System*. Office of the High Commissioner for Human Rights, United Nations Office www.un.org/development/desa/indigenouspeoples/about-us.html

Jackson, K., Roberts, R., & McKay, R. (2019). Older people's mental health in rural areas: Converting policy into service development, service access and a sustainable workforce. *Australian Journal of Rural Health, 27*(4), 358–365. https://doi.org/10.1111/ajr.12529

Jacobs, R., & Morris, S. (2016). *National lesbian, gay, bisexual, transgender and intersex mental health and suicide prevention strategy: A new strategy for inclusion and action*. National LGBTI Health Alliance.

Jetten, J., Dane, S., Williams, E., Liu, S., Haslam, C., Gallois, C., & McDonald, V. (2018). Ageing well in a foreign land as a process of successful social identity change. *International Journal of Qualitative Studies on Health and Well-Being, 13*(1), 1. https://doi.org/10.1080/17482631.2018.1508198

Joseph, A. (2019). Constituting 'lived experience' discourses in mental health: The ethics of racialized identification/representation and the erasure of intergeneration colonial violence. *Journal of Ethics in Mental Health. 10* https://jemh.ca/issues/v9/documents/JEMH%20Inclusion%20i.pdf

Kaphle, S., Hungerford, C., Blanchard, D., Doyle, K., Ryan, C., & Cleary, M. (2022). Cultural safety or cultural competence: How can we address inequities in culturally diverse groups? *Issues in Mental Health Nursing, 43*(7), 698–702. https://doi.org/10.1080/01612840.2021.1998849

Kewley, C., Hazelton, M., & Newman, L. (2018). Reconciling incommensurate world health views and explanatory models of mental illness: A New model of integrated mental health care for culturally diverse populations (Conference Abstract). *International Journal of Integrated Care, 18*(s2), 308. http://doi.org/10.5334/ijic.s2308

Khawaja, N., Kamo, R., & Ramirez, E. (2021). Building resilience in transcultural adults: Investigating the effect of a strength-based programme. *Australian Psychologist, 56*(4), 324–334. https://doi.org/10.1080/00050067.2021.1919489

Kiely, K., Brady, B., & Byles, J. (2019). Gender, mental health and ageing. *Maturitas, 129*, 76–84.

Kilicaslan, J., & Petrakis, M. (2019). Heteronormative models of health-care delivery: Investigating staff knowledge and confidence to meet the needs of LGBTIQ+ people. *Social Work in Health Care, 58*(6), 612–632. https://doi.org/10.1016/j.maturitas.2019.09.004

Kirmayer, L., Adeponle, A., & Dzokoto, V. (2018). Varieties of global psychology: Cultural diversity and constructions of the self. In S. Fernando & R. Moodley (Eds.), *Global psychologies* (pp. 21–37). Palgrave Macmillan.

Krakouer J Wise, S., & Connolly, M. (2018). 'We live and breathe through culture': Conceptualising cultural connection for Indigenous Australian children in out-of-home care. *Australian Social Work, 71*(3), 265–276. https://doi.org/10.1080/0312407X.2018.1454485

Lebaron, V. (2018). What is the rural cultural perspective? *Oncology Nursing Forum, 45*(6), 683–685. https://doi.org/10.1188/18.ONF.683-685

LeBlanc, M., Petrie, S., Paskaran, S., Carson, D., & Peters, P. (2020). Patient and provider perspectives on eHealth interventions in Canada and Australia: A scoping review. *Rural and Remote Health, 20*(3), 1–11. https://doi.org/10.22605/RRH5754

Leininger, M. (1997). Transcultural nursing research to transform nursing education and practice: 40 years on. *Journal of Nursing Scholarship, 29*(4), 341–347. https://doi.org/10.1111/j.1547-5069.1997.tb01053.x

Leininger, M (Ed.). (1988). *Care: The essence of nursing and health*. Wayne State University Press.

Levine, M., & Levine, A. (1970). *A social history of helping services: Clinic, court, school and community*. Appleton-Century-Crofts.

Lewis, T., Hill, A., Bond, C., & Nelson, A. (2017). Yarning: Assessing proppa ways. *Journal of Clinical Practice in Speech-Language Pathology, 19*(1), 14–18. www.speechpathologyaustralia.cld.bz/JCPSLP-Vol-19-No-1-March-2017/16

LGBTQIA Resource Centre. (2019). *LGBTQIA Resource Centre Glossary*. University of California. www.lgbtqia.ucdavis.edu/educated/glossary

LGBTIQ+ Health Australia. (2021). *Snapshot of mental health and suicide prevention statistics for LGBTIQ+ People.* www.lgbtiq health.org.au/statistics

Life in Mind. (2023). *Effective suicide prevention strategies. Everymind.* https://lifeinmind.org.au/about-suicide/suicide-prevention/effective-suicide-prevention-strategies

Loganathan, S., & Varghese, M. (2019). Formative research on devising a street play to create awareness about mental illness: Cultural adaptation and targeted approach. *International Journal of Social Psychiatry, 65*(4), 279–288. https://doi.org/10.1177/0020764019838306

Malatzky, C., & Glenister, K. (2019). Talking about overweight and obesity in rural Australian general practice. *Health and Social Care in the Community, 27*(3), 599–608. https://doi.org/10.1111/hsc.12672

Markwick, A., Ansari, Z., Clinch, D., & McNeil, J. (2019). Perceived racism may partially explain the gap in health between Aboriginal and non-Aboriginal Victorians: A cross-sectional population based study. *SSM — Population Health, 7*, 100310. https://doi.org/10.1016/j.ssmph.2018.10.010

Martin, R., Fernandes, C., Taylor, C., Crow, A., Headland, D., Shaw, N., & Zammit, S. (2019). 'We don't want to live like this': The lived experience of dislocation, poor health, and homelessness for Western Australian Aboriginal people. *Qualitative Health Research, 29*(2), 159–172. https://doi.org/10.1177/1049732318797616

Mbuzi, V., Fulbrook, P., & Jessup, M. (2018). Effectiveness of programs to promote cardiovascular health of Indigenous Australians: A systematic review. *International Journal for Equity in Health, 17*(1). https://doi.org/10.1186/s12939-018-0867-0

McBride, K., Franks, C., Wade, V., King, V., Rigney, J., Burton, N., Dowling, A., Howard, N. J., Paquet, C., Hillier, S., Nicholls, S. J., & Brown, A. (2021). Good heart: Telling stories of cardiovascular protective and risk factors for aboriginal women. *Heart, Lung & Circulation, 30*(1), 69–77. https://doi.org/10.1016/j.hlc.2020.09.931

McCallum, K., & Waller, L. (2017). Indigenous media studies in Australia: traditions, theories and contemporary practices. In J. Budarick & G. S. Han (Eds.), *Minorities and media* (pp. 105–124). Palgrave Macmillan.

McDermott, E., Hughes, & Rawlings, V. (2018). Norms and normalisation: Understanding lesbian, gay, bisexual, transgender and queer youth, suicidality and help-seeking. *Culture, Health & Sexuality, 20*(2), 156–172. https://doi.org/10.1080/13691058.2017.1335435

McGough, S., Wynaden, D., & Wright, M. (2018). Experience of providing cultural safety in mental health to Aboriginal patients: A grounded theory study. *International Journal of Mental Health Nursing, 27*(1), 204–213. https://doi.org/10.1111/inm.12310

McPhail-Bell, K., Appo, N., Haymes, A., Bond, C., Brough, M., & Fredericks, B. (2018). Deadly choices empowering Indigenous Australians through social networking sites. *Health Promotion International, 33*(5), 770–780. https://doi.org/10.1093/heapro/dax014

Meijer, E., Schout, G., & Abma, T. (2019). Family Group Conferencing in coercive psychiatry: On forming partnership between the client, social networks and professionals. *Issues in Mental Health Nursing, 40*(6), 459–465. https://doi.org/10.1080/01612840.2018.1563254

Michaelson, V., Pickett, W., & Davison, C. (2018). The history and promise of holism in health promotion. *Health Promotion International, 34*(4), 824–832. https://doi.org/10.1093/heapro/day039

Minas, H. (2018). Mental health in multicultural Australia. In D. Moussaoui, D. Bhugra, & A. Ventriglio (Eds.), *Mental health and illness worldwide: Mental illness in migration* (pp. 1–30). Springer.

Mirza, A., Birtel, M., Pyle, M., & Morrison, A. (2019). Cultural differences in psychosis: The role of causal beliefs and stigma in white British and South Asians. *Journal of Cross-Cultural Psychology, 50*(3), 441–459. https://doi.org/10.1177/0022022118820168

Moleiro, C., Freire, J., Pinto, N., & Roberto, S. (2018). Integrating diversity into therapy processes: The role of individual and cultural diversity competences in promoting equality of care. *Counselling & Psychotherapy Research, 18*(2), 190–198. https://doi.org/10.1002/capr.12157

Mollah, T., Antoniades, J., Lafeer, F., & Brijnath, B. (2018). How do mental health practitioners operationalise cultural competency in everyday practice? A qualitative analysis. *BMC Health Services Research, 18*, 480. https://doi.org/10.1186/s12913-018-3296-2

Molloy, L., Walker, K., Lakeman, R., & Lees, D. (2019a). Encounters with difference: Mental health nurses and Indigenous Australian users of mental health services. *International Journal of Mental Health Nursing, 28*(4), 922–929. https://doi.org/10.1111/inm.12592

Molloy, L., Walker, K., Lakeman, R., & Lees, D. (2019b). Mental health nursing practice and Indigenous Australians: A multi-sited ethnography. *Issues in Mental Health Nursing, 40*(1), 21–27. https://doi.org/10.1080/01612840.2018.1488902

Moran, A., Haines, H., Raschke, N., Schmidt, D., Koschel, A., Stephens, A., Opie, C., & Nancarrow, S. (2019). Mind the gap: Is it time to invest in embedded researchers in regional, rural and remote health services to address health outcome discrepancies for those living in rural, remote and regional areas? *Australian Journal of Primary Health, 25*(2), 104–107. https://doi.org/10.1071/PY18201

Muir-Cochrane, E., O'Kane, D., McAllister, M., Levett-Jones, T., & Gerace, A. (2018). Reshaping curricula: Culture and mental health in undergraduate health degrees. *International Journal of Mental Health Nursing, 27*(2), 652–661. https://doi.org/10.1111/inm.12350

Mulder, C., Debassige, D., Gustafson, M., Slater, M., Eshkawkogan, E., & Walker, J. (2022). Research, sovereignty and action: lessons from a first nations–led study on aging in Ontario. *Healthcare Quarterly, 24*, 93–97. https://doi.org/10.12927/hcq.2022.26767

Mullins, C., & Khawaja, N. (2018). Non-Indigenous psychologists working with Aboriginal and Torres Strait Islander people: Towards clinical and cultural competence. *Australian Psychologist, 53*(5), 394–404. https://doi.org/10.1111/ap.12338

National Rural Health Alliance. (2017). *Mental health in rural and remote Australia: Fact sheet.* www.ruralhealth.org.au/sites/default/files/publications/nrha-mental-health-factsheet-dec-2017.pdf

Nickerson, A., Liddell, B., Bryant, R., Hadzi-Pavlovic, D., Keegan, D., Edwards, B., Felmingham, K., Forbes, D., O'Donnell, M., Silove, D., Steel, Z., McFarlane, A., & van Hooff, M. (2019). Longitudinal association between trust, psychological symptoms and community engagement in resettled refugees. *Psychological Medicine, 49*(10), 1661–1669. https://doi.org/10.1017/S0033291718002246

Padmanabhan, D. (2017). From distress to disease: A critique of the medicalisation of possession in DSM-5. *Anthropology and Medicine*, *24*(3), 261–275. https://doi.org/10.1080/13648470.2017.1389168

Parajuli, J., & Horey, D. (2019). How can health care professionals address poor health service utilisation among refugees after resettlement in Australia? A narrative systematic review of recent evidence. *Australian Journal of Primary Health*, *25*(3), 205–213. https://doi.org/10.1071/PY18120

Parfitt, B. (2018). *Working across cultures: Study of expatriate nurses working in developing countries in primary health care*. Routledge Revivals.

Passi, N. (2018). Looking forward, looking back: An Indigenous trainee perspective. *Emergency Medicine Australasia*, *30*(6), 862–863. https://doi.org/10.1111/1742-6723.13195

Pennay, A., McNair, R., Hughes, T., Leonard, W., Brown, R., & Lubman, D. (2018). Improving alcohol and mental health treatment for lesbian, bisexual and queer women: Identity matters. *Australian and New Zealand Journal of Public Health*, *42*(1), 35–42. https://doi.org/10.1111/1753-6405.12739

Perales, F. (2019). The health and wellbeing of Australian lesbian, gay and bisexual people: A systematic assessment using a longitudinal national sample. *Australian and New Zealand Journal of Public Health*, *43*(3), 281–287. https://doi.org/10.1111/1753-6405.12855

Perales, F., & Todd, A. (2018). Structural stigma and the health and wellbeing of Australian LGB populations: Exploiting geographic variation in the results of the 2017 same-sex marriage plebiscite. *Social Science & Medicine*, *208*, 190–199. https://doi.org/10.1016/j.socscimed.2018.05.015

'Pienaar, K., Murphy, D., Race, K., & Lea, T. (2018). Problematising LGBTIQ drug use, governing sexuality and gender: A critical analysis of LGBTIQ health policy in Australia. *International Journal of Drug Policy*, *55*, 187–194. https://doi.org/10.1016/j.drugpo.2018.01.008

Poon, A., & Lee, J. (2019). Carers of people with mental illness from culturally and linguistically diverse communities. *Australian Social Work*, *72*(3), 312–324. https://doi.org/10.1080/0312407X.2019.1604300

Porter, L., Jackson, S., & Johnson, L. (2018). Indigenous communities are reworking urban planning, but planners need to accept their history. *The Conversation*. www.theconversation.com/indigenous-communities-are-reworking-urban-planning-but-planners-need-to-accept-their-history-92351

Power, T., Virdun, C., Gorman, E., Doab, A., Smith, R., Phillips, A., & Gray, J. (2018). Ensuring Indigenous cultural respect in Australian undergraduate nursing students. *Higher Education Research & Development*, *37*(4), 837–851. https://doi.org/10.1080/07294360.2018.1440537

Queensland Transcultural Mental Health Centre. (2019). *For health professionals*. Queensland Government. www.metrosouth.health.qld.gov.au/qtmhc/for-health-professionals

Renfrew, M., Morton, D., Northcote, M., Morton, J., Hinze, J., & Przybylko, C. (2021). Participant perceptions of facilitators and barriers to adherence in a digital mental health intervention for a nonclinical cohort: Content analysis. *Journal of Medical Internet Research*, *23*(4), e25358. https://doi.org/10.2196/25358

Rhodes, L. (2020). The Colonising effect of western mental health discourses. *Social Work & Policy Studies: Social Justice, Practice and Theory*, *2*(2). Student edition. www.openjournals.library.sydney.edu.au/index.php/SWPS/article/view/14182

Ringland V (2019) Indigenous trauma healing: A modern model. *Australian Counselling Research Journal*, *13*(1). www.acrjournal.com.au/resources/assets/journals/Volume-13-Issue-1-2019/Manuscript1%20-%20Indigenous%20Trauma%20Healing%20A%20Modern%20Model.pdf

Royal Australian & New Zealand College of Psychiatrists. (2016). *Aboriginal and Torres Strait Islander mental health workers*. www.ranzcp.org/news-policy/policy/policy-and-advocacy/position-statements/aboriginal-torres-strait-islander-mh-workers

Salch, N. (2020). *How the stigma of mental health is spread by mass media*. Verywell Mind. www.verywellmind.com/mental-health-stigmas-in-mass-media-4153888

Samuel, S., Advocat, J., & Russell, G. (2018). Health seeking narratives of unwell Sri Lankan Tamil refugees in Melbourne Australia. *Australian Journal of Primary Health*, *24*(1), 90–97. https://doi.org/10.1071/PY17033

Schultz, R., & Cairney, S. (2017). Caring for country and the health of Aboriginal and Torres Strait Islander Australians. *Medical Journal of Australia*, *207*(1), 8–10. https://doi.org/10.5694/mja16.00687

Secretariat of the Permanent Forum on Indigenous Issues. (2009). *State of the world's indigenous peoples*. United Nations Press. www.un.org/development/desa/indigenouspeoples/publications/state-of-the-worlds-indigenous-peoples.html

Shand, F., Mackinnon, A., O'Moore, K., Ridani, R., Reda, B., Hoy, M., Heard, T., Duffy, L., Shanahan, M., Pulver, L., & Christensen, H. (2019). The iBobbly Aboriginal and Torres Strait Islander app project: Study protocol for a randomised controlled trial. *Trials*, *20*(1). https://doi.org/10.1186/s13063-019-3262-2

Shawyer, F., Enticott, J., Block, A., Cheng, I., & Meadows, G. (2017). The mental health status of refugees and asylum seekers attending a refugee health clinic including comparisons with a matched sample of Australian-born residents. *BMC Psychiatry*, *17*(1), 76. https://doi.org/10.1186/s12888-017-1239-9

Shen, Y., Radford, K., Daylight, G., Cumming, R., Broe, T., & Draper, B. (2018). Depression, suicidal behaviour, and mental disorders in older Aboriginal Australians. *International Journal of Environmental Research and Public Health*, *15*(3), 447. https://doi.org/10.3390/ijerph15030447

Schout, G. (2022). Into the swampy lowlands. Evaluating family group conferences. *European Journal of Social Work*, *25*(1), 41–50. https://doi.org/10.1080/13691457.2020.1760796

Silove, D., Ventevogel, P., & Rees, S. (2017). The contemporary refugee crisis: An overview of mental health challenges. *World Psychiatry*, *16*(2), 130–139. https://doi.org/10.1080/10.1002/wps.20438

Smith, S., Sim, J., & Halcomb, E. (2019). Nurses' experiences of working in rural hospitals: An integrative review. *Journal of Nursing Management*, *27*(3), 482–490. https://doi.org/10.1111/jonm.12716

St Clair, M., & Murtagh, D. (2019, August 12-14). Barriers to telehealth uptake in rural, regional, remote Australia: What can be done to expand telehealth access in remote areas? *Health Informatics Conference*, *266*, 174–182. https://doi.org/10.3233/SHTI190791

Stanley, S., Laugharne, J., Chapman, M., & Balaratnasingam, S. (2019). The physical health of Indigenous people with a mental illness in the Kimberley: Is ongoing monitoring effective? *Australasian Psychiatry*, *27*(4), 358–361. https://doi.org/10.1177/1039856219833776

Stodart, K., & Kai, T. (2018). Cultural knowledge enhances care. *Nursing New Zealand*, *24*(4), 12–13. www.aihw.gov.au

Strobel, N. (2019). *Improving the health and wellbeing of Aboriginal and Torres Strait Islander children in Australia. Unpublished doctoral dissertation*. Australian National University. https://openresearch-repository.anu.edu.au/handle/1885/155692

Sutherland, C. R., Chur-Hansen, A., & Winefield, H. (2017). Experiences of fly-in, fly-out and drive-in, drive-out rural and remote psychologists. *Australian Psychologist*, *52*(3), 219–229. https://doi.org/10.1111/ap.12194

Taylor, K., & Guerin, P. (2019). *Health care and Indigenous Australians: Cultural safety in practice* (4th ed.). Red Globe Press.

Temple, J., Kelaher, M., & Paradies, Y. (2019). Experiences of racism among older Aboriginal and Torres Strait Islander People: Prevalence, sources, and association with mental health. *Canadian Journal on Aging/La Revue Canadienne du Vieillissement*, 1–12. https://doi.org/10.1017/S071498081900031X

Thompson, N. (2018). *Mental health and well-being: Alternatives to the Medical Model*. Routledge.

Titov, N., Schofield, C., Staples, L., Dear, B., & Nielssen, O. (2019). A comparison of Indigenous and non-Indigenous users of MindSpot: An Australian digital mental health service. *Australasian Psychiatry*, *27*(4), 352–357. https://doi.org/10.1177/1039856218789784

Tomasi, A., Slewa-Younan, S., Narchal, R., & Rioseco, P. (2022). Professional mental health help-seeking amongst Afghan and Iraqi Refugees in Australia: Understanding predictors five years post resettlement. *International Journal of Environmental Research and Public Health*, *19*(3). https://doi.org/10.3390/ijerph19031896

Transcultural Mental Health Centre. (2019). *Cross-cultural mental health care*. NSW Government. www.dhi.health.nsw.gov.au/transcultural-mental-health-centre-tmhc/health-professionals/cross-cultural-mental-health-care-a-resource-kit-for-gps-and-health-professionals/cross-cultural-mental-health-care-resource-kit

Triandis, H. (2018). *Individualism and collectivism*. Routledge.

Tseris, E. (2019). *Trauma, women's mental health, and social justice: Pitfalls and possibilities*. Routledge.

Valibhoy, M., Szwarc, J., & Kaplan, I. (2017). Young service users from refugee backgrounds: Their perspectives on barriers to accessing Australian mental health services. *International Journal of Human Rights in Health care*, *10*(1), 68–80. https://doi.org/10.1108/IJHRH-07-2016-0010

Vallesi, S., Wood, L., Dimer, L., & Zada, M. (2018). 'In their own voice'. Incorporating underlying social determinants into Aboriginal health promotion programs. *International Journal of Environmental Research and Public Health*, *15*(7). https://doi.org/10.1514.10.3390/ijerph15071514

Van Spijker, B., Salinas-Perez, J., Mendoza, J., Bell, T., Bagheri, N., Furst, M., Reynolds, J., Rock, D., Harvey, A., Rosen, A., & Salvador-Carulla, L. (2019). Service availability and capacity in rural mental health in Australia: Analysing gaps using an Integrated Mental Health Atlas. *Australian and New Zealand Journal of Psychiatry*, *53*(10), 1000–1012. https://doi.org/10.1177/0004867419857809

Vasefi, S. (2019, August 25). 'Australia is a bigger cage': The ongoing trauma of Nauru's child refugees. *The Guardian*. www.theguardian.com/australia-news/2019/aug/25/australia-is-a-bigger-cage-the-ongoing-trauma-of-naurus-child-refugees

Villalonga-Olives, E., Wind, T., Armand, A., Yirefu, M., Smith, R., & Aldrich, D. (2022). Social-capital-based mental health interventions for refugees: A systematic review. *Social Science & Medicine*, *301*, 11478. https://doi.org/10.1016/j.socscimed.2022.114787

Wamwayi, M., Cope, V., & Murray, M. (2019). Service gaps related to culturally appropriate mental health care for African immigrants. *International Journal of Mental Health Nursing*, *28*(5), 1110–1118. https://doi.org/10.1111/inm.12622

Ward, R. (1958). *The Australian legend*. Oxford University Press.

Wendt, C. (2017). Closing the gap between Aboriginal and non-Aboriginal health workers through story telling. *Women & Birth Supplement*, *1*(30), 36–36. https://doi.org/10.1016/j.wombi.2017.08.093

Wesch, M. (2018). *The Art of Being Human: A textbook for cultural anthropology*. New Prairie Press.

White, R. (1981). *Inventing Australia: Images and identity 1688–1980*. Allen and Unwin.

Wicks, J., Cubillo, C., Moss, S., Skinner, T., & Schumann, B. (2018). Intensive child-centered play therapy in a remote Australian Aboriginal community. *International Journal of Play Therapy*, *27*(4), 242–255. https://doi.org/10.1037/pla0000075

Wilson, C., & Cariola, L. (2020). LGBTQI+ Youth and Mental Health: A Systematic Review of Qualitative Research. *Adolescent Research Review*, *5*, 187–211. https://doi.org/10.1007/s40894-019-00118-w

Wilson, T., Temple, J., Lyons, A., & Shalley, F. (2020). What is the size of Australia's sexual minority population? *BMC Research Notes*, *13*, 535. https://doi.org/10.1186/s13104-020-05383-w

Williams, R. (1963). *Title culture and society, 1780–1950*. Harmondsworth Penguin in association with Chatto & Windus.

Wolf, K., Umland, K., & Chai, L. (2019). The current state of transcultural mental health nursing: A synthesis of the literature. *Annual Review of Nursing Research*, *37*(1), 209–222. https://doi.org/10.1891/0739-6686.37.1.209

Wood, N., Charlwood, G., Zecchin, C., Hansen, V., Douglas, M., & Pit, S. (2019). Qualitative exploration of the impact of employment and volunteering upon the health and wellbeing of African refugees settled in regional Australia: A refugee perspective. *BMC Public Health*, *19*(1), 1–15. https://doi.org/10.1186/s12889-018-6328-2

World Health Organization. (2020). *Enhancing mental health pre-service training with the mhGAP Intervention Guide: Experiences and lessons learned*. www.who.int/publications/i/item/9789240007666

World Health Organization. (2019). *Refugee and migrant health*. www.who.int/health-topics/refugee-and-migrant-health

World Health Organization. (n.d.). *Social determinants of health*. www.who.int/health-topics/social-determinants-of-health

World Health Organization. (1997). Jakarta declaration on leading health promotion into the 21st century. In *Fourth International Conference on Health Promotion: New Players for a New Era — Leading Health Promotion into the 21st Century*. www.who.int/teams/health-promotion/enhanced-wellbeing/fourth-conference/jakarta-declaration

World Health Organization. (1986). Ottawa charter for health promotion. *First International Conference on Health Promotion*. www.who.int/teams/health-promotion/enhanced-wellbeing/first-global-conference

World Population Review. (n.d.). *What languages do people speak in australia?* www.worldpopulationreview.com/countries/australia/language

Wright, A., Briscoe, K., & Lovett, R. (2019). A national profile of Aboriginal and Torres Strait Islander Health Workers, 2006–2016. *Australian and New Zealand Journal of Public Health*, *43*(1), 24–26. https://doi.org/10.1111/1753-6405.12864

Yick, A., & Daines, Λ. (2019). Data in–data out? A metasynthesis of interpreter's experiences in health and mental health. *Qualitative Social Work*, *18*(1), 98–115. https://doi.org/10.1177/1473325017707027

Yu, N. (2019). Interrogating social work: Australian social work and the Stolen Generations. *Journal of Social Work*, *19*(6), 736–750. https://doi.org/10.1177/1468017318794230

ACKNOWLEDGEMENTS

Photo: © Ariel Skelley / Getty Images

Photo: © LittlePanda29 / Shutterstock.com

Photo: © Ian Waldie / Getty Images

Photo: © Holli / Shutterstock.com

Photo: © coffeehuman / Shutterstock.com

Photo: © mastersky / Shutterstock.com

Photo: © Byronsdad / Getty Images

Photo: © uslatar / Adobe Stock

Photo: © fizkes / Shutterstock.com

Photo: © polkadot_photo / Shutterstock.com

Photo: © lightscience / Adobe Stock

Common reactions to stressful situations

This chapter will:

5.1 explain the difference between stress and distress

5.2 identify the most common physical, emotional and behavioural reactions to stressful situations

5.3 examine the major factors that influence the way people respond to stress

5.4 describe the main priorities when supporting people through stressful situations

5.5 outline the importance of facilitating and providing information that meets the needs of the person, carer or family and community

5.6 consider the different ways that health professionals can self-care.

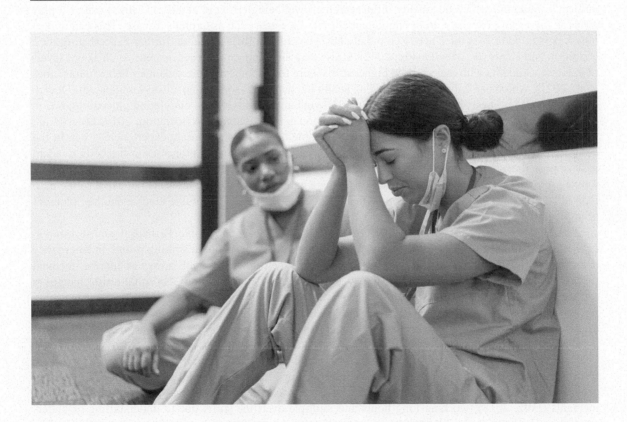

Introduction

There is no single 'normal' or routine **reaction** to the stress or distress that accompanies experiences of illness, injury, events, disaster, incapacitation, hospitalisation or rehabilitation. Different people will feel or exhibit different physical, emotional, behavioural and interpersonal reactions at different times and for longer periods. That said, there are a number of common reactions that people are likely to experience in stressful situations.

This chapter examines the reactions of people when they encounter stressful situations in health-related contexts and describes how health professionals can best support people who experience stress. The chapter commences by explaining the difference between stress and distress, then moves on to describe the more common physiological, emotional and behavioural reactions of people to stressful situations. The major factors that influence the way in which people react to stress are also considered, including the person's age, background, culture, coping style, context and setting, locus of control, protective factors, level of resilience and the type of support they receive. Following this, the chapter moves on to explain the main priorities for health professionals who provide care to people who experience stressful situations. Finally, the chapter identifies the need for health professionals to self-care and outlines strategies to help them to manage their own positive wellbeing and levels of stress.

5.1 Stress reactions

LEARNING OBJECTIVE 5.1 Explain the difference between stress and distress.

Stress occurs when a person's physiological balance or homeostasis is disturbed, presenting a challenge to their emotional, social or psychological wellbeing (Port & Last, 2018). Stress is caused by a **stressor** — that is, an event, situation or condition that precipitates stress reactions in a person. The COVID-19 pandemic, for example, generated different kinds of stressors for college students, including educational, economic and environmental, which negatively influenced their wellbeing (Hoyt et al., 2021). Stress can also play a role in increasing or reactivating ongoing or chronic illnesses, such as Crohn's disease. This can impact how a person addresses their needs on a daily basis or reduces their self-care, further exacerbating their condition and stress (de Dios-Duarte, 2022). Stress may also impact self-care in areas, such as our levels of exercise. Students who experienced higher stress were found to have more sedentary behaviours (Lines et al., 2021), which can cause longer-standing health impacts. Stressors are not always unpleasant (Quelch & Knoop, 2018). For example, exercise increases sympathetic activity and circulating glucocorticoids in the same way as pain or other adverse events (American Psychological Association, 2019; Oster et al., 2017). Similarly, drinking coffee — which many people describe as a pleasant experience — can fit the definition of a stressor as the caffeine activates a variety of physiological processes in the body to adapt to or oppose the action of caffeine (James et al., 2018). Likewise, buying a new house, starting a new job, moving to a new country, getting married or having a baby may all be joyful events but can also increase individual and family stress. All stressors, then, produce stress reactions of one kind or another, pleasant or unpleasant.

Examples of stressors for people who access health services are innumerable. Perhaps the most common of these stressors are illness or injury. Other less obvious stressors include waiting rooms in emergency departments, health professionals who use jargon, high-tech machines with arrays of alarms, medical procedures, loss of personal control and dignity, being forced to share a room in a hospital ward, changes in routine, worry about the future, ongoing pain and discomfort and being told bad news. No less disturbing for many people are the health-related stressors located in the community context, where the experiences of altered health states include chronic illness and pain, worry about the future, adjustment to disability, loss and grief (O'Connor & McConnell, 2018).

Health professionals will also encounter stress and stressors in their place of work. These arise from busy, fast-paced or unpredictable work environments, including unrealistic expectations regarding deadlines and time pressures (Dubale et al., 2019), ever-increasing caseloads or dealing with critical incidents (Folz, 2018), working long hours and multiple overtime shifts due to understaffing or under-resourcing (Birhanu et al., 2018) and supporting people who may present as angry or aggressive (Beattie et al., 2019). For example, emergency nurses were thought to be at increased risk of burnout and PTSD during the COVID-19 pandemic (Yang et al., 2022). During the pandemic, possible stressors include the need to wear restrictive personal protective equipment (PPE), increased sudden and severe morbidity, supporting individuals who couldn't have family visits within health care settings and increased mortality rates. Employment-related stress isn't unique to health professionals, unfortunately. Increasing work intensity or hearing about/witnessing fatalities were positively associated with PTSD for rail workers in the UK as higher job satisfaction was identified with reduced levels of PTSD (Carnall et al., 2022). The Perceived Occupational Stress (POS) scale may be helpful in establishing a comprehensive understanding of work-related stress in different roles and settings (Marcatto et al., 2021).

UPON REFLECTION

A stress epidemic?

Stress has been described as the 'health epidemic of the twenty-first century' (Soleil, 2017). Reasons for increased feelings of stress include:

- higher costs of living, such as mortgage interest rates, utility bills and foods leading to worry over 'making ends meet'
- pressure (internal and external) to 'get ahead' or 'have it all and have it now', leading to a constant juggling of work/study/family/social commitments, with nutrition, sleep and rest times, hobbies and interests often taking second place
- worry over the future, including the world political climate, wars and violence, crime, pandemics and the effects of climate change
- being 'online' and available 24/7 through social media, alongside exposure to a 24-hour news cycle that plays and re-plays troubling local, national and international events
- working at home in isolation from colleagues with the continuing demands of workplace productivity.

QUESTIONS

1. How stressed do you feel right now? How does this compare to your levels of stress one year ago? Five years ago? Ten years ago?
2. What are your individual stressors or triggers for stress?
3. What strategies do you use to manage your levels of stress?

When people — patients, carers or health professionals — experiences stress, their bodies produce a range of physiological and, as part of this, emotional and behavioural responses to help them adapt to or cope with the situation, and return to their pre-stressed state (Centre for Studies on Human Stress, 2019; Moore, 2018). This pre-stressed state is called **homeostasis**; that is, the tendency in systems (including the human body's systems) to maintain balance or stability and thereby support the systems' wellbeing. Homeostasis is achieved through stress reactions, which are also called coping or adaptive mechanisms (Centre for Studies on Human Stress, 2019).

Coping or adaptive mechanisms are stressor-specific; consequently, the processes by which homeostasis or wellbeing is restored will differ according to the stressful experience (Dewe & Cooper, 2017). For example, viral or bacterial infection, threat of physical harm, drugs, exercise, sexual activity, high altitude, restraint, hunger and thirst will each generate quite different stress responses and adaptive mechanisms in a person. Some of these mechanisms may be beneficial to the person in the long term because they promote longevity and good health (e.g. stress responses to fight infection). Other stress reactions have the potential to be harmful (e.g. stress responses to prolonged thirst). Some stress reactions may be quite varied, affecting people in different ways. For example, a literature review focusing on stress effects on older adults found stress adversely impacted their verbal fluency, with no significant impact on their executive functioning while actually enhancing their working memory performance (Mikneviciute et al., 2022).

The terms 'stress' and 'distress' are often used interchangeably. However, over the years, the evidence has shown that there are differences between a healthy adaptive stress response and the potentially harmful state of distress (Ghawadra et al., 2019; Selye, 1976). **Distress** is the result of acute, severe or prolonged stressors or multiple and cumulative stressful events (Riley et al., 2018). For example, people become distressed when they are unable to adapt to or cope with stressful situations, leading to a compromise of their wellbeing. Also, a person may continue to be distressed, even if they appear to recover rapidly after the removal of the stressor or the conclusion of the procedure. Periods of prolonged distress (e.g. homelessness, flooding, fires) can generate long-lasting harmful physiological, emotional and behavioural impacts for individuals, even when a situation has been resolved.

The transition from stress to distress depends on several factors; the first and perhaps most important is the duration and intensity of the stress (Centre for Studies on Human Stress, 2019). For example, a person may adapt well to high levels of pain or discomfort in the short term; however, if the stressor is prolonged, the person will begin to show signs of distress. Other factors that differentiate stress from distress are predictability and controllability. If a person can predict the onset of stress and/or control its duration, the impact of the stressor will be minimised. This is why a full explanation of a medical or health-related procedure needs to be provided to a person before its commencement. Armed with knowledge of what is going to happen, when and why, the person will more likely be able to predict and prepare for the stressful event, feel more in control of their situation and thereby feel less stressed (Visser et al., 2019).

IN PRACTICE

Different reactions to stressful situations

Scenario 1

Dorothy is a 60-year-old female who needed to visit the busy city hospital for a scan to investigate a lump in her right breast. She found the lump while taking a shower three months ago but delayed going to the local doctor. Her older sister died of breast cancer five years ago, aged 62. Her daughter has driven her to the hospital. The journey was very busy, taking 45 minutes longer than expected. Parking the car was difficult at the hospital because there is currently building work, so the number of car parking spaces is limited. Dorothy was running late for her scan appointment. On arrival at the medical imaging department, Dorothy starts to cry. She reports she is experiencing palpitations, having trouble breathing and feeling very anxious. The health professional provides instruction to Dorothy to sit down, but Dorothy is pacing around. She states she is worried she might be dying like her sister, leaving her husband of 35 years, adult children aged 33 and 30 and four grandchildren.

Scenario 2

A 15-year-old female presents to the community mental health team for assessment and support. Her local doctor referred her, stating she had been feeling sad and becoming increasingly withdrawn. When meeting with the mental health team, she explained how a recent situation made her anxious, overwhelmed, hurt and betrayed. She disclosed that she had told a friend whom she thought she could trust that she was questioning her sexuality. She's worried that her friend may have disclosed their conversation to someone else in the class. She desperately doesn't want her parents to find out, as she doesn't feel ready to let them know yet. She wants more time to reflect on how she felt first and to find the words to express herself to them.

Scenario 3

Joan is a Registered Nurse who works in a busy emergency department (ED) in a tertiary-level facility. Joan finds her work stressful, particularly on evening shifts over the weekend, when the demands are high and the environment hectic. There's often more aggression and agitation with more people present after consuming alcohol and substances during the weekend evening shifts.

One busy Saturday evening, the paramedics brought in a 24-year-old male, who required assessment and treatment after a car crash. He was under police guard after being charged with driving under the influence of alcohol and causing a serious traffic offence, which has injured four other people. His injuries are thought to be life threatening. The extent of the injuries of the four other people remains unknown. Joan recognises the man, as he is her best friend's son. Her best friend has been experiencing low mood in recent months after getting a divorce. Joan is feeling confused, overwhelmed and deeply troubled by the situation. She knows the Accident and Emergency doctor is calling her best friend and the families of the other injured parties.

....

QUESTIONS

1. Identify the different stressors people may experience in the scenarios. Discuss the different reactions to stress that each of the people in these scenarios, including health professionals, may be experiencing.
2. What presumptions are being made by each of the people in these scenarios?
3. As a health professional, what are some of the strategies you could use to support people in these situations?

5.2 Physical, emotional and behavioural reactions

LEARNING OBJECTIVE 5.2 Identify the most common physical, emotional and behavioural reactions to stressful situations.

Different people will react to stress in diverse — physical, emotional or behavioural ways. In this section, we consider each of these reactions in turn and consider how health professionals can support people who are reacting to stress. Of particular note are the strategies that can be used by health professionals to support the person who is feeling angry or displaying aggressive behaviours.

Physiological reactions

Physiological adaptive mechanisms can include activation of the sympathetic nervous system and adrenal medulla, secretion of glucocorticoids and prolactin, and mobilisation of the immune system (O'Connor & McConnell, 2018). These mechanisms work to manage stressors, such as an infection, giving rising to the biochemicals that give rise to the emotions.

Another significant and more observable physiological adaptive mechanism is called 'acute stress reaction'. Any person may have an **acute stress reaction**, particularly after experiencing a highly stressful or traumatic event (Baumeler et al., 2017). Interestingly, it is not necessary for the person to have been physically involved in a trauma to experience such a reaction (Jeronimus et al., 2019). For example, a person may experience an acute stress reaction after witnessing the sudden collapse of a family member and/or the frantic attempts by first responders to resuscitate that family member.

Acute stress reactions are usually self-limiting and in most cases do not require any specific biomedical treatments, for example, medications (Bryant et al., 2019). Even so, the symptoms can be severe and distressing for the person, and may include a range of experiences:

- anxiety (e.g. sweating, increased heart rate, flushing of the face, shaking)
- an initial state of 'daze'
- reduced levels of consciousness
- agitation or over-activity
- withdrawal.

These symptoms usually occur within a few minutes of the stressful event and disappear within hours or days.

An essential part of the health care of a person experiencing an acute stress reaction includes supporting the person, treating the symptoms and providing explanations and information about the event. Treating the symptoms usually involves first-aid measures. For example, if someone is shivering, the health professional will provide them with a blanket or other covering. Health professionals can also give explanations to support the process of **normalising** the experience for the person, including reassurance that the person is experiencing a common physical reaction to a stressful situation. While providing such support, it is helpful to ask if the person would like family or significant others, informed and involved. Additional support can be helpful for the person experiencing the stress reaction and for family or significant others who may be feeling concerned about the way the person is reacting.

If symptoms of acute stress reaction persist in their frequency and severity for longer than four weeks, then the condition may develop into a **post-traumatic stress disorder (PTSD)** (Zhou et al., 2018). According to the Phoenix Australia — Centre for Posttraumatic Mental Health (2019), 5–10 per cent of people will experience PTSD at some time in their lives. PTSD is a less common stress response and so is not described in detail in this chapter. In general terms, however, the condition is diagnosed in those who have survived specific types of trauma, such as war, terrorist attacks, rape or other assault, disaster, refugee experiences, the sudden unexpected death of a loved one, significant or traumatic medical events or those who experience highly stressful situations over a prolonged period (Gluff et al., 2017). PTSD has ongoing lifestyle and adjustment implications and requires referral to specialised mental health professionals for support.

Emotional and behavioural reactions

Emotional responses include any feeling that is produced in a stressful situation (Zerbe et al., 2017). Emotional responses are closely connected to physiological and behavioural mechanisms, which are stimulated through activation of the sympatho-adrenomedullary (SAM) system and give rise to rapid increases in blood flow to the muscles and glucose levels (Chrousos et al., 2013). Behavioural reactions work to enhance the person's capacity for 'fight, flight, freeze or fawn'. In this section, the emotional and behavioural reactions are considered together because the two are so closely connected. For example, a person who is feeling strong emotions will often behave in a particular way, driven by those emotions (Petitta et al., 2018). A person may feel sad and isolate from others or feel angry and behave aggressively.

The more common of the negatively valorised emotions and behaviours produced in the health context are now considered in turn: anger, anxiety, denial, fear, grief and tearfulness. Strategies for dealing with the less common or complex reactions or behaviours that health professionals may encounter, such as aggression and violence, can be found in the chapter that discusses people displaying challenging behaviours.

What are emotions?

Emotions are integral to personhood, along with the physical, psychological, social, sexual, cultural, spiritual, environmental and functional aspects of being (Greenberg, 2017; Cohen & Stern, 2017). Emotions are perhaps best defined by the synonyms 'feelings', 'moods', 'sensations' or 'passions'. Related words describe emotions in subjective terms, such as 'happy', 'sad' or 'angry'. Although subjective in nature, emotions nevertheless have a neurological and chemical basis (Beatty, 2019). Emotions are generated spontaneously in response to a thought, behaviour or experience. Once generated, they are given meaning cognitively and expressed either behaviourally (e.g. crying or avoidance of situations) or through language (e.g. 'I'm feeling sad!'). This suggests that the emotional, behavioural and cognitive capacities in humans are inextricably connected and influence one another (Furtak, 2018).

There are many theories about emotions, including those related to their classification, intensity, cause and effect. For example, some describe the **prime emotions** as the simplest emotions, the building blocks of all feelings (Burton, 2019). It can be important to name these emotions to help people understand the intensity and confusing composite of sensations or reactions they may sometimes feel. Some suggest that there are only two prime emotions — love and fear — with all feelings a combination of one or both of these emotions (Corey, 2017). Others have identified up to seven of the more negatively valorised prime emotions: fear, helplessness, hopelessness, hurt, sadness, worthlessness and aloneness (Greenberg, 2017). Regardless of the number or nature of the negatively valorised prime emotions, it is important to remember that they drive all human reactions to stress and they have the potential to harm health and wellbeing (Burton, 2019).

The causes and effects of emotions are equally debatable. For example, advocates of cognitive behavioural therapy support the view that emotions are the outcome of thoughts and behaviours (Corey, 2017). On the other hand, advocates of emotion-focused therapy suggest that thoughts and behaviours are an outcome of the emotions (Greenberg, 2017; Wilsonisa, 2019). Since there has been less empirical research conducted to support the notion that emotions drive our behaviours, at this point in time the former view has found greater acceptance. One reason for this situation is that the emotions fall outside the parameters of the science-driven biomedical model that underpins the delivery of contemporary health services.

Another reason is that the emotions are difficult to measure empirically. Arguably, there are many observable or measurable expressions of emotion. For example, externally, there is laughing, sweating, shaking, flushing, trembling and increased energy; internally, there is pain, tense muscles, diarrhoea, rapid pulse, changes in brainwave patterns and increased respiration. Each of these expressions of emotion can be measured to some degree. Even so, the inherently subjective nature of emotions presents challenges to scientific researchers, and suggests one reason why human emotions are sometimes described as 'unreliable' (Barrett et al., 2019).

To exemplify, people can demonstrate a split between their thoughts and feelings (Otis, 2019). This is expressed through sentences, such as 'I know that to be true in my head, but I don't feel that way'. Also, when people are in intense emotional stress, reason, judgement and volition can often reduce. This explains why descriptions, such as 'she's just being emotional' or 'that's a very emotional response' often have quite negative connotations and should be avoided where possible. Although the emotions may be viewed by some as unreliable, all people — regardless of gender — can be described as 'reliably' emotional because how they feel is real for them.

Individual variation in the expression of emotions is based on a range of factors. In particular, when a person is either physically unwell or they are experiencing mental health concerns, their capacity to think, feel, make decisions and behave as expected may change (Crum et al., 2017). Consequently, health professionals must have some knowledge of the emotions that are most commonly experienced by people in stressful situations, and the factors that can influence the way a person reacts to stressful situations. Such knowledge will allow the health professional to gauge how best to support the person who is stressed.

Suppression and repression

Pleasant emotions can engender exciting and expressive experiences; people may be motivated and energised. Unpleasant emotions, on the other hand, can have a quite different outcome. This explains why some people may shut down or minimise their unpleasant emotions by:

- labelling the emotions as irrational and ignoring them
- distancing themselves from their feelings through work, exercise, music
- displacing their feelings onto other people or things (projection)
- compensating for the emotions (e.g. through eating, spending money, increased hours of work or using alcohol or other substances).

Behaviours that shut down or minimise the emotions are learned. The extent to which a person exhibits these kinds of behaviours will vary, depending on a range of factors. These factors are described in more detail later in this chapter.

People are often aware of their emotions and are comfortable to feel or express them, appropriate to setting, context and culture (Beatty, 2019). Indeed, emotions are meant to be felt or expressed (Cohen & Stern, 2017). However, there will be times when suppressing an emotion will help a person to cope with a particularly stressful event: in the short term, the **suppression** of emotions is a coping strategy to help a person through a difficult time. If emotions are suppressed over a long period of time, however, they can immobilise or exhaust the person, or influence them to behave in a way that is unusual for them (Chervonsky & Hunt, 2017). Unpleasant emotions that are suppressed long-term become repressed emotions.

Repression of emotions will affect the way a person reacts to stress. For example, an event may occur in the present that is similar to a past event. Emotions that belong to the past event are triggered. A **trigger** is a word, comment, event or other experience that produces an instantaneous and often uncontrollable feeling or reaction within a person (Middaugh, 2018). The environment, smells, sights and people associated with the event may for example by triggers. When a current event triggers an emotion or behaviour that belongs to a past event, the reaction is often far stronger than is appropriate in the 'here and now'. This is because past and present emotions join together and the reactions are intensified (O'Brien et al., 2019).

Stress and the emotions

People who experience stressful situations can feel and exhibit a range of emotional reactions that translate into behaviours (Wilsonisa, 2019). These reactions can be further intensified by factors, such as illness, injury, tiredness and feelings of isolation or helplessness (Petitta et al., 2018). In combination, strong emotions may be expressed by the person who is stressed in ways that may be considered inappropriate by the health professional. For example, the emotions may be inappropriate to the event, place or context to the health professional. For example, some health professionals may view loud and apparently hysterical laughter followed by uncontrollable crying as concerning, especially if this reaction is prompted by an event or issue that health professionals view as relatively minor. The health professional may react to such behaviours by referring the person for assessment by a mental health professional — rather than, perhaps more appropriately, accepting that the person is experiencing a strong reaction to a stressful situation and helping the person by listening to their concerns and supporting them where they can.

There may also be times when the health professional feels unappreciated, uncomfortable, belittled by a person they encounter in their workplace or feel physically threatened and unsafe (Beattie et al., 2019). These feelings may be justified, especially if the person with the health issue is invading personal space, angry or has resorted to aggression or violence. On the other hand, the health professional's reaction may be the result of their own personal triggers (Middaugh, 2018). For example, a health professional may feel uncomfortable because a person is crying and the health professional does not like the strong and inexplicable feelings this may arouse. Rather than allowing the person to express their feelings, the health professional may unhelpfully react by:

- changing the subject to divert the attention of the person
- over talking so the person doesn't get space to express their own emotions
- using sedatives or other medications to 'calm down' the person.

By curtailing the expression of the emotion by the person, the health professional is in essence serving to reduce their own feelings of discomfort. The person, on the other hand, is left feeling frustrated, anxious, unheard and misunderstood by the health professional.

In the health context, any number and range of emotions are experienced or demonstrated by people of all ages with different backgrounds and cultures. Those who attend a health facility are generally unwell, injured or supporting another person who is unwell or injured. In short, these people are experiencing stressful situations. The most common emotions generated by such experiences of stress include anger, anxiety, denial, fear, grief and loss. These emotions are now discussed in turn.

Anger

Becoming angry is one way by which people protect themselves emotionally (Benjamin, 2018). Generally, anger hides other emotions, such as frustration, anxiety, fear, helplessness or hopelessness. As a person struggles to work through a stressful situation, anger may be the outward expression of these feelings. In addition, becoming angry can temporarily shift the focus away from the issues at hand and onto external objects or subjects. This provides the person with a way to distance or 'externalise' the situation, as they work to come to terms with what is happening to or around them (Appignanesi, 2018).

It is vital that health professionals understand these dynamics so they are less likely to presume that the anger a person expresses is aimed at them. Moreover, if health professionals help the person who is angry to appropriately express their true feelings, the anger will often diminish. This means that health professionals are best not to dismiss the anger as 'just venting', but rather acknowledge the specific concerns of the person and take suitable actions to address the content of their concerns, for example, assure them that their concerns will be taken seriously and pass on complaints to relevant managers for investigation to clarify if further action if needed and feedback to the person.

Health professionals who work in any environment can help the person who is angry or upset to express themselves safely through a process called 'de-escalation' (Price et al., 2018). **De-escalation** is an approach that is often used to assist a person to express their anger in a safe context. Figure 5.1 outlines the steps that a health professional can take to de-escalate a situation. These steps include providing a safe environment and supporting the person to express their feelings.

FIGURE 5.1	De-escalating a person who is angry

To 'de-escalate' the person who is angry, the health professional needs to take the following steps.

1. Always treat the person with dignity and respect. It can be helpful to introduce yourself and use the person's name when talking to them for example. Offer to sit with the person to talk further providing it is safe to do so.
2. Appear calm, confident and patient.
   - Stand slightly to the side of and at an angle to the person.
   - Keep hands in front of the body and in an open position.
   - Do not fold arms across the chest.
3. Use suitable direct eye contact — do not try to 'stare down' a person who is angry but rather use eye contact to create a connection with the person.
4. Allow the person adequate personal space.
5. Use active listening skills and offer empathic responses.
6. Allow the person to talk or ventilate.
   - Do not personalise any of the comments made by the person who is angry.
   - Consider the safety of the person, yourself and others around you if the person is expressing threats.
   - Remember that the person needs to express themselves. If the health professional enables the person to express themselves verbally, the anger will most often dissipate.
7. Try to see things from the person's point of view (e.g. 'It must be a worry for you, with your child unwell and no-one is sure why.').
8. Do not be judgemental, threatening, accusing, give advice or suggest to the person that they are wrong or highly emotional. Generally, this will only incite the person to more anger.
9. Be honest — do *not* make promises that cannot be kept. Rather, ask the person what would be most helpful and supportive for them at the time.
10. Speak firmly, slowly and clearly, and maintain this approach for as long as it takes the person to say what they want/need to say.

A general attitude of goodwill also helps to de-escalate such situations.

It is unrealistic for any health professional to expect to be able to de-escalate a situation without practice. It is recommended that health professionals engage with colleagues, away from the clinical front-line, to practise their skills in de-escalation (Snorrason & Biering, 2018). Similarly, health professionals must develop awareness of their own personal triggers, and remove themselves from the situation if they feel intense emotion or the urge to react inappropriately when interacting with a patient or consumer.

What are my 'triggers'?

There will be occasions when you, as a health professional, will find yourself feeling distressed by a word, event or situation that is relatively benign. Examples could include a colleague or service user who markedly irritates, angers or offends you with stories that other colleagues seem to find amusing, or events where you feel threatened or upset for no obvious reason. This kind of situation is usually the result of memories, conscious or unconscious, of something that occurred in the past, with the current situation 'triggering' the unpleasant emotions from the past. It is helpful for health professionals to have strategies and supportive people in place for debriefing after being involved in these situations. Knowing what these strategies are and who and where support people are located in advance is helpful for when heightened emotional situations may occur.

QUESTIONS

1. Consider a situation where you have felt suddenly angry because of something that was said or done by a friend or colleague. Was your response the result of a personal 'trigger'? If so, what influences do you think have contributed to the development of this 'trigger'?
2. Consider a time when you were feeling angry and a friend or colleague supported you. How did their support influence your emotions? How did you react?
3. Consider a time when someone insulted you or said something offensive to you. How did you react? What could you do, as a health professional, to manage your reactions to this kind of situation in an occupational setting?

Anxiety as an emotion

Anxious reactions are common in people who are facing uncertainty about the situation or event they are experiencing (Moore, 2018). For example, the process of attending or being admitted to hospital, with its unfamiliar environment and routines, can be a source of considerable anxiety for some people (Benjamin, 2018). Others, such as the older person or an Indigenous Australian, may associate hospitals with death because they have known relatives or friends who have been admitted to hospital to receive health care, only to die soon after. People with these kinds of experiences may feel reluctant to share their feelings about the situation with health professionals. There is a need, then, to engage with the person's family members or significant others so that they can help with identifying the source of the anxiety. Ensure consent is established from the person prior to approaching the family and others.

Anxiety can manifest itself in a variety of ways, including an increased sense of panic, unease and apprehension, along with feelings of irritability, impatience and agitation (Moore, 2018). Similarly, feelings of anxiety may reduce the person's tolerance to pain and increase levels of physical discomfort and muscular tension. Other common symptoms include palpitations, breathlessness, loss of appetite, insomnia and tightness in the chest (Hensch, 2017). Some people, especially those with a history of acute cardiac events, may misinterpret these symptoms as an exacerbation of their coronary condition. This in turn can lead to the vicious cycle of further anxiety and chest pain, necessitating additional investigations that result in delays to rehabilitation and recovery (Webster et al., 2017). Alternatively, people assume their experiences, such as breathlessness and chest pain are manifestations of anxiety and delay assessment, when the symptoms may be associated with their physical health.

A number of strategies and interventions can be useful to help the person who is anxious (Hensch, 2017). For all health professionals, an important means of supporting people to manage their anxiety is to provide them with information about what is happening to them or what they can expect will happen to them. Such information may be enough to reassure the person and reduce their anxiety levels (Brown et al., 2017). Other people may require more specific interventions, such as undertaking diversional activities (e.g. taking a warm bath, talking, engaging in a practical task or having a warm drink) or learning relaxation techniques (Benjamin, 2018). A low stimulating environment with less noise, activity and visual distractions may be helpful for some people experiencing anxiety. If a person has a diagnosed anxiety disorder, they would best be referred on to a specialist health professional for assistance.

Denial

When people are first faced with a stressful event, the suppression of emotions (transitory denial) is a common reaction (Chervonsky & Hunt, 2017). This defence mechanism, usually unconscious, provides a way to limit and manage otherwise overwhelming emotions. For this reason, the defence mechanism needs to be viewed as part of the overall process of coping and adapting to the situation (Shahar et al., 2019).

Denial is not necessarily a problem in itself, but rather a short-term strategy that is commonly used to deal with pain or incapacity. Consequently, it is more appropriate for the health professional to explore the fears or anxieties that lie beneath the denial by talking with the person and asking them how they are feeling. The denial or related behaviour(s) will most often resolve over time, depending on the level of support that is available to the person, together with the quality of their interpersonal or family relationships at that time (Raymond et al., 2019).

There may be occasions when a person continues to deny the fact that they are feeling acutely stressed or distressed. This can give rise to a number of situations, including an appearance of overt optimism in the face of issues that, from the point of view of the health professional, need to be dealt with more realistically (Furtak, 2018). Ongoing denial of this nature may lead to long-term repression of emotion, and eventually give rise to mental health issues (Beatty, 2019). In such circumstances, health professionals are advised to refer the person to a specialist for assessment.

Fear

The events or moments that generate fear in someone are usually very personal, but can also arise from socio-cultural norms (Furedi, 2018). Fear can be the result of a lack of trust in others or the very appropriate reaction to an uncertain, threatening or hostile situation (Seele, 2017). Illness or injury can lead to pain or death; it is understandable, then, that people who are seriously unwell will have fears for the future. Likewise, the health interventions received for some health conditions can be painful — an unpleasant experience for most people — and so it is appropriate that people view some health interventions with a degree of fear (France & France, 2019).

There are times when fear can be a useful emotion; for example, in dangerous situations, fear triggers the release of adrenaline, which enables a person to prepare to fight or flee (Furedi, 2018). On the other hand, fear can 'paralyse' a person cognitively, keeping them from making necessary decisions (Gomes et al., 2019). Such scenarios provide reasons why health professionals may sometimes be called upon to actively support a person through a fearful experience, including coaching the person or their significant others to come to a decision about the best treatment or support options at that moment in time (Berger-Höger et al., 2019).

It is necessary for health professionals to explore whether the person is harbouring unrealistic fears about their diagnosis or prognosis. To illustrate, a person may fear that a diagnosis of cancer will inevitably be life-limiting or that all of the health interventions available for the condition will cause hair loss. Checking what it is that the person fears provides a valuable means by which the health professional can support the person with reassurance. Quite often, a reduction in the level of intensity of the emotion may be achieved by allowing the person to talk about the fear and providing them with accurate information that helps them to understand what is happening to them and why (Brown et al., 2017).

On the other hand, the person may not be able to identify the underlying cause of their fear. Instead, they may feel an abstract fear of 'the unknown' that comprises a composite of the many possibilities ahead of them (Furedi, 2018). In this case, the health professional is best to encourage the person to talk about their situation, rather than the emotion, and provide relevant and regular information and explanations as the health interventions progress (Nguyen, 2019).

Another key strategy to help people to manage their fear is relaxation therapy or 'mindfulness', which helps people to recognise what they feeling or thinking and accept that the moment is temporary (Sanford et al., 2019). The ways in which an individual relaxes or practices mindfulness are very personal — some people enjoy lying back and listening to music, others prefer an activity, such as drawing or painting. The health professional can help by talking to the person about their usual meaningful activities and hobbies to identify which are suitable and helpful at that time. Likewise, health professionals may recommend muscular relaxation, breathing and meditation to the person. These strategies are most often taught by a specialist, so it is recommended that health professionals have the relevant information on hand about how to access these specialists.

Grief and loss

Many people are familiar with the seminal work of Kübler-Ross and her model of the five stages of grief. These were first posited in 1969 in her book *On death and dying*. Since that time, Kübler-Ross has applied the model to other grief experiences, including loss of income, divorce and illness (Kübler-Ross & Kessler, 2014).

According to Kübler-Ross, the five stages of grief include the following.
1. *Denial* — 'This can't be happening to me!'
2. *Anger* — 'Why me? It's not fair! Who can I blame?'
3. *Bargaining* — 'If I can just have a little longer, I promise . . .'
4. *Depression* — 'What's the point of even trying?'
5. *Acceptance* — 'I'm ready for what lies ahead.'

These stages do not necessarily follow the same order in each and every person; nor are all steps experienced by all people. Sometimes people will oscillate between stages; others may never reach the acceptance stage.

Knowledge of these stages of grief and how different people may react when they are grieving will assist health professionals to understand why a person is reacting in a particular way (Rodgers & DuBois, 2018). Such knowledge will help health professionals to accept that grieving is a very human and healthy process (Bui, 2018). Health professionals can support the person through the grief process by listening, showing empathy and providing explanations. Details on how to provide such explanations are outlined later in this chapter. Offering or facilitating practical support may also be helpful dependent on the person's situation.

Reactions of families and carers

The previous section outlined the more common emotions that are exhibited by individuals who are unwell, injured, or experiencing a change in health status. This section considers how family members or carers will, in turn, react when supporting loved ones in health settings. For example, a partner or significant other will generally feel upset or anxious when they see their loved one in pain, unwell or incapacitated (Tabootwong & Kiwanuka, 2019). In addition, there is stress or distress attached to dealing with the changes to their lifestyles that may occur as a result of the illness or injury of a loved one (Breisinger et al., 2018). Such changes may include additional responsibilities for the family, adjusting to a disruption in routines and relationships, and learning to deal with feelings of uncertainty, fear or helplessness (Petrinec, 2017).

It is the role of health professionals to support, not only the person with the health condition, but also their partner, carer, family members, including children or friends. This support will help the person's significant others to move through the process of renegotiating the roles in their relationships due to the experience of illness. Research suggests that the quality or closeness of relationships between a person and those with whom they are in a relationship is a major factor in influencing their levels of stress when they are unwell (e.g. Isik et al., 2019). By supporting those involved through the process of adjustment or adaptation, health professionals can enable the best possible outcomes for all (Gomes et al., 2019).

The type of support health professionals can provide may include listening, following through with requests wherever possible, sourcing information or allowing the family members to spend time with the person (Ates et al., 2018; Nguyen, 2019), and linking the families or carers to support services, such as Centrelink, community health centres and support groups (Yu et al., 2019). Health professionals can also refer families and carers on to specialists for more focused interventions, such as interpersonal therapy.

Interpersonal therapy (IPT) is an approach that focuses on a person's current relationships with peers and family members, and the way in which that person perceives themselves in those relationships (Weissman et al., 2017). The goals of IPT are to reduce relationship difficulties and improve social adjustment by helping people to identify and modify interpersonal problems; and to understand and manage relationship problems (Landström et al., 2019). The issues most often explored in IPT are unresolved grief, role disputes, role transitions and interpersonal concerns.

IN PRACTICE

Stress and diverse cultures

Uma is a 20-year-old female living in Sydney, New South Wales, Australia. She moved to Australia from India five years ago with her family. Although it took a while for Uma to settle into the Australian culture, she feels like she has adapted well. She used to feel anxious and embarrassed having a conversation with others who speak English, but after attending English language and speaking classes, she now feels comfortable. Uma and her family continue to hold Hindu values and practices; for example, they avoid eating beef.

Uma was admitted into hospital for observation after visiting Accident and Emergency at the local hospital with acute onset of severe pain in her abdominal area. The ward staff administered painkillers and rehydration. On day three after admission, at 2.30 pm, Uma was beginning to feel better and wanted to eat lunch. She asked the nurse if she could have a sandwich or something light to eat. The nurse checked the ward supplies. There was a beef sandwich and a banana left in the fridge. Uma explained that she didn't eat beef and asked for any other non-meat varieties. The nurse quietly explained that she only had beef available and that would have to do. Uma tried to say that she does not want to eat beef because of cultural reasons, but the nurse raised her voice and put her hand up in a way that Uma felt silenced. Uma became upset and started to cry. She had spent three days in severe pain, felt worried and anxious about her physical health, been away from her family and was finding the nurse's approach uncomfortable and disrespectful. She simply could not eat the sandwich as it would be disrespectful to the animal, her culture and her family, but she felt so very hungry and weak.

QUESTIONS

1. Consider the behaviour of the nurse. Is this behaviour ethical and helpful for Uma? Consider the ethical principles of beneficence, nonmaleficence, autonomy and justice when formulating your answer. Could the nurse's approach be considered culturally sensitive and patient centred? Justify your answer.
2. How can health professionals better support people from culturally and linguistically diverse backgrounds, including Indigenous Australians, in health settings?

Communication with families and carers

The levels and quality of communication between partners, carers, family members or friends will vary, depending on the established interpersonal patterns of behaviour that have developed between them over years and possibly decades (Healy, 2018). It is extremely unlikely that such interpersonal patterns will suddenly improve when one member of a couple or family becomes unwell. It is more likely that stressful situations will test interpersonal patterns and exacerbate a person's sense of distress (O'Toole, 2016). It is important that health professionals take this likelihood into account when interacting with a person who is experiencing stress and adapt their own communication patterns accordingly (Jo et al., 2019).

Relevant discussions with carers, family members and significant others need to include how the health issue or injury is affecting them (Kynoch et al., 2017). In the same way, it is vital to explore how they can cope with or manage the physical, psychological and social demands of the situation more effectively (Chan, 2017). Questions and concerns about an unexpected health issue may include:

- how the health issue came about
- whether anyone did something to cause it or if anyone is 'to blame'
- whether something could have been done to prevent it
- whether it is contagious or can be inherited
- treatment options and prognosis
- what supports are available in the community to help the person and their family.

In cases of sudden injury or trauma, concerns may include:

- how long the person could be in hospital
- who will pay the medical expenses
- what the family needs to do in the short term
- when the family can expect to 'get back to normal'.

The health professional has a key role, then, in supporting and guiding the person and family members through their quest for knowledge about the health issue and its possible consequences (Nguyen, 2019).

There is also a need for health professionals to be aware of the high rates of depression in individuals who care for a person with chronic health issues (Lacerda et al., 2017). Caring for a partner, family member or friend with chronic health issues inevitably involves long-term stress for the carer, social restrictions, limitations on the choices open to them, financial constraints and physical demands. Regularly checking with carers about their own health status, including their social and emotional wellbeing, is a necessary part of providing comprehensive health care to the individual.

Finally, in certain instances — particularly those involving chronic illness, palliative care or death — discussions about advance care agreements, wills and other family arrangements are crucial (Otani et al., 2017). In these circumstances, significant others may be equally struggling with their family member's physical changes due to the illness or anticipated loss of their loved one. First and foremost, the health professional must listen to the person and allow them to express their feelings. As previously explained, grief is a common and quite reasonable reaction experienced by people located in the health context. An empathetic health professional will understand this and give people the time, space and acceptance they need to work through their feelings (Appignanesi, 2018).

In some instances, it may be appropriate for the health professional to convey the message that it is possible to live life more fully in the present and enjoy the 'here and now' rather than postpone fulfilment based on an illusion of infinite time (Brighton et al., 2019). For example, those close to the person who is unwell can be encouraged to make the most of the time they have left with the person by planning some special activities to share together. In situations such as these, however, it is advised that health professionals refer the person on to specialist support services for assistance, including the palliative care team, counsellors or chaplains (Sawin et al., 2019).

Managing occupational stress

Health settings can be stressful for patients and health professionals alike. Examples of situations in which health professionals may feel upset or stressed include the following.

- As a first responder, you are called out four times in one evening for matters that can only be described as minor, for example, a blister on a toe, a minor cut, a headache. This is a common occurrence and you and your colleagues are at your wits end as such call-outs take away from your emergency work. You know that an emergency call was made for a person experiencing severe chest pain while you were engaging with a person who called with minor ailments. The person with the chest pain went into cardiac arrest and died awaiting the arrival of the emergency service.
- You have been working in the community with a patient for several months. You've been doing your best to support the person, although they had rejected your support on several occasions. During a home visit the person's family members suggest that you are responsible for the person's limited recovery progress and that your practice is somehow lacking and threaten to report you to your manager.
- A health professional contacts the on-call medical practitioner about a patient's deteriorating health status. The medical practitioner questions the health professional in a way that suggests they think the health professional is incompetent and should not have made the call.
- A colleague's ongoing behaviour suggests that they are not handling the stress of working as a health professional. They are irritable, lacking energy and motivation in work and seem to be making concerning decisions about patients' care. You are finding it difficult to cooperate with them as a team member. You approach the person to ask how they are doing and if they feel okay but they are dismissive of your concern. The colleague insists that everything is 'just fine'.

....

QUESTIONS

Consider each of the scenarios in light of the following questions.

1. What could you do to help identify and manage your reactions to such situations in the workplace?
2. What strategies could teams put in place to help members who are experiencing stressful situations in the workplace?
3. What could you do to help patients and families to manage the stress they may be experiencing in the health setting?

5.3 Factors that influence stress reactions

LEARNING OBJECTIVE 5.3 Examine the major factors that influence the way people respond to stress.

Most people feel stressed when they experience significant and adverse changes in their levels of health. An experience of illness or injury may be new, unpredictable or uncontrollable, and will invariably involve a degree of change and loss. The impact of such events will be very much influenced by the person's perception of what is happening to them, and what the experience means for them (Lovallo, 2016; Ogden, 2019). A person's past health and service use experiences will also influence their views about their current situation. Similarly, the way in which a health professional reacts to a stressful situation will depend on many factors, including the systems and structures that frame their work, their understanding of how people cope and adapt to stressful situations, and their own personal beliefs about the expression of emotions (Dewe & Cooper, 2017; Riley et al., 2019). Their sense of emotional and physical safety and supports within the workplace can influence a health professional's stress reactions also. In this section, the factors and influences that shape the way people react and respond to stress are examined. These factors and influences include the age of the person, their background and culture, their individual coping style, the context and/or setting in which they are situated, their locus of control and levels of resilience, together with the way in which the health professional provides supports.

Age

People from across the lifespan — children, adolescents, adults and older people — tend to respond in different ways to stressful situations (Cheetham-Blake et al., 2019; Non et al., 2019). For example, toddlers and preschool-age children who are stressed typically demonstrate increased attachment to their parents, high levels of crying, developmental regression, distress when left alone, eating difficulties and an acute sensitivity to their immediate environment (Ogden, 2019). In early to middle childhood (5–11 years), behaviours of children who are stressed commonly include problems associated with sleeping, gastrointestinal irritation, avoidance of social interaction, regressive reactions, such as bed-wetting or thumb sucking, learning difficulties at school and general withdrawal. Early adolescents may exhibit a continuation of avoiding social interactions (often in their relationships with friends and family); while stressed adolescents (14–18 years) may experience nightmares and/or excessive sleeping, difficulty focusing on tasks, and symptoms, such as skin irritations and headaches (Jolley et al., 2018).

Likewise, older people will react differently to children and adults in stressful situations (Ogden, 2019). For example, older people often exhibit fewer physiological or emotional reactions because their previous life experiences, including hardship or difficult times, have given them the opportunity to develop coping skills and resilience (Rainville, 2018). On the other hand, older people may have physical limitations that add to the difficulties experienced in a stressful situation. For example, a deteriorating health status can lead to reductions in mobility and, consequently, levels of independence (Shao et al., 2019). Further, they may experience multiple deaths of people at similar age to them within their family or social group, resulting in a multitude of experiences, such as intense grief, possible feelings of isolation and worry for their own health and death.

Age, then, is a necessary consideration when helping people through stressful situations. Younger people and older people alike will need additional understanding and support to minimise the effects of stress.

Background

A person's background, including their gender, educational level, attitude, personality traits, culture and religious beliefs will influence the way they respond to stressful situations (Keramat Kar et al., 2019; Liddon et al., 2018). For example, the dominant culture in Australia tends to discourage the expression of painful emotions, among men for example. This has developed from the 'stiff upper lip' Anglo tradition of the first white settlers, who needed to be strong, indomitable and 'in control' in a country that seemed so hostile. This view is also celebrated as part of the ANZAC tradition (Pickard, 2017). Certainly, there have been changes to this tradition due to the influences of multiculturalism, postmodernism, the questioning of traditional norms and generational and gender differences (Liddon et al., 2018; Zhao & Zhang, 2018). Even so, generally speaking, many people who live in contemporary Australia continue to believe that showing emotion is a sign of weakness; or that those who struggle to deal with stressful situations should just 'get over it' or 'get a hold of themselves'. Thus, the socio-cultural background of the person who experiences stress will play a large role in the way they perceive and respond to stress (Rzeszutek et al., 2017).

The many different factors involved in shaping the way a person responds to stress are outlined in figure 5.2 and include social, psychological and family factors, as well as health beliefs and values.

The extent to which each of these factors affects the person will be determined by:
• the degree to which the person feels 'in control' of what is happening to them
• the person's current interpersonal, social, cultural and spiritual contexts
• the person's resilience or repertoire of personal coping skills or techniques
• the way the person has dealt with past stressful situations and life events.

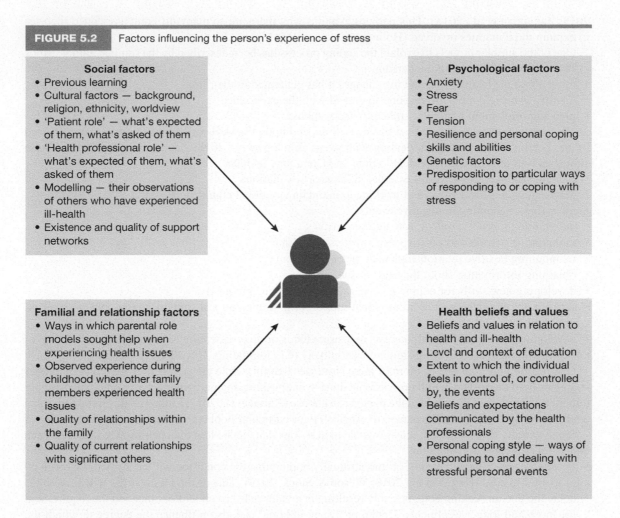

FIGURE 5.2 Factors influencing the person's experience of stress

Social factors
- Previous learning
- Cultural factors — background, religion, ethnicity, worldview
- 'Patient role' — what's expected of them, what's asked of them
- 'Health professional role' — what's expected of them, what's asked of them
- Modelling — their observations of others who have experienced ill-health
- Existence and quality of support networks

Psychological factors
- Anxiety
- Stress
- Fear
- Tension
- Resilience and personal coping skills and abilities
- Genetic factors
- Predisposition to particular ways of responding to or coping with stress

Familial and relationship factors
- Ways in which parental role models sought help when experiencing health issues
- Observed experience during childhood when other family members experienced health issues
- Quality of relationships within the family
- Quality of current relationships with significant others

Health beliefs and values
- Beliefs and values in relation to health and ill-health
- Level and context of education
- Extent to which the individual feels in control of, or controlled by, the events
- Beliefs and expectations communicated by the health professionals
- Personal coping style — ways of responding to and dealing with stressful personal events

People will most often move within and between their family and social contexts, drawing on any number of social, psychological and familial factors, as well as their beliefs about the situation (Crum et al., 2017; Lovely et al., 2018). This makes it difficult to reduce a person's reactions to stress into a single, cause-and-effect relationship that is easily 'fixed' or addressed (Hanna et al., 2019). Indeed, for the health professional to do this would be to minimise the richness and diversity of the person's life, relationships, situation and circumstances (Lovallo, 2016).

To provide the most appropriate and comprehensive care, the health professional needs to consider the complex factors that have made the consumer the person they are. This can be achieved by the health professional talking to the person about the way in which these background factors affect them and working with the person to determine the best options to support them through the stressful experience.

Coping style

A person's reactions to stress will also be influenced by their individual style of coping (Scott, 2017). For example, some people will cope with a stressful experience by limiting the amount of information they receive. This is demonstrated by behaviours such as not asking questions or avoiding discussion of the implications or effects of the health issue. Others may deal with their stressful experience by actively seeking out information or repeatedly requesting reassurance and explanations from health professionals.

The coping process

People may experience a range of stressful events or situations that affect their health, including accidents and injury, disasters, acute or chronic illness, ongoing treatment or health interventions, hospitalisation, rehabilitation and extended recovery. The process of coping with such situations is complex (Lovely et al.,

2018; Zamanian et al., 2018). This perhaps explains why there are so many different associated theories to explain the dynamics involved (Holmgreen et al., 2017; Moore, 2018).

One of the simpler models to explain the coping process has been described by the seminal author, Moos (1984) and includes helping the person to:

- think about the health issue and the changes it has generated in their life
- identify ways to cope with, respond to or deal with the experience
- plan and implement particular strategies and responses.

The **strategies** that are used by a person will depend upon the skills or actions that have been utilised by the person in the past when dealing with stress (Liddon et al., 2018; Zamanian et al., 2018). These strategies will differ from individual to individual, and may include:

- reducing or changing harmful external influences or situations
- decreasing emotional stress and working to maintain emotional equilibrium
- tolerating or adapting to negative events
- maintaining a positive self-image and esteem
- maintaining helpful and positive relationships with others
- maintaining positive relationships with the environment
- obtaining information about the health issue
- developing new skills for coping (e.g. yoga or relaxation techniques)
- seeking out practical, social or emotional support (e.g. joining a local support group, consumer forum or church/spiritual group)
- developing new or additional interests to distract focus or divert attention (e.g. gardening)
- expressing distressing feelings more constructively (e.g. journaling, artwork or counselling).

One person may find one or more of these strategies helpful, while the next person may find that other strategies help them. The health professional must avoid pushing any particular activity onto a person, but rather provide options from which the person can choose (Kartal et al., 2017; Liddon et al., 2018; Zamanian et al., 2018) and work with the person to establish their particular hobbies, interests and activities.

Some people, when stressed, may gravitate to activities that can be less than helpful. Examples of such unhelpful strategies may include:

- ignoring or denying symptoms, or unrealistically hoping that the condition will go away or be resolved of its own accord (Hanna et al., 2019; Wilson & Stock, 2019). This dealing with stress will sometimes delay the person seeking help, possibly resulting in greater risks to self and/or other and the requirement for more and longer treatments. Denial or 'living in hope' can also influence the degree to which the individual and their family are able to collaborate and cooperate with decisions around the health care received (e.g. pharmacological interventions)
- using 'transference' to externalise the issue or shift attention from the real issues (Bapat & Bojarski, 2019; Buxton, 2017). This can include behaviours such as blaming someone or something else when there is no legitimate reason for doing so or focusing excessively upon specific symptoms or deficits caused by the experience, to the extent that health gains are adversely affected. One example of this is a focus on possible side effects of pharmacological treatments. The person may wish to reduce the amount or frequency of their medications or stop the medication before they had originally planned to.

Health professionals are well placed to help the person examine the ways in which they are coping and discuss how useful their coping strategies may be (Zamanian et al., 2018). Figure 5.3 provides a diagrammatic summary of the coping process for those who are experiencing health issues, and outlines the influence of context, the type of change in health status and the different ways of coping and adapting.

A person's choice of coping strategies is unlikely to be a conscious one. It is only when a person becomes aware of the coping strategies they tend to use 'automatically' that they will be able to think about developing more helpful ways of coping, if this is required.

Context and setting

Contextual factors and the setting(s) in which a person is located will affect that way in which the person copes with stress. For example, people with strong family or social supports will cope with a stressful situation better than those who are isolated (Halligan, 2017; Lee, 2018; Keramat Kar, Whitehead & Smith, 2019). Likewise, people who are part of cohesive communities will cope better with challenging situations than those who live in fragmented or disconnected communities (Szabo et al., 2017).

FIGURE 5.3 The process of coping with health issues

Contextual factors influencing the person's response
- Social and interpersonal issues — relationships, employment, role in social network (e.g. is the person the main income generator?)
- Family dynamics and communication
- Societal response and perception of the health issue (e.g. stigma)

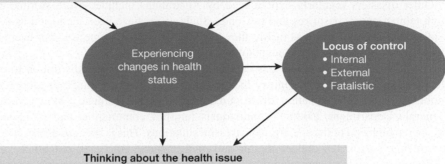

Experiencing changes in health status

Locus of control
- Internal
- External
- Fatalistic

Thinking about the health issue
- How serious is it?
- How will I cope?
- What will happen to me and other people (e.g. my family)?
- What do I want (e.g. do I want treatment)?
- Who will help me/us?

Outcomes

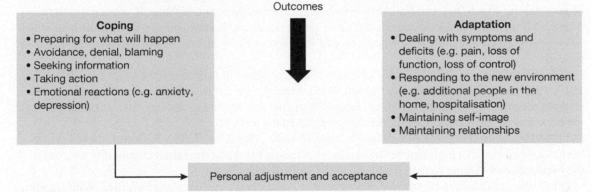

Coping
- Preparing for what will happen
- Avoidance, denial, blaming
- Seeking information
- Taking action
- Emotional reactions (e.g. anxiety, depression)

Adaptation
- Dealing with symptoms and deficits (e.g. pain, loss of function, loss of control)
- Responding to the new environment (e.g. additional people in the home, hospitalisation)
- Maintaining self-image
- Maintaining relationships

Personal adjustment and acceptance

Source: Adapted from Ogden (2019)

UPON REFLECTION

Stress and Indigenous Australians

Indigenous Australians report higher levels of stress and distress than non-Indigenous Australians (McNamara et al., 2018). Reasons include lower socio-economic status, higher levels of morbidity, disability and functional limitations, and lower levels of social support. Of particular concern is the high level of distress experienced by older Indigenous Australians who also experience increased levels of morbidity and disability.

QUESTIONS

1. How does lower social-economic status contribute to stress and distress?
2. How can community connectivity help to reduce levels of stress and distress in Indigenous communities?
3. How can family communications help to reduce levels of stress and distress?

Social networks and cohesive communities are particularly important in Australia today, with many people experiencing stress from climate change. Research suggests that the negative health outcomes of climate change is on the increase, particularly in relation to heatwaves, which have the highest mortality rates of all extreme weather events (Mora et al., 2017), as well as drought, flood, fire and rising sea levels

(Cooper, 2018; Gibson et al., 2019). In the next section, stress and coping is discussed in the context of the increasing number of extreme weather events and other disasters being experienced by people worldwide.

Disasters

Australia was known for its challenging environments as far back as 1904, when Dorothea Mackellar wrote her famous poem *My country* ('I love a sunburnt country'). In this poem, she refers to ongoing droughts and flooding rains.

Other disasters regularly experienced by Australians include severe storms, episodes of prolonged high temperatures, bushfires and cyclones. Such events have been identified as disasters because of the widespread damage and loss of life they generate — with extreme weather events now on the increase, due to the effects of climate change (Woodward & Samet, 2018).

The Australian Government has defined a **disaster** as a serious disruption to community life, which threatens or causes death or injury in that community and/or damage to property, and requires special mobilisation and organisation of resources (Australian Emergency Management Institute, Attorney-General's Department, 2011). For individuals, families, communities and the nation as a whole, disasters fall on the high end of the spectrum of stressful situations. This is because disasters can have significant and detrimental personal, social, economic and environmental outcomes, potentially affecting the health and wellbeing of people and communities for many years afterwards. For example, recent flooding across areas of New South Wales resulted in people experiencing distress while waiting for rescue from their homes, being relocated to temporary accommodation, surveying damage and loss of personal items and property and being unable to contact loved ones and removed from their sense of community. When disasters occur, often whole communities are impacted; therefore, people and organisations who were their usual supports often become unavailable as they too are impacted by the disaster. People may also be living with a sense of uncertainly, which they can find very distressing. Lismore, New South Wales is one such community living with uncertainty, as they await decisions about relocating homes and the town from land which has recently experienced multiple floods. One of the most obvious adverse health outcomes of a disaster is death.

Historically, the type of disaster that has caused the most deaths in Australia is the heatwave (1911, 1912, 1913, 1926, 1939, 2009) (Gissing & Coates, 2018). Many people express surprise when they learn of this statistic because they are unaware of, or underestimate, the stresses and associated risks of prolonged high temperatures on the human body, particularly for the young and old.

There have been a number of extreme heatwaves since 2009 (Cox, 2019). However, these heatwaves have not given rise to a high number of deaths. One reason for this is the raised community awareness of the importance of staying hydrated and staying indoors during a heatwave.

Other types of disasters commonly experienced in Australia are cyclones and bushfires. With regard to death toll, cyclones in 1911, 1912 and 1935 caused the most deaths, ranging from 122 to 178; and the 2009 Black Saturday bushfires in Victoria, which caused 173 deaths and 414 injuries (Productivity Commission, 2014). Several areas around New South Wales, including the North Coast, Hunter region, Hawkesbury, Blue Mountains, Illawarra and the South Coast, Riverina and Snowy Mountains, experienced major fires in 2019, lasting several months through to 2020. The fires were the worst recorded in New South Wales, resulting in the deaths of 20 civilians and six fire workers. The Australian Institute for Disaster Resilience (n.d.) reported that 2448 homes were destroyed. Although the death tolls of Cyclone Tracy (65 deaths) and the 1983 Ash Wednesday bushfires (75 deaths) are likewise significant, they are not in the 10 worst Australian disasters in terms of death toll.

Disasters include 'man-made' accidents. For example, the 1977 Granville (Sydney) rail crash caused 83 deaths. Equally, bus crashes can have a disastrous toll in terms of death and injury, with the 1989 Kempsey bus crash killing 35 people and injuring 41; and the 1989 Grafton (NSW) bus crash killing 21 people and injuring 22. While the number of deaths is of course important to consider, it's also critical to think about short- and longer-term physical, psychological, emotional, cultural, spiritual and financial impacts on communities. Land and property that holds significant historic value to communities and cultural groups may be damaged, generating a very personal sense of loss for many. The sense of 'belonging' to a group of people or location may be forever changed or the feelings of physical safety may be reduced, leaving people with ongoing worry and fear.

Disaster events also affect first responders and other health professionals who provide health care to those affected by the trauma, with some health professionals reporting high levels of stress and symptoms of PTSD (Paton et al., 2017). Stress experienced by first responders and health professionals can also impact their own families as they return home tired and fatigued, possibly disengaging from family life, activities and communications in order to sustain their own mental and emotional health. Given this, it is important that organisations plan, organise and train their workers to manage both the actual disaster and the impacts on the organisations, teams and individuals (Gregg et al., 2022, Keim, 2022).

The number of natural and man-made disasters worldwide, including in Australia, is increasing (Benevolenza & DeRigne, 2019). While the reasons for the increase in natural disasters are generally connected to climate change, the reasons for an increase in human-made disasters may include population growth and technology issues. The Australian Disaster Resilience (https://knowledge.aidr.org.au), a federal government initiative, gives access to information about the disasters that have occurred in Australia over the years, including the date, location, type of disaster and name of the disaster. It also provides details of available assistance for current disasters. On the website, 'Disaster type' includes bushfires, cyclones, earthquakes, floods and other natural occurrences, as well as influenza and terrorist attacks. Interestingly, heatwaves are not included, despite them, as already noted, resulting in more deaths than any other extreme weather event or drought.

Australians are also affected by overseas disasters. For example, the 2004 Indian Ocean tsunami killed over 270 000 people across numerous countries (including 20 Australians), with many others injured or experiencing adverse health outcomes (Johannesson et al., 2011). In a more recent overseas natural disaster, the majority of those killed in the 2019 volcanic eruption on Whakaari (White) Island in New Zealand were Australian (BBC News, 2019). Additionally, emergency services and military personnel from Australia assisted in the retrieval response, including transporting a number of casualties to Australia for specialised health care.

Likewise, acts of terror can have disastrous consequences, with 28 Australians killed in the shooting down of the Malaysia Airlines flight MH17 in 2014 and 88 Australians dying in the 2002 Bali bombing (Chim et al., 2007). Many casualties from the Bali bombing were transported to Darwin to receive health care by Australian health professionals, while a large contingent of Australian health professionals travelled to Bali to assist in 2002 and again in 2005, when there were further bombings (Mallett & Evison, 2017). Australians have also been injured and killed during the invasion of Ukraine. People born in Ukraine and currently living in Australia have been worried about family members who may be fighting for Ukraine or caught up in areas of bombings and violence. People living in Australia who have travelled from Ukraine are also deeply distressed about the damage to their homeland and the recovery process. Regardless of their country of origin, people living in Australia are affected by hearing and watching the stories of displacement and violence towards others.

Hand-in-hand with the increase in the number of disasters have been improvements in the ways in which Australia manages its responses to disasters. These improvements have been supported by the development of a relatively new health discipline, **disaster health**, in response to the health needs of individuals and communities who experience disasters (Reifels et al., 2019). Related research includes an examination of the way in which first responders provide and coordinate health care, follow-up post-disaster, as well as support one another during the disaster itself (Horrocks et al., 2019; Howard et al., 2018).

Indeed, there is a growing expectation that health professionals in Australia will be suitably prepared to respond to national and international disasters (Demorest et al., 2019; Griggs et al., 2017). For example, the Australian Department of Foreign Affairs and Trade (2019) notes that impacts of disasters, including humanitarian crises, are the greatest in the Indo-Pacific region. The aid provided to affected populations by Australia includes millions of dollars in funds along with Australian health professionals, emergency services personnel and care workers travelling from Australia to the affected locations to assist.

Disaster preparedness includes giving consideration to how health professionals can best provide appropriate support to people who are affected by stress as a result of a disaster (Irons & Paton, 2017; Sweileh, 2019). For example, while many people show great courage and resilience during and after a disaster, others report a long lasting impact on their mental health (Hiromi et al., 2017). Immediate stressors include near-death escapes; being unable to save family or friends and watching them die; watching houses and possessions being swept away or burned, with family or friends losing everything they have in an instant; and generally experiencing high levels of emotion (Australian Emergency Management Institute, Attorney-General's Department, 2011). Ongoing stressors include the difficult task of dealing with the practical aspects of daily life after the disaster, including obtaining water, food and shelter; living in crowded temporary accommodation; cleaning up the physical damage; dealing with insurance companies and a bewildering range of community services; and constant reminders of the personal and community loss (Bandla et al., 2019). Moreover, PTSD and depression can emerge in people months later, placing additional strains on relationships and giving rise to family and relationship conflicts. This distress is further compounded if the person is dislocated from their local community or has experienced breakdown in their usual support networks (Zhou et al., 2018).

It is also important that health professionals consider how to develop or build their own disaster resilience (Paton et al., 2017). This includes working within health systems and teams to ensure disaster preparedness in terms of plans, education and skills development; together with building individual resilience to withstand the additional expectations that will be placed upon them to deliver health care during a disaster (Tyer-Viola, 2019).

Disaster resilient Australia

Every year, Australian communities face devastating losses caused by disasters, including heatwaves, bushfires, floods and storms. The associated consequences of these disasters have significant impacts on communities, the economy, infrastructure and the environment.

The Australian Department of Home Affairs oversees efforts across Australia to respond to and recover from disasters and emergencies. While state and territory governments manage emergency responses in their jurisdictions, the federal government coordinates physical and financial support for disasters and emergencies. Another important aspect of the work of this department is the collaboration with the Bureau of Meteorology and Geoscience Australia to provide the Australian Tsunami Warning System (www.bom.gov.au/tsunami/about/atws.shtml).

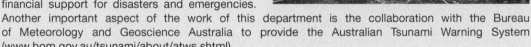

The work undertaken by the Department of Home Affairs is framed by the United Nations International Strategy for Disaster Reduction (UNISDR) and supported by the Australian Institute for Disaster Resilience (AIDR), which aims to build the resilience of Australian people, families and communities through the National Strategy for Disaster Resilience (NSDR).

The Australian NSDR has described the attributes of disaster resilience in communities as:
- functioning well under stress
- successfully adapting to change
- being self-reliant
- having social capacity and support systems.

The AIDR works towards achieving these outcomes by developing, maintaining and sharing knowledge with individuals and communities through conferences and other events, education programs, providing scholarships for those seeking to develop their capabilities, in particular emerging leaders and developing risk guidelines (Australian Institute for Disaster Resilience [AIDR], 2018).

Other key messages disseminated by the AIDR include the following.

Disasters will happen.

Natural disasters are inevitable, unpredictable and significantly impact communities and the economy.

Disaster resilience is your business.

Governments, businesses, not-for-profit organisations, communities and individuals all have a role to play and need to be prepared.

Connected communities are resilient communities.

Connected communities are ready to look after each other in times of crisis when immediate assistance may not be available.

Know your risk.

Every Australian should know how to prepare for any natural disaster.

Get ready — then act.

Reduce the effects of future disasters by knowing what to do.

Learn from experience.

We reduce the effects of future disasters by learning from past experiences.

Health professionals can support the development of a disaster resilient Australia by considering each of these key messages in turn, in particular how to apply them in practice.

Source: Australian Institute for Disaster Resilience (2019)

Locus of control

Experiences of illness and injury can often result in the person feeling that they have lost control. One way these feelings may be explained is through the seminal psychological approach known as the health locus of control theory, first introduced in the 1960s (Rotter, 1966), then further developed since that time (Ning Hou et al., 2017; Schultz & Schultz, 2017; Wallston et al., 1978). The term 'locus of control' describes the extent to which a person believes they can control the events that affect them. A person's locus of control can be influenced in how they experience the event and their adjustment and recovery process. In the health context, the **health locus of control** theory explains the degree to which a person believes that their health is controlled by internal, external or fatalistic factors (Spector, 2017). In short:

- *internal factors* include those that are the direct result of the person's own behaviour or actions (e.g. smoking cigarettes, eating fatty foods, playing high-impact sports)
- *external factors* include powerful others (e.g. employers, health professionals), peer pressure (e.g. 'everyone does it!'), genetics, culture, age or gender
- *fatalistic factors* include influences, such as fate, luck, chance or God (Ning Hou et al., 2017; Schultz & Schultz, 2017).

The impact of these beliefs upon a person's capacity to change are outlined in table 5.1.

TABLE 5.1   **Health locus of control and its impact on people**

Perspective	Description	Possible impact on recovery
Internal health locus of control	People who believe health is determined and influenced by their own behaviours and actions	More likely to take personal responsibility for their health and wellbeing View themselves as working in collaboration with the health professional to overcome health issues More likely to assimilate health promotion messages and to act on these; for example, adopting a healthier lifestyle to prevent ill-health or to aid recovery
External health locus of control	Individuals who believe health and illness or injury is something that has occurred or has happened to them as a result of external factors, such as an epidemic, genetics or family history, significant or traumatic experiences and relationships.	Likely to demonstrate a passive response to illness or injury Unlikely to take the initiative in determining how they will overcome or deal with their health issues
Fatalistic perspective	An extended example of an external locus of control Occurs when a person believes that health and illness or injury is largely influenced by factors, such as fate, luck or God	Likely to demonstrate a fatalistic view of what has happened or is likely to happen to them May appear indifferent towards health promotion information or advice given by health professionals May not implement changes in lifestyle designed to reduce risk, as they believe such changes are unlikely to make a difference May demonstrate this type of belief system with statements such as, 'Well, it's got to happen to someone' Unlikely to take responsibility for initiating strategies to promote or enhance recovery

Source: Adapted from Grady and Wallston (1988); Morrison and Bennett (2016); Schultz and Schultz (2017); Wallston et al. (1978).

The health professional who understands a person's individual locus of control can help the person to recognise the facilitators of their reactions or behaviours. At the same time, however, there is a need to understand that the health locus of control theory is only one of many perspectives to consider, when helping people who are experiencing health issues. In practice, reactions and behaviours are the result of a complex interplay between the various physiological, social, historical, psychological and interpersonal factors that will influence how anyone reacts to, copes with and adapts to a significant change in health status (American Psychological Association, 2019; Moore, 2018). As a result, adapting to an experience of injury or illness can be described as a dynamic process that is influenced by any or all of the internal, external or fatalistic perspectives held by the person.

Finally, it is important to iterate that, while psychological models for explaining the way people respond to stress provide a useful means by which health professionals can unpack the dynamic processes involved, there is a greater need for health professionals to turn their attention to the individuals or people involved (Healy, 2018). This includes actively listening to the person, meeting their immediate needs during a crisis or stress event and addressing longer term issues related to locus of control at a later time.

Resilience

Resilience is an abstract concept that is difficult to pin-down. It involves a person's capacity to function well following a stressful event (Hensch, 2017). It includes the inner strengths, assets or stamina/endurance of the person, not only to endure stressful experiences, but also to cope with and adapt to changed circumstances and, in so doing, continue to develop as people (Aldrich, 2018). Generally, people who are resilient are able to:
- think optimistically
- build and maintain meaningful and trusting relationships
- set realistic goals and carry them through
- have a clear set of values
- open themselves to new experiences
- accept what they cannot change and/or adapt to change.

Resilience then, relates to the way a person thinks, acts and feels about themselves, others, and the world around them (Bourbeau, 2018).

The Australian government has funded programs for children, in states and territories across the nation, to support development of the inner qualities needed to withstand or adapt to stressful situations across the lifespan (Department of Education, 2019). The many different programs that have been made available involve educators, as well as health professionals, working with students, from preschool through to university, to develop the skills they need to manage the difficult times people will experience at some stage in their lives (Singh et al., 2019). In the same way, there is a need for health professionals who work in health settings to encourage people to develop or draw upon the internal and external resources required to deal constructively with the stressful health-related situations (Cheetham-Blake et al., 2019; Southwick & Charney, 2018).

UPON REFLECTION

The ethics of humour

People who experience stressful situations often report feelings of anger, anxiety, fear and grief. Others, including health professionals, report using laughter as a means of managing stress and trauma (Westman & Chen, 2017). Research also suggests that humour is the 'glue' that enables teams of first responders and health professionals to continue working together in very stressful circumstances (Sliter et al., 2017).

Humour can make light of events that are serious or socially 'off limits' for discussion. For example, some health professionals use humour to cope with the traumatic events to which they are exposed by joking about what has occurred in the privacy of their staff rooms. This can help the health professional to normalise the situation or feel more able to control their feelings of distress or vulnerability.

QUESTIONS

1. How can health professionals use humour to reflect upon their own workplace emotions?
2. Consider a time when you have used humour to help you to manage a difficult situation. In what way did it help you? What were the reactions of those around you to your use of humour?
3. How can the use of humour in the workplace be helpful or unhelpful for health professionals and the people who use their services?

Type of support received

Ensuring that people receive the right support at the right time can be challenging. For example, the way health professionals think about and approach their practice, including how they support people who are feeling stressed or distressed, will be constrained by their roles as health professionals and by the setting(s) in which they work (Holmgreen et al., 2017).

All health professionals practice within the systems and structures by which the employer operates. For example, the Australian health system presents many challenges to health professionals who are committed to providing person-centred, biopsychosocial or comprehensive 'all-of-health' care to a person. This is because the health system is dominated by the biomedical model of health care, which can focus on physical symptoms in isolation at times, with the social and emotional aspects of a person often overlooked or dismissed as peripheral to the disease process (Walker & Peterson, 2017). Consequently, many people with health issues who are also experiencing stress do not receive the support they need.

Other factors that frame the type of support people receive include the location in which they are situated, the referral systems and criterion and focus of the health professional's role (i.e. scope of practice). For example, the health professional who works as a 'first responder' will take one approach when helping people; nurses or allied health professionals who work in acute, subacute or rehabilitation inpatient settings will take other approaches to helping people; those who work in the community setting will take different approaches again. Some health professionals may work with brief interventions with a focus on assessment and crisis intervention, while others have a longer-term view concentrating on quality of life and social integration. This can work against the person with health issues, with some needs being overlooked in some settings. A person's risk areas such as harm to self and/or others may be neglected, calling into question the health professional's role and responsibilities.

Systems and settings that overlook or minimise the emotional or social aspects of the person can also work against the health professionals themselves. For example, a health professional who feels stressed by a situation at work where biomedical imperatives are most important may be less likely to report their stress or take action to address what they are feeling in case they are labelled as 'unable to manage the work' (Udod et al., 2017). In such situations, there is an increased risk of the health professional experiencing burn out (Rodríguez-Rey et al., 2019), which may negatively impact emotional engagement with patients or consumers and reduce productivity.

UPON REFLECTION

'Not my job'

Consider the following statements made by health professionals who work in various contexts.

- 'My job as a first responder, first and foremost, is to save lives. Once the person is physically safe, my job is done!'
- 'There are other health and social care professionals, to deal with someone's emotions.'
- 'It is unfair of the patients to complain that we don't support them emotionally. I spend a lot of time chatting to them as I take their vital signs and give them their medications. I'm not sure what else I can do.'
- 'We have so much paperwork to fill in these days, it is impossible to spend time with the clients. The managers put so much focus on having the paperwork completed on time because of the professional issues.'
- 'We shouldn't spend too much time talking to patients, we don't want them to develop a dependency on the health service. Surely they can talk to their families and have their own friends.'

QUESTIONS

1. In the context of these statements, what can a health professional do to balance the provision of social and emotional support with the more tangible or 'practical' tasks often expected of them?
2. Why is it important to make time to talk to the people you are helping?

5.4 Priorities when supporting people through stressful situations

LEARNING OBJECTIVE 5.4 Describe the main priorities when supporting people through stressful situations.

There are a number of priorities for health professionals to consider when supporting people who experience stressful situations. For example, many health professionals work in an environment that is task-oriented, with the sheer volume of work they are required to complete each day overwhelming (Nayak, 2018). In addition, they experience pressures to deal with emergencies, reduce response times, wait times and/or lengths of stay in hospital. Further, there is rarely a 'quick fix' for a person who is feeling stressed. This can be frustrating for health professionals who are often committed to saving lives, alleviating pain with timely action or medication. As a consequence, some health professionals may choose to avoid the person in need of emotional support, rather than find the time or resources to help them (Karanikola & Mpouzika, 2018).

As members of the caring professions, health professionals must consider the competing priorities they face in the workplace and decide which of these priorities is the most important for the person with health needs (Nayak, 2018). Of course, there will be times when these priorities change, depending on the setting, situation and circumstances. Generally, however, there are five main priorities for health professionals who provide support to the person or people who are experiencing stressful situations.

The first of these priorities is to engage with the person and their carers or family members, and establish a positive and supportive connection. The second priority for the health professional is to form a therapeutic relationship with the person, to enable them to work with an ethos of partnership. The third priority relates to assessment and care planning, which involves the health professional assessing the person's situation and needs and discuss a way forward with them and their family to develop a clear plan for all to follow. The fourth priority is to help the person understand their situation. This may involve listening to the person as they verbalise and work through their experiences and options or providing information to assist the person in understanding the situation. The final priority occurs if or when the health professional does not have the relevant skills needed to provide the most appropriate or effective help to the person and their significant others. In such cases, health professionals must make a formal referral to a specialist service that enables the person to access the assessment and care they need.

Four of these five priorities are now discussed: engagement and collaboration, relationship, care planning and referral. The priority of facilitating and providing information is described in more detail in the final section of the chapter.

Engagement and collaboration

The active participation of consumers and carers in the planning, development and provision of health services is a feature of western health systems across the world (Abelson et al., 2019). Australia is no different, with health policy ensuring that engagement and collaboration occur at all levels of health service delivery (Westman & Chen, 2017).

Consumer and carer involvement is vital as it enables engagement with and ownership of the process of recovery, higher rates of satisfaction, and better health outcomes for consumers and carers (Rainville, 2018). Consequently, the health professional is responsible for ensuring that they involve each person, and those close to them, in decisions about the health interventions and services that best meet their health needs and preferences (Haines et al., 2017).

Health professionals should respectfully seek consent from the person prior to involving family members in their health care. This reinforces the ethos of partnership and working alongside the consumer. Of course, in some circumstances, a consumer may request that family members are not informed of the specific details of their health care, and these wishes need to be respected (see the chapter on the legal and ethical context of mental health care for further details). Even so, such requests can provide a useful opportunity for discussion. For example, the health professional may ask the person about their anxieties and the concerns that have led them to make this decision, the emotions that may be influencing them, and the likely consequences of keeping information from those who are best positioned to support their recovery journey (Cody et al., 2018). For example, an 18-year-old visiting the Accident and Emergency department for mental health-related assistance may verbalise they do not want their parents informed of their situation. However, the person's parents may be waiting in the Accident and Emergency department, feeling very distressed and confused about their teenager's presentation. This may create ethical concerns for the health professional, as the young person has explicitly expressed their wishes, which the health professional should respect, but feeling that they also have a responsibility to the parents. Discussions with the young person about their anxieties about their parents' involvement in their care and offering to facilitate positive family conversations may increase the family support for the young person while also helping to reduce the parents' anxieties and possible fear.

Similarly, health professionals must consider the context, including the resources that may be available, for the person's significant others. Individual circumstances will vary. In particular, time and financial constraints will always determine the ability of family members to be involved (Feinberg, 2019). Even so, the health professional must not make presumptions about a person's preferences or availability. Instead, every effort must be made to engage with those close to the person, at a time that suits them; and that invitations are extended according to their needs and preferences, rather than those of the health professional.

Therapeutic alliance or relationship

The reactions and responses of people to stressful situations will vary. To provide effective support to those with health issues and their family members or carers, health professionals need to make effective use of the therapeutic alliance or relationship (Thompson et al., 2018). The elements that are critical for establishing an effective therapeutic relationship are outlined in the chapter on assessment in the mental health context. In short, health professionals need to:

- be aware of verbal and non-verbal communication (e.g. introduce yourself, ask how the person would like to be addressed, welcome people with emotional warmth, consider facial expressions, use appropriate eye contact, tone of voice and body posture, speak calmly and confidently)
- use active listening when talking with the person (e.g. avoid excessive note taking during an interview or conversation, paraphrase back what you understand that they are saying, allow for silence for the person to gather their thoughts)
- use open-ended questions (e.g. 'What is troubling you?', 'In what way has this issue affected you?') as a means of encouraging people to talk and to clarify problems. Consider use of closed questions for the very short term if a person may be struggling to articulate their thoughts
- make empathic comments (e.g. 'This seems to be a really difficult time for you.')
- respond to verbal and non-verbal cues (e.g. if the person becomes guarded when discussing a particular subject, it may be appropriate to pick up on this, 'You seem to find it uncomfortable when we talk about this relationship. Is it something that you find distressing?')
- observe for any possible contextual, relationship and family issues (e.g. what is the person's health history, what is their family's health history?); and ask how family members perceive the problem and/or how the current problem is affecting other members of the family (e.g. children)
- identify the person's unique concerns. While these may be relatively straightforward, they may also be causing some distress to the family member or significant other (e.g. how will the person's partner get to hospital to visit them if they cannot drive? How will their partner cope while they're in hospital? Who will feed their pet while they are in hospital?). As with all other aspects of the person's health care, social and emotional support needs to be addressed systematically. If a systematic approach is not taken, the need for social and emotional support can easily be overlooked, which means the care provided is not comprehensive
- use appropriate reassurance. Providing reassurance to those who are experiencing stress or distress is a necessary activity for health professionals. However, clichéd phrases, such as 'everything is going to be just fine', 'it will all work out for the best, I'm sure', 'there's every hope' or 'there's nothing to worry about' will have a quite empty ring in the face of very real fears. Instead, health professionals need to listen carefully, respond openly and as honestly as possible to the person's questions
- identify the actions required to meet the needs of the person. This would include following up on questions that you are unable to answer or issues that the person has raised, and reporting back to the person in a timely way.

Other important aspects of building and maintaining the therapeutic alliance is to focus on working with the person and their family members or carers to develop a **care plan**.

Care plans

Care plans are written documents (paper or electronic) that are developed collaboratively by the health professional, the person with a health issue and, wherever possible, the person's carer or family members (Wilson et al., 2018). Care plans are sometimes called treatment plans or recovery plans, with each type of plan taking a slightly different focus. For example, the care plan focuses on the individualised care received by the person and their family; the treatment plan focuses on the treatment provided to the person; the recovery plan is developed around the goals of the person and the steps they need to take to achieve recovery. The overall purpose of each of these types of plans is to support the person who is experiencing health issues to achieve improved levels of health (Australian Commission on Safety and Quality in Health Care, 2019; Queensland Health, 2018) and optimum quality of life. This includes:

- ensuring the person and their family members understand their health needs and the range of health care options and services available to them
- giving the person and their family members a voice about the type and time of care or treatment they receive
- clearly documenting the preferences of the person, and their family members or carers, in relation to the health care and support they receive
- recording the information, with a copy for the person so they are actively involved and receive consistent health care from all the health professionals who support them
- recording the progress made by the person towards achieving their goals.

Because the care plan is written in collaboration with the person and, wherever possible, their carer or family members, it can be a very powerful tool to assist the health professional to engage and develop a strong therapeutic relationship with the person. For example, focussed discussion with the person about their health needs and preferences provides the health professionals with the opportunity to talk with the person and build trust (Fernandes dos Santos Lima et al., 2017). The discussion also enables health professionals to ascertain the expectations of the person and their carers or family members and respond to requests for information and advice on health interventions or options. At the same time, health professionals can show that they are willing to consider the person's underlying health beliefs, consider their coping style(s) and check the person's understanding of what can be expected to happen next. This would ideally include the use of a brief written summary for the person and their partner, carer, family members (Yalcinturk et al., 2018).

While care plans can take different forms, dependent upon the health context or settings and type of plan being developed (Wilson et al., 2018), they generally contain the following four components.

1. *Goals*, where the overall goal of or for the person is identified. These should be timely and realistic for the person. They should identify both short- and longer-term goals to help provide direction and hope for the person.
2. *Objectives*, which include the steps to be taken to achieve these goals.
3. *Interventions*, actions to address the biopsychosocial needs of the person.
4. *Progress*, including any challenges encountered (e.g. side effects of medications) and ways or means of overcoming these challenges.

Care plans must be updated regularly — several times a day, if need be — as the needs and preferences of the person changes (Castellà-Creus et al., 2019). Because they form part of the person's medical records, this updating must be timely and accurate — and, of course, undertaken in collaboration with the person. Providing the person with this ongoing information will assist them to manage the stress they may feel as part of their experience of illness.

Chronic illness and collaborative care plans

I am 25 years old and have lived with endometriosis for 10 years. I've had crushing period pains to the point that I can't walk at times. My periods are so heavy. It's so embarrassing going to university. I sit in class with this sense of dread of standing up and moving around the room. I managed to get a part-time office job to help fund my studies. I'm thinking I may need to give it up because I feel so anxious getting on the bus to go to the office in case I bleed and others can see it on my clothes. I get bloating and struggle with constipation because of the side effects of hormones and painkillers. It feels like it takes so much energy to do anything. It took me

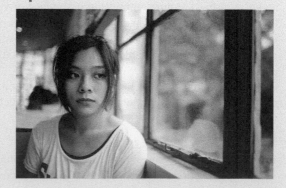

3 years to get properly diagnosed with endometriosis, despite several visits to both my local doctor and emergency department. The doctors kept saying it was my normal periods and I was too young for endometriosis. I feel like I can't remember what life was like without pain and anxiety. The doctors have told me that there is no cure for my endometriosis. It's an inflammatory condition that I will most likely need hormonal treatment to reduce the development of new sites, pain medications, surgery, lifestyle changes to reduce stress and I will need to think about an anti-inflammatory diet.

My boyfriend tells me not to worry and that things will get better, but I can't help wondering if things will. It frightens me that endometriosis can sometimes cause fertility issues. How will I know if that will happen to me and what will I say to my boyfriend if he wants children? I know I will need more surgery again. During the last surgery, the surgeon took eight biopsies of areas of inflammation. All of them were confirmed as endometriosis sites. Having endometriosis is very stressful. I always have to think about the things I eat and what I do in case it sets off an flare-up within the following days.

My mum had endometriosis that seemed to calm down a little once she reached menopause. I'm 25 years old, I don't know if I can keep on with how I'm going at the moment. My mum says she feels guilty because she thinks she gave endometriosis to me. She feels upset and says she doesn't know how to get the support and treatments I need. The doctor at the health centre said he can get someone for me to talk to. I think he means a counsellor. I think the doctor realises I need some help and support. He said he'll refer me to a pain specialist because some of my pain killers are addictive and he's worried about how many I'm needing to take. I said I need a physiotherapist as well. I was reading an article on the Internet that mentioned that pelvic physiotherapy can be really helpful for endometriosis. I'm at the point where I'll give anything a go. It just means that there's going to be quite a lot of appointments for me with seeing the doctor, counsellor, pain specialist and physiotherapist. I'll have to look at how much they all cost. I'm not sure if the services will be covered and how many sessions Medicare will pay for.

Referral

There may be occasions when a health professional decides that the person who is experiencing a stressful situation requires the support of health professionals from another discipline. There are many support services in the health and community contexts that can assist people who need support to cope with stressful situations. For example, multi-disciplinary support may better address the longer standing issues people with rheumatic disease are struggling with as a result of the COVID-19 pandemic (Duculan et al., 2022). It is recommended that health professionals familiarise themselves with the variety of options available so they can make appropriate referrals, including the counselling, psychotherapy, pastoral care or social support services provided by health services, community-managed organisations and faith-based organisations (Scott, 2017). These services may incorporate approaches, such as engaging with the person to develop strategies for relaxation and building more effective levels of resilience (Aldrich, 2018).

Building networks with staff across different services will help to enable timely and supportive consultations and referral pathways. Referral is a vital tool that all health professionals can use to ensure that people who are experiencing stressful situations receive the health care they need (Brisson, 2019). Referral can be made verbally or in writing. Some health professionals feel that making a referral to another health professional reflects upon their own skills set, but this is not the case. The best multidisciplinary team is one where health professionals trust one another to ensure people achieve the best possible health outcomes.

UPON REFLECTION

Community paramedicine

Community paramedicine is a relatively new model of care that extends on the traditional emergency response and transportation model of paramedicine. It has been tried and tested in countries, such as Canada and the United States (Ontengco, 2019) and is emerging in Australia (O'Meara & Duthie, 2018). The new model is focussed on primary health care and community capacity building, including the prevention of emergency situations (such as falls in older people) and the promotion of good health (such as managing stress), particularly in smaller rural communities. A focus of the community paramedicine model is developing and maintaining good relationships with community members so that they can develop local plans to prepare for — or prevent — emergencies. Community paramedicine provides a solution to the ageing population and stretched health systems.

▶

QUESTIONS

1. What steps can be taken by paramedics to develop a therapeutic alliance or relationship with the people they assist?

2. What other models of care could be developed by health and social services to deliver timely support for rural communities?

5.5 Providing information

LEARNING OBJECTIVE 5.5 Outline the importance of facilitating and providing information that meets the needs of the person, carer or family and community.

This section emphasises the importance of providing information to people, particularly those who are feeling stressed or experiencing a challenging situation. In the past, information was provided to a person based on what health professionals deemed the person needed to know. This often included limiting the information from patients and their families because 'they wouldn't understand anyway' or 'they would only worry'. In contemporary health settings, however, information needs to be provided in a way and at a time that is driven by the person(s) with health needs (Weishaar et al., 2019). It may be helpful for the health professional to facilitate the person sourcing accurate information at times, as opposed to the health professional providing all of the information. This may be a positive way to help engage the person, so they are active as opposed to passive travellers in their own health care.

Information about a health condition or the situation in which a person finds themselves helps to alleviate confusion and enable people with health issues to feel more in control of the situation, thereby reducing their levels of stress (Robotin et al., 2017). Information can also act as a form of reassurance and emotional support for the person (Lesselroth & Monkman, 2019). Perhaps most importantly, with good information, people are able to make the best possible decisions or choices about their health and are thereby empowered (De Vries et al., 2019).

The provision of information to educate people about their health and ill-health has now become a key sub-specialty for health professionals (Nguyen, 2019). Health literacy, including **mental health literacy**, is discussed in detail in the chapter on mental health service delivery, and includes helping people to become more 'literate' or knowledgeable about health issues. To assist a person to develop health or mental health literacy, the health professional must:

- provide information that explains how to seek out accurate information
- explain potential benefits, risk factors, options for self-treatment or self-management, and where to go for other professional help if required
- promote attitudes that improve recognition and appropriate help-seeking.

This kind of support is valuable for helping people to understand when to seek help, how to seek help, where to go for help and what services are available (Robotin et al., 2017).

Many people with health needs may feel uncertain about what information they need. Remember, people do not know what they do not know. For example, a health professional may ask, 'Is there anything else that you would like to know?', but quite often a person will have no idea of what to ask (Matas & Bronstein, 2018). Consequently, health professionals are advised to give the person some general information at the outset, then return to the person later to ask them more specifically about which aspects of the situation they are finding the most difficult and whether they may need more information about them.

Understanding information in stressful situations

When people are stressed they will often feel overwhelmed and struggle to keep pace with what is happening around them (Krans et al., 2018). Health professionals may relay information and assume the information has been understood by the person. However, even under normal circumstances, only 30 per cent of the information a person receives is retained (Ousseine et al., 2019). Moreover, there is evidence that people retain far less information in stressful situations, such as when they are given an unwelcome diagnosis (Hobson, 2018). For example, family members of people who are treated in the hospital context will often say that they have not been given information, despite health professionals documenting that it has indeed been provided. Consequently, it is recommended that health professionals clarify a person's understanding of their situation and provide relevant information more than once.

When checking that the person has an understanding of the information that has been provided, the health professional needs to consider if the person's health status allows them to:

- understand what they are being told
- retain the information
- weigh up options on the basis of the information given
- make a clear decision with an understanding of the short- and longer-term implications of that decision.

It is also important to remember that a person will only develop an understanding of what is happening, in relation to their context and individual circumstances, over time (MacWilliams et al., 2017). This is why health professionals must make use of techniques such as:

- checking that the person has understood the information by making the time to sit down with the person and asking them to repeat what was communicated
- making audio recordings or leaving written information with the person and their family or significant others
- documenting that the information has been provided
- following up with the person and their family to answer any questions, discuss any issues and provide more information if required.
- This approach ensures that the dialogue continues for as long as is necessary and the person receives adequate and appropriate support (Lesselroth & Monkman, 2019).

Preparing information

When considering how to provide information, it is worth finding out who will be involved in the activity. How many people will be in attendance? Will there be partners, carers, family, friends or children? What are their learning preferences (written, visual, verbal)? And who is best placed to provide the information? Some people may prefer the medical practitioner to provide the information; others may feel they share an affinity with another member of the multidisciplinary team and prefer to interact with them (Crompton & Hardy, 2018). There may even be times when the person prefers to speak to a student health professional, perhaps because they are less intimidating or have more time to spend with them (Johnson et al., 2018).

Initially, even before thinking about what information to give the person, there must be clarity regarding the reasons the information is being provided (Rapchak et al., 2018). As noted earlier, there was a time when health professionals routinely withheld information, believing it to be damaging for the person to be told what is happening to them (e.g. Oken, 1961). However, approaches to providing health care have now shifted from paternalism to consumer-centred models. In contemporary health settings, information is provided as a matter of course (MacWilliams et al., 2017). Providing timely and accurate information is a fundamental part of gaining consent for treatment from health care consumers. It is vital, then, to give the person the opportunity to express their views about what information they might wish to receive, how they would like to receive it and who they would like to be in attendance.

The clarity of what is said, the way in which it is said, and the environment in which the discussion takes place, will likewise have a significant impact on relationships between the health professional and those to whom they provide a service (Crompton & Hardy, 2018). Questions the health professional may ask could include the following.

- 'What do you know about your situation?'
- 'How do you feel about your current situation?'
- 'What do you think will happen with your health issue?'

Each of these questions seeks to explore the person's ideas and feelings or interpretations regarding their condition, which may be very different from the situation as it is understood by the health professional.

There may also be times when a person asks a surprise question and the health professional feels unable to respond. Rather than inventing an answer, it is better for the health professional to request that the person waits while the correct information is located, and return to discuss the matter at the earliest opportunity.

Table 5.2 provides a summary of dos and don'ts to consider when facilitating and providing information to a person. This table is a useful tool for health professionals to guide them to provide the most appropriate information, at the best time and in the most suitable manner.

TABLE 5.2   A summary of dos and don'ts when providing information

Do	Don't
Be guided by what the person has said they want to know about their health issue.	Provide information that is irrelevant or not required.
Think through and prepare carefully what it is that needs to be communicated, including body language and non-verbal cues as well as verbal cues.	Rush into providing the person with information because the opportunity seems to present itself or you have been asked an awkward question.
Find out what the person already knows about their health issues and how they understand the information.	Assume you know what the person already knows.
Have written information available about the person's health issue, including different options for addressing the issue.	Begin the discussion without adequately preparing.
Invite partners, carers, family members or significant others to attend.	Begin without knowing who is in the room, whether the person wants everyone who is in the room to be there, or if there is someone else the person wants to be present who has not been invited.
Prepare the physical environment in which the dialogue will take place.	Allow interruptions, such as pagers, mobile phones or colleagues 'wanting a moment'.
Use simple language with as little jargon as possible.	Use jargon.
Actively listen to the person, their partner, carer, family members or significant others.	Disregard or selectively listen to the feedback provided.
Find out the person's agenda and align yourself, without giving up the need to provide information.	Trivialise the information or the person's experience (e.g. 'Everything will be all right' or 'I'm sure you'll cope very well').
Lead up to the key points you would like to impart.	Become defensive or critical of other health professionals or service providers who are involved in the person's health care.
Clarify the person's understanding of what has been said.	Make glib promises that you may not be able to keep (e.g. telling the person 'I promise you, everything will be okay', or 'There's no need to worry').
Use reiteration.	Make assumptions.
Use and tolerate short silences.	Allow insufficient time for the discussion.
Explore the person's feelings and reactions.	Leave the meeting without having checked what ongoing support the person and their partner, carer or family thinks they may need.
Use open questions, always listening for cues from the person.	Use closed questions, which don't give the person the option to talk freely.
Use diagrams to illustrate difficult technical concepts or anatomical information.	Assume the person always understands what is being said, particularly if the information is complex.
Leave written information for the person, their partner, carer, family members or significant others to read in their own time.	Assume the person has absorbed all the information in a single meeting.
Tell the person about other sources of information (e.g. reputable internet sites, self-help organisations and leaflets).	Limit the information or choices, nor assume the person can find the information themselves.
Assure those involved that you will get back to them with answers to questions to which you don't know the answer.	Invent answers to questions to which you don't know the answer.

Follow up with the person, their partner, carer, family members or significant others — particularly if you have told them you will get back to them.	Leave following up with the person to someone else, or forget about it altogether.
Document, in detail, what has been discussed and feedback to the multidisciplinary team.	Underestimate the importance of clear communication.
Follow up the initial discussion with further discussions.	Assume that you will only need to provide the information once.

UPON REFLECTION

Brochures: 'the good, the bad and the ugly'

Many health professionals use brochures, flyers or pamphlets to provide information to consumers and their families. Brochures, flyers or pamphlets can be useful as they outline essential information and address frequently asked questions, in an easily accessible format.

However, consumers and their significant others often complain that health professionals hand them brochures without explanation. This approach is not helpful and most often the brochure, flyer or pamphlet ends up in the rubbish bin. Also, information presented in this format doesn't cater for the person's individual experiences of a health condition for example and assumes a standard basis of knowledge and understanding of health for all people.

QUESTIONS

1. Consider the last time you were handed a brochure by someone. Did you read all of the information in detail or skip over some?
2. How could brochures, flyers or pamphlets be used more effectively to communicate health information to people across different cultural groups?

5.6 Self-care

LEARNING OBJECTIVE 5.6 Consider the different ways that health professionals can self-care.

Health professionals will experience many and varied stressful situations in the course of their work including onerous caseloads, overtime and under-resourcing, constant interruptions, aggression and violence, bullying, moral distress, trauma and death (Christie et al., 2017). It is also important to acknowledge that health professionals are people with their own emotions, experiences, agendas and idiosyncrasies (Ghawadra et al., 2019). It can therefore be very difficult for them leave their personal beliefs about health behind them as they walk into their place of work.

For example, a health professional may have had personal experience of domestic abuse, physical assault or relatives dying, and may therefore feel stressed when re-exposed to events at work that are reminiscent of these personal experiences. Another health professional may have years of experience of dealing with people who are angry or aggressive and, in so doing, have developed a hard, protective shell. Every experience across the years of service adds another dimension to the way in which a health professional views a situation or event, and also to their overall development as a practitioner. Similarly, past experiences will affect the way in which a health professional responds to stressful situations.

Awareness of their own reactions to stress, and the experiences that have shaped these reactions, will enable health professionals to respond more appropriately to any given situation in the workplace (Butler et al., 2019). Indeed, health professionals who have developed an acceptance of who they are — both as individuals and in their relationships with others — will be more able to understand and accept the beliefs, perceptions and reactions of other people (Sanford, Hofmann & Carpenter, 2019). This understanding and acceptance will in turn enable the health professional to more effectively provide support and engage emotionally with the person who is experiencing stress.

Some health professionals may not know where to begin to gain this kind of personal awareness (Rasheed et al., 2019). The sections that follow provide steps in the process of awareness-raising.

In addition, it is recommended that health professionals read relevant self-help books, attend suitable courses or seek the help of a specialised health professional to develop their skills and capabilities in this area of practice.

Reflective practice

The first step for health professionals in managing their reactions to stressful situations is to explore the feelings that are engendered by the stressful situation. This will involve a degree of self-reflection (Richard et al., 2019). Questions health professionals could ask of themselves are as follows.

- What name could I give these emotional reactions? (e.g. anxiety, anger, fear)
- Why am I experiencing these particular emotions?
- Am I able to manage these emotions myself or should I seek support because of the nature and intensity of how I feel?

It is important for the health professional to consider the cause of the emotional reaction. For example, each time a health professional attends a call-out of the medical emergency team (MET), they may feel tightness in the stomach. This health professional would be wise to put some time aside to consider that tightness in the stomach and what it means. Is it adrenaline/excitement? Or is it anxiety? Fear? If the latter, what factors have given rise to this anxiety or fear? What steps could the health professional take to reduce the level of this emotion?

Another common myth in our society is that other people are responsible for making us feel a certain way. For example:

- 'He frightened me.'
- 'You make me feel anxious when you do that.'
- 'It makes me so angry when they don't listen!'

When a health professional lays the blame for a feeling on another person, they displace their personal responsibility and ownership of their own emotions. However, effective health professionals accept that feelings are an inevitable part of a stressful situation (Parissopoulos, 2019).

It is important that health professionals identify these feelings and deal with them as they arise. For example, health professionals may ask, 'What is going on for me that I am having such an intense reaction to that person yelling?' When they allow themselves to explore what is happening within, they learn more about their emotions. This, in turn, provides them with insight regarding how to manage or deal with their emotions.

The key for health professionals is to understand that feelings are meant to be felt. When they are ignored, suppressed or dismissed, there is a build-up of emotional energy (Chervonsky & Hunt, 2017). Of course, in the workplace there will often be times when health professionals are required to delay feeling the emotions until a more suitable time, that is, after they have dealt with the situation at hand. However, when the occasion arrives and they can give full attention to the feelings or reactions, health professionals may then ask themselves questions such as the following.

- What thoughts, feelings and actions was I experiencing during that stressful situation?
- What will happen if I allow myself to sit with the unpleasant feelings right now?
- This strategy will help the health professional to feel the emotions and thereby reduce their intensity.

Finally, it is not uncommon for people, including health professionals, to find that they are unable to perform this self-caring work without assistance. It is therefore recommended that a health professional talk to a colleague about the situation or seek advice from a trusted friend, colleague, counsellor or specialised mental health practitioner who will teach them the skills they need to manage their own reactions on an ongoing basis.

Another way the health professional can reflect upon their practice is through the process of journaling (Spence, 2017). Some health professionals use journaling as a tool to consider practice issues or personal interactions that may be troubling them. Journaling can increase self-awareness, provide opportunities for a person's growth and help them to achieve their goals (Monk & Maisel, 2021). Specific questions that the health professional could ask themselves might include the following.

- What assumptions are being made by me or others in this stressful health-related situation?
- What are the factors contributing to the stressful situation?
- What and how could I do things differently in future?

Regularly journaling in this way, while being mindful of consumer confidentiality can help the health professional to reflect upon stressful situations and think about ways to improve their practice.

Other health professionals may prefer to participate in practice reflection by verbalising. This can be achieved by identifying another health professional and forming a mutually trusting peer relationship that enables both participants to explore professional issues and practices in a safe environment (McDermott et al., 2018). Such informal discussions can also be undertaken in groups. A more formal arrangement to participate in practice reflections is called 'clinical supervision'.

Clinical supervision

In the health context, **clinical supervision** is a formal and ongoing process of giving and receiving professional support through reflective practice (Pollock et al., 2017). It provides a useful means by which health professionals can access professional support and education. Clinical supervision, which can be received one-to-one or in a group, enables health professionals to formally reflect upon and discuss ways of developing their practice (Dickie et al., 2019).

In some health settings, the term 'clinical supervision' is used in the medical sense to describe the supervisory relationship between the expert practitioner and student who is practising their skills in a 'real world' context (e.g. Witney et al., 2018). This appropriation of the term by the medical fraternity is unfortunate because it has created some confusion. Clinical supervision, however, is not about precepting, facilitating or supervising students in a clinical context. Nor is it about line management or performance appraisal as it is often associated with (Masamha et al., 2022). Rather, clinical supervision is about helping the health professional to consider their practice and discuss insights or issues with another (senior) health professional, with a view to improving their knowledge and competence (Vandette & Gosselin, 2019).

There are two broad aims for clinical supervision. The first is to provide health professionals with a confidential, safe and supportive environment to critically reflect upon their professional practice and improve their self-awareness (Wubbolding, 2017). The second is to improve the mental health practice of health professionals and, as a consequence, outcomes for consumers and their families (White, 2017). Outcomes of clinical supervision include supporting the practice and mental health of health professionals, safeguarding practice standards and improving the quality of care that is being provided (Pollock et al., 2017).

In Australia, health professionals who work in all areas of health care provision are encouraged to participate in clinical supervision on a regular basis (Russell et al., 2017). In particular, those who work in stressful workplaces have found clinical supervision to be a useful tool that enables them to examine situations that are challenging. It is important to consider both problem- and emotional-focused strategies to reduce psychological distress (Lorente et al., 2020). Further, it can be advantageous for health professionals to cognitively consider an event or situation as opposed to experiencing intense emotions for long periods. Similarly, health professionals who participate in clinical supervision have higher levels of satisfaction with their work and are less likely to 'burn out' (Macdonald, 2019).

It is critical that health professionals feel supported — and, indeed, *are* supported — in their workplace. Clinical supervision provides one way this can occur. Health professionals are encouraged to ask their manager how they can regularly receive clinical supervision from a suitably qualified health professional. It is important that health professionals feel comfortable with the supervisor also. A study with medical students found they were more likely to engage with the process of clinical supervision when they felt psychological safe (Thyness et al., 2022).

Time out

Health professionals work in a very demanding field. Many health professionals find the nature of their work to be stressful and may leave their work in the health context for less demanding work. It is crucial, then, that health professionals undertake pleasurable self-caring activities that can be equated with 'time out'. The nature of these activities will vary according to personal preference. As a general rule, however, the following activities are recommended for those who work in stressful occupations.

• Balance time alone for quiet reflections and activities with others.
• Pursue other personal/individual/group activities that give pleasure.
• Develop or pursue significant positive relationships with others (personal, social, spiritual, cultural).
• Ensure regular sleep, preferably eight hours per day.
• Participate in regular exercise which is enjoyable for the individual.
• Minimise alcohol, nicotine and caffeine intake.
• Ensure regular, healthy eating and keep hydrated.
• Plan for and take regular breaks.

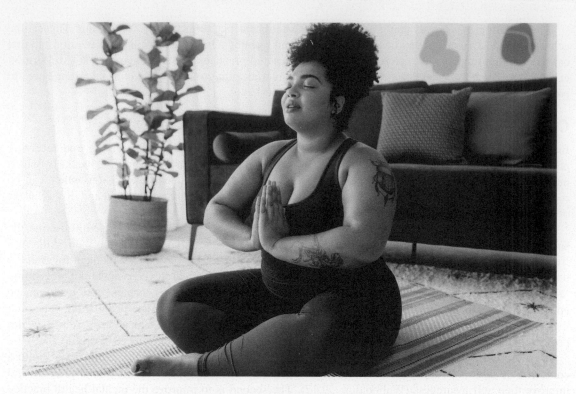

Health professionals must also ensure that they manage their own general health and wellbeing. Many practitioners are so busy assessing the health status of other people that they forget about, ignore or continually postpone thinking about their own health. They must make regular visits to a GP or other health professional to assess their general health and wellbeing (Tackett, 2018).

Health professionals who regularly self-care will be better able to manage their reactions to stressful situations as they arise. Equally, they will be better able to respond to stressful situations in a considered way.

UPON REFLECTION

'To feel or not to feel' — that is the question

There are times, especially in emergency situations, when health professionals cannot allow themselves to feel their emotions, but instead must deal with the situation-at-hand. Such situations could include providing health care to a child who has life threatening injuries or experiencing violent or aggressive behaviour by a consumer.

Other situations may be less urgent and provoke strong emotions in health professionals. For example, Vaclavik et al. (2018) discuss the impact of the moral distress experienced by health professionals who find themselves working in situations they feel are wrong. The common situation was some health professionals offering false hope to people with life-limiting health conditions. Continuing active and distressing treatments when a person's prognosis or life-expectancy are very limited is another example.

Such situations raise the question of whether it is appropriate, or even 'professional', for health professionals to express what they are feeling in an occupational setting.

There is no doubt that many health professionals find it useful to suppress their emotions until they are in a more appropriate time and location, to process what has occurred. Problems arise when health professionals either express strong and intense emotions in the clinical setting when it is not suitable to do so or continue to deny their feelings, are not aware of what is happening for them and do not learn appropriate strategies for dealing with their stress.

QUESTIONS

1. What are your current strategies to identify and manage stress?

2. Who are the people who support you when you are experiencing stress?

3. What strategies do you use to support others who are experiencing stress?

SUMMARY

This chapter outlined the physiological, emotional and behavioural reactions most often experienced by people in stressful situations. Such reactions include the acute stress reaction; as well as emotional and behavioural responses, such as anger, anxiety, denial, fear, grief and loss.

There are factors that influence the way people react to stress and stressful situations, for example, a person's age, background, coping style and locus of control. The chapter also identified context and setting as influencing factors. Specifically, people and communities that experience a disaster will often experience high levels of emotion. Likewise, a person who is in a hospital setting may react quite differently to another person in the same situation or differently to a person who is in a community setting.

The chapter then considered the main priorities for health professionals who support people who are experiencing stress. Subsequent to this, the need for health professionals to find the time to support people through stressful situations was discussed. In addition, it was recommended that health professionals work to engage with the person and their significant others to establish connections and form therapeutic relationships. Recommendations were then made for health professionals to refer the person on to a specialist for assistance when appropriate.

An essential focus of the chapter was the provision of information, including how and when to provide information to people who are stressed. This includes a description of how to prepare the information. Finally, the chapter identified the value of self-caring activities for health professionals, outlining some strategies to support health professionals to this end.

All health professionals have a unique role to play in helping to bridge the gap between the biological, psychological, emotional, social, spiritual and functional elements of care. An improved understanding of the impact of ill-health or injury upon a person, and the way the person is most likely to react, ensures health professionals develop the confidence to reclaim this essential aspect of health care.

KEY TERMS

acute stress reaction A transient psychological anxiety condition that develops physiologically in response to a traumatic event; usually begins within minutes of the event and disappears after hours or days.

care plan Written document developed by the health professional in collaboration with the patient — and, wherever possible, family members — outlining the patient's overall health or treatment goals, the objectives or steps to be taken to achieve these goals, the specific health interventions to be implemented and ongoing progress.

clinical supervision A formal and ongoing process of giving and receiving professional support through reflective practice.

de-escalation The process by which a person's strong feelings or reactions are reduced in intensity.

disaster health An interdisciplinary approach to the prevention of, preparedness for, response to, and recovery from the various health issues that arise from a disaster.

disaster A sudden event, such as an accident or a natural catastrophe, that causes great damage or loss of life.

distress Where a person's wellbeing is compromised due to an inability to adapt to acute, severe or prolonged stressors, or multiple and cumulative stressful events.

health locus of control The extent to which a person believes that their health is controlled by internal, external or fatalistic factors.

homeostasis The tendency in systems, including the human body systems, to maintain the balance, stability or wellbeing of those systems.

interpersonal therapy (IPT) A time-limited therapeutic approach that aims to improve social adjustment by focusing on interactions that occur in current relationships, and the way a person perceives themselves in those relationships.

mental health literacy The knowledge and understanding about mental health and illness that assists people to prevent, recognise, manage mental health issues and associated recovery.

normalising The process of reframing a person's feelings or perceptions of an event or situation so that these feelings or perceptions become more acceptable to that person.

post-traumatic stress disorder (PTSD) A diagnosed mental health condition characterised by the development of a long-lasting anxiety reaction following a traumatic or catastrophic event.

prime emotions Emotions in their simplest form. They cannot be divided into more than one particular feeling.

reaction The immediate or instantaneous feeling, action, movement or tendency within a person that is caused by a stimulus of some kind.

repression An unconscious long-term process where feelings are minimised or ignored.

resilience The psychological and emotional strengths, assets, stamina and endurance of a person to adapt to changed circumstances.

strategies The actions taken by a particular person after due consideration has been given to the possible and/or actual affects and outcomes of a stimulus.

stress The physical, emotional, psychological, social or spiritual reaction that is stimulated in a person in response to a situation, event or condition.

stressor Any event or circumstance that precipitates a stress reaction in a person.

suppression The process by which the person consciously puts feelings aside so he or she can cope with an event.

trigger A word, comment, event or other experience that produces an immediate or instantaneous feeling or reaction within a person; a trigger is most often linked to a past event or experience.

REVIEW QUESTIONS

1 What is the difference between stress and distress? In what situations are people more likely to experience distress?

2 What is an acute stress reaction and how would you support a person who is experiencing this kind of reaction to stress?

3 What are some common emotional reactions to stressful situations that people may exhibit in health settings such as in and out-patients clinic, while visiting Accident and Emergency or in a palliative care unit? As a health professional, what strategies would you take to support a person who is experiencing a common reaction to a stressful situation?

4 What are the major factors that influence the way people respond to stress?

5 Outline the steps required to 'de-escalate' a person who is angry.

6 Describe the key messages from the AIDR to support communities to develop disaster resilience.

7 Define 'resilience' and explain how health professionals can help support people to improve their levels of resilience.

8 What are the most important aspects of a care plan and how can they be used to help people with health issues to better understand and manage their levels of stress?

9 Identify the main steps taken by health professionals to facilitate and provide information to people who are experiencing stressful situations.

10 Identify four ways in which health professionals can self-care.

11 Identify five possible symptoms of anxiety.

12 What are some suppression and repression strategies which people may use to manage their emotions?

DISCUSSION AND DEBATE

1 The term 'stress' is used in our everyday language. How might the understanding of stress differ across cultures and communities?

2 Children react quite differently than adults when experiencing stressful situations. As a health professional, name three strategies you can use to support children who are experiencing high levels of stress. How might the strategies differ when supporting parents who may also be experiencing high levels of stress?

3 What is 'disaster resilience'? What can health professionals do to help people develop 'disaster resilience'?

4 Consider the importance of the care plan or treatment plan or recovery plan. What challenges must be overcome to ensure that such plans are truly collaborative? What steps can be taken to ensure consumers are actively engaged in their own health assessment and care planning?

5 What are the different factors that attract people to work in the health professions? How can these factors promote longevity in health care employment?

6 What strategies can health professionals use to positively engage with consumers and their families?

7 What are some of the possible benefits of clinical supervision for health professionals?

8 How can timely information be helpful for people when they are affected by a disaster?

PROJECT ACTIVITY

Go to the Emergency Management Australia podcasts provided by the Australian Government, Attorney-General's department: www.buzzsprout.com/19389

These podcasts cover a range of issues related to the emergency management of bushfires, cyclones, earthquakes and tsunamis. They also cover policy development and program delivery issues.

Select at least five podcasts, listen to them and take notes on the points that most catch your attention.

1 What are the major issues identified in emergency management and/or disaster preparedness in Australia for individuals, families and communities?

2 What are the major issues related to the provision and delivery of services during a disaster?

3 Why do we need national policies and programs to oversee emergency management, including disasters?

4 How prepared are you to assist in a disaster or other emergency? What can you do to increase your disaster preparedness?

WEBSITES

1 The World Health Organization provides a range of resources and documents to guide first responders and other emergency personnel who give mental health and psychosocial support in emergencies: https://www.who.int/news-room/fact-sheets/detail/mental-health-in-emergencies. Their Building Back Better publication focuses on sustainable mental health care after emergencies: https://apps.who.int/iris/bitstream/handle/10665/96378/WHO_MSD_MER_13.1_eng.pdf?sequence=8. There is also the World Health Organisation Special Initiative for Mental Health 2019–2023 which seeks to provide access to quality and affordable mental health care for all: www.who.int/initiatives/who-special-initiative-for-mental-health.

2 The Australian Centre for Grief and Bereavement is an independent, not-for-profit organisation which opened in January 1996 and is the largest provider of grief and bereavement education in Australia. Registered as a public benevolent institution, the centre receives operational funding through the state cancer and palliative care program of the Victorian Department of Health: www.grief.org.au.

3 Disaster Assist is an Australian government initiative that provides details of the assistance available for current disasters, as well as link to assistance and responses to previous disasters that have affected Australians, both in Australia and overseas: www.disasterassist.gov.au.

4 Helpguide is a not-for-profit resource providing free information to help empower people with knowledge, support and hope to improve their mental health: www.helpguide.org.

5 Lifeline provides access to crisis support, suicide prevention and mental health support services. People call Lifeline's 24-hour crisis support service, 13 11 14, about many things, including anxiety, depression, loneliness, abuse and trauma, physical or mental wellbeing, suicidal thoughts or attempts, stresses from work, family or society, and information for friends and family. Lifeline also provides national services and campaigns that promote emotional wellbeing, encourage help-seeking and address suicide prevention and awareness: www.lifeline.org.au.

6 'Get Healthy' is a NSW Health initiative offering up to 13 phone calls over a 6-month period. The program provides basic information and tools for people to start making healthier changes. This includes information on eating better, being active, limiting alcohol, maintaining a healthy weight and managing stress: www.gethealthynsw.com.au.

7 Mental Health Australia is the peak, national non-government organisation representing and promoting the interests of the Australian mental health sector, committed to achieving better mental health for all Australians: www.mhaustralia.org.

REFERENCES

Abelson, J., Tripp, L., Kandasamy, S., & Burrows, K. (2019). Supporting the evaluation of public and patient engagement in health system organizations: Results from an implementation research study. *Health Expectations*, *22*(5), 1132–1143. https://doi.org/10.1111/hex.12949

Aldrich, R. (2018). *Resilience*. American Library Association.

American Psychological Association. (2019). *Stress effects on the body*. www.apa.org/helpcenter/stress-body

Appignanesi, L. (2018). *Everyday madness: On grief, anger, loss and love*. HarperCollins.

Ates, M., Dogru, B., Yesilbalkan, O., Karadakovan, A., & Akman, P. (2018). Educational needs of caregivers of patients hospitalized in a neurology clinic: Results of questionnaire. *International Journal of Caring Sciences*, *11*(2), 968–976. www.internationaljournalofcaringsciences.org/docs/38_yesilbakan_original_10_2.pdf

Australian Commission on Safety and Quality in Health Care. (2019). *Action 5.12: Developing the comprehensive care plan*. www.safetyandquality.gov.au/standards/nsqhs-standards/comprehensive-care-standard/developing-comprehensive-care-plan/action-512

Australian Emergency Management Institute, Attorney-General's Department. (2011). *Disaster health: Handbook 1*. Commonwealth of Australia.

Australian Institute for Disaster Resilience. (2018). *AIDR Strategy 2018–2021. AIDR*. https://knowledge.aidr.org.au/media/5708/aidr-strategy.pdf

Australian Institute for Disaster Resilience. (2019). *National strategy for disaster resilience: Companion booklet*. AIDR. https://knowledge.aidr.org.au/media/2154/nationalstrategyfordisasterresilience-companionbooklet.pdf

Australian Institute for Disaster Resilience. (n.d.). *Disaster map*.

Bandla, S., Nappinnai, R., & Gopalasamy, S. (2019). Psychiatric morbidity in December 2015 flood-affected population in Tamil Nadu, India. *International Journal of Social Psychiatry*, *65*(4), 338–344. https://doi.org/10.1177/0020764019846166

Bapat, A., & Bojarski, E. (2019). Transference and countertransference in palliative care. *Journal of Palliative Medicine*, *22*(4), 452–453. https://doi.org/10.1089/jpm.2019.0042

Barrett, L., Adolphs, R., Marsella, S., Martinez, A., & Pollak, S. (2019). Emotional expressions reconsidered: Challenges to inferring emotion from human facial movements. *Psychological Science in the Public Interest*, *20*(1), 1–68. https://doi.org/10.1177/1529100619832930

Baumeler, L., Gürber, S., Grob, A., Surbek, D., & Stadlmayr, W. (2017). Antenatal depressive symptoms and subjective birth experience in association with postpartum depressive symptoms and acute stress reaction in mothers and fathers: A longitudinal path analysis. *European Journal of Obstetrics & Gynecology & Reproductive Biology*, *215*, 68–74. https://doi.org/10.1016/j.ejogrb.2017.05.021

BBC News. (2019, December 17). White Island: NZ Police complete identification of volcano victims. *BBC News*. www.bbc.com/news/world-asia-50818622

Beattie, J., Griffiths, D., Innes, K., & Morphet, J. (2019). Workplace violence perpetrated by clients of health care: A need for safety and trauma-informed care. *Journal of Clinical Nursing*, *28*(1/2), 116–124. https://doi.org/10.1111/jocn.14683

Beatty, A. (2019). *Emotional worlds: Beyond an anthropology of emotion*. Cambridge University Press.

Benevolenza, M., & DeRigne, L. (2019). The impact of climate change and natural disasters on vulnerable populations: A systematic review of literature. *Journal of Human Behavior in the Social Environment*, *29*(2), 266–281. https://doi.org/10.1080/10911359.2018.1527739

Benjamin, L. (2018). *Interpersonal reconstructive therapy for anger, anxiety and depression: It's about broken hearts, not broken brains*. American Psychological Association.

Berger-Höger, B., Liethmann, K., Mühlhauser, I., Haastert, B., & Steckelberg, A. (2019). Nurse-led coaching of shared decision-making for women with ductal carcinoma in situ in breast care centers: A cluster randomized controlled trial. *International Journal of Nursing Studies*, *93*, 141–152. https://doi.org/10.1016/j.ijnurstu.2019.01.013

Birhanu, M., Gebrekidan, B., Tesefa, G., & Tareke, M. (2018). Workload determines workplace stress among health professionals working in Felege-Hiwot Referral Hospital, Bahir Dar, Northwest Ethiopia. *Journal of Environmental Public Health*, *2018*, 6286010. https://doi.org/10.1155/2018/6286010,

Bourbeau, P. (2018). *On resilience: Genealogy, logistics and world politics*. Cambridge University Press.

Breisinger, L., Bires, A., & Cline, T. (2018). Stress reduction in postcardiac surgery family members: Implementation of a postcardiac surgery tool kit. *Critical Care Nursing Quarterly*, *41*(2), 186–196. https://doi.org/10.1097/CNQ.0000000000000198

Brighton, L., Selman, L., Bristowe, K., Edwards, B., Koffman, J., & Evans, C. (2019). Emotional labour in palliative and end-of-life care communication: A qualitative study with generalist palliative care providers. *Patient Education & Counseling*, *102*(3), 494–502. https://doi.org/10.1016/j.pec.2018.10.013

Brisson, G. (2019). Colleagues unknown — how peer evaluation could enhance the referral process. *New England Journal of Medicine*, *381*(14), 1303–1305. www.nejm.org/doi/10.1056/NEJMp1905524

Brown, T., Dyck, I., Greenhough, B., Raven-Ellison, M., Dembinsky, M., Ornstein, M., & Duffy, S. (2017). Fear, family and the placing of emotion: Black women's responses to a breast cancer awareness intervention. *Social Science & Medicine*, *195*, 90–96. https://doi.org/10.1016/j.socscimed.2017.10.037

Bryant, R., Stein, M., & Hermann, R. (2019). Acute stress disorder in adults: Epidemiology, pathogenesis, clinical manifestations, course, and diagnosis. *UptoDate*. www.uptodate.com/contents/acute-stress-disorder-in-adults-epidemiology-pathogenesis-clinical-manifestations-course-and-diagnosis

Bui, E. (2018). Grief: From normal to pathological reactions. In E. Bui (Ed.), *Clinical handbook of bereavement and grief reactions* (pp. 85–101). Springer International Publishing.

Burton, N. (2019). What are basic emotions? *Psychology Today*. www.psychologytoday.com/au/blog/hide-and-seek/201601/what-are-basic-emotions

Butler, L., Mercer, K., McClain-Meeder, K., Horne, D., & Dudley, M. (2019). Six domains of self-care: Attending to the whole person. *Journal of Human Behavior in the Social Environment, 29*(1), 107–124. https://doi.org/10.1080/10911359.2018.1482483

Buxton, D. (2017). Why are patients difficult for staff? *Journal of Palliative Medicine, 20*(10), 1170. https://doi.org/10.1089/jpm.2017.0210

Carnall, L. A., Mason, O., O'Sullivan, M., & Patton, R. (2022). Psychosocial hazards, posttraumatic stress disorder, complex posttraumatic stress disorder, depression, and anxiety in the U.K. rail industry: A cross-sectional study. *Journal of Traumatic Stress, 35*(5), 1460–1471. https://doi.org/10.1002/jts.22846

Castellà-Creus, M., Delgado-Hito, P., Casanovas-Cuellar, C., Tàpia-Pérez, M., & Juvé-Udina, M. (2019). Barriers and facilitators involved in standardised care plan individualisation process in acute hospitalisation wards: A grounded theory approach. *Journal of Clinical Nursing, 28*(23/24), 4606–4620. https://doi.org/10.1111/jocn.15059

Centre for Studies on Human Stress. (2019). *Biology of stress.* https://humanstress.ca/stress/what-is-stress/biology-of-stress

Chan, Z. (2017). A qualitative study on communication between nursing students and the family members of patients. *Nurse Education Today, 59*, 33–37. https://doi.org/10.1016/j.nedt.2017.08.017

Cheetham-Blake, T., Turner-Cobb, J., Family, H., & Turner, J. (2019). Resilience characteristics and prior life stress determine anticipatory response to acute social stress in children aged 7–11 years. *British Journal of Health Psychology, 24*(2), 282–297. https://doi.org/10.1111/bjhp.12353

Chervonsky, E., & Hunt, C. (2017). Suppression and expression of emotion in social and interpersonal outcomes: A meta-analysis. *Emotion, 17*(4), 669–683. https://doi.org/10.1037/emo0000270

Chim, H., Yew, W., & Song, C. (2007). Managing burn victims of suicide bombing attacks: Outcomes, lessons learnt, and changes made from three attacks in Indonesia. *Critical Care, 11*, R15. https://doi.org/10.1186/cc5681

Christie, C., Bidwell, S., Copeland, A., & Hudson, B. (2017). Self-care of Canterbury general practitioners, nurse practitioners, practice nurses and community pharmacists. *Journal of Primary Health Care, 9*(4), 286–291. https://doi.org/10.1071/HC17034

Chrousos, G., Loriaux, D., & Gold, P. (2013). *Mechanisms of physical and emotional stress.* Springer Science & Business Media.

Cody, S., Sullivan-Bolyai, S., & Reid-Ponte, P. (2018). Making a connection: Family experiences with bedside rounds in the intensive care unit. *Critical Care Nurse, 38*(3), 16–26. https://doi.org/10.4037/ccn2018128

Cohen, A., & Stern, R. (2017). *Thinking about the emotions: A philosophical history.* Oxford University Press.

Cooper, R. (2018). Perspectives on the holiday season from a California psychiatrist: No joy for the world. *Psychiatric Times, 35*(12).

Corey, G. (2017). *Theory and practice of counseling and psychotherapy* (10th ed.). Cengage.

Cox, L. (2019, January 17). Extreme heatwave: All-time temperature records fall across parts of Australia. *The Guardian.* www.theguardian.com/australia-news/2019/jan/17/extreme-heatwave-all-time-temperature-records-fall-across-parts-of-australia

Crompton, H., & Hardy, S. (2018). Preparing to improve access for young people's mental healthcare. *Practice Nursing, 29*(12), 600–605. https://doi.org/10.12968/pnur.2018.29.12.600

Crum, A., Akinola, M., Martin, A., & Fath, S. (2017). The role of stress mindset in shaping cognitive, emotional, and physiological responses to challenging and threatening stress. *Anxiety, Stress & Coping, 30*(4), 379–395. https://doi.org/10.1080/10615806.2016.1275585

de Dios-Duarte., J, M., Arias, A., Durantez-Fernández, C., Virtudes Niño, M., Olea, E., Barba-Pérez, M., Pérez-Pérez, L., Cárdaba-García, R. M., & Barrón, A. (2022). Flare-ups in Crohn's disease: Influence of stress and the external locus of control. *International Journal of Environmental Research and Public Health, 19*(20), 13131. https://doi.org/10.3390/ijerph192013131

De Vries, M., Jansen, J., Van Weert, J., & Holland, R. (2019). Fostering shared decision making with health informatics interventions based on the boosting framework. *Studies in Health Technology & Informatics, 263*, 109–121. https://doi.org/10.3233/SHTI190116

Demorest, S., Spengeman, S., Schenk, E., Cook, C., & Weston, H. (2019). The nurses climate challenge: A national campaign to engage 5,000 health professionals around climate change. *Creative Nursing, 25*(3), 208–215. https://doi.org/10.1891/1078-4535.25.3.208

Department of Education. (2019). *Student resilience and wellbeing resources.* Australian Government. www.education.gov.au/student-resilience-and-wellbeing/student-resilience-and-wellbeing-resources

Department of Foreign Affairs and Trade. (2019). *Humanitarian preparedness and response.* Australian Government. https://dfat.gov.au/aid/topics/investment-priorities/building-resilience/humanitarian-preparedness-and-response/Pages/humanitarian-preparedness-and-response.aspx

Dewe, P., & Cooper, C. (2017). *Work stress and coping: Force of change and challenges.* SAGE.

Dickie, R., Bartle, E., Jackman, K., & Bonney, D. (2019). Clinical supervisors' experiences of using an interprofessional clinical supervision model in an acute care setting. *Journal of Interprofessional Care, 33*(6), 812–815. https://doi.org/10.1080/13561820.2019.1594728

Dubale, B., Friedman, L., Chemali, Z., Denninger, J., Mehta, D., Alem, A., Fricchione, G., Dossett, M., & Gelaye, B. (2019). Systematic review of burnout among healthcare providers in sub-Saharan Africa. *BMC Public Health, 19*(1), 1247. https://doi.org/10.1186/s12889-019-7566-7

Duculan, R., Jannat-Khah, D., Wang, X. A., & Mancuso, C. A. (2022). Psychological stress reported at the start of the COVID-19 pandemic and subsequent stress and successful coping in patients with rheumatic diseases: A longitudinal analysis. *Journal of Clinical Rheumatology, 28*(5), 250–256. https://doi.org/10.1097/RHU.0000000000001846

Feinberg, L. (2019). Paid family leave: An emerging benefit for employed family caregivers of older adults. *Journal of the American Geriatrics Society, 67*(7), 1336–1341. https://doi.org/10.1111/jgs.15869

Fernandes dos Santos Lima, M., de Santana Carvalho, E., Marques dos Santos, L., & Martins Júnior, D. (2017). Nursing diagnoses of the 'coping/tolerance to stress' domain, identified in women with leg ulcers. *Journal of Nursing UFPE, 11*(Suppl. 3), 1365–1374.

Folz, E. (2018). Implementation of a critical incidence stress management program at a tertiary care hospital. *Canadian Journal of Critical Care Nursing, 29*(2), 37–38.

France, C., & France, J. (2019). Estimating the risk of blood donation fainting for self versus others: The moderating effect of fear. *Transfusion*, *59*(6), 2039–2045. https://doi.org/10.1111/trf.15225

Furedi, F. (2018). *How fear works: Culture of fear in the twenty-first century*. Bloomsbury.

Furtak, R. (2018). *Knowing emotions: Truthfulness and recognition in affective experience*. Oxford University Press.

Ghawadra, S., Abdullah, K., Choo, W., & Phang, C. (2019). Mindfulness-based stress reduction for psychological distress among nurses: A systematic review. *Journal of Clinical Nursing*, *28*(21/22), 3747–3758. https://doi.org/10.1111/jocn.14987

Gibson, K., Haslam, N., & Kaplan, I. (2019). Distressing encounters in the context of climate change: Idioms of distress, determinants, and responses to distress in Tuvalu. *Transcultural Psychiatry*, *56*(4), 667–696. https://doi.org/10.1177/1363461519847057

Gissing, A., & Coates, L. (2018, January 18). *Heatwaves are Australia's deadliest natural hazard and many of us are unprepared. The Conversation*. www.abc.net.au/news/2018-01-18/heatwaves-australias-deadliest-hazard-why-you-need-plan/9338918

Gluff, J., Teolis, M., Moore, A., & Kelly, D. (2017). Post-traumatic stress disorder (PTSD): A webliography. *Journal of Consumer Health on the Internet*, *21*(4), 389–401. https://doi.org/10.1080/15398285.2017.1377539

Gomes, B., Dowd, B., & Sethares, K. (2019). Attitudes of community hospital critical care nurses toward family-witnessed resuscitation. *American Journal of Critical Care*, *28*(2), 142–148. https://doi.org/10.4037/ajcc2019162

Grady, K., & Wallston, B. (1988). *Research in health care settings*. Sage.

Grainger, S., Vanman, E., Matters, G., & Henry, J. (2019). The influence of tears on older and younger adults' perceptions of sadness. *Psychology & Aging*, *34*(5), 665–673. https://doi.org/10.1037/pag0000373

Greenberg, L. (2017). *Emotion-focused therapy* (revised.ed.). American Psychological Society.

Gregg, H. R., Restubog, S. L., Dasborough, M., Xu, C., Deen, C. M., & He, Y. (2022). When disaster strikes! An interdisciplinary review of disasters and their organizational consequences. *Journal of Management*, *48*(6), 1382–1429. https://doi.org/10.1177/01492063221076808

Griggs, C., Fernandez, A., & Callanan, M. (2017). The impact of healthcare on global warming and human health: Connecting the dots. *British Journal of Healthcare Assistants*, *11*(7), 348–353. https://doi.org/10.12968/bjha.2017.11.7.348

Haines, K., Kelly, P., Fitzgerald, P., Skinner, E., & Iwashyna, T. (2017). The untapped potential of patient and family engagement in the organization of critical care. *Critical Care Medicine*, *45*(5), 899–906. https://doi.org/10.1097/CCM.0000000000002282

Halligan, S. (2017). How can informal support impact child PTSD symptoms following a psychological trauma? *Emergency Medicine Journal*, *34*(12):A894. https://emj.bmj.com/content/34/12/A894.1

Hanna, J., McCaughan, E., & Semple, C. (2019). Challenges and support needs of parents and children when a parent is at end of life: A systematic review. *Palliative Medicine*, *33*(8), 1017–1044. https://doi.org/10.1177/0269216319857622

Healy, K. (2018). *The skilled communicator in social work: The art and science of communication in practice*. Palgrave.

Hensch, D. (2017). *Positively resilient: 5½ secrets to beat stress, overcome obstacles and defeat anxiety*. The Career Press.

Hiromi, T., Yoshiyuki, T., Makiko, O., & Takashi, I. (2017). Intervention for post-traumatic stress disorder in children after disaster: A literature review. *International Journal of Child & Adolescent Health*, *10*(1), 7–15.

Hobson, N. (2018). *Why your brain on stress fails to learn properly. Psychology Today*. www.psychologytoday.com/us/blog/ritual-and-the-brain/201804/why-your-brain-stress-fails-learn-properly

Holmgreen, L., Tirone, V., Gerhart, J., & Hobfoll, S. (2017). Conservation of resources theory: Resource caravans and passageways in health contexts. In L. C. Cooper & J. Campbell Quick (Eds.), *The handbook of stress and health: A guide to research and practice* (pp. 443–460). Wiley and Sons.

Horrocks, P., Hobbs, L., Tippett, V., & Aitken, P. (2019). Paramedic disaster health management competencies: A scoping review. *Prehospital & Disaster Medicine*, *34*(3), 322–329. https://doi.org/10.1017/S1049023X19004357

Howard, A., Agllias, K., Bevis, M., & Blakemore, T. (2018). How social isolation affects disaster preparedness and response in Australia: Implications for social work. *Australian Social Work*, *71*(4), 392–404. https://doi.org/10.1080/0312407X.2018.1487461

Hoyt, L. T., Cohen, A. K., Dull, B., Maker Castro, E., & Yazdani, N. (2021). "Constant stress has become the new normal": Stress and anxiety inequalities among U.S. college students in the time of COVID-19. *Journal of Adolescent Health*, *68*(2), 270–276. https://doi.org/10.1016/j.jadohealth.2020.10.030

Irons, M., & Paton, D. (2017). Social media and emergent groups: The impact of high functionality on community resilience. In D. Paton & D. Johnston (Eds.), *Disaster resilience: An integrated approach* (2nd ed., pp. 194–212). Charles C Thomas Publisher.

Isik, A., Soysal, P., Solmi, M., & Veronese, N. (2019). Bidirectional relationship between caregiver burden and neuropsychiatric symptoms in patients with Alzheimer's disease: A narrative review. *International Journal of Geriatric Psychiatry*, *34*(9), 1326–1334. https://doi.org/10.1002/gps.4965

James, J., Baldursdottir, B., Johannsdottir, K., Valdimarsdottir, H., Heiddis, B., & Sigfusdottir, I. (2018). Adolescent habitual caffeine consumption and hemodynamic reactivity during rest, psychosocial stress, and recovery. *Journal of Psychosomatic Research*, *110*, 16–23. https://doi.org/10.1016/j.jpsychores.2018.04.010

Jeronimus, B., Snippe, E., Emerencia, A., Jonge, P., & Bos, E. (2019). Acute stress responses after indirect exposure to the MH17 airplane crash. *British Journal of Psychology*, *110*(4), 790–813. https://doi.org/10.1111/bjop.12358

Jo, M., Song, M., Knafl, G., Beeber, L., Yoo, Y., & Van Riper, M. (2019). Family-clinician communication in the ICU and its relationship to psychological distress of family members: A cross-sectional study. *International Journal of Nursing Studies*, *95*, 34–39. https://doi.org/10.1016/j.ijnurstu.2019.03.020

Johannesson, K., Lundin, T., Frojd, T., Hultman, C., & Michel, P. (2011). Tsunami-exposed tourist survivors: Signs of recovery in a 3-year perspective. *Journal of Nervous & Mental Disease*, *199*(3), 162–169. https://doi.org/10.1097/NMD.0b013e31820c73d1

Johnson, R., Clark, R., & O'Brien, T. (2018). Improving family nurse practitioner students' confidence for clinical decision making and presenting patient information to the preceptor. *Journal of Doctoral Nursing Practice*, *11*(2), 114–118. https://doi.org/10.1891/2380-9418.11.2.114

Jolley, S., Kuipers, E., Stewart, C., Browning, S., Bracegirdle, K., Basit, N., Gin, K., Hirsch, C., Corrigall, R., Banerjea, P., Turley, G., Stahl, D., & Laurens, K. (2018). The Coping with Unusual Experiences for Children Study (CUES): A pilot randomized controlled evaluation of the acceptability and potential clinical utility of a cognitive behavioural intervention package for young people aged 8–14 years with unusual experiences and emotional symptoms. *British Journal of Clinical Psychology, 57*(3), 328–350. https://doi.org/10.1111/bjc.12176

Karanikola, M., & Mpouzika, M. (2018). Time to create a healthy work environment in ICU: A review of current evidence and commentary. *CONNECT: The World of Critical Care Nursing, 12*(2), 44–47. https://connect.springerpub.com/content/sgrwfccn/12/2/44

Kartal, Y., Oskay, U., & Umran, Y. (2017). Anxiety, depression and coping with stress styles of pregnant women with preterm labor risk. *International Journal of Caring Sciences, 10*(2), 716–725. https://www.internationaljournalofcaringsciences.org/docs/9_kartal_original_10_2.pdf

Keim, M. (2022). *Disaster planning: A practical guide for effective health outcomes.* Cambridge University Press.

Keramat Kar, M., Whitehead, L., & Smith, C. (2019). Characteristics and correlates of coping with multiple sclerosis: A systematic review. *Disability & Rehabilitation, 41*(3), 250–264. https://doi.org/10.1080/09638288.2017.1387295

Krans, J., Brown, A., & Moulds, M. (2018). Can an experimental self-efficacy induction through autobiographical recall modulate analogue posttraumatic intrusions? *Journal of Behavior Therapy & Experimental Psychiatry, 58,* 1–11. https://doi.org/10.1016/j.jbtep.2017.07.001

Kübler-Ross, E., & Kessler, D. (2014). *On grief and grieving: Finding the meaning of grief through the five stages of loss.* Simon and Schuster.

Kynoch, K., Crowe, L., McArdle, A., Munday, J., Cabilan, C., & Hines, S. (2017). Structured communication intervention to reduce anxiety of family members waiting for relatives undergoing surgical procedures. *ACORN: The Journal of Perioperative Nursing in Australia, 30*(1), 29–35. https://doi.org/10.26550/2209-1092.1013

Lacerda, M., Cirelli, M., de Barros, L., & Lopes, J. (2017). Anxiety, stress and depression in family members of patients with heart failure. *Revista da Escola de Enfermagem da USP, 51,* 1–8. https://doi.org/10.1590/S1980-220X2016018903211

Landström, C., Levander, L., & Philips, B. (2019). Dynamic interpersonal therapy as experienced by young adults. *Psychoanalytic Psychotherapy, 33*(2), 99–116.https://doi.org/10.1080/02668734.2019.1641834

Lee, S. (2018). Understanding the dynamics among acculturative stress, coping, and growth: A grounded theory of the Korean immigrant adolescent experience. *Children & Youth Services Review, 94,* 105–114. https://doi.org/10.1016/j.childyouth.2018.09.030

Lesselroth, B., & Monkman, H. (2019, August 23–24). Narratives and stories: Novel approaches to improving patient-facing information resources and patient engagement. Lille, France. *Context Sensitive Health Informatics (CSHI) Conference, Studies in Health Technology & Informatics, 265,* 175–180. https://doi.org/10.3233/SHTI190159

Liddon, L., Kingerlee, R., & Barry, J. (2018). Gender differences in preferences for psychological treatment, coping strategies, and triggers to help-seeking. *British Journal of Clinical Psychology, 57*(1), 42–58. https://doi.org/10.1111/bjc.12147

Lines, R. L. T., Ducker, K. J., Ntoumanis, N., Thøgersen-Ntoumani, C., Fletcher, D, D. F., & Gucciardi,. (2021). Stress, physical activity, sedentary behavior, and resilience—The effects of naturalistic periods of elevated stress: A measurement-burst study. *Psychophysiology, 58*(8), e13846. https://doi.org/10.1111/psyp.13846

Lorente, L., Vera, M., & Peiró, T. (2020). Nurses´ stressors and psychological distress during the COVID-19 pandemic: The mediating role of coping and resilience. *Journal of Advanced Nursing, 77*(3), 1335–1344. https://doi.org/10.1111/jan.14695

Lovallo, W. (2016). *Stress and health:Biological and psychological interactions* (3rd ed.). Sage.

Lovely, A., Linu, G., & Tessy, J. (2018). Stress, coping and lived experiences among caregivers of cancer patients on palliative care: A mixed method research. *Indian Journal of Palliative Care, 24*(3), 313–319. https://doi.org/10.4103/IJPC.IJPC_178_17

Macdonald, B. (2019). Restorative clinical supervision: A reflection. *British Journal of Midwifery, 27*(4), 258–264. https://doi.org/10.12968/bjom.2019.27.4.258

MacWilliams, M., Lunar, E., & Denzen, E. (2017). An innovative educational program for international hematopoietic cell transplant pediatric patients. *Journal of Cancer Education, 32*(2), 401–405. https://doi.org/10.1007/s13187-016-0989-2

Mallett, X., & Evison, M. (2017). Critical issues in the historical and contemporary development of forensic anthropology in Australia: An international comparison. *Forensic Science International, 275,* e1–314. e8. 314. https://doi.org/10.1016/j.forsciint.2017.03.019

Marcatto, F., Di Blas, L., Luis, O., Festa, S., & Ferrante, D. (2021). The perceived occupational stress scale: A brief tool for measuring workers' perceptions of stress at work. *European Journal of Psychological Assessment: Official Organ of the European Association of Psychological Assessment, 38*(4), 293–306. https://doi.org/10.1027/1015-5759/a000677

Masamha, R., Alfred, L., Harris, R., Bassett, S., Burden, S., & Gilmore, A. (2022). Barriers to overcoming the barriers': A scoping review exploring 30 years of clinical supervision literature. *Journal of Advanced Nursing, 78*(9), 2678–2692. https://doi.org/10.1111/jan.15283

Matas, H., & Bronstein, J. (2018). A qualitative inquiry of old people's health literacy in situations of health uncertainty. *Health Information & Libraries Journal, 35*(4), 319–330. https://doi.org/10.1111/hir.12234

McDermott, H., Husbands, A., & Brooks-Lewis, L. (2018). Collaborative team reflective practice in trauma service to improve health care. *Journal of Trauma Nursing, 25*(6), 374–380. https://doi.org/10.1097/JTN.0000000000000404

McNamara, B., Banks, E., Gubhaju, L., Joshy, G., Williamson, A., Raphael, B., & Eades, S. (2018). Factors relating to high psychological distress in Indigenous Australians and their contribution to Indigenous–non-Indigenous disparities. *Australian & New Zealand Journal of Public Health, 42*(2), 145–152. https://doi.org/10.1111/1753-6405.12766

Middaugh, D. (2018). Delusion of control: Pushing buttons. *MEDSURG Nursing, 27*(6), 399–400.

Mikneviciute, G., Ballhausen, N., Rimmele, U., & Kliegel, M. (2022). Does older adults' cognition particularly suffer from stress? A systematic review of acute stress effects on cognition in older age. *Neuroscience and Biobehavioral Reviews, 132,* 583–602. https://doi.org/10.1016/j.neubiorev.2021.12.009

Monk, L., & Maisel, E. (2021). (Monk, & E. Maisel (Eds.), *Transformational journaling for coaches, therapists, and clients: A complete guide to the benefits of personal writing.* Routledge.

Moore, K. (2018). *Stress and anxiety: Theories and realities.* Logos Verlag.

Moos, R. (1984). *Coping with physical illness: New perspectives.* Plenum Press.

Mora, C., Counsell, C., Bielecki, C., & Louis, L. (2017). Twenty-seven ways a heatwave can kill you: Deadly heat in the era of climate change. *Circulation: Cardiovascular Quality & Outcomes, 10*(11), 1–3. https://doi.org/10.1161/CIRCOUTCOMES.117.004233

Morrison, V., & Bennett, P. (2016). *An introduction to health psychology* (4th ed.). Pearson.

Nayak, S. (2018). Time management in nursing — hour of need. *International Journal of Caring Sciences, 11*(3), 1997–200. www.internationaljournalofcaringsciences.org/docs/72_nayak_special_11_3_2.pdf

Nguyen, J. (2019). Educating patients. In M. Rawe, K. Nahm, & J. Tomedia (Eds.), *A Practice guide to therapeutic communication for health professionals* (2nd ed., pp. 36–54). Elsevier.

Ning Hou, A., Johnson, B., & Chen, Y. (2017). Locus of control. In L. C. Cooper & J. Campbell Quick (Eds.), *The handbook of stress and health: A guide to research and practice* (pp. 283–298). Wiley and Sons.

Non, A., León-Pérez, G., Glass, H., Kelly, E., & Garrison, N. (2019). Stress across generations: A qualitative study of stress, coping, and caregiving among Mexican immigrant mothers. *Ethnicity & Health, 24*(4), 378–339. https://doi.org/10.1080/13557858.2017.1346184

O'Connor, M., & McConnell, M. (2018). Grief reaction: A neurobiological approach. In E. Bui (Ed.), *Clinical handbook of bereavement and grief reactions* (pp. 45–62). Springer International Publishing.

O'Toole, G. (2016). *Communication: Core interpersonal skills for health professionals* (3rd ed.). Elsevier.

O'Brien, K., O'Keeffe, N., Cullen, H., Durcan, A., Timulak, L., & McElvaney, J. (2019). Emotion-focused perspective on generalized anxiety disorder: A qualitative analysis of clients' in-session presentations. *Psychotherapy Research, 29*(4), 524–540. https://doi.org/10.1080/10503307.2017.1373206

Ogden, J. (2019). *Health psychology* (6th ed.). MacGraw-Hill Education.

Oken, D. (1961). What to tell cancer patients: a study of medical attitudes. *Journal of the American Medical Association, 175,* 1120–1128. https://doi.org/10.1001/jama.1961.03040130004002

O'Meara, P., & Duthie, S. (2018). Paramedicine in Australia and New Zealand: A comparative overview. *Australian Journal of Rural Health, 26*(5), 363–368. https://doi.org/10.1111/ajr.12464

Ontengco, J. (2019). Increasing referrals to a community paramedicine fall prevention program through implementation of a daily management system. *Journal of Trauma Nursing, 26*(1), 50–58. https://doi.org/10.1097/JTN.0000000000000415

Oster, H., Challet, E., Ott, V., Arvat, E., Kloet, R., Dijk, D., Lightman, S., Vgontzas, A., & Van, Cauter E. (2017). The functional and clinical significance of the 24-hour rhythm of circulating glucocorticoids. *Endocrine Reviews, 38*(1), 3–45. https://doi.org/10.1210/er.2015-1080

Otani, H., Yoshida, S., Morita, T., Aoyama, M., Kizawa, Y., Shima, Y., Tsuneto, S., & Miyashita, M. (2017). Meaningful communication before death, but not present at the time of death itself, is associated with better outcomes on measures of depression and complicated grief among bereaved family members of cancer patients. *Journal of Pain & Symptom Management, 54*(3), 273–279. https://doi.org/10.1016/j.jpainsymman.2017.07.010

Otis, L. (2019). *Banned emotions: How metaphors can shape what people feel.* Oxford University Press.

Ousseine, Y., Durand, M., Bouhnik, A., Smith, A., & Mancini, J. (2019). Multiple health literacy dimensions are associated with physicians' efforts to achieve shared decision-making. *Patient Education & Counseling, 102*(11), 1949–1956. https://doi.org/10.1016/j.pec.2019.05.015

Parissopoulos, S. (2019). Reflection and reflective practice: A cornerstone value for the future of nursing. *Rostrum of Asclepius, 18*(3), 200–203.

Paton, D., Moss, S., Violanti, J., De Leon, J., & Morrissey, H. (2017). Responding to critical incidents and disasters: Facilitating resilidence in high risk professions. In D. Paton & D. Johnston (Eds.), *Disaster resilience: An integrated approach* (2nd ed., pp. 308–322). Charles C Thomas Publisher.

Petitta, L., Hartel, C., Ashkanasy, N., & Zerbe, W. (2018). *Individual, relational, and contextual dynamics of emotions.* Emerald Publishing.

Petrinec, A. (2017). Post intensive care syndrome in family decision makers of long term acute care hospital patients. *American Journal of Critical Care, 26*(5), 416–422. https://doi.org/10.4037/ajcc2017414

Phoenix Australia – Centre for Posttraumatic Mental Health. (2019). *Australian PTSD resources.* www.phoenixaustralia.org/australian-guidelines-for-ptsd

Pickard, S. (2017). *Going over the top: ANZAC stoicism, sacrifice and the constriction of Australian values. ABC Religion and Ethics.* www.abc.net.au/religion/going-over-the-top-anzac-stoicism-sacrifice-and-the-constriction/10095838

Pollock, A., Campbell, P., Deery, R., Fleming, M., Rankin, J., Sloan, G., & Cheyne, H. (2017). A systematic review of evidence relating to clinical supervision for nurses, midwives and allied health professionals. *Journal of Advanced Nursing, 73*(8), 1825–1837. https://doi.org/10.1111/jan.13253

Port, M., & Last, J. (2018). *A dictionary of public health.* Oxford University Press.

Price, O., Baker, J., Bee, P., Grundy, A., Scott, A., Butler, D., Cree, L., & Lovell, K. (2018). Patient perspectives on barriers and enablers to the use and effectiveness of de-escalation techniques for the management of violence and aggression in mental health settings. *Journal of Advanced Nursing, 74*(3), 614–625. https://doi.org/10.1111/jan.13488

Productivity Commission. (2014). *Natural disaster funding arrangements: Productivity Commission inquiry report: volume 2: Supplement.* Australian Government.

Queensland Health. (2018). *Mental health pathways.* https://www.qld.gov.au/health/mental-health/get-started/mental-health-pathways

Quelch, J., & Knoop, C. (2018). *Compassionate management of mental health in the modern workplace.* Springer International Publishing.

Rainville, G. (2018). Public religious activities, stress, and mental well-being in the United States: The role of religious reframing in coping. *Mental Health, Religion & Culture, 21*(3), 288–303. https://doi.org/10.1037/rel0000251

Rapchak, M., Nolfi, D., & Turk, M. (2018). Implementing an interprofessional information literacy course: Impact on student abilities and attitudes. *Journal of the Medical Library Association, 106*(4), 464–470. https://doi.org/10.5195/jmla.2018.455

Rasheed, S., Younas, A., & Sundus, A. (2019). Self-awareness in nursing: A scoping review. *Journal of Clinical Nursing*, *28*(5/6), 762–774. https://doi.org/10.1111/jocn.14708

Raymond, C., Marin, M., Juster, R., & Lupien, S. (2019). Should we suppress or reappraise our stress? The moderating role of reappraisal on cortisol reactivity and recovery in healthy adults. *Anxiety, Stress & Coping*, *32*(3), 286–297. https://doi.org/10.1080/10615806.2019.1596676

Reifels, L., Dückers, M., & Blashki, G. (2019). Examining the national profile of chronic disaster health risks in Australia. *Prehospital & Disaster Medicine*, *34*, s5–s5. https://doi.org/10.1017/S1049023X19000293

Richard, A., Gagnon, M., & Careau, E. (2019). Using reflective practice in interprofessional education and practice: A realist review of its characteristics and effectiveness. *Journal of Interprofessional Care*, *33*(5), 424–436. https://doi.org/10.1080/13561820.2018.1551867

Riley, J., Collins, D., & Collins, J. (2019). Nursing students' commitment and the mediating effect of stress. *Nurse Education Today*, *76*, 172–177. https://doi.org/10.1016/j.nedt.2019.01.018

Riley, R., Spiers, J., Buszewicz Taylor, A., Thornton, G., & Chew-Graham, C. (2018). What are the sources of stress and distress for general practitioners working in England? A qualitative study. *BMJ Open*, *8*, e017361. https://doi.org/10.1136/bmjopen-2017-017361

Robotin, M., Porwal, M., Hopwood, M., Nguyen, D., Sze, M., Treloar, C., & George, J. (2017). Listening to the consumer voice: Developing multilingual cancer information resources for people affected by liver cancer. *Health Expectations*, *20*(1), 171–182. https://doi.org/10.1111/hex.12449

Rodgers, R., & DuBois, R. (2018). Grief reactions: A sociocultural approach. In Bui. E (Ed.), *Clinical handbook of bereavement and grief reactions* (pp. 1–18). Springer International Publishing.

Rodríguez-Rey, R., Palacios, A., Alonso-Tapia, J., Pérez, E., Álvarez, E., Coca, A., Mencía, S., Marcos, A., Mayordomo-Colunga, J., Fernández, F., Gómez, F., Cruz, J., Ordóñez, O., & Llorente, A. (2019). Burnout and posttraumatic stress in paediatric critical care personnel: Prediction from resilience and coping styles. *Australian Critical Care*, *32*(1), 46–53. https://doi.org/10.1016/j.aucc.2018.02.003

Rotter, J. (1966). Generalised expectancies for internal vs external control of reinforcement. *Psychological Monographs*, *80*(1), 1–26.

Russell, K., Alliex, S., & Gluyas, H. (2017). The influence of the art of clinical supervision program on nurses' knowledge and attitude about working with students. *Journal for Nurses in Professional Development*, *33*(6), 307–315. https://doi.org/10.1097/NND.0000000000000400

Rzeszutek, M., Oniszczenko, W., & Kwiatkowska, B. (2017). Stress coping strategies, spirituality, social support and posttraumatic growth in a Polish sample of rheumatoid arthritis patients. *Psychology, Health & Medicine*, *22*(9), 1082–1088. https://doi.org/10.1080/13548506.2017.1280174

Sanford, J., Hofmann, S., & Carpenter, J. (2019). The effect of a brief mindfulness training on distress tolerance and stress reactivity. *Behavior Therapy*, *50*(3), 630–645.

Sawin, K., Montgomery, K., Dupree, C., Haase, J., Phillips, C., & Hendricks-Ferguson, V. (2019). Oncology nurse managers' perceptions of palliative care and end-of-life communication. *Journal of Pediatric Oncology Nursing*, *36*(3), 178–190. https://doi.org/10.1177/1043454219835448

Schultz, D., & Schultz, S. (2017). *Theories of personality* (11th ed.). Cengage Learning.

Scott, M. (2017). *Towards a mental health system that works: A professional guide to getting psychological health*. Routledge.

Seele, P. (2017). *Stand up to stigma: How we reject fear and shame*. Berrett-Koehler Publishers.

Selye, H. (1976). Stress without distress. In G. Serban (Ed.), *Psychopathology of human adaptation* (pp. 137–146). Springer Science.

Shahar, B., Kalman-Halevi, M., & Roth, G. (2019). Emotion regulation and intimacy quality: The consequences of emotional integration, emotional distancing, and suppression. *Journal of Social & Personal Relationships*, *36*(11–12), 3343–3361. https://doi.org/10.1177/0265407518816881

Shao, J., Yang, H., Weiping, L., & Zhang, Q. (2019). Commonalities and differences in psychological adjustment to chronic illnesses among older adults: A comparative study based on the stress and coping paradigm. *International Journal of Behavioral Medicine*, *26*(2), 143–153. https://doi.org/10.1007/s12529-019-09773-8

Singh, N., Minaie, M., Skvarc, D., & Toumbourou, J. (2019). Impact of a secondary school depression prevention curriculum on adolescent social-emotional skills: Evaluation of the resilient families program. *Journal of Youth & Adolescence*, *48*(6),1100–1115. https://doi.org/10.1007/s10964-019-00992-6

Sliter, M., Jones, M., & Devine, D. (2017). Funny or funnier? A review of the benefits (and detriments) of humor in the workplace. In L. C. Cooper & J. Campbell Quick (Eds.), *The handbook of stress and health: A guide to research and practice* (pp. 523–537). Wiley and Sons.

Snorrason, J., & Biering, P. (2018). The attributes of successful de-escalation and restraint teams. *International Journal of Mental Health Nursing*, *27*(6), 1842–1850. https://doi.org/10.1111/inm.12493

Soleil, G. (2017, July 1). *Workplace stress: The health epidemic of the 21st century*. *Huffington Post*. www.huffpost.com/entry/workplace-stress-the-heal_b_8923678

Southwick, S., & Charney, D. (2018). *Resilience: The science of mastering life's greatest challenges* (2nd ed.). Cambridge University Press.

Spector, P. (2017). Puppet or puppeteer? The role of resource control in the occupational stress process. In P. Perrewe & C. Rosen (Eds.), *Power, politics and political skills in job stress* (pp. 137–158). Emerald.

Spence, D. (2017). Supervising for robust hermeneutic phenomenology: reflexive engagement within horizons of understanding. *Qualitative Health Research*, *27*(6), 836–842. https://doi.org/10.1177/1049732316637824

Sweileh, W. (2019). A bibliometric analysis of health-related literature on natural disasters from 1900 to 2017. *Health Research Policy & Systems*, *17*(1), 18. https://doi.org/10.1186/s12961-019-0418-1

Szabo, A., English, A., Zhijia, Z., Jose, P., Ward, C., & Jianhong, M. (2017). Is the utility of secondary coping a function of ethnicity or the context of reception? A longitudinal study across Western and Eastern cultures. *Journal of Cross-Cultural Psychology*, *48*(8), 1230–1247. https://doi.org/10.1177/0022022117719158

Tabootwong, W., & Kiwanuka, F. (2019). Family caregivers for older adults with a tracheostomy during hospitalization: Psychological impacts and support. *International Journal of Caring Sciences*, *12*(2), 1244–1250. https://www.internationaljournalofcaringsciences.org/docs/75_1-tabootwong_special_12_2.pdf

Tackett, S. (2018). Stigma and well-being among health care professionals. *Medical Education*, *52*(7), 683–685. https://doi.org/10.1111/medu.13604

Thompson, N., Fiorillo, D., Rothbaum, B., Ressler, K., & Michopoulos, V. (2018). Coping strategies as mediators in relation to resilience and posttraumatic stress disorder. *Journal of Affective Disorders*, *225*, 153–159. https://doi.org/10.1016/j.jad.2017.08.049

Thyness, C., Steinsbekk, A., & Grimstad, H. (2022). Learning from clinical supervision - a qualitative study of undergraduate medical students' experiences. *Medical Education Online*, *27*(1), 2048514–2048514. https://doi.org/10.1080/10872981.2022.2048514

Tyer-Viola, L. (2019). Grit: The essential trait of nurses during a disaster. *Journal of Perinatal & Neonatal Nursing*, *33*(3), 201–204. https://doi.org/10.1097/JPN.0000000000000416

Udod, S., Cummings, G., Care, W., & Jenkins, M. (2017). Role stressors and coping strategies among nurse managers. *Leadership in Health Services*, *30*(1), 29–43. https://doi.org/10.1108/LHS-04-2016-0015

Vaclavik, E., & Staffileno, B. &Carlson, E. (2018). Moral distress: Using mindfulness-based stress reduction interventions to decrease nursing perceptions of distress. *Clinical Journal of Oncological Nurses*, *22*(3), 326–332. https://doi.org/10.1188/18.CJON.326-332

Vandette, M., & Gosselin, J. (2019). Conceptual models of clinical supervision across professions: A scoping review of the professional psychology, social work, nursing, and medicine literature in Canada. *Canadian Psychology*, *60*(4), 302–314. https://doi.org/10.1037/cap0000190

Ven, N., Meijs, M., & Vingerhoets, A. (2017). What emotional tears convey: Tearful individuals are seen as warmer, but also as less competent. *British Journal of Social Psychology*, *56*(1), 146–160. https://doi.org/10.1111/bjso.12162

Visser, L., Tollenaar, M., van Doornen, L., de Haes, H., & Smets, E. (2019). Does silence speak louder than words? The impact of oncologists' emotion-oriented communication on analogue patients' information recall and emotional stress. *Patient Education & Counseling*, *102*(1), 43–52. https://doi.org/10.1016/j.pec.2018.08.032

Walker, C., & Peterson, C. (2017). Multimorbidity: A sociological perspective of systems. *Journal of Evaluation in Clinical Practice*, *23*(1), 209–212. https://doi.org/10.1111/jep.12599

Wallston, K., Wallston, B., & Devellis, R. (1978). Development of multidimensional health locus of control (MHLC) scales. *Health Education Monographs*, *6*(2), 160–170. https://doi.org/10.1177/109019817800600107

Webster, R., Thompson, A., Norman, P., & Goodacre, S. (2017). The acceptability and feasibility of an anxiety reduction intervention for emergency department patients with non-cardiac chest pain. *Psychology, Health & Medicine*, *22*(1), 1–11. https://doi.org/10.1080/13548506.2016.1144891

Weishaar, H., Hurrelmann, K., Okan, O., Horn, A., & Schaeffer, D. (2019). Framing health literacy: A comparative analysis of national action plans. *Health Policy*, *123*(1), 11–20. https://doi.org/10.1016/j.healthpol.2018.11.012

Weissman, M., Markowitz, J., & Klerman, G. (2017). *The guide to interpersonal psychotherapy* (Expanded, updated ed.). Oxford University Press.

Westman, M., & Chen, S. (2017). Crossover of burnout and engagement from managers to followers: The role of social support. In C. L. Cooper & J. Campbell Quick (Eds.), *The handbook of stress and health: A guide to research and practice* (pp. 236–251). Wiley and Sons.

White, E. (2017). Claims to the benefits of clinical supervision: A critique of the policy development process and outcomes in New South Wales, Australia. *International Journal of Mental Health Nursing*, *26*(1), 65–76. https://doi.org/10.1111/inm.12292

Wilson, B., Woollands, A., & Barret, D. (2018). *Care planning: A guide for nurses*. Routledge.

Wilson, C., & Stock, J. (2019). The impact of living with long-term conditions in young adulthood on mental health and identity: What can help? *Health Expectations*, *22*(5), 1111–1121. https://doi.org/10.1111/hex.12944

Wilsonisa, A. (2019). Emotion-focused therapy: Coaching clients to work through their feelings. *Therapy Today*, *30*(7), 51–51.

Witney, M., Isaac, V., Playford, D., Walker, L., Garne, D., & Walters, L. (2018). Block versus longitudinal integrated clerkships: Students' views of rural clinical supervision. *Medical Education*, *52*(7), 716–724. https://doi.org/10.1111/medu.13573

Woodward, A., & Samet, J. (2018). Climate change, hurricanes, and health. *American Journal of Public Health*, *108*(1), 33–35. https://doi.org/10.2105/AJPH.2017.304197

Wubbolding, R. (2017). *Reality therapy and self-evaluation: The key to client change*. John Wiley & Sons.

Yalcinturk, A., Dissiz, M., & Kurt, N. (2018). Nursing diagnoses of the patients who have been treated in acute psychiatry clinics in the recent year. *International Journal of Caring Sciences*, *11*(3), 1736–1742. https://internationaljournalofcaringsciences.org/docs/46._dissiz_original_11_3.pdf

Yang, B., Yen, C., Lin, S., Huang, C., Wu, J., Cheng, Y., Hsieh, C., & Hsiao, F. (2022). Emergency nurses' burnout levels as the mediator of the relationship between stress and posttraumatic stress disorder symptoms during COVID-19 pandemic. *Journal of Advanced Nursing*, *78*(9), 2861–2871. https://doi.org/10.1111/jan.15214

Yu, M., Brown, T., & Thyer, L. (2019). The association between undergraduate occupational therapy students' listening and interpersonal skills and performance on practice education placements. *Scandinavian Journal of Occupational Therapy*, *26*(4), 273–282. https://doi.org/10.1080/11038128.2018.1496272

Zamanian, H., Poorolajal, J., & Taheri-Kharameh, Z. (2018). Relationship between stress coping strategies, psychological distress, and quality of life among hemodialysis patients. *Perspectives in Psychiatric Care*, *54*(3), 410–415. https://doi.org/10.1111/ppc.12284

Zerbe, W., Hartel, C., Ashkanasy, N., & Petitta, L. (2017). *Emotions and identity*. Emerald Publishing.

Zhao, S., & Zhang, J. (2018). The association between depression, suicidal ideation and psychological strains in college students: A cross-national study. *Culture, Medicine & Psychiatry, 42*(4), 914–928. https://doi.org/10.1007/s11013-018-9591-x

Zhou, B., Boyer, R., & Guay, S. (2018). Dangers on the road: A longitudinal examination of passenger-initiated violence against bus drivers. *Stress & Health: Journal of the International Society for the Investigation of Stress, 34*(2), 253–265. https://doi.org/10.1002/smi.2779

Zhou, X., Wu, X., & Zhen, R. (2018). Self-esteem and hope mediate the relations between social support and post-traumatic stress disorder and growth in adolescents following the Ya'an earthquake. *Anxiety, Stress & Coping, 31*(1), 32–45. https://doi.org/10.1080/10615806.2017.1374376

ACKNOWLEDGEMENTS

Photo: © Fly View Productions /E+ / Getty Images

Photo: © Daria Nipot / Shutterstock.com

Photo: © Lewis Tse / Shutterstock.com

Photo: © Julia Amaral / Adobe Stock

Extract © Australian Institute for Disaster Resilience. (2019). *National strategy for disaster resilience: Companion booklet.* Victoria: AIDR.

People displaying challenging behaviours

LEARNING OBJECTIVES

This chapter will:

6.1 explore the nature of challenging behaviours

6.2 define reasonable and unreasonable behaviour

6.3 identify the most common causes and triggers of challenging behaviour

6.4 describe challenging behaviours exhibited by health professionals

6.5 explain the clinical, legal and ethical principles to follow when addressing challenging behaviours

6.6 outline the process of risk assessment and management strategies.

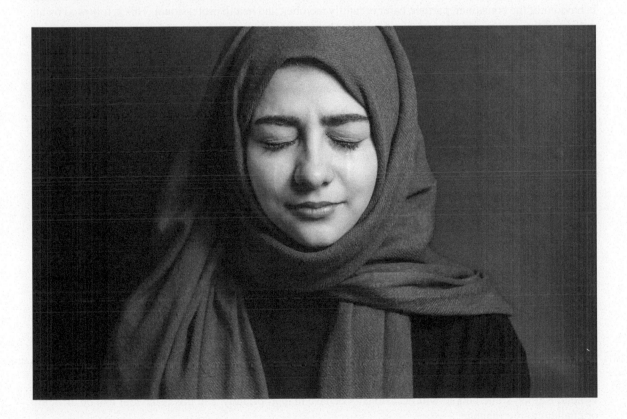

Introduction

The chapter that looks at common reactions to stressful situations explained that different people will have different reactions to the stress they experience in the health context. It noted that the provision of effective care involves health professionals practicing acceptance, respect and a commitment to listen. Indeed, fraught situations can most often be effectively managed by health professionals who allow consumers to express their feelings, deal appropriately with the consumers' complaint, issue or feedback, and provide consumers with information. There will occasionally be times, however, when a consumer does not respond to this approach, and their behaviour becomes challenging for the individual health professional, the multidisciplinary team, health service managers and the health organisation as a whole.

Challenging behaviours are not necessarily the consequence of a mental health problem. Significantly, however, people with challenging behaviours often end up in the mental health system, and are labelled accordingly. But such a label is a misnomer. This is because challenging behaviours can be the consequence of any number of factors, such as emotional, psychological, communication or systemic. Challenging behaviours are only occasionally related to symptoms of mental illness.

Challenging behaviours can include aggression and violence, assault and property damage; behaviours related to intoxication by alcohol or withdrawal from drugs; and staff splitting. Many health professionals also view self-harming behaviours as challenging (discussed further in the chapter on caring for a person who has self-harmed), together with the behavioural and psychological symptoms of dementia (see the chapter that focuses on caring for an older person with mental illness). Others find the behaviours that are often associated with borderline personality disorder difficult to manage.

The focus of this chapter is the *un*common reactions or challenging behaviours exhibited by people, and how health professionals can best manage these behaviours. The nature of challenging behaviours is explored, and the terms 'the difficult patient' and 'manipulative behaviour' considered. The context in which challenging behaviours occur is discussed, including external factors that can influence the behaviour of the consumer, partner, carer or family member, and health professional. This is followed by an outline of the causes and triggers of challenging behaviours. Risk assessment and management strategies are identified as vital to the process of providing care to the person with challenging behaviour. The chapter concludes with a debate about the proactive methods of addressing the issues involved, including ways and means of minimising the negative impact of the behaviour on all those involved.

6.1 The nature of challenging behaviours

LEARNING OBJECTIVE 6.1 Explore the nature of challenging behaviours.

Health services across Australia have adopted **zero tolerance** of aggression, violence, assault, bullying or any other act of violence in the workplace. Quite rightly, governments, industrial organisations and health services are upholding the right of all staff to work in a violence-free workplace (Department of Home Affairs, 2019). Consumers and their partners, carers, families and friends also have the right to receive health care or visit a health care setting that is free from risks to their personal safety.

This section discusses the nature of behaviours that are a risk to health professionals and others in the workplace. Wherever possible, the term 'challenging' behaviour is used in preference to 'violent' behaviour. This is because 'violence' has many negative connotations. In Australia, violence is understood as the use or expression of force — physical, psychological or emotional — against one or more people for ends that are selfish or regardless of basic human rights. In the health setting, violence and aggression most often, although not exclusively, involves the behaviour of consumers towards health professionals.

It is interesting to note that different people have different views of what constitutes a violent act. Indeed, notions of violence are often culturally, even politically, constructed. For this reason, the discussion in this chapter is based upon the premise that people, apart from a few rare exceptions, are not inherently violent. Rather, some people will occasionally behave inappropriately, and this behaviour can be difficult or challenging to manage.

Responding to violence

Immediate response options

Every effort should be made, via the risk management process, to prevent violence from occurring. However, in the event that a violent incident does eventuate, it is important that staff are aware that they do have a range of response options. These responses will depend on a number of factors, including the nature and severity of the event; whether it is a consumer, visitor or intruder who exhibits violent behaviour; and the skills, experience and confidence of the staff member/s involved. Responses may include calling for backup, security or local police.

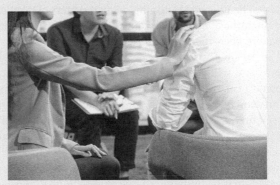

When a consumer becomes violent, consideration should always be given to the possible clinical aspects of the behaviour. A violent outburst by a consumer waiting to be seen by a doctor in the emergency department may be secondary to a number of medical conditions. After ensuring staff and other consumers' safety, initial clinical assessment and prompt treatment should be of primary concern.

Health services will have local procedures and protocols in place to support the range of available options. Procedures must be communicated to staff, and staff should be provided with training to enable them to exercise the options appropriately and effectively, particularly those involving clinical restraint.

Post-incident response

When the incident is concluded, staff should be provided with clear guidelines regarding support services (if they have not already been provided), and the option of time out from duties. Appropriate psychological and operational debriefing should be set up and coordinated. In addition, a management review of the incident by appropriate staff and experts, such as a security consultant, should be included. The purpose of a review is to critically analyse, without attributing blame, how the incident was managed with a view to setting new standards for management of future incidents.

Incident reporting

Violent incidents must be reported and recorded using the appropriate local format; for example, an employee incident form, or database, and forwarded to the manager or supervisor and work health and safety personnel. In most states and territories, depending on the nature of the incident, it may also be necessary to report significant events especially when harm has been caused, to external agencies such as Workcover, WorkSafe, the Australian Federal Police or other appropriate external organisations.

Incident investigation

The most effective way to prevent a recurrence of an incident is to determine why it happened and if it was preventable. The Western Australian government states that the principles of incident investigations include transparency, accountability, probity/fairness, open just culture, obligation to act and prioritisation of events (WA Health, 2019). SafeWork SA (2018) also recommends incident investigations follow these steps.

- *Investigate as soon as possible after the incident.* Collect evidence when it is still available, when the people involved can remember events and the order in which they happened.
- *Collect information.* Find out: what happened, where it happened and why it happened. Collect information by conducting interviews and reviewing written reports, patient histories, training records, workplace plans and before-and-after photographs.
- *Look for causes.* Did the response systems work? Look at all aspects of the incident — the environment, equipment, people, responses.
- *Review risk control measures.* Do the risk control measures work as intended? How could they be improved?
- *Identify new control measures.* The main reason for conducting an investigation is to prevent future incidents. The investigation should lead to improved preventative measures and response processes.
- *Outcomes.* The results of an investigation should be documented and communicated to all relevant parties and affected workers. The investigation report should outline what happened, what has been done, and what will be done.

6.2 Reasonable and unreasonable behaviour

LEARNING OBJECTIVE 6.2 Define reasonable and unreasonable behaviour.

Notions of 'reasonable' and 'unreasonable' were discussed in the chapter on the legal and ethical context of mental health care, outlining the parameters of providing health care to people with a mental illness. In this section, these notions are considered again, this time in the context of managing challenging behaviours that are occasionally exhibited in the health context.

In an ideal world, people will behave reasonably. For example, in the ideal health setting, people who seek help will politely and courteously accept the assistance they are given. They may even express their thanks. Likewise, health professionals will treat one another with courtesy and equity. This is not an unreasonable expectation. Unfortunately, however, the ideal health setting does not exist.

Defining the difference between reasonable and unreasonable behaviour is not easy. The seminal playwright and author George Bernard Shaw once noted that 'The reasonable man adapts himself to the world; the unreasonable one persists in trying to adapt the world to himself. Therefore, all progress depends on the unreasonable man'. The point of Shaw's observation is that it is often only by challenging the status quo — that is, by being unreasonable — that improvements can be made. This philosophy applies to all occupations, professions and settings, including those in health-related fields.

Unreasonable behaviour, then, can sometimes lead to change for the better. Similarly, behaviour that seems unreasonable but in fact, has a purpose, may be viewed as reasonable in the long term or according to context. As noted in the chapter on common reactions to stressful situations, people in the health context who are fearful or angry may behave in ways that are reasonable when considered in light of the given situation, but which would be inappropriate in a different context. For example, it may be quite reasonable for someone who is concerned about a partner or family member who has been seriously injured to make emotional demands for information from health professionals about the person's condition. However, it would be unreasonable for that person to physically or verbally assault health professionals in the process of obtaining this information. Furthermore, Sundler et al. (2022) found that consumers who had difficulties coping with changes, waiting times or adversities considered by others to be harmless, are those with anxiety, phobias or autism, for example.

This raises a number of questions. For example, where is the line between reasonable and unreasonable behaviour, between anger and aggression, between common and uncommon reactions, between acceptable and challenging behaviours? **Challenging behaviour** is defined as behaviour that is so intense, frequent or lasting that it threatens the quality of life and/or physical safety of the individual or others (Gleeson, 2019, p. 12). Adding to this, Gleeson states:

> Any behaviour ... which is considered challenging or inappropriate by others, or which gives rise to reasonable concern, may be considered as challenging. However, the use of the term challenging should be understood in terms of the social context in which behaviour occurs, rather than a symptom of individual pathology.

This definition highlights that risk covers many areas in the health context, not just the physical dimension. For this reason, in this text, behaviours are defined as challenging when they are of such intensity, frequency or duration that the physical, emotional or social/relational safety of a person or persons are at risk.

Figure 6.1 is an infographic that illustrates the range of challenging behaviours from property damage to physical assault. These behaviours threaten the physical and emotional safety of health care staff and hinder safe delivery of care to consumers.

| FIGURE 6.1 | Challenging behaviour spectrum |

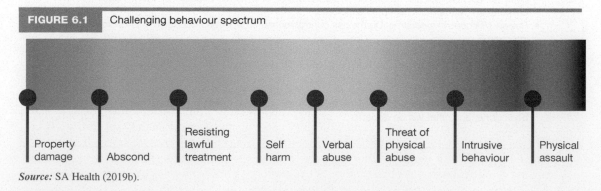

Source: SA Health (2019b).

Balancing person-centred approaches in a work place environment

Consider what workplace practices are frequently questioned by consumers. Which of these practices regularly result in consumers feeling frustrated, who may then display behaviours that are challenging? Examples are issues regarding caffeinated versus decaffeinated coffee, television viewing hours, set meal times, removal of potential 'at risk' personal items, restrictive use of mobile phone or social media platforms, leave provision.

QUESTIONS

1. Which practices are supported by evidence-informed policy and which are workplace practices that perhaps do not have empirical evidence to support them?
2. Are the non-policy practices more convenient for staff or genuinely in the best interest of consumers? Explain your answer.
3. What would be some possible outcomes if these restrictive practices were to change? What operational strategies could you put in place to support staff and consumers with these proposed practice changes?
4. How could you best utilise a consumer consultant or the peer workforce to assist you in addressing these issues?

Challenging behaviours in children

While this chapter focuses on adults who display challenging behaviours, there may be occasions when a child or adolescent displays behaviours that are considered unreasonable or unacceptable in a health care context. Many challenging behaviours of children are considered normal and part of expected developmental pathways. For this reason, specialists in child and adolescent services should be consulted when children or adolescents present with ongoing disruptive behaviours that cannot be adequately managed in a health care setting.

The Australian government Department of Health website (www.health.gov.au) also has a number of fact sheets available to parents, carers and health professionals on the management of challenging child behaviours.

The 'difficult patient'

According to Zoboli et al. (2016), the 'difficult patient' is a well-known figure in the everyday primary health context. Melville (2016) writes that the term 'difficult patient' is often used to describe a 'person who engages in disruptive behaviours, in comparison with patients who engage in neutral, or undisruptive behaviours, regardless of clinical presentation complexity'. Behaviours that some health professionals may perceive as 'difficult' include:

- constant complaints against staff members
- 'splitting' and/or 'staff splitting' (see figure 6.3)
- non-adherence to investigations or treatment
- a lack of improvement in the consumer's health status, for example, someone whose pain cannot be controlled or who presents a new set of symptoms as soon as a previous set of symptoms has resolved
- sexual disinhibition
- non-cooperation with staff requests
- discrimination (gender, sexuality, race, religion)
- silence and/or withdrawal
- asking too many questions
- dependence, which can manifest itself through constant demands for attention from health professionals or an insatiable desire to be noticed
- confusion, wandering
- self-harm.

In light of these characteristics, it would seem that notions of 'difficult' are mostly defined by a health professional's perception of how much or to what degree the person is complying with the traditional role of the 'ideal patient'; that is, someone who is patient, passive, compliant and grateful. In short, if the person is demanding, active, non-compliant and ungrateful, they do not meet the health professional's expectations of how the recipient of a health service 'should' behave. This, in turn, may lead to a perception by the health professional, conscious or unconscious, that the consumer does not deserve their attention or care. As a result, the health outcomes for that consumer are challenged.

Knaak et al. (2017) go on to suggest that health care professionals can display stigmatising attitudes and behaviours towards consumers they identify as difficult or manipulative, and therefore the term 'difficult patient' also has a stigmatising influence. This term also suggests that the health professional knows what is best for the person, and disregards what the relationship between the person and the health professional is like. Health professionals may experience challenging relationships with consumers, but they must remember that there is more than one person in the interaction; thus, to resolve these situations, all involved parties need to be active in addressing the issues.

The term 'difficult patient', then, needs to be avoided by health professionals as it labels and stereotypes (Cerit et al., 2020). It also negates the principle, described in the chapter on common reactions to stressful situations, that each person is unique and complex, a product of their upbringing, experiences, culture, education and circumstances. Indeed, some behaviours that seem unacceptable may actually be the consequence of unusually challenging situations. Given a particular set of circumstances, every person is capable of behaviour that may be considered inappropriate. Before labelling a person's behaviour, then, it may be helpful for the health professional to stop and consider how they themselves might react in a similar situation (Ali, 2018).

Koekkoek and colleagues (2006) go on to identify four categories of 'difficult' behaviours:
1. withdrawn and hard to reach
2. demanding and claiming
3. attention seeking and manipulating
4. aggressive and dangerous.

Although these terms are broadly self-explanatory, the term 'manipulating' needs some explanation. The *Macquarie Dictionary* defines the word 'manipulate' as 'to handle, manage, or use, especially with skill, in some process of treatment or performance'. Significantly, this dictionary meaning is neutrally valorised. In Australian society, however, the term 'manipulative' tends to have a negative connotation. Indeed, 'manipulating' is seen as the way a person manages, uses or even orchestrates a situation for their own ends. The consumer whose behaviour is manipulating, then, is often viewed as self-seeking, to the detriment of others.

Based on a comprehensive research project spanning 35 years, Koekkoek and colleagues (2006) identified three separate subgroups of 'difficult' behaviours. These are:
1. unwilling care avoiders who do not consider themselves to be ill and resent 'interference' by health professionals
2. ambivalent care seekers who have a serious illness but are unable to maintain a relationship with caregivers
3. demanding care claimers who may not need long-term care but who could benefit from short-term care (Koekkoek et al., 2006).

The general characteristics of each of these are outlined in more detail in table 6.1. It is interesting to note that consumers who exhibit these general characteristics are either relegated to the mental health services, the forensic services, or excluded from service or treatment altogether. In short, due to the challenging behaviour, health outcomes are challenged.

TABLE 6.1 **Characteristics of the 'difficult patient'**

	'Types' of 'difficult patients'		
Characteristic	Unwilling care avoider (Group 1)	Ambivalent care seeker (Group 2)	Demanding care claimer (Group 3)
Diagnosis	Psychotic disorder	Depressive disorders	Substance use disorder
	Personality disorder, cluster A, especially paranoid personality disorder	Personality disorder, clusters B and C, especially borderline personality disorder	Depressive disorders
			Personality disorder, cluster B, especially antisocial personality disorder and narcissistic personality disorder

Gender	Male	Female	Male
Difficult behaviours	Withdrawn	Demanding	Attention seeking
	Hard to engage	Claiming	Manipulating
	Aggressive	Self-destructive	Aggressive and destructive
		Dependent	
Acceptance of sick role: • by the consumer • by the health professional.	No Yes ('mad')	Yes Alternating ('mad' or 'bad')	When opportune and expedient No ('bad')
Prevailing discourse	Medical psychiatric	Mixed	Social-moral
	Difficult to treat the consumer	Difficult consumer	Difficult non-consumer
Probable treatment setting	Mental health care	Usually mental health care, risk of no care	Justice or forensic health

Source: Adapted from Koekkoek et al. (2006).

While avoiding the use of labels is considered good professional practice, table 6.1 does in fact highlight that from a diagnostic perspective, a number of psychiatric disorders are more commonly associated with consumers who exhibit challenging behaviours for health care practitioners. Of particular importance, the literature is laden with articles related to the management of Personality Disorders, particularly Cluster B types, identified in both Group 2 and Group 3 of Koekkoek's subgroups of difficult behaviours.

Table 6.2 explains the three personality disorder clusters as described by the American Psychiatric Association *Diagnostic and Statistical Manual of Mental Disorders version 5 (DSM-5)*.

TABLE 6.2   Personality disorder clusters

Cluster type	Description	Grouped disorders generally displaying behaviours that are:
Cluster A	Paranoid personality disorder Schizoid personality disorder Schizotypal personality disorder	Odd and eccentric
Cluster B	Antisocial personality disorder Borderline personality disorder Histrionic personality disorder Narcissistic personality disorder	Dramatic, erratic and unpredictable
Cluster C	Avoidant personality disorder Dependent personality disorder Obsessive–compulsive personality disorder	Anxious and fearful

Source: APA (2013).

Within cluster B, borderline personality disorder has received the most attention. Chapman et al. (2022) report borderline personality disorder has a general population prevalence rate of 1.6 per cent, increasing to 20 per cent for the inpatient psychiatric population. The DSM-5 outlines specific criteria for diagnosing borderline personality disorder which are: 'a pervasive pattern of instability of interpersonal relationships, self-image, and affects, and marked impulsivity, beginning by early adulthood and present in a variety of contexts', as indicated by five (or more) of the behaviours detailed in figure 6.2.

1. Frantic efforts to avoid real or imagined abandonment. (*Note:* Do not include suicidal or self-mutilating behaviour covered in Criterion 5.)
2. A pattern of unstable and intense interpersonal relationships characterised by alternating between extremes of idealisation and devaluation.
3. Identity disturbance: markedly and persistently unstable self-image or sense of self.
4. Impulsivity in at least two areas that are potentially self-damaging (e.g. spending, sex, substance abuse, reckless driving, binge eating). (*Note:* Do not include suicidal or self-mutilating behaviour covered in Criterion 5.)
5. Recurrent suicidal behaviour, gestures, or threats, or self-mutilating behaviour.
6. Affective instability due to a marked reactivity of mood (e.g. intense episodic dysphoria, irritability or anxiety usually lasting a few hours and only rarely more than a few days).
7. Chronic feelings of emptiness.
8. Inappropriate, intense anger or difficulty controlling anger (e.g. frequent displays of temper, constant anger, recurrent physical fights).
9. Transient, stress-related paranoid ideation or severe dissociative symptoms.

Source: Headspace (2022).

Health care professionals must understand the diagnostic criteria for personality disorders, implications of labelling a person based solely on a diagnosis, and potential behaviours that people diagnosed with personality disorders may display. Outcomes of labeling, unconscious behaviours, splitting, staff splitting and issues of control and power will now be discussed.

Outcomes of labelling

When managing challenging behaviours, avoiding labels is especially important because they tend to target the person rather than the action or behaviour, thereby perpetuating notions that the person rather than the behaviour is the problem. Outcomes targeting the person are rarely positive.

Indeed, the impact of labelling on a person who exhibits challenging behaviours, and on their partner or carer and family members, is always detrimental (Nyblade et al., 2019). One reason for this is the negative attitudes of health professionals that labels perpetuate. For example, a consumer may be labelled 'difficult' by a health professional shortly after they present to the health service for assistance. The perception of 'difficult' could be due to any numbers of reasons; for example, the consumer does not fit the role of a 'good patient' for this particular health professional because they asked too many questions in a demanding tone of voice. The label of 'difficult' is then passed on or handed over by the health professional to the next health professional, and then the next health professional again. Consequently, all of the health professionals concerned have preconceptions about the person that are based upon little more than the original health professional's idealised personal values system. These preconceptions go on to influence the way all of the health professionals interact and engage with the consumer.

Significantly, there is an emerging shift within the literature suggesting that the term 'behaviour that challenges' more accurately reflects the difficulties that health practitioners experience. Behaviour that challenges suggests that the (perceived) challenging behaviour is not necessarily measured by the acuity or intensity of the behaviour, but rather by whether health professionals have the skills and resources to manage their interactions; for example, see National Institute for Health and Care Excellence (NICE, 2015a). Indeed, labelling various types of behaviour as 'challenging' often comes down to the degree of the behaviour and to what is considered reasonable or acceptable behaviour in a particular setting. For example, a man who has spent several hours in a hospital emergency department might raise his voice to express concern about the fact that his wife has not yet been attended to. In this case, the health professional has to decide whether this behaviour could escalate to physical violence (NICE, 2015b). While the raised voice should be viewed as a 'risk factor', the intensity or degree of the person's frustration or anger must also be considered. As noted in the chapter on common reactions to stressful situations, anger can most often be de-escalated by a health professional by allowing the person to vent in a safe environment, treating them with unconditional positive regard, listening to and addressing their concerns, and practising empathy.

Defence mechanisms

Defence mechanisms refer to a way of theorising about how people unconsciously respond to threats or anxiety when faced with unpleasant thoughts, feelings or behaviours. Defence mechanisms are used by everyone from time to time to deal with stressful situations; they are one of the many coping strategies used by people to help them deal with the challenging aspects of their daily lives.

Projection is one example of a defence mechanism used by an individual to protect themselves against the fear, anxiety or other emotion generated in reaction to a challenging situation. Projection can reduce the emotions involved by allowing the individual to unconsciously express their unwanted unconscious impulses or desires by 'externalising' them. For example, an individual may be feeling guilty because they are partly responsible for a family member being injured. To help them to cope with their feelings, they blame other people, including the health professional. This behaviour can easily be interpreted by the health professional, who may feel attacked by the individual, as 'challenging'.

Splitting is another defence mechanism that often challenges health professionals. As with all defence mechanisms, splitting is a strategy that any person might employ given a certain set of circumstances, in particular when they are stressed or feeling vulnerable. Splitting occurs when an individual unconsciously separates notions of 'good' and 'bad' in situations that evoke powerful feelings, which can lead to the individual viewing people and situations in a polarised way — for example, with feelings of either love or hate, attachment or rejection. At the same time, the person is unable to accept or integrate equally their own positive and negative qualities (Vater et al., 2015). In reality, however, situations or circumstances that involve people are almost never black and white, but rather a complex mix of many feelings and perceptions. The individual who is splitting, however, is unable to accept this.

An example of splitting is the child who is abused by the father she depends on for love and protection. She separates the father who abuses her from the father she depends upon. This allows her to preserve an image of a 'good' father, but this comes at great cost. The child is left identifying herself as 'bad' in order to make sense of the abuse. In turn, as she grows up, she is unable to reconcile these two parts — nor the idea that no one is all good or all bad. As an adult, this may become a problem when she feels stressed or vulnerable. She may view the situation as all good or all bad. Likewise, she divides health professionals into categories of good or bad, and seeks to gain support for her views from other service users and even other staff members. This becomes the challenging behaviour known as 'staff splitting'.

Staff splitting

Staff splitting is a known phenomenon in health care and manifests itself when a consumer asks different members of staff for the same thing until they get what they want. This dynamic is often viewed as 'manipulating' behaviour. Staff splitting is also evident when a clinical team or specific discipline group loses their professional unitedness and splits into strongly opposing perspectives of the consumer presentation (Green, 2018). The process of staff splitting is particularly evident when the multidisciplinary team has suggested treatment options or management strategies and the consumer is ambivalent about these options or strategies. Consequently, the consumer may move from health professional to health professional, testing their commitment to the treatment options and making judgements about the health professional based upon their response to the consumer's requests. This can be reminiscent of a child playing one parent against the other.

Another example of staff splitting is when a consumer is struggling to deal with the stress of illness, injury or even hospitalisation. To protect themselves against the anxiety or other feelings that the stress has generated, the consumer finds a health professional who seems responsive and willing to meet their needs. The consumer then begins to idealise this health professional, and criticise other health professionals. The idealised health professional finds it difficult to resist the temptation of being viewed as 'special' and begins to treat the consumer, likewise, as 'special'. Such treatment may include meeting the consumer's needs regardless of the circumstances or setting, by going that extra mile or, on occasion, bending the rules of the health service to suit the consumer. This leads to tensions in the workplace between members of the multidisciplinary team (Novac et al., 2014).

In the previous example, however, the health professional will inevitably betray the consumer's idealisation — health professionals are human, with human frailties. When this happens, the consumer, overcome by the anxiety this generates, turns on the health professional and attacks them physically, emotionally or personally. The consumer then moves on to find another health professional to idealise and use as a means of coping with the anxiety or other feelings the situation is provoking in them. The first health professional is left feeling demeaned, humiliated and attacked; and so the process continues.

The dynamic of staff splitting is further exemplified diagrammatically in figure 6.3, which shows how splitting may affect relationships between consumers and health professionals, and between health professionals themselves on the multidisciplinary team. By way of explanation, the behaviours and communication of the consumer and health professional B are negative, reinforcing the consumer's worst feelings about him or herself. On the other hand, the behaviours and communications of the consumer and health professional A are far more positive. These two health professionals then replicate the consumer's own internal 'split' in their own discussion and enact the consumer's internal conflicts as they cannot agree about the consumer's behaviour and health care needs.

FIGURE 6.3 The process of staff splitting

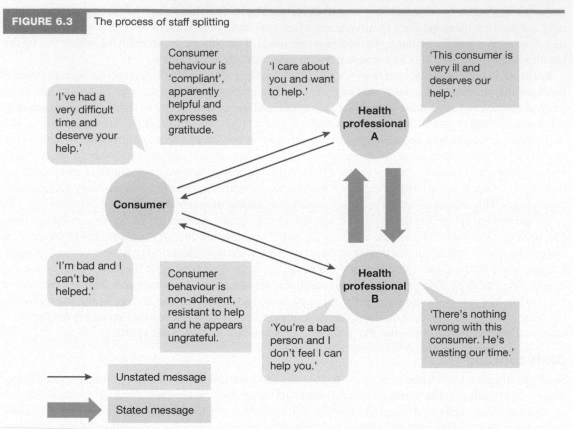

Source: Adapted from Perlin (2001).

Challenging the process of staff splitting can be difficult for the health professional and the multidisciplinary team. In general, the subsequent steps must be followed.

- Clear communication between the multidisciplinary team about the care and treatment decisions made with the consumer.
- Understanding of and regular communication between the multidisciplinary team about the dynamic of staff splitting.
- Ongoing support and clinical supervision provided to all members of the multidisciplinary team when caring for a consumer with these behaviours.

It is also important to note that health professionals who demonstrate respect, professional integrity, skills competency and a willingness to provide the consumer with meaningful control and choice in their own care, are more likely to be effective in their interactions with the consumer.

On the other hand, many health professionals may project an authoritarian attitude or demeanour towards a person they perceive to be 'manipulative' or 'difficult'. Such an attitude may help the health professional feel more in control of the situation, but it is actually counterproductive. As noted by Thibeault (2016), an authoritarian attitude will most often lead to a power struggle between the consumer and health professional, with neither players benefiting in the long term.

Control and power

Many consumers have felt helpless, powerless or overlooked when dealing with health professionals (Clough, 2018, p. 13). There is an obvious irony in this, as many health professionals ascribe great power

---

or control to individuals engaged in challenging behaviours, demonstrated by the health professional's intense emotional reactions to the challenging behaviours of the consumer, and expressed by language such as 'He makes me feel like . . .' As noted in the chapter on common reactions to stressful situations, such language suggests one way the health professional blames the other person, displacing their personal responsibility and walking away as the 'innocent victim'. In reality, however, it is the health professional who holds the balance of power.

Indeed, challenging behaviours often result in a struggle for control or a series of responses from health professionals that do not address the problem, but instead establish a conflictive relationship (Thibeault, 2016). These forms of response merely perpetuate the problem and increase levels of frustration, since all parties involved are likely to become dissatisfied with the way they interact and with the outcome of the conflict. Bowers and colleagues (2015) found that improved staff–consumer relationships reduce episodes of conflict in acute psychiatric wards. Gender also plays a part, as discovered by Edward and colleagues (2016) when conducting a meta-analysis with data spanning more than 50 years. These researchers found that female health care workers are statistically more likely to experience verbal abuse than their male colleagues; however, male workers are more likely than females to be involved in physically abusive incidents (Edward et al., 2016).

It can sometimes be easier for a health professional to focus on the task at hand rather than to make an effort to interact on a personal level with an individual who is exhibiting challenging behaviours. This is especially true when the health professional has made a negative assumption about the person. Instead, health professionals need to recognise that people react and respond to both verbal and non-verbal cues. In short, body language is just as important as verbal messages (Tasmanian Public Health Services, 2018). People will react to what the health professional says and to the way they say it. If the health professional holds preconceived ideas, expectations or negative perceptions about a particular 'type' of consumer, it is very difficult for them to conceal it. Their attitudes will almost always be betrayed through the language they use or the attitudes they display. It is therefore critical for the health professional to be aware of their belief system and personal judgements about people who are exhibiting challenging behaviours; and challenge attitudes that are counterproductive (Aggarwal, 2016). A more detailed explanation of how the health professional can develop self-awareness is provided in the chapter on common reactions to stressful situations.

The next sections consider further the power imbalance between consumers and health professionals, and how this power imbalance can affect the behaviour of the consumer. The discussion is undertaken in light of the causes and triggers of challenging behaviours. Prior to this, brief consideration is given to the influence of the health professional in determining the nature of a challenging interaction.

The influence of health professionals

There is now a growing body of literature that supports the suggestion that aggression, violence and other challenging behaviours are mediated by the levels of education and training, and skills or competence of the health professional, as well as their attitude towards the consumer (Black, 2021; NICE, 2015a). The quality of the relationship between the consumer and health professional is also significant to decreasing aggressive incidents. For this reason, it is important that health professionals consider the role they have played after an aggressive incident has occurred. Questions they may ask themselves may include the following.

- 'Who is it that finds this behaviour unpleasant, difficult or problematic?'
- 'What is it about this person's behaviour that is specifically difficult to manage?'
- 'From the person's point of view, is it legitimate and understandable?'

As noted, the influence of control and power when dealing with the consumer is important. Just as influential is the attitude, behaviour, the internal world and the situational context of the health professional at the time of the incident. For example, what has been happening to or for the particular health professional in the time leading up to an incident that made the interaction challenging?

Such practice reflection would ideally include the health professional participating in regular in-service education about managing people who exhibit challenging behaviours, and regular clinical supervision (see the chapters on common reactions to stressful situations, and mental health service delivery). Indeed, it is accepted that this kind of practice reflection leads to optimal patient care and outcomes, while supporting professional and wellbeing needs of health professionals (Health Victoria, 2019).

Clinical supervision is 'a formally structured professional arrangement between a supervisor and one or more supervisees. It is a purposely constructed regular meeting that provides for critical reflection on the work issues brought to that space by the supervisee(s)' (Australian College of Mental Health Nurses

[ACMHN], Australian College of Midwives, and Australian College of Nursing, 2019a). The Australian Clinical Supervision Association (2018) also states that the benefits gained from clinical supervision will be 'determined by your input into the process'. It is through clinical supervision that health professionals are helped to consider their practice and discuss insights or issues with another health professional, with a view to improving knowledge and competence. The Clinical Supervision for Nurses and Midwives Position Statement declares there are significant positive outcomes for clinical supervisees and these include increased competence, confidence, self-efficacy and professional accountability; increased self-awareness, including insights into the use of self in the work and improved coping at work and general well-being; improved identification of, and access to supports; and reduced stress, anxiety and burnout, which can be a consequence of dealing with the challenging behaviours. (ACMHN et al., 2019a).

UPON REFLECTION

The use of labelling ...

The impact of labelling a person who exhibits behaviour that is challenging as 'difficult' is usually detrimental to that person and has the potential to interfere with therapeutic alliance.

QUESTIONS

1. Consider an occasion when another health professional indicated that a particular consumer was 'difficult'. Given this information, did you change your behaviour or approach towards the consumer? 'Did you unconsciously adopt a non-therapeutic role to cope with the situation?' Was the approach you took genuine, non-confrontational and person-centred? What was the outcome of the interaction?
2. What strategies could you use to address 'difficult patient' labelling within your discipline or clinical area?
3. What training or education needs do you and/or your team require in order to support your strategies?

6.3 Causes and triggers of challenging behaviour

LEARNING OBJECTIVE 6.3 Identify the most common causes and triggers of challenging behaviour.

Although challenging behaviours may have their origins in the more extreme reactions and responses of people to the stress they experience in the context of receiving health care, it is important to give wider consideration to the issues involved. Feelings of vulnerability and powerlessness can arise from the experience of illness and the need to seek help (Aggarwal, 2016).

First and foremost, consideration needs to be given to whether the challenging behaviour has been precipitated by an organic cause. For example, aggression in an older person may be due to a delirium or dementia (see the chapter that looks at caring for an older person with mental illness). In particular, a delirium can be life threatening and must be immediately assessed by a medical officer. Again, the challenging behaviour of an apparently intoxicated person may not be alcohol related at all, but rather due to a head injury that has not been identified.

Alternatively, challenging behaviour can often be perpetuated by extenuating circumstances (Ali, 2018). A systematic review of prevalence and risk factors regarding aggression in psychiatric wards conducted by Weltens et al., (2021) highlights three main categories identified as antecedents to violent behaviour. These domains were as follows.

1. *Ward factors.* Important risk factors identified in psychiatric wards were (i) high bed occupancy, (ii) busy ward areas, (iii) walking rounds, (iv) an unsafe environment, (v) a restrictive environment, (vi) lack of structure in the day, (vii) smoking and (viii) a lack of privacy.
2. *Staff factors.* Recognised staff risk factors included (i) male gender, (ii) unqualified or temporary staff, (iii) job strain, (iv) dissatisfaction with the job or management, (v) burnout and (vi) the quality of the interaction between consumers and staff.
3. *Patient factors.* Identified patient risk factors were: (i) diagnosis of psychotic disorder or bipolar disorder, (ii) substance abuse, (iii) a history of aggression and (iv) younger age.

Indeed, access problems, treatment and care issues and many staff-related factors have also been reported by consumers and carers as the basis for formal complaints in mental healthcare systems (Sundler et al., 2022).

As previously identified, challenging behaviours may be the result of the power imbalance that is inherent within the relationship between the health professional and the person they are assisting (Aggarwal, 2016). Indeed, many consumers feel powerless and open to exploitation simply by presenting themselves to a health service for assistance. Reasons for this can include the experience of illness itself, including feeling weak, nauseous and generally unwell. These feelings are often exacerbated when faced by a bureaucratic health care system with long waiting times, where health professionals often seem more concerned with maintaining routines than with helping people. Numerous contributing personal and social determinants of health influences may lead to consumers being vulnerable to poor outcomes. The Consumer Policy Research Centre (CPRC) has identified a range of potentially vulnerable circumstances, which fall under four broad headings. These are:

- health and disabilty
- resilience
- life events
- capabilty (Consumer Policy Research Centre, 2020).

Effective health professionals will consider these factors when helping a person with challenging behaviours, and explore ways and means by which the person can be empowered. These will include actively preserving the dignity of the consumer by practising kindness and unconditional positive regard, and by being aware that the consumer may be feeling vulnerable and powerless.

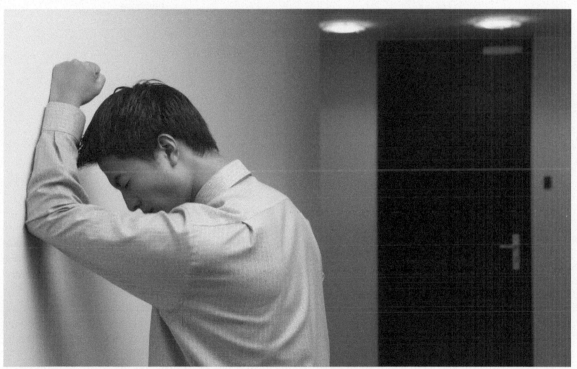

Feelings of vulnerability and powerlessness can arise from the experience of illness.

Communication and challenging behaviours

Lim et al. (2019) interviewed 27 mental health nurses who identified a correlation between highly aroused or distressed consumer behaviours on admission with an increased risk of aggression. Figure 6.4 illustrates the process of communication involved. An external stimulus is received and the person tries to make sense of it by placing the event or situation into context. However, this is mediated by their personal or individual experiences and perceptions. The cognitive process overlaps with the emotional responses and the impulse to act is based upon the judgement reached.

It may well be argued, then, that challenging behaviours are often used to communicate what the individual has otherwise been unable to articulate. If this is the case, it is unlikely that the person with the challenging behaviour has any conscious or developed understanding of the process; that is, they are unaware that there are more constructive and effective ways of communicating. For the health professional, the use of validation, empathy, reframing the situation and refocusing the therapeutic alliance are ways to manage the situation more effectively (Black, 2021).

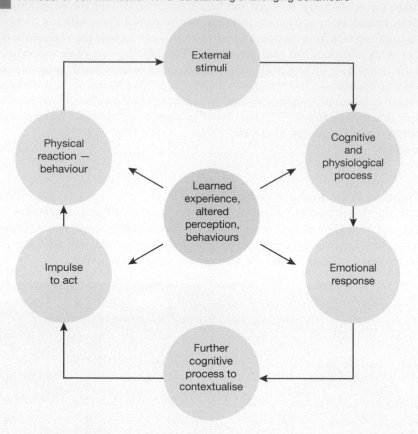

General assessment

An assessment by the health professional of what has triggered or caused the challenging behaviour will begin with a biographical and social history. Engaging with the person and encouraging them to tell their story will enable the health professional to identify their current issues, which will provide some context to the person's current issues and problems. If a clear pattern emerges of, for example, difficulty in dealing with or responding to others constructively, health professionals need to take this into account during future interactions. Such patterns also provide the health professional with the opportunity to discuss issues related to the behaviour in the health context. Alternatively, the health professional may find that the person is someone with a higher than usual need for information or an inbuilt critical approach to problems. Again, this will enable the health professional to adapt the way they respond to the person.

Another option may be that the consumer has grown into the role of a 'difficult patient' as a result of past experiences when they received poor or disappointing treatment. In this case, the health professional will be positioned by the consumer as the 'bad health professional', in a role reversal of sorts, with resultant interactions difficult. At the same time, the health professional also needs to consider the current experience of ill-health or injury and its progression. For example, a consumer with chronic illnesses or conditions, especially those that involve great pain, will often have a lower threshold for coping with additional stress.

An example of a challenging behaviour exhibited by a person who lacks skills in communicating effectively is provided in the following 'In practice' box. In this narrative, the woman's perceptions and understanding of the situation are limited by her past experiences and the way in which these experiences have shaped the person she is when she becomes unwell. She is unable to describe her emotions and acts out her feelings instead.

Understanding the causes of challenging behaviour

Cindy-Lee was admitted to a medical ward several days ago following a self-harm episode, and is being cared for in a single room. Cindy-Lee presented to the medical ward staff as chatty and cheerful, right up until she was informed that she would be transferred to the psychiatric inpatient unit as soon as a bed became available. Cindy-Lee instantly became irritable, unwilling to have her vital sign observations taken and recorded and refusing her medication.

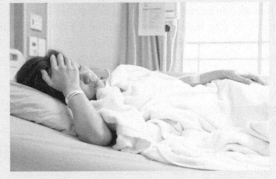

From Cindy-Lee's perspective, she simply does not want to go to the psychiatric unit as she very much likes her single room on the medical ward and she would prefer to stay where she is so she can keep company with the good friends she has made over the past two days. There are a series of confrontations between Cindy-Lee and the frustrated staff. It is only when a nurse from the mental health consultation liaison team meets with Cindy-Lee that she articulates these troubled thoughts and feelings. Cindy-Lee then begins to communicate her feelings and the extremely negative image she has constructed of the psychiatry unit, including one time when she was secluded following an incident with another consumer. Conversing with the liaison team enables Cindy-Lee to share her thoughts and feelings about her previous traumatic experiences, and her preferences regarding her treatment regimen and ongoing care for her injuries.

QUESTIONS

1. What communication strategies would you utilise to effectively engage Cindy-Lee?
2. What advice could you provide to the ward staff to assist them to manage Cindy-Lee's behaviour?
3. What Recovery Focused Care principles would best suit your engagement with Cindy-Lee?
4. As a health professional, what strategies could you employ to help manage your feelings about Cindy-Lee's behaviour?

Older people and challenging behaviours

Other causes of challenging behaviours may be associated with Alzheimer's disease and related dementias (see the chapter on caring for an older person with mental illness). These challenging behaviours could include restlessness, pacing and wandering, and repetitive calling or questioning (see the chapter on caring for an older person with mental illness). Previous research reported that psychotropic medication was prescribed to approximately 80 per cent of people diagnosed with dementia in Australian aged care facilities, with the sole purpose of controlling behavioural and psychological symptoms of dementia (BPSD) (Alzheimer's Australia, 2014, p. 8). To address this staggering issue, the Aged Care sector has adopted very rigid processes to mitigate the overuse of medication prescribing to control behaviours. A 'behaviour support plan' is now required for any residents exhibiting any behaviours of concern or changed behaviours; or who have restrictive practices incorporated into their treatment and care (Aged Care Quality and Safety Commission, n.d).

This streamlined practice supports that even in a person with dementia, the condition itself may not be the cause of the challenging behaviour. For example, the person may be experiencing physical pain due to a toothache. The side effects of some pain reducing medication can also cause behavioural disturbance, including confusion and agitation. Physical discomfort can also give rise to challenging behaviours in older people, for example, constantly needing to go to the toilet. Finally, the person with a toothache may also be less inclined to drink. This could lead to dehydration, which can cause dizziness, headaches, dry skin, infection, cramps, constipation, urinary problems and increased confusion, all of which can result in disturbed behaviour.

For this reason, challenging behaviour can sometimes be the only way a person is able to communicate discomfort, pain or that there is something 'not quite right'. This includes occasions when the person has a psychotic illness or a personality disorder. Health professionals may think they cannot respond effectively to someone who is thought disordered or has a psychosis, as the meaning of the conversation may be inaccessible. However, the health professional needs to be open to 'listening' to the expression on the person's face or their body language.

It is also important to note that anger and aggression are a response to the same physiological sensations that prompt the fight-or-flight response. For this reason, leaving any person in an anxious or frightened state may lead to an escalation of behaviour as they try to communicate their feelings through their behaviour. The following 'In practice' box describes the experience of an older male person who is exhibiting anxious and frightened behaviours.

IN PRACTICE

Communicating with the older person

During a public health infectious diseases crisis, an 88-year-old man who resides in a nursing home arrives in the emergency department (ED). For the past four days, Mr King was treated for a urinary tract infection, a high temperature, nausea and diarrhoea. However, Mr King has deteriorated over the past 24–48 hours, with nursing home staff recording incontinence, low fluid intake, unstable vital signs, and intermittent agitation and confusion. During the transfer to ED, it becomes obvious that Mr King is missing his hearing aid and walking stick. Since arriving in the ED, Mr King is constantly calling out for his wife, Selina, and for Mocha, his beloved Maltese cross fox terrier. Mr King is regularly attempting to get out of bed, and he becomes physically and verbally aggressive when staff attempt to contain him. He continues to yell out for Selina, saying he urgently needs her help and for her to come quickly. Mr King has not been able to give a coherent description of his circumstances since arriving in the ED.

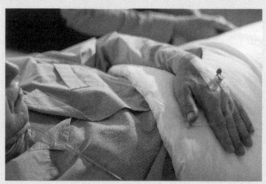

QUESTIONS

1. What is your provisional diagnosis in this scenario? Does theorising a diagnosis help you to consider the situation, or hamper you?
2. What are the best strategies to put in place in relation to reducing the stimulation in ED for Mr King? Are these strategies realistic and attainable?
3. In this public health emergency, all staff (clinical and non-clinical) are wearing masks, face visors and other personal protective equipment. What impact do you think this unfamiliar attire has when attempting to engage with Mr King?
4. What methods of communication are likely to give the best responses from Mr King?
5. What specific questions could you ask the nursing home staff to obtain further information regarding Mr King's presentation?

6.4 Challenging behaviours exhibited by health professionals

LEARNING OBJECTIVE 6.4 Describe challenging behaviours exhibited by health professionals.

Significantly, a toxic workplace environment is more likely to experience workplace stress (Wang et al. (2020) and negative consequences on staff wellbeing, consumer safety and organisational outcomes are associated with unprofessional behaviours of health care practitioners (Pavithra et al., 2022). On the other hand, positive work environments have been found to support good consumer care and mitigate adverse events (Maassen et al., 2021). This provides a good basis for suggestions that health professionals must work to build and maintain cohesive relationships with managers, consumers and colleagues within the multidisciplinary team and be committed to supporting one another in the workplace.

It is a sad fact that many health professionals, despite being members of the caring profession, are not immune from workplace bullying. The phrase 'horizontal violence' is one term used to describe the bullying behaviour of a health professional towards a colleague.

Bullying has been identified as one of the most concerning forms of aggression experienced by health professionals, with health workers being the occupational group with the third highest reported rate of serious mental health condition claims (6 per cent), after high-risk occupations such as defence force members, firefighters and police (9 per cent) and school teachers (8 per cent) (Safe Work Australia, 2019). Vento and colleagues further identifies the highest risk work places as the emergency department, mental health units, drug and alcohol settings, ambulance services and remote Health Posts with insufficient security and single health care workers (Vento et al., 2020). The Fair Work Ombudsman (2022) states that a worker is bullied at work if:

- a person or group of people repeatedly act unreasonably towards them or a group of workers
- the behaviour creates a risk to health and safety.

In this definition, unreasonable behaviour includes behaving aggressively towards others, teasing or playing practical jokes, pressuring someone to behave inappropriately, excluding someone from work-related events and unreasonable work demands.

Bullying behaviour can range from very obvious verbal or physical assault to very subtle psychological abuse. This behaviour may include but is not limited to:

- abusive, insulting or offensive language or comments
- aggressive and intimidating conduct
- belittling or humiliating comments
- victimisation
- practical jokes or initiation
- unjustified criticism or complaints
- deliberately excluding someone from work-related activities
- withholding information that is vital for effective work performance
- setting unreasonable timelines or constantly changing deadlines
- setting tasks that are unreasonably below or beyond a person's skill level
- denying access to information, supervision, consultation or resources to the detriment of the worker
- spreading misinformation or malicious rumours
- changing work arrangements such as rosters and leave to deliberately inconvenience a particular worker or workers.

Workplace bullying, then, is more than rudeness and incivility. Although it can include behaviours such as overt aggression or threats of violence, it more commonly involves subtle or covert acts such as belittling, blaming and public humiliation. Significantly, bullying has been reported from health care students during undergraduate education, in both clinical and academic settings (Averbuch et al., 2021; Gamble Blakey et al., 2019).

Many health professionals, regardless of their discipline area or professional loyalties, will be bullied at some time in their working life, with such experience even considered to be part of the job. Research has identified that of all professions, nursing has one of the highest rates of workplace bullying (Johnson, 2021), as does paramedics (State of Victoria, 2021, p. 5). Additional to this, despite the overall national prevalence of bullying reports declining over the past decade, Australia still ranks in the top three countries when compared to Europe for workplace bullying statistics (Dollard et al., 2021).

Although some bullies may have personality characteristics that predispose them to this behaviour, bullying does not continue unless the workplace climate condones, or even rewards this kind of behaviour (Suskind, 2022). It seems that some work environments in Australia, including health care environments, have a long way to go before the practice of bullying and workplace violence carried out by health professionals is recognised as being detrimental, not only to the victim, but to those witnessing the incidents.

Even so, there are a number of essential strategies that can be utilised by the health professional to combat bullying in the workplace. Many of these strategies relate to conflict management and include:

- acknowledging that conflict exists
- listening
- being non-judgemental
- creating an atmosphere where health professionals are committed to working to solve problems.

As noted at the beginning of the chapter, the development of a zero tolerance approach to workplace violence is being actively promoted by the Commonwealth Department of Health, and Departments of

Health in all states and territories and is further supported by the principles in the *Fair Work Act 2009* and the *Fair Work Amendment (COVID-19) Bill 2020*. It is the responsibility of each and every health professional to work to support these initiatives and play a role in combating the challenging behaviour exhibited by colleagues. This is discussed in more detail in the following section.

UPON REFLECTION

Seeking help . . .

Given the prevalence of workplace bullying behaviours, it is likely that most health professionals will experience, or know someone who has experienced, some form of horizontal violence.

....

QUESTIONS

1. What formal reporting pathways are available to health professionals who are experiencing workplace bullying?
2. Alternatively, what informal options are available to those facing such situations?
3. From a professional perspective, how could you support a colleague who is experiencing bullying in the workplace?
4. From a personal perspective, what (adaptive) strategies can you take to reduce the likelihood of experiencing bullying behaviour from colleagues and others?

6.5 Addressing challenging behaviours

LEARNING OBJECTIVE 6.5 Explain the clinical, legal and ethical principles to follow when addressing challenging behaviours.

This section discusses the different ways the challenging behaviours of a consumer are addressed in Australian health services. This includes a description of organisational responses, risk assessment and some practice strategies that can be used by the health professional. Consideration is also given to the use of seclusion and restraint.

Organisational responses

The Australian Commission on Safety and Quality in Health Care developed the *Australian Charter of Healthcare Rights*, which was then endorsed by Australian health ministers in July 2008. After wide consultation, this charter was updated in 2019 and specifies the key rights of consumers when seeking health care services. The second edition further emphasises the principle of person-centred care and strengthens support for consumers to be active participants in their own health journey. These rights are:
• access
• safety
• respect
• partnership
• information
• privacy
• give feedback (Australian Commission on Safety and Quality in Health Care [ACSQHC], 2019).

All of these rights are equally important. However, the right to receive open, timely and appropriate communication about the health care being provided, and in a way the consumer can understand, is particularly relevant for health professionals who are caring for someone with challenging behaviours (ACSQHC, 2019). In response to the charter of rights, zero tolerance strategies have now been established in virtually every public service across Australia. As already noted, behaviours such as aggression, violence, assault, bullying or any other acts of violence are unacceptable and actively discouraged in the workplace. Governments, industrial unions, professional bodies and managers alike are upholding the right of all staff to work in a violence-free workplace; and consumers, partners, carers, families and friends also have the right to receive health care or visit their partner, relative or friend in a therapeutic environment free from risks to their personal safety.

Even so, research has identified that health professionals are more vulnerable to occupational violence than other professional groups (Chataway, 2021). At the extreme, 56-year-old Gayle Woodford (RN) was working as a Remote Area Nurse (RAN) when she was raped and murdered in March 2016 by a community member in the remote Anangu Pitjantjatjara Yankunytjatjara Lands in South Australia. The tragic death of Gayle Woodford illustrated the immediate need for improved security and protection of all nurses, but particularly for those who were classified as RANs and other sole health care practitioners in very remote areas. After her death and the successful social media campaign #GaylesLaw, which called for the federal and SA governments to introduce improved protective safety laws for isolated workers, the SA Parliament passed the *Health Practitioner Regulation National Law (South Australia) (Remote Area Attendance) Amendment Act 2017*, more commonly referred to as 'Gayle's Law'. This law stipulates that remote area health care practitioners must work in pairs when attending an out-of-hours or unscheduled callout (SA Health, 2019a).

On the global front, in rare but rising circumstances, the murder of a health professional has occurred (Lorettu et al., 2021; Noble, 2022), and on other occasions, health care workers have been wounded, kidnapped, arrested and inadvertently killed due to an attack being perpetrated on a health care facility, rather than on the individual level (Safeguarding Health in Conflict Coalition, 2021). In the Australian context, results from an online survey of more than 3600 NSW nurses and midwives found that 80 per cent reported being exposed to at least one form of patient aggression (including verbal abuse and swearing) on at least one occasion in the preceding six months (Pich, 2018, p 3). Although verbal abuse and swearing usually results in little or no physical injury, the psychological responses can be significant. Such responses reported by health professionals in the study, indicate that 28 per cent of workers self-identify as having sustained a psychological or physical injury following the violent episode (Pich, 2018). Specifically, female health care workers and those who feel responsible for the incident are most likely to develop higher psychological distress and impact (Van Gerven et al., 2016). Perhaps most worrying is the fact that, despite awareness of workplace violence, health professionals continue to accept that the violence they receive from consumers is a regular part of their work (Stephens, 2019; Jubb & Baack, 2019). However, it is hardly surprising that this fatalistic thinking exists when reports of the risk of assault to nurses working in mental health settings is close to 100 per cent (Havaei, 2021).

Such research raises questions about the effectiveness of the zero tolerance policies and strategies being implemented nationally and across all states and territories. For example, why are these policies so difficult to enforce in practice? Another important factor is the role of the police, who are often reluctant to intervene in a hospital or other health care environment, particularly if there is any suspicion that those involved may have mental health issues. It is also important to consider workloads and the levels of stress of health professionals. Increases in expectations to meet key performance indicators and complete outcome measures have led to increases in levels of frustration, resentment and stress in health professionals.

Although the notion of zero tolerance is commendable, its widespread application in health settings remains complex. To be effective, anti-violence policies need to include higher levels of clinical staff, more effective training and more appropriate facilities, with the use of restraint and a zero tolerance approach being last-resort measures (NSW Health, 2015).

Education and training

The UK National Institute for Health and Care Excellence (NICE) *Violence and Aggression: Short-term Management in Mental Health, Health and Community Settings* guideline (NICE, 2015b) suggests that health professionals working with people who exhibit challenging behaviours, need specific training on how to anticipate and reduce violence and aggression. Likewise, the Australian College of Mental Health Nurses (2019b, p. 14) supports the use of induction and ongoing training as a means of educating health professionals to effectively manage aggression and violence in the workplace, including competency in de-escalation techniques to avoid inadvertently escalating the conflict. Furthermore, research has demonstrated that undergraduate nurses also benefit from aggression management training (Searby et al., 2019). Conversely, health agencies have engaged in social media and television advertising to educate the community on acceptable community behaviours when seeking health care services, for example, the highly effective 2015 SA Health social media campaign Hands off our Ambos (Association for Data-driven Marketing and Advertising, 2017). From the global perspective, the World Health Organization (WHO) launched a new Charter in 2020 called 'Health Worker Safety: a priority for patient safety', dedicated to all health workers, particularly those who worked through the initial stages of the COVID-19 pandemic.

The Charter further advocates for all health-related agencies to pledge commitment to developing urgent and sustainable actions to ensure health worker safety and patient safety (WHO, 2020).

The NICE guideline proposes de-escalation strategies intended to inform staff to:

- recognise the early signs of agitation, irritation, anger and aggression
- understand the likely causes of aggression or violence, both generally and for each service user
- use techniques for distraction and calming, and ways to encourage relaxation
- recognise the importance of personal space
- respond to a service user's anger in an appropriate, measured and reasonable way and avoid provocation (NICE, 2015b).

There are many different aggression management training programs available across Australia. One such program — PART (predict, assess, respond to) — has been legally tested in the United States, and is recommended for all health professionals who are at high risk of encountering a person who is aggressive or violent. Generally, the training is run over two to three days and provides health professionals with a comprehensive and systematic approach to predicting, assessing and responding to aggressive or challenging behaviour. The program emphasises problem-solving principles to defuse potentially dangerous situations, thereby avoiding the possibility of physical restraint. It works to minimise risk and increase staff confidence in responding safely and effectively to challenging situations. Health professionals across Australia are encouraged to approach their line manager about attending this training, or an equivalent occupational violence management program, in their local area.

One concern about the zero tolerance policies being rolled out across Australia relates to the levels of insight of the person who is exhibiting the challenging behaviour. Some consumers may not be aware that their behaviour is perceived as aggressive. In particular, the person with a mental health problem may have lost touch with reality to the point where they cannot be held responsible. In such cases, the recommended approach is to manage the behaviour of these consumers and ensure that nobody is injured, rather than taking the stand that aggression or violence will not be tolerated, regardless of the cause, triggers or context (NSW Health, 2015). Indeed, although health professionals have every right to a safe work environment, they also have a duty of care to provide the best-evidence treatment to the consumer who is displaying challenging behaviours (see the chapter on the legal and ethical context of mental health care). This will always include undertaking an assessment of risk.

6.6 Risk assessment

LEARNING OBJECTIVE 6.6 Outline the process of risk assessment and management strategies.

As previously discussed, when addressing challenging behaviours, it is important to know the reasons behind the behaviours, as this can help to identify the problem that needs to be addressed (Jubb & Baack, 2019). Table 6.3 lists some factors to consider.

TABLE 6.3   **Factors to consider when assessing challenging behaviours**

Factors to consider before assessment	Where will the assessment be carried out?
	Is it safe for those involved?
	If not, what steps need to be taken to ensure everyone's safety?
What has prompted the assessment at this time?	What recent event(s) precipitated or triggered this presentation or made you think an assessment was necessary now?
	Does the person pose an immediate (i.e. within the next few minutes or hours) risk with specific plans to self-harm or perpetrate aggression/violence towards you or others?
	Is there any suggestion, or does it appear likely, that the person may try to abscond?
What is the actual problem?	Is there a clear description of the behaviour and understanding of why it is a problem?
	For whom is it a problem?
	Is there a pattern to this behaviour?
	Is there an underlying cause (e.g. organic, drug and/or alcohol intoxication or withdrawal, mental illness)?
	Has anything worked in the past to reduce or stop the behaviour?

Past history	Does the person have a history of violence?
	Is there a history of self-harm?
	Does the person have a personality disorder with a behavioural component?
	Does the person have a mental illness?
Perceptions	Does the person have a psychotic disorder that is contributing to the problem? (See the chapter on caring for a person with a serious mental illness.)
	What is the person's perception of the problem?
	Does the person feel they have any control over the situation?
Cognition	Does the person have the capacity to consent? (Can the person understand and retain information, and then make balanced judgements based on an evaluation of his or her options?)
Risk	What are the risks?
	How immediate is the risk?
	What would be the likely impact of any actions if the person were to act upon their ideas?
Formulation	What is your understanding of the issues the person has described?
	What is the level of risk?
	Is immediate action required (e.g. action to make the situation safe, such as calling a 'threat code', rapid tranquillisation, involving security staff or contacting the police)?
	Is a referral to the mental health liaison team necessary and, if so, how urgent is it?

It is vital to identify both the actual and potential risks of the behaviour. For this reason, a specific risk assessment is required. The risk assessment needs to be focused on the behaviour, but it must also incorporate a wider perspective. For example, although the behaviour might be occurring in the health context, if the consumer leaves that context, what could be the risk to others? The health professional must consider this as part of the assessment, and discuss options with the multidisciplinary team.

In the event that the situation escalates and it is decided to remove or relocate the individual who is displaying the challenging behaviours to ensure the safety of other consumers and staff, local policies, procedures and legal requirements must be considered (see the chapter on the legal and ethical context of mental health care). These may include liaising with police, ambulance, other emergency service personnel, other health services and various medical officers. It is likely that the consumer will require sedation to further reduce the risks. This is described in more detail in the following section.

IN PRACTICE

Using a risk assessment framework

The use of a clinical or actuarial risk assessment framework can be useful and informative for many health professionals. The use of such a tool can assist in the development of a tailored management plan to meet specific clinical and legal needs of each consumer.

In the current political climate of health care, some health professionals believe that there is an over-emphasis on risk management practices, and that some risk management strategies are really about social control measures.

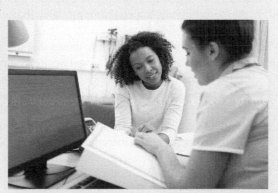

▶

Working with people with challenging behaviours

The most important aspect of managing challenging behaviours in consumers is the therapeutic alliance or relationship. As noted in the chapter that looks at assessment in the mental health context, a positive therapeutic alliance or relationship is an essential ingredient in providing high-quality health care and can be achieved only through person-centred or therapeutic communication. In particular, it is important that health professionals practise **empathy** (Rodriguez & Lown, 2019), which is an ability to perceive and reason as well as the ability to communicate understanding of the other person's feelings and their attached meanings. Further, Rodriguez and Lown (2019) report that displaying empathy and compassion promotes a positive work environment. Mindfulness and communication skills training are also reported to reduce aggressive incidents (Baby et al., 2019). Indeed, while environmental, educational and organisational factors are enablers, it is the therapeutic relationship that is going to minimise the problems and disruption attributed to challenging behaviour.

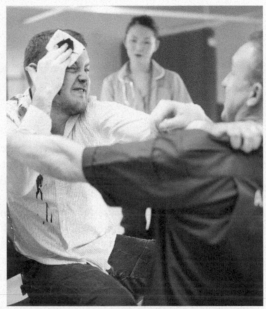
Paramedics deal with challenging behaviours.

For this reason, health professionals need to employ the range of skills and attributes that are integral to building and maintaining the therapeutic alliance and relationship. This includes engaging the person in a meaningful negotiation about the care and treatment they are to receive. This is not to suggest there will never be problems, but challenging behaviour can be a symptom of someone who is unsure of what is happening.

Many of the integral skills and attributes that are required to engage with a consumer are discussed in the chapter on assessment in the mental health context. The attributes that are more specific to the issues of caring for a person who is displaying a challenging behaviour as follows.

- Provide a consistent framework of care and treatment.
- Minimise staff splitting by keeping the same health professionals working with the person and using treatment and care plans that have been negotiated and collaboratively developed by all stakeholders.
- Explore reasons for non-adherence and address these with the consumer.
- Set clear limits, but emphasise what is available if the person stays within them.
- Give positive rewards for non-challenging behaviour, but do not react to challenging behaviour unless necessary and then do so consistently.
- Look at previous negative experiences and work with the consumer to see if he or she can identify differences from his or her current treatment and care.
- Take an unbiased look at the person's requirements and criticisms.

- Acknowledge the feelings of the consumer.
- Demonstrate empathy (see the chapter on assessment in the mental health context).
- Employ anxiety management techniques (as anxiety will underlie most challenging behaviours).
- Teach new behaviours, such as assertiveness and interpersonal effectiveness.
- Provide more information, if that is what the consumer is seeking and there is information to give.
- Make use of regular clinical supervision (reflective practice) provided by a trained facilitator.

Conflict resolution

Conflict resolution has also been recognised as a key skill when working with people with challenging behaviours. The approaches chosen will depend on the skills of the health professional and the attributes of the person with the challenging behaviour. Techniques can include:
- withdrawal from the source of conflict
- suppression or 'smoothing over' of the conflict
- the use of authority to contain the situation
- compromise or negotiation
- integration or collaboration.

The last technique is usually the most successful in the health context, with the emphasis on partnership and trying to solve the problem at hand, rather than on defending particular positions or factions (Aged Care Quality and Safety Commission, n.d.). The other techniques run the risk of apparently resolving the conflict but leaving one or both parties dissatisfied, which can be grounds for further conflict in the future, even if this isn't acknowledged.

The use of the 'third-person' de-escalation technique may also be useful during formal and informal conflict resolution. A **third-person intervention** occurs when a third person is introduced into the conflict dynamic to assist in resolving the situation. The third person is most often identified as a neutral person not previously involved with the conflict, and a trained mediator who can facilitate the communication between both parties to achieve the best possible outcome.

Planning ahead

When dealing with people who exhibit challenging behaviours, it is essential that all those involved are aware of, know or understand the notion of boundaries. The term **boundary** is often bandied around in the health context and refers to the limits of acceptability or appropriateness in a human interaction. Boundaries mark the point beyond which people are not expected to go, and are often differentiated when an individual says, 'He has just stepped over the line!' However, this differentiation can be problematic because often those involved are not aware of where the line is or what the rules are. In the health context especially, boundaries should be clear and clearly communicated (Medical Indemnity Protection Society, 2022). One way this can be achieved is by outlining the expectations of the organisation that provides the health service to the consumer. The expectation of the health professionals involved also need to be flagged. Being informed of the boundaries or 'rules' can be an important means by which people feel safe in a new or unfamiliar context. Boundaries are also a means by ensuring appropriate care and protection for consumers (Australian College of Nursing, 2020).

In addition to being informed about the kind of behaviours that are and are not acceptable in a particular context, it is also necessary for health professionals to outline the consequences to the consumer when the boundaries are crossed. It needs to be noted, however, that a one-size-fits-all approach to every situation is not appropriate (see the chapters on mental health care in Australia, and mental health service delivery). Indeed, such approaches assume that every situation is the same and over-simplify the complexity of human relationships and health care provision. One-size-fits-all approaches also suggest that the health professional is reacting after an incident has occurred, rather than responding in a measured way to a new situation as it occurs.

What is needed, then, is a proactive approach that addresses the person's clinical needs and the organisational needs of health professionals. Figure 6.5 outlines the three stages in the clinical management process to minimise challenging behaviours, including the proactive stage where the consumer is provided with information; the intermediate stage, where health professionals are provided with training in risk assessment and managing challenging behaviours; and the crisis stage, where tools and training are used to ensure staff are adequately equipped to deal with challenging situations.

Stage 1: Proactive
- Maintain an environment that is as calm and as peaceful as possible.
- Provide the consumer with information and materials to relieve boredom.
- Maintain effective systems of open communications.
- Identify health professionals and support staff as people, rather than 'anonymous' staff.
- Offer flexibility within clear boundaries.
- Take an attentive approach, both in listening and in communicating.
- Prioritise time to get to know the consumer's individual needs.
- Have ongoing training and education programs, particularly around de-escalation techniques and communication, and mental health issues in general settings.
- Hold multidisciplinary team reviews of all consumers and routinely involve consumers in collaborative decisions about their treatment and care.
- Provide clinical supervision (reflective practice).
- Develop and use problem-solving forums (e.g. shared governance committees).

Stage 2: Intermediate
- Provide regular training in risk assessment, de-escalation techniques and conflict transformation.
- Have access to specialist clinical management around particular consumers and/or situations (this is a service that most mental health liaison teams can deliver — see the chapter that looks at approaches to mental health service delivery).

Stage 3: Crisis
- Have up-to-date and effective alarm and personal duress systems.
- Have staff trained in de-escalation techniques and in safe procedures for managing violence and aggression.
- Ensure clinicians are aware of the seclusion, sedation or rapid tranquillisation policies for their context.
- Utilise security officers or the police when required.

Perhaps most important of all is the provision of workplace support to health professionals. Such support will influence the quality of the care and communication that the consumer receives. If health professionals feel confident and able to achieve their goals and have some perspective on their work, with as little organisational conflict as possible, they will be better equipped to address internal conflicts and any conflicts that occur with consumers or other stakeholders.

Contracts

Another way in which boundaries or limit setting can be utilised is through the 'contract'. A **contract**, also known as a 'voucher agreement' or 'patient-controlled admission' between a consumer and health professional can be written or verbal, and stands as an agreement between the parties that they will conform to mutually agreed-upon behaviours (Nyttingnes et al., 2021). Failure to conform will give rise to consequences, which are also mutually agreed upon. Achievement in meeting the requirements of the contract will likewise generate mutually agreed-upon benefits.

Such contracts can identify specific ways to help people with challenging behaviours to stay physically and emotionally safe. The contracts are developed with the consumer during the times when the consumer is feeling calm, behaviour is appropriate, and the consumer is ready to engage, participate and negotiate. Language used in the contract must be simple, and provide clear behaviour responses to manage unsafe feelings or behaviours. For example, 'When I feel like hurting myself, I will ...', 'When I feel like destroying property, I will ...'

Contractual and collaboratively negotiated admissions, sometimes referred to as 'brief admissions' have been shown to create a means by which consumers are able to take responsibility for their treatment, care and behaviour and work with health professionals to achieve positive outcomes (Eckerström et al., 2020).

UPON REFLECTION

Considerations for utilising an admission contract

The use of contractual admissions is often afforded to people with borderline personality disorder. This strategy gives the person a sense of control, and they can determine the best time for them to seek support when subjectively distressed. This process can void situations where objective symptomatology would ordinarily not meet admission criterion.

QUESTIONS

1. What benefits are likely to occur for consumers when they are able to negotiate an inpatient admission on their own terms?
2. What types of 'rules' need to be considered when negotiating such contracts? For example, is there a maximum number of days the person can be admitted, and a total number of days across a specific time period?
3. Are there any foreseeable difficulties with this practice? Are the difficulties for the consumer, the organisation or your own practice?
4. What strategies could be implemented to mitigate these potential ramifications from occurring?
5. In your place of work, is there a systematic process for the monitoring and review of contract usage and outcomes? If not, how do you think you can address this issue?

Seclusion and restraint

Seclusion refers to the 'confinement of a person alone in a room or area where they are prevented from free exit' (AIHW, 2022). Restraint is defined as 'the restriction of a person's freedom of movement by physical or mechanical means' (AIHW, 2022).

Under jurisdictional mental health legislation, seclusion is cited as a restrictive intervention, and the strict rationale for the initial and ongoing use of seclusion are prescribed, for example, *Mental Health Act 2015*. Seclusion may be initiated by either health care professionals or individuals receiving care (AIHW, 2022). However, outside of mental health legislation, seclusion and restraint may be practised by community services or National Disability Insurance Scheme (NDIS) registered providers when managing community-based people with an intellectual or cognitive deficit. On occasions, and only following thorough assessment and approval processes, can challenging behaviour considered so extreme result in the individual being restrained, whether through the use of medication, mechanical or manual restraint, seclusion, or a combination of one or more of these methods (Queensland Department of Seniors, Disability Services and Aboriginal and Torres Strait Islander Partnerships, 2021). While seclusion and restraint are primarily used for safety and containment purposes, they nonetheless may cause harm and/or distress to consumers, staff and others present. Due to negative cultural and historical factors and experiences, Aboriginal and Torres Strait Islander peoples may also require additional social and emotional wellbeing support and monitoring during mental health inpatient episodes of care, inclusive of periods of seclusion and restraint (Molloy et al., 2021). Given the potential harm of this type of intervention, the use of seclusion and restraint is heavily monitored and is reportable across all states and territories. Furthermore, all health sectors are continuously working towards the reduction and elimination of these restrictive practices, in line with the national safety priorities for mental health services (National Mental Health Commission (2022). It is notable that legislative, policy and clinical practice modifications have resulted in significantly reducing national rates of seclusion by almost half over the past 10 years. However, rates of physical restraint remain unchanged (AIHW, 2022).

Additionally, there are different cultural views in relation to seclusion and restraint practices (ACMHN, 2019b, p. 21). For example, generally health professionals in the United States view pharmacological (or chemical) restraint (i.e., providing a consumer who is exhibiting challenging behaviours with a sedative) as more restrictive than physical restraint. In contrast, in Australia the physical restraint of consumers located in mental health facilities is being actively discouraged, with sedatives viewed as the less restrictive alternative (see the chapter on the legal and ethical context of mental health care). For this reason, the seclusion method of managing challenging behaviour in the health context is less commonly used in contemporary Australia. The NICE guideline states that 'restrictive interventions may be used only if de-escalation and other preventive strategies, including PRN medication, have failed and there is potential for harm to the service user or other people if no action is taken'. It is also recommended not to 'use restrictive interventions to punish, inflict pain, suffering or humiliation, or to establish dominance' (NICE, 2015a, pp. 30–31).

Furthermore, although some health professionals consider the use of seclusion or restraint practices to be necessary, they would welcome a reduction in the use of this practice — with the ultimate aim of elimination. SA Health, for example, have developed a toolkit underpinned by best available evidence, to support the minimisation of seclusion and restraint practices, which includes alternatives to seclusion and restraint. Alternate strategies include the use of personal safety and prevention plans, effective limit setting and sensory modulation opportunities (SA Health, 2015b).

LIVED EXPERIENCE

A catastrophic story of restraint ... this is our story

You may not know us, but we want to tell you about something very personal that shattered our lives and changed our family forever.

...

Seni was just 23 years old — an IT graduate — when he died in hospital on 3 September 2010. He died because of prolonged restraint, when he was held down by 11 police officers while he was a patient in a mental health hospital.

Seni had never had any mental health issues before, but over that bank holiday weekend in 2010 he seemed agitated and his behaviour became odd. We took him to A&E and, after an assessment, we were told to take him to Bethlem Royal Hospital. We took him there, to what we thought would be the best place for him to get help.

Seni agreed to stay overnight at the hospital as a voluntary patient. We were asked to leave him at the end of visiting hours, and we did so reluctantly. Shortly afterwards, he became agitated when he was stopped from leaving the hospital because he wanted to come home. The hospital staff 'sectioned' him and called the police who came and agreed to take Seni to a seclusion room in the hospital. He was co-operative until he stopped at the threshold of the seclusion room. As soon as he stopped, the police officers pushed him inside and forced him face down to the floor.

The police officers held Seni face down, shackled his hands with two sets of handcuffs and put his legs in two sets of restraints. They held him down like that over a period of some 45 minutes altogether, in a restraint they knew was dangerous, until he went limp. And even then, instead of treating him as a medical emergency, they simply walked away: they believed he was faking it! They left our son on the floor of a locked room, all but dead. All of this happened in the presence of hospital staff including nurses and a doctor who stood by and looked on, unable or unwilling to intervene. Seni never regained consciousness and died four days later. That is how we lost our beloved son.

At the inquest into his death, the jury found Seni died as a result of excessive, disproportionate and unreasonable restraint and force. To this day, we struggle to comprehend that our son died as he did, simply because those who were responsible for his care — police officers and medical staff alike — failed in their duty to treat him with the respect that he deserved as a human being.

In a signed statement after these events, one doctor described how the officers treated our son: 'I felt like it wasn't a human being that they were trying to restrain ... it was like trying to contain an animal ... after they had tied him up with the straps it seemed like when a hunter has tied the animal ... it was an uneasy feeling that I had that it was not a human being that they were restraining'. That is how he was seen and treated at that point: as an animal, rather than a petrified young man, terrified at the prospect of being put in a padded seclusion room.

We don't want anyone else to go through this. We have been fighting for over eight years to get answers and justice for Seni. Now, through initiatives in his name — such as Seni's Law, a parliamentary bill with cross party support designed to open up the system to greater transparency and accountability to stop the disproportionate use of force and restraint — we feel that our son may not have died in vain. If we can make sure this never happens to anyone else, that would be an amazing legacy for Seni.

That is why we are really pleased to see the publication of these new standards, but this must be just the beginning. There is so much more to do in view of the increasing number of deaths in the context of restraint. In addition to health, education and social care services, we need to get law enforcement agencies involved in these standards concerning the use of restraint. We need to ensure these standards are not just implemented, but also regulated. And we need to make sure that the use of force and restraint is not just reduced but prevented altogether when dealing with vulnerable individuals who may find themselves in Seni's position in the future.

Source: Aji & Conrad Lewis cited in Ridley and Leitch (2019).

Rapid tranquillisation

Rapid tranquillisation is the 'use of medication by the parenteral route (usually intramuscular or, exceptionally, intravenous) if oral medication is not possible or appropriate and urgent sedation with medication is needed' (Cookson, 2018).

As noted in the chapter on the legal and ethical context of mental health care, to protect the client, community members and health professionals from physical harm, a decision can sometimes be made to sedate a consumer who is exhibiting a challenging behaviour. This sedation may be provided very quickly, in a process called 'rapid tranquillisation'. Pharmacological options are both a valuable and suitable management option when a person's behaviour places either themselves or others at a significant immediate risk, especially if the aetiology of the behaviour is mental health related. In some states and territories in Australia, paramedics are now involved in this process in the community however, this would occur only in an emergency. In most cases, rapid tranquillisation would occur in a hospital context. According to Queensland Health (2021), the short-term management of disturbed/violent behaviour in psychiatric inpatient settings and emergency departments will include the use of droperidol, with ketamine, olazapine and diazepam being second-line agents.

Health professionals in Australia are strongly advised to obtain the policy and procedures for rapid tranquillisation that have been developed by their state or territory government, or local employer prior to participating in a rapid tranquillisation and to undertake the relevant training. In the absence of local documents, NICE have developed suggested guidelines to follow when dealing with violent or disturbed behaviour in a psychiatric inpatient setting or in the emergency department of hospitals. These guidelines provide direction in assessing the risk, diffusing a possible volatile situation and managing violence should it occur. A comprehensive risk assessment should be conducted with clear management procedures in place. Staff should receive regular training on how to recognise threatening behaviour and how to manage their reactions in these situations. It is vital to ensure that education trainers have the requisite knowledge, skills, competency and experience required to deliver the training (Ridley & Leitch, 2019).

Rapid tranquillisation, physical restraint and seclusion should only be used when all other strategies have been unsuccessful, and the staff who are responsible for administering these controls should be trained in appropriate life support techniques such as resuscitation and the use of defibrillators. NICE advises that physical restraint should be conducted as a group with one staff member responsible for the support of the head and neck of the patient to ensure their airway is kept clear and that the patient's vital signs are continuously monitored. NICE also suggests that any service members that are at risk of exposure to violent or disturbed behaviour should be given an opportunity to complete a living will to ensure their needs and wishes are recorded.

The use of restraints for older people with challenging behaviours

The Aged Care Royal Commission findings (2018–2020) and the introduction of the Aged Care Quality Standards (2019), resulted in Australian aged care providers being under much governance monitoring and public scrutiny, including in relation to the use of restraint practices. Part of this reform included the Australian Government implementing a Mandatory Quality Indicator Program for physical restraint, which is a prescriptive reporting loop for all approved aged care providers (see www.health.gov.au/sites/default/files/documents/2020/09/use-of-physical-restraint-quick-reference-guide-national-aged-care-mandatory-quality-indicator-program_0.pdf). Challenging older resident behaviour may include 'at risk behaviours' such as harm to self or others, loss of dignity, or property damage. Physical restraints have been used on older people with a dementing or mental illness who are considered to be in danger of falling or wandering, with restraints being a way of life for some residents in aged care facilities (Borello, 2019). While much of the literature relates to the use of physical restraints in aged care facilities, these restraints are also used on older people with behavioural disturbances who are being cared for in an acute care setting.

Perhaps not surprisingly, given the negative impact coercion can have on the therapeutic relationship, and feedback received from the Aged Care Royal Commission, there is a significant move away from the automatic use of restraints and the perceived over-reliance on safety considerations (Commonwealth of Australia, 2019). In support of a restraint-free environment, the Australian government has a number of resources available to support this goal. Resources and information include the identification of individualised psychosocial interventions to manage challenging behaviours in nursing homes, as opposed to the regular use of physical restraint. There are a number of effective non-pharmacological interventions for behavioural disorders in dementia, including aggressive behaviour in older adults, that may have favourable outcomes in terms of reducing aggressive behaviour. These strategies include provision of suitable social activities and companionship, increased observation, and reducing noisy and over-stimulated environments for consumers (Department of Health and Aging, 2012).

Regardless of the age of the consumer, restraints should be used to manage physical behaviour only as a last resort. As already noted, health professionals who focus on engaging with consumers, forging a therapeutic alliance and developing this into a relationship, are far better placed to work effectively with consumers who exhibit challenging behaviours. Practising unconditional positive regard is likewise essential to providing high-quality health care and can be achieved only when the health professional is committed to supporting the improvement of health outcomes for all consumers, regardless of their behaviour.

Aged Care Quality Standards outcome

In 2019, the Commonwealth Government introduced the Aged Care Quality Standards, with the sub-theme 'engage, empower, safeguard'. The aim of the Standards is to improve the quality and safety of care provided to older Australians who receive services from a government-funded aged care provider — either at home or in an aged care facility. The eight Standards are listed in figure 6.6.

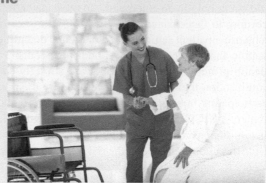

FIGURE 6.6   The Aged Care Quality Standards

1. Consumer dignity and choice.
   - *Consumer outcome:* I am treated with dignity and respect, and can maintain my identity. I can make informed choices about my care and services, and live the life I choose.
2. Ongoing assessment and planning with consumers.
   - *Consumer outcome:* I am a partner in ongoing assessment and planning that helps me get the care and services I need for my health and wellbeing.
3. Personal care and clinical care.
   - *Consumer outcome:* I get personal care, clinical care, or both personal care and clinical care, that is safe and right for me.
4. Services and supports for daily living.
   - *Consumer outcome:* I get the services and supports for daily living that are important for my health and well-being and that enable me to do the things I want to do.
5. Organisation's service environment.
   - *Consumer outcome:* I feel I belong and I am safe and comfortable in the organisation's service environment.
6. Feedback and complaints.
   - *Consumer outcome:* I feel safe and am encouraged and supported to give feedback and make complaints. I am engaged in processes to address my feedback and complaints, and appropriate action is taken.
7. Human resources.
   - *Consumer outcome:* I get quality care and services when I need them from people who are knowledgeable, capable and caring.
8. Organisational governance.
   - *Consumer outcome:* I am confident the organisation is well run. I am a partner in improving the delivery of care and services.

Source: My Aged Care (2019).

QUESTIONS

1. In broad terms, in what ways did the COVID-19 pandemic impact on the aged care sector?
2. As a direct result of the declared Public Health Emergency, what were the consequences that older people experienced? Consider direct and indirect consequences.
3. Given that these Standards were developed to enhance the delivery of care and safety for older people, were practices adopted by service providers aligned with the Standards, and which practices did not?
4. Were the human rights of older people in aged care facilities upheld during the Public Health Emergency?
5. In which Standards did aged care facilities generally perform well during the pandemic, and achieve the desired consumer outcomes as stated?

SUMMARY

People exhibit challenging behaviours in the health context for many reasons. They are not necessarily the outcome of a mental health problem. Rather, challenging behaviours can be the result of the power imbalance that is inherent within the relationship between the health professional and the person they are assisting. At other times, the triggers are situational, such as ill-health or injury, pain, the unfamiliar health context, requiring assistance with personal care, belonging to a marginalised group, or experiencing a loss of self-determination. Feelings of vulnerability and powerlessness that lead to challenging behaviours can also arise from the health system itself or the wider social context.

This chapter discusses the nature of challenging behaviours and notes that defence mechanisms are used by everyone from time to time. They are one of the many means of coping that can help people to manage the challenging situations that make up their daily lives. The causes or triggers of challenging behaviours are considered, such as the demands being made by the health professional on the consumer, the health professional's negative attitude to the consumer, and disputes between the health professional and the consumer. The need to conduct a general and risk assessment is also identified, as well as the problem of bullying in the workplace between health professionals. The section describes health service organisational responses to bullying and other challenging behaviours in the workplace. The need for higher levels of education and training is identified and an explanation is provided of some techniques that can be used by health professionals to manage challenging behaviour in the workplace.

To be effective, health professionals must consider the many contributing factors that may lead to a person exhibiting challenging behaviours in the health context. This consideration will include identifying and practising ways and means of empowering the consumer. Such strategies can be highly specialised, but also include, quite simply, actively preserving the dignity of the consumer by practising kindness and unconditional positive regard.

KEY TERMS

boundary The limits of acceptability or appropriateness in a human interaction.

challenging behaviour Behaviour of such intensity, frequency or duration as to threaten the quality of life and/or the physical safety of the individuals or others and is likely to lead to responses that are restrictive, aversive or result in exclusion.

clinical supervision A formal and ongoing process of giving and receiving professional support through reflective practice.

contract The written or verbal agreement between the consumer and health professional or health service provider that involves both the consumer and health professional or health service provider agreeing to conform to mutually agreed-upon behaviours.

defence mechanisms A normally unconscious mental process that can help to reduce potentially negative feelings such as anxiety, shame or fear.

empathy A human quality demonstrated by a person that shows they are able to identify with the thoughts, feelings or experiences of another person.

projection The process in which one person assigns (or projects) their uncomfortable thoughts or feelings onto another person.

splitting Where an individual is unable to see that people are complex beings with both positive and negative attributes who may behave differently according to context. Instead, the individual reduces people and behaviours into simplistic and often polarised categories.

staff splitting A defence mechanism that occurs when a consumer idealises a health professional and manipulates them to meet their own needs; this behaviour challenges consistency of care and creates tension in the multidisciplinary team.

third-person intervention The practice of using a third person during formal and informal conflict resolution to de-escalate perceived or actual conflict.

zero tolerance A work health and safety principle that proscribes workplace violence. This includes physical and non-physical violence that may result in physical harm or psychological harm.

REVIEW QUESTIONS

1 Name the four categories of 'difficult' behaviour as identified by Koekkoek and colleagues (2006).
2 Describe the principles of clinical supervision.
3 Identify the main factors to consider when assessing challenging behaviours.
4 What steps can multidisciplinary teams take to reduce the risk of staff splitting occurring?
5 What is the definition of zero tolerance?
6 Name the seven principles of the Australian Charter of Health Care Rights.
7 What are four key skills that are helpful to improve engagement with people displaying challenging behaviours?
8 What are the three stages of clinical management that are determined to minimise challenging behaviours?
9 What techniques are often used in conflict resolution?
10 What governance systems exist to protect consumers from unlawful seclusion and restraint practices?
11 What is the definition of 'professional boundary'?
12 What are the eight Aged Care Quality Standards, and who do they apply to?

DISCUSSION AND DEBATE

1 Think of a time when you lost your temper or became anxious (e.g. flight cancelled, long queue, lost child at shops, unhelpful staff, wallet or keys missing). How did you react to this event emotionally and behaviourally? What physiological changes did you notice in yourself? How did you treat others who were attempting to assist you during your distress? Were there other things happening that clouded your judgement? Was there anyone who was helpful during this incident? If so, what was it that person said or did that helped you? As you think about this experience, does it arouse any unresolved feelings from the past? What can you learn about yourself from this event?
2 Review the social media campaign Hands off our Ambos. Discuss the advantages and disadvantages of this footage. How could you adopt this strategy to suit your own profession/context?
3 What term do you think better conceptualises the notion of difficult interactions: 'challenging behaviour' or 'behaviours that challenge'? Provide a rationale for your preference.
4 As a health professional, what actions could you implement in your workplace to minimise bullying behaviours? What training is available in your workplace or university regarding this issue? How does your discipline-specific professional code of conduct reinforce the acceptable behaviours of your profession?
5 How important is non-verbal communication/body language, during our interactions with others? What signs and signals can you observe in others? What is likely to obstruct a health care professional's ability to be open and receptive towards another person? How can health care professionals increase their level of knowledge in relation to non-verbal communication?
6 Given the contemporary language and behaviour we see in our daily lives, on social media and on television/films and so on, how realistic is the concept of 'zero tolerance' in the workplace? Give reasons for your answer.
7 Discuss the notion of 'rapid tranquillisation'. Consider the issue from a safety perspective, from a human rights perspective, from a legal perspective and from a professional/ethical perspective? In which quadrant do you most align with. Provide an explanation for your viewpoint.
8 The rates of seclusion and restraint have reduced significantly over recent years. Is it possible to completely eliminate these practices given the prevalence of challenging behaviors and occupational violence in healthcare, and in the context of community norms? Discuss.

PROJECT ACTIVITY

The Australian College of Nursing (ACN) supports all health care practitioners and consumers to develop and maintenance appropriate professional boundaries. Their website features an overview describing how to maintain a professional relationship, and also provides scenarios for when professional boundary transgressions may occur.

Access the flyer via www.acn.edu.au/wp-content/uploads/career-hub-resources-maintaining-professio nal-boundaries.pdf. Read the eight scenarios and then select one to further unpack. Answer the questions posed and then consider the following.

1 What clinical issues were raised in the vignette?
2 How could you address the concerns raised in the vignette in your workplace?
3 What practices could you put in place to minimise this situation occurring in your practice?
4 Identify your training needs in order to fully understand your professional obligations in relation to social media participation and potential boundary issues.
5 What policy and procedure development needs to occur to ensure that you are protected from potential boundary violations in the workplace?

WEBSITES

1 The Restraint Reduction Network website provides informative resources to protect human rights and reduce restrictive practices for health, education and social services settings: www.restraintreduction network.org.
2 The Phoenix Australia Centre for Posttraumatic Mental Health at the University of Melbourne undertakes world-class trauma-related research, policy advice, service development and education. Its innovative services help organisations and health professionals who work with people affected by traumatic events: www.phoenixaustralia.org.
3 The Australian Government Comcare site contains much information regarding zero tolerance and professional workplace bullying: www.comcare.gov.au.
4 The Mental Health Professional Online Development website has two useful modules: (i) Reducing and eliminating seclusion and restraint and (ii) Working with People with Borderline Personality Disorder: www.mhpod.gov.au.
5 The Project Air Strategy for Personality Disorders is an internationally recognised leader in research, education and treatment. Project Air partners with health, justice, education, communities, families and individuals and has a number of resources and e-learning modules related to borderline personality disorder, narcissistic personality disorder, antisocial personality disorder, and paranoid, schizoid, schizotypal, histrionic, avoidant, dependent and obsessive-compulsive personality disorders: www. uow.edu.au/project-air.
6 The National BPD Training Strategy provides a five module e-learning package, Effective Psychological Treatment for Borderline Personality Disorder, with information on borderline personality disorder: www.bpdfoundation.org.au/learning-modules.php.
7 Bullying. No way! is a site to help keep children and young people safe from bullying. The site provides information and ideas for students, teachers, parents and community leaders: www.bullyingnoway. gov.au.
8 The Clinical Practice Guidelines portal is an initiative of the Australian National Health and Medical Research Council (NHMRC) and is freely available to all clinicians. The site provides links to numerous health-related clinical guidelines used in Australia, including for the management of Borderline Personality Disorder: www.clinicalguidelines.gov.au.
9 The Department of Health website hosts numerous publications relevant to this chapter, including fact sheets on managing challenging child behaviours: www.health.gov.au.
10 White Ribbon Australia provides an eLearning course for those who want to expand their understanding of violence against women, and how to prevent it. The Prevntion of Violence Against Women for Workplaces: www.whiteribbon.org.au/Learn-more/Learning.
11 The Aged Care Quality Standards website provides comprehensive information for each of the eight standards: www.agedcare.health.gov.au/quality/aged-care-quality-standards.
12 The Fair Work Ombudsman website has two useful tutorials to assist with difficult conversations. One is primarily for managers and the other for employees: www.fairwork.gov.au/employee-entitlements/ bullying-and-harassment#what-is-bullying.

REFERENCES

Aged Care Quality and Safety Commission. (n.d.). *Overview of restrictive practices*. Commonwealth of Australia www.agedcarequality.gov.au/resources/overview-restrictive-practices

Aggarwal, N. (2016). Empowering people with mental illness within health services. *Acta Psychopathologica*, 2(36).

Ali, M. (2018). Communication skills 6: Difficult and challenging conversations. *Nursing Times*, 114(4), 51–53.

Alzheimer's, Australia. (2014). *The use of restraints and psychotropic medications in people with dementia. Paper 38.* Alzheimer's Australia.

American Psychiatric Association. (2013). *Diagnostic and statistical manual of mental disorders* (5th ed.). American Psychiatric Association.

Association for Data-driven Marketing and Advertising. (2017). *AC&E awards. Most Effective Use of Content.* Showpony Advertising, Hands Off Our Ambos, SA Health www.adma.com.au/events/2016/acandeawards/winners/case-studies/hands-off-our-ambos-showpony-advertising

Australian Clinical Supervision Association. (2018). *Definitions of clinical supervision.* https://clinicalsupervision.org.au/wp-content/uploads/2022/08/ACSA-Definitions-CS-2015.pdf

Australian College of Mental Health Nurses, Australian College of Midwives, and Australian College of Nursing. (2019a). Position statement: Clinical supervision for nurses & midwives. *ISBN: 978-1-925913-58-3 (e-book).*

Australian College of Mental Health Nurses. (2019b). *Safe in care, safe at work. Ensuring safety in care and safety for staff in Australian mental health services.* ACMHN.

Australian College of Nursing. (2020). *Career Hub. Maintaining professional boundaries.* www.acn.edu.au/wp-content/uploads/career-hub-resources-maintaining-professional-boundaries.pdf

The Australian Commission on Safety and Quality in Health Care. (2019a). *Australian Charter of Healthcare Rights.* ACSQHC. https://www.safetyandquality.gov.au/sites/default/files/migrated/Charter-PDf.pdf

Australian Institute of Health and Wellbeing. (2019b). *Mental health services in Australia.* AIHW. www.aihw.gov.au/reports/mental-health-services/mental-health-services-in-australia-in-brief-2019/summary

Australian Institute of Health and Wellbeing. (2019c, March 22). *Use of restrictive practices in mental health facilities continues to fall. Media release.* www.aihw.gov.au/news-media/media-releases/2019/march/use-of-restrictive-practices-in-mental-health-faci

Australian Institute of Health and Wellbeing. (2022). *Mental health services in Australia.* Restrictive Practices in Mental Health Care. www.aihw.gov.au/reports/mental-health-services/mental-health-services-in-australia/report-contents/restrictive-practices/seclusion

Averbuch, T., Eliya, Y., & Van Spall, H. G. C. (2021). Systematic review of academic bullying in medical settings: dynamics and consequences. *BMJ Open*, 11, e043256 https://doi.org/10.1136/bmjopen-2020-043256

Baby, M., Gale, C., & Swain, N. (2019). A communication skills intervention to minimise patient perpetrated aggression for healthcare support workers in New Zealand: A cluster randomised controlled trial. *Health and Social Care in the Community*, 27(1), 170–181.

Black, D. (2021). Managing 'difficult' patient encounters. *Current Psychiatry*, 20(7), 12–19. https://doi.org/10.12788/cp.0144

Borello, E. (2019). *Aged care royal commission to examine use of restraints on patients after cases in NSW, Victoria. ABC News.* www.abc.net.au/news/2019-01-17/aged-care-royal-commission-to-review-use-of-restraint-in-homes/10720672

Bowers, L., James, K., Quirk, A., Simpson, A., SUGAR Stewart, D., & Hodsoll, J. (2015). Reducing conflict and containment rates on acute psychiatric wards: The Safewards cluster randomised controlled trial. *International Journal of Nursing Studies*, 52(9), 1412–1422.

Bully Zero Australia Foundation. (2016). *Workplace bullying.* www.bullyzero.org.au/workplace-bullying

Cerit, K., Karataş, T., & Ekici, D. (2020). Behaviours of healthcare professionals towards difficult patients: A structural equation modelling study. *Nursing Ethics*, 27(2), 554–566. https://doi.org/10.1177/0969733019858694

Chapman, J., Jamil, R. T., & Fleisher, C. (2022). *Borderline personality disorder.* StatPearls [Internet]. StatPearls Publishing. www.ncbi.nlm.nih.gov/books/NBK430883

Chataway, M. (2021). *Occupational violence against healthcare professionals: Applying a criminological lens. Centre for Justice Briefing Paper.* Queensland University of Technology. ISSN 2652-5828 (Print), 2652-6441 (Online)

Clough, R. (2018). *Making a noise: 40 years of consumer health advocacy in the ACT.* Health Care Consumers' Association.

Commonwealth of Australia. (2019). *Royal commission. Restrictive Practices in residential Aged Care in Australia. Background Paper 4.* The Royal Commission into Aged Care Quality and Safety. www.agedcare.royalcommission.gov.au/sites/default/files/2019-12/background-paper-4.pdf

Comorbidity Guidelines. (2022). *What are the different types of personality disorders?.* Australian Government, Department of Health. https://comorbidityguidelines.org.au/what-are-personality-disorders/what-are-the-different-types-of-personality-disorders

Consumer Policy Research Centre. (2020). *Exploring regulatory approaches to consumer vulnerability – A report for the Australian Energy Regulator* (pp. 29–35). Australian Energy Regulator.

Cookson, J. (2018). Rapid tranquillisation: The science and advise. *British Journal of Psychiatric Advances*, 24(5), 346–358. https://doi.org/10.1192/bja.2018.25.

Department of Health Aging. (2012). *Decision-making tool: Supporting a restraint free environment in residential aged care.* Commonwealth of Australia.

Department of Home Affairs. (2019). *Working in Australia. Workers rights and restrictions.* https://immi.homeaffairs.gov.au/visas/working-in-australia/work-rights-and-exploitation

Dollard, M. F., Owen, M., Afsharian, A., & Potter, R. (2021). *Bullying and Harassment in Australian Workplaces 2021: Australian Workplace Barometer Fact Sheet.* University of South Australia, Psychosocial Safety Climate Global Observatory. www.safeworkaustralia.gov.au/system/files/documents/1702/the-australian-workplace-barometer-report.pdf

Eckerström, J., Flyckt, L., Carlborg, A., Jayaram-Lindström, N., & Perseius, K. I. (2020). Brief admission for patients with emotional instability and self-harm: A qualitative analysis of patients' experiences during crisis. *International Journal of Mental Health Nursing*, *29*(5), 962–971. https://doi.org/10.1111/inm.12736 PMID: 32406168

Edward, K. L., Stephenson, J., Ousey, K., Lui, S., Warelow, P., & Giandinoto, J. A. (2016). A systematic review and meta-analysis of factors that relate to aggression perpetrated against nurses by patients/relatives or staff. *Journal of Clinical Nursing*, *25*(3–4), 289–299.

Fair Work Ombudsman. (2022). *Bullying in the Workplace*. www.fairwork.gov.au/employment-conditions/bullying-sexual-harassment-and-discrimination-at-work/bullying-in-the-workplace.

Gamble Blakey, A., Smith-Han, K., Anderson, L., Collins, E., Berryman, E., & Wilkinson, T. J. (2019). Interventions addressing student bullying in the clinical workplace: A narrative review. *BMC Medical Education*, *19*. https://doi.org/10.1186/s12909-019-1578-y

Gleeson. (2019). *Restrictive practices policy*. Icare Insurance and Care NSW.

Green, H. (2018). Team splitting and the 'borderline personality': A relational reframe. *Psychoanalytical Psychotherapy*, *32*(3), 1–18.

Havaei, F. (2021). Does the type of exposure to workplace violence matter to nurses' mental health? *Healthcare (Basel)*, *9*(1), 41. https://doi.org/10.3390/healthcare9010041 PMID: 33466294; PMCID: PMC7824770

Headspace. (2022). *Clinical toolkit. Clinical Tips: Criteria for Diagnosing Borderline Personality Disorder*. www.headspace.org.au/professionals-and-educators/health-professionals/resources/treatment-guidelines/bpd-0

Health Victoria. (2019). *Allied health workforce*. Department of Health & Human Services, State Government of Victoria. www2.health.vic.gov.au/health-workforce/allied-health-workforce

Johnson, S. L. (2021). Workplace bullying in the nursing profession. In P. D'Cruz, E. Noronha, L. Keashly, & S. Tye-Williams (Eds.), *Special topics and particular occupations, Professions and Sectors. Handbooks of Workplace Bullying, Emotional Abuse and Harassment* (Vol. 4)). Springer. https://doi.org/10.1007/978-981-10-5308-5_14

Jubb, J. M., & Baack, C. J. (2019). Verbal de-escalation for clinical practice safety. *American Nurse Today*, *14*(1), 5–7.

Knaak, S., Mantler, E., & Szeto, A. (2017). Mental illness-related stigma in healthcare. Barriers to access and care and evidence-based solutions. *Healthcare Management Forum*, *30*(2), 111–116.

Koekkoek, B., van Meijel, B., & Hutschemackers, G. (2006). Difficult patients in mental health care: A review. *Psychiatric Services*, *57*(6), 795–802.

Lim, E., Wynaden, D., & Heslop, K. (2019). Changing practice using recovery-focused care in acute mental health settings to reduce aggression: A qualitative study. *International Journal of Mental Health Nursing*, *28*, 237–246.

Lorettu, L., Nivoli, A. M. A., Daga, I., Milia, P., Depalmas, C., Nivoli, G., & Bellizzi, S. (2021). Six things to know about the homicides of doctors: a review of 30 years from Italy. *BMC Public Health*, *21*, 1318. https://doi.org/10.1186/s12889-021-11404-5

Maassen, S. M., van Oostveen, C., Vermeulen, H., & Weggelaar, A. M. (2021). Defining a positive work environment for hospital healthcare professionals: A Delphi study. *PLoS ONE*, *16*(2), e0247530. https://doi.org/10.1371/journal.pone.0247530

Medical Indemnity Protection Society. (2022). *Keeping within Professional Boundaries*. https://support.mips.com.au/home/keeping-within-professional-boundaries

Melville, N. (2016). *'Difficult' patients more likely to be medically misdiagnosed*. Medscape Medical News. www.medscape.com/viewarticle/860495

Molloy, L., Guha, M. D., Scott, M. P., Beckett, P., Tran Merrick, T., & Patton, D. (2021). Mental health nursing practice and Aboriginal and Torres Strait Islander people: An integrative review. *Contemporary Nurse*, *57*(1-2), 140–156. https://doi.org/10.1080/10376178.2021.1927773

My Aged Care. (2019). *Quality indicator — use of physical restraint*. Commonwealth of Australia. www.myagedcare.gov.au

National Institute for Health and Care Excellence. (2015a). *Challenging behaviour and learning disabilities: Prevention and interventions for people with learning disabilities whose behaviour challenges*. NICE guideline [NG11] www.nice.org.uk/guidance/ng11

National Institute for Health and Care Excellence. (2015b). *Violence and aggression: Short-term management in mental health, health and community settings. NICE guideline [NG10]*. www.nice.org.uk/guidance/ng10

National Mental Health Commission. (2022). *Reducing restrictive practices*. www.mentalhealthcommission.gov.au/lived-experience/contributing-lives,-thriving-communities/reducing-restrictive-practices

Noble, N. (2022). *Oklahoma gunman killed 4 people, including surgeon who treated him. June, Reuters World News*, *3*. 2022 www.reuters.com/world/us/oklahoma-police-say-gunman-chose-site-shooting-deliberately-2022-06-02

Novac, A., McEwan, S., & Bota, R. G. (2014). Negative rumor: Contagion of a psychiatric department. *Primary Care Companion CNS Disorders*, *16*(2), CC.13br01614.

NSW Health. (2015). *Principles for safe management of disturbed and /or aggressive behaviour and the use of restraint*. Document number PD2015_004. Clinical Excellence Commission, Ministry of Health NSW. www1.health.nsw.gov.au/pds/ArchivePDSDocuments/PD2015_004.pdf

Nyblade, L., Stockton, M. A., Giger, K., Bond, V., Ekstarnd, M. L., McLean, R., Mitchell, E. M. H., Nelson, L. E., Sapag, J. C., Siraprapasiri, T., Turan, J., & Wouters, E. (2019). Stigma of health facilities: Why it matters and how we can change it. *BMC Medicine*, *17*, 25.

Nyttingnes, O., Šaltytė Benth, J., & Ruud, T. (2021). Patient-controlled admission contracts: a longitudinal study of patient evaluations. *BMC Health Serv Res*, *21*, 36. https://doi.org/10.1186/s12913-020-06033-4

Pavithra, A., Sunderland, N., Callen, J., & Westbrook, J. (2022). Unprofessional behaviours experienced by hospital staff: Qualitative analysis of narrative comments in a longitudinal survey across seven hospitals in Australia. *BMC Health Services Research*, *22*, 410. https://doi.org/10.1186/s12913-022-07763-3

Perlin, C. K. (2001). Social responses and personality disorder. In G. W. Stuart & M. T. Laraia (Eds.), *Principles and practice of psychiatric nursing* (pp. 439–60). Mosby.

Pich, J. (2018). *Violence in nursing and midwifery in NSW*. NSW Nurses' and Midwives' Association and UTS. www.nswnma.asn.au/wp-content/uploads/2019/02/Violence-in-Nursing-and-Midwifery-in-NSW.pdf

Queensland Department of Seniors,Disability Services, and Aboriginal and Torres Strait Islander Partnerships. (2021). *Publications and resources*. Restrictive Practice requirements. Queensland Government. www.dsdsatsip.qld.gov.au/our-work/disability-services/disability-connect-queensland/positive-behaviour-support-restrictive-practices/publications-resources

Queensland Health. (2021). *Management of patients with acute severe behavioural disturbance in emergency departments*. Queensland Emergency Department Strategic Advisory Panel. Department of Health Guideline. QH-GDL-438:2016 www.health.qld.gov.au/__data/assets/pdf_file/0031/629491/qh-gdl-438.pdf

Ridley, J., & Leitch, S. (2019). *The Restraint Reduction Network training standards 2019* (1st ed.). British Institute of Learning Disabilities.

Rodriguez, A. M., & Lown, B. A. (2019). Measuring compassionate healthcare with the 12-item Schwartz Center Compassionate Care Scale. *PLoS One, 14*(10), e0220911.

Safe Work Australia. (2019). *Infographic: Workplace mental health*. www.safeworkaustralia.gov.au/system/files/documents/1704/infographic-mental-disorders.pdf

SA Health. (2019a). *Gayle's Law. Department for Health and Ageing, Government of South Australia*. www.sahealth.sa.gov.au/wps/wcm/connect/public+content/sa+health+internet/about+us/legislation/gayles+law

SA Health. (2019b). *Taking care of challenging behaviour*. Department for Health and Ageing, Government of South Australia.

SA Health. (2015a). *Preventing and responding to challenging behaviour, violence and aggression policy guideline PUBLIC: I1-A1*. Department for Health and Ageing, Government of South Australia.

SA Health. (2015b). *Restraint and seclusion in mental health services policy guideline*. Department for Health and Ageing, Government of South Australia.

Safeguarding Health in Conflict Coalition. (2021). *UNRELENTING VIOLENCE: Violence against health care in conflict 2021*. SHCC. www.icn.ch/system/files/2022-05/SHCC%202021%20Unrelenting%20Violence.pdf

SafeWork SA. (2018). *Work-related violence. Preventing and responding to work-related violence*. Government of South Australia. www.safework.sa.gov.au/__data/assets/pdf_file/0008/136358/Preventing-and-responding-to-work-related-violence.pdf

Searby, A., Snipe, J., & Maude, P. (2019). Aggression management training in undergraduate nursing students: A scoping review. *Issues in Mental Health Nursing, 40*(6), 503–510.

State of Victoria. (2021). *Independent review into workplace equality in Ambulance Victoria volume 1*. Victorian Equal Opportunity and Human Rights Commission www.humanrights.vic.gov.au/legal-and-policy/research-reviews-and-investigations/ambulance-victoria-review/final-report

Stephens, W. (2019, May 12). *Violence against healthcare workers: A rising epidemic. American Journal of Managed Care*. In Focus Blog. www.ajmc.com/focus-of-the-week/violence-against-healthcare-workers-a-rising-epidemic

Sundler, A. J., Raberus, A., Carlsson, G., Nilsson, C., & Darcy, L. (2022). Are they really allowed to treat me like that?'– A qualitative study to explore the nature of formal patient complaints about mental health care services in Sweden. *International Journal of Mental Health Nursing, 31*, 348–357. https://doi.org/10.1111/inm.12962bs_bs_banner

Suskind, D. (2022). *Bully-wise. Work Shouldn't Hurt: How to eliminate workplace abuse. Three steps organizations can take to stop workplace bullying*. www.psychologytoday.com/au/blog/bully-wise/202206/work-shouldnt-hurt-how-eliminate-workplace-abuse

Tasmanian Public Health Services. (2018). *Responding to emotions and communicating effectively*. Tasmanian Department of Health and Human Services. www.dhhs.tas.gov.au/publichealth/about_us/health_literacy/health_literacy_toolkit/responding_to_emotions

Thibeault, C. (2016). An interpretation of nurse–patient relationships in inpatient psychiatry: Understanding the mindful approach. *Global Qualitative Nursing Research, 3*, 1–10.

Van Gerven, E., Bruyneel, L., Panella, M., Euwema, M., Sermeus, W., & Vanhaecht, K. (2016). Psychological impact and recovery after involvement in a patient safety incident: A repeated measures analysis. *British Medical Journal Open, 6*(8), 1–11.

Vater, A., Schröder-Abé, M., Weißgerber, S., Roepke, S., & Schütz, A. (2015). Self-concept structure and borderline personality disorder: Evidence for negative compartmentalization. *Journal of Behaviour Therapy and Experimental Psychiatry, 46*, 50–58.

Vento, S., Cainelli, F., & Vallone, A. (2020). Violence against healthcare workers: A worldwide phenomenon with serious consequences. *Front Public Health, 8*, 570459. https://doi.org/10.3389/fpubh.2020.570459 PMID: 33072706; PMCID: PMC7531183

WA Health. (2019). *Clinical incident management guideline* (Appendix 3, p. 31). WA Department of Health. ww2.health.wa.gov.au/-/media/Files/Corporate/Policy-Frameworks/Clinical-Governance-Safety-and-Quality/Policy/Clinical-Incident-Management-Policy-2019/Supporting/Clinical-Incident-Management-Guideline-2019.pdf

Wang, Z., Zaman, S., Rasool, S. F., Zaman, Q. U., & Amin, A. (2020). Exploring the Relationships between a toxic workplace environment, workplace stress, and project success with the moderating effect of organizational support: Empirical evidence from Pakistan. *Risk Management and Healthcare Policy, 13*, 1055–1067. https://doi.org/10.2147/RMHP.S256155

Weltens, I., Bak, M., Verhagen, S., Vandenberk, E., Domen, P., van Amelsvoort, T., & Drukker, M. (2021). Aggression on the psychiatric ward: Prevalence and risk factors. A systematic review of the literature. *PLoS One, 16*(10), e0258346. https://doi.org/10.1371/journal.pone.0258346 PMID: 34624057; PMCID: PMC8500453+

World Health Organization. (2020). Charter: Health worker safety: a priority for patient safety. World Health Organization (WHO). ISBN: 978 92 4 001159 5 www.who.int/publications/i/item/9789240011595

Zoboli, E. L. C. P., Santos, D. V., & Schveitzer, M. C. (2016). Difficult patients in primary health care: Between care and order. *Interface (Botucatu), 20*(59). [ePub]

ACKNOWLEDGEMENTS

Figure 6.1: © SA Health. (2019). *Taking care of challenging behaviour.* Department for Health and Ageing, Government of South Australia.

Figure 6.2: © Headspace. (2022). *Clinical Toolkit. Clinical Tips: Criteria for Diagnosing Borderline Personality Disorder.* © headspace National Youth Mental Health Foundation Ltd.

Figure 6.5: © From Federal Register of Legislation (Schedule 2 - Aged Care Quality Standards, Quality of Care Principles 2014), hwww.legislation.gov.au. Licensed under CC BY 4.0

Extract 6A: © SafeWork SA. (2018). *Work-related violence. Preventing and responding to work-related violence.* Government of South Australia. Retrieved December 6, 2019 from www.safework.sa.gov.au/sites/default/files/resources/workrelatedviolence.pdf. Licensed under CC BY 3.0.

Extract 6B: © Ridley J & Leitch S. (2019). *The Restraint Reduction Network training standards 2019* (1st ed.). Birmingham: British Institute of Learning Disabilities.

Photo: © Tutatamafilm / Shutterstock.com

Photo: © Shutter2U / Adobe Stock

Photo: © PanoramaStock RF / Getty Images

Photo: © jeep5d / Shutterstock.com

Photo: © Photographee.eu / Shutterstock.com

Photo: © Monkey Business Images / Shutterstock.com

Photo: © sturti / Getty Images

Photo: © michaeljung / Shutterstock.com

Depression, anxiety and perinatal mental health care

This chapter will:

7.1 explain the prevalence, contributing factors and experiences of depression

7.2 discuss anxiety and its impact on people

7.3 identify the recovery-oriented interventions for adults with depression and anxiety

7.4 describe how to support women and their families with perinatal mental health concerns

7.5 explore the issues for young people with depression or anxiety.

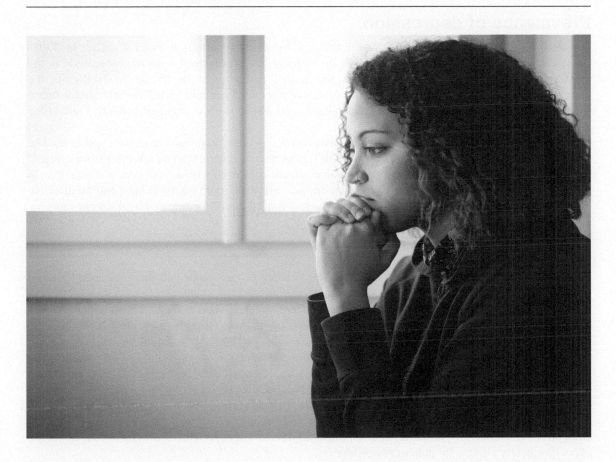

Introduction

Depression and anxiety are the most commonly reported mental illnesses. Approximately one in ten Australians experienced depression, and over 13 per cent reported anxiety-related conditions in 2017–18 (Australian Bureau of Statistics [ABS], 2018). Depression and anxiety are leading causes of disability worldwide and major contributors to the global disease burden. Depression is also a risk factor for suicide.

The focus of this chapter is depression and anxiety. The chapter begins by exploring the prevalence, symptoms, causes, types and assessment of the two conditions, followed by a section on the main interventions used to support people who experience depression and anxiety, including non-pharmacological, pharmacological and brain stimulation therapies. There is also a section on perinatal mental health conditions, including how to support the woman, her baby, partner and family. The chapter concludes by explaining depression and anxiety in young people, including early identification and the best treatment options to support young people in their recovery journey.

7.1 Depression

LEARNING OBJECTIVE 7.1 Explain the prevalence, contributing factors and experiences of depression.

According to the World Health Organization (2021), 5 per cent of adults globally experience depression. Depression is a leading cause of disability worldwide and a major contributor to the global burden of disease. In addition, depression can lead to suicide. This section focuses on depression, including the **prevalence** and experience of anxiety in Australia, the most common forms of depression, and how health professionals can support people with depression on their recovery journey.

Prevalence of depression

The Australian National Study of Mental Health and Wellbeing reported on mood disorders in 2020–21 and found that almost 5 per cent of adults in Australia had experienced a depressive episode in the previous 12 months (ABS, 2022). In addition, just under 2 per cent met the criteria for **dysthymia**, the term used to describe persistent but mild depression, and just over 2 per cent for bipolar affective disorder. These statistics translate to 1.5 million Australians aged 16–85 with a mood or **'affective' disorder** (ABS, 2022).

Women experienced higher rates of affective disorders (8.5 per cent) compared to men (6.2 per cent). The ABS (2022) also reported that 30 per cent of LGBTQIA+ people experienced an **affective disorder**; and over 5 per cent of females experienced a depressive episode compared with 3.8 per cent of males. People without a permanent place to live at some time in their life were more likely to have had an affective disorder in the previous 12 months than people who had not (17 per cent compared with 6.4 per cent).

Experiences of depression

Everyone experiences depression in different ways. Moreover, there are different types of depression, each with different presentations and characteristics. Health professionals call these presentations and characteristics 'signs and symptoms'.

The signs and symptoms of the different types of depression are listed in the two most widely utilised classification systems for diagnosing mental disorders: the DSM-5 (American Psychiatric Association [APA], 2013) and the ICD-11 (World Health Organization [WHO], 2019). Medical practitioners and psychologists commonly use one or the other of these classification systems during their work. While some people equate a diagnosis to a stigmatising 'label', a diagnosis can also enable health professionals to work with the person to develop more targeted interventions for recovery.

Depression frequently co-occurs with anxiety (Black Dog Institute, n.d.) and substance misuse (Lai et al. 2015, Hunt et al. 2020). This co-occurrence means that the experience of depression is not always straightforward. Generally, however, a person who is depressed will experience some or all of the following every day, nearly all day, for at least two weeks:

- feelings of sadness or an irritable mood *or* loss of interest in usual activities, including those that were once pleasurable (one or the other of these symptoms is essential for a diagnosis)
- unplanned weight loss
- insomnia or hypersomnia
- psychomotor disturbance

- reduced energy
- feelings of guilt
- poor concentration/indecisiveness
- recurrent thoughts of death or suicidal ideation (National Institute of Mental Health [NIMH], 2021).

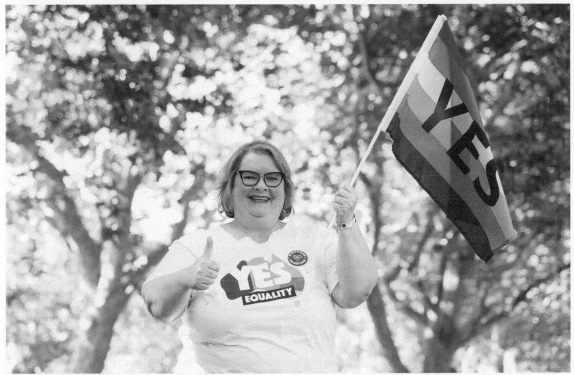

Magda Szubanski, actor, comedian, best-selling author and LGBTQIA+ advocate, has spoken publicly about her depression.

Due to diverse experiences, people with depression find it difficult to undertake their usual activities of daily living, leading to decreased quality of life (Cho et al., 2019).

It is important to note that some symptoms of depression are ordinary or everyday experiences for many people. The presence of one or two of these symptoms does not necessarily imply a diagnosis of depression. Instead, a diagnosis of depression can be made only after a comprehensive assessment.

This comprehensive assessment will include physical tests ordered by the medical practitioner to rule out the presence of a physical illness (e.g. a thyroid condition) that may mimic depressive symptoms. Assessment for depression also considers the person's risk.

UPON REFLECTION

Depression and stigma

Attitudes towards depression have changed in Australia in recent years due to the ongoing work of organisations such as the Black Dog Institute, Beyond Blue and Headspace. Even so, many people with depression do not seek care or treatment.

One reason for this situation is the stigma that continues to be associated with mental health concerns (Yokoya et al., 2018), particularly in some culturally and linguistically diverse populations, Indigenous Australians and LGBTQIA+ groups (Morgan et al., 2021). Stigma and the associated reluctance to seek treatment may contribute to the unacceptably high suicide rate among people who experience depression.

QUESTIONS

1. What more can health services organisations do to reduce the stigma of mental illness, including depression, in diverse populations?
2. What more could you do to reduce the stigma of mental illness, including depression, in diverse populations?

Risk factors for depression

There is no single cause of depression. Instead, various risk factors can contribute to a person developing depression. According to the Black Dog Institute (2022), these factors are interrelated and include:

- genetics and family history, with around 30 per cent of the predisposition for developing depression due to genetics
- biochemical factors, including mood-regulating neurotransmitters not functioning normally, with research continuing to occur in this area
- physical illness and/or chronic pain, with some physical conditions closely associated with low mood
- personality style and/or temperament, such as a 'self-critical', 'personality reserved', 'socially avoidant' or 'anxious worrying' types
- ageing, including dementia, mini-strokes
- stress, including abusive relationships, bullying and work-related stress and stressful or traumatic events
- depression occuring during pregnancy and the postnatal period, due to hormonal changes and adjustment challenges.

Table 7.1 outlines some of the more common factors contributing to a person developing depression. Health professionals are encouraged to be familiar with these factors and how they will affect the care and treatment options for a person with depression.

TABLE 7.1   Overview of the possible causes of depression

Perspective	Commentary
Biological	Biochemical mechanisms underlying depression are complex and poorly understood, although one hypothesis is that certain neurotransmitters are imbalanced within the brain. Two neurotransmitters, serotonin (5-HT) and noradrenaline (NA)[1], have been the focus of much research. In all types of depression, the transmission of serotonin is likely reduced or disrupted. With more severe depression, other neurotransmitter pathways are likely to be functioning abnormally (such as those for noradrenaline and dopamine). Subsequently, medications targeting these neurotransmitter systems have been developed and are among Australia's most commonly prescribed medications.
	Endocrine disorders are associated with an increased risk of depression. Depression may also occur in families, with hereditary factors evident.
	Birth trauma, physical deprivation, physical illness and chronic pain have been found to play a role in the development of depression.
	Depression can be related to substance use. Substances implicated include alcohol, benzodiazepines, opioids, amphetamines, hallucinogens and inhalants, while cannabis has since been identified as a possible contributor to mental disorders like depression.
Psychological	The concept of loss is central to the psychodynamic understanding of depression. Loss may be experienced as the result of bereavement, relationship issues or work-related.
	Life events, even those considered to be 'positive' events, can precipitate a depressive episode: childbirth, children leaving home and job promotions all have the potential to trigger depression in vulnerable individuals.
	Early life experiences and the impact of parental role models, the development of particular cognitive schema (thinking patterns) and attribution styles are considered influential; for example, core beliefs, low self-esteem and negative thinking patterns.
Social	Impact of gender and social status; for example, depression is more common in women than men and more common in people with employment problems (e.g. long-term unemployment or ongoing work stress), housing difficulties, financial problems and lack of supportive social networks.
	There are high rates of depression in individuals who consume excessive amounts of alcohol and/or drugs; significant social sequelae related to substance use can contribute to depression.

[1]. Noradrenaline and norepinephrine can be used interchangeably to refer to the same neurotransmitter.

Source: Hunt et al. (2020); Lai et al. (2015); Black Dog Institute (2022); WHO (2021).

In addition, a range of general risk factors can affect whether a person develops depression. These factors are closely related to the risk factors for all mental health issues outlined in the chapter that discusses mental health service delivery. Of particular concern for developing depression is the risk factor of physical illness, including cardiovascular disease, degenerative neurological disorders, epilepsy, brain tumour, metabolic conditions, endocrine disorders and some cancers (NIMH, 2021).

Depression and physical illness

Depression increases the likelihood of developing physical health conditions, such as heart disease, stroke, diabetes and Alzheimer's disease; moreover, people with depression and a physical illness have more severe symptoms of both illnesses (NIMH, 2021). Reasons for this are unclear but may relate to changes in how different body systems function that may impact physical health, including increased inflammation, abnormalities in stress hormones and metabolic changes (NIMH, 2021).

If a person is physically ill for an extended period, especially with a chronic disease such as cardiac, neurological, cancer, autoimmune, diabetes or pain, they are more likely to develop depression (Tully et al., 2021; Zambrano et al., 2020). Again, the reasons for this connection are unclear. In some conditions (e.g. stroke), there may be changes in the brain. Anxiety and stress related to the illness can also trigger depression, as can some medications used to treat the physical illness (NIMH, 2021). Of particular note are the following.

- *Pain.* This can directly influence a person's mood. Both depression and anxiety can affect an individual's perception and tolerance of pain. Anxiety is discussed later in this chapter.
- *Loss and grief.* People who experience physical illness very often experience a sense of loss and grief related to (e.g.) losing a way of life, the loss of limb or organ and loss of privacy and self-determination. Feelings of loss and grief are common reactions to stressful situations (see the chapter that discusses the common reactions to stressful situations). However, there may be times when a person is unable to process these feelings, which can contribute to the development of depression.
- *Prescription medication.* Some prescribed medications can lead to the development of depressive symptoms.
- *Alcohol and illicit or non-prescription medication.* These substances also need to be considered in determining the possible cause or complicating factors of depression. Although alcohol has a depressant effect on the central nervous system, its short-lived **anxiolytic** effect can be a factor leading to excessive consumption. A person with a physical illness needs to be asked about substance use as part of the comprehensive assessment provided by the health professional (refer to the chapter that focuses on substance use disorders).
- *Cognitive impairment.* Cognitive impairment, such as poor recall and impaired concentration, can be a symptom of depression, particularly in older people. However, it can mask other depressive symptoms. For example, people with dementia are at a higher risk of depression, but this often goes unnoticed (refer to the chapter that looks at caring for an older person with a mental illness).
- *Self-perception.* It has been suggested that people prone to depression often have a negative belief system that adversely influences their perceptions of the self (Beck, 1970/2006). Rogers (1951) described this phenomenon as a basic mismatch between the individual's 'ideal and actual self'. Depression may occur when individuals consistently set themselves ideals and goals that they cannot hope to achieve. People with a physical illness often struggle to achieve goals that were once achievable but are no longer so, leading them to question their self-perception.
- *Coping mechanisms.* It is usual for people to experience some fluctuation in the way they feel day-to-day. This fluctuation may be directly related to their physical health, environment, stress level, how the person feels about themselves and other social and interpersonal factors. How a person responds to and deals with life's many challenges is determined by their confidence level and ability to cope, problem solve, make decisions and be supported. Sometimes it is difficult to discern the difference between someone who is not coping and someone who is depressed, particularly if the person is also experiencing anxiety or stress.

Regardless of the **contributing factors** to depression, it is clear that the condition reduces a person's capacity to manage a physical illness which, in turn, limits their overall health outcomes. Hence, health professionals who care for people who are physically unwell — especially people with chronic physical conditions — must take an approach to care that includes the person's biological or physical, psychological or mental health and social facets.

Types of depression

There is a need to understand the different types of depression so that the person receives the most appropriate care. The Australian Government's Healthdirect (2020b) lists the different types of depression.

- *Major depression.* Characterised by low mood and loss of interest in activities that were once considered pleasurable. The low mood persists for at least two weeks and is experienced on most days. There are two sub-types of major depression. Melancholic depression is a severe form of depression that includes physical and emotional symptoms. Psychotic depression includes a pervasive and unremittingly low mood, with delusional thinking. For example, the person believes they are completely worthless and deserves to be dead, or they believe they have already died. Perceptual disturbances may also be a feature of psychotic depression.
- *Bipolar affective disorder* (previously known as 'manic depression'). This condition is characterised by variations or 'swings' in mood, from elevation, **hypomania** and **mania** to depression (for more information, see the chapter that looks at caring for a person with a serious mental illness).
- *Seasonal affective disorder.* This condition can be a depression or mania that has a seasonal pattern. Most often, the depressive symptoms commence in winter and fade in spring.
- *Perinatal or postnatal depression.* This depressive disorder occurs during pregnancy or after the birth of a baby and affects up to 1 in every 5 women in Australia. Perinatal mental health conditions are discussed in a later section of this chapter.
- *Organic mood disorders.* These usually occur secondary to a physical or organic abnormality (e.g. brain tumour) or metabolic disturbance (e.g. electrolyte imbalance) affecting the brain. The mood changes may appear the same or similar to depression or other mental illnesses.
- *Cyclothymia.* An illness in the bipolar spectrum of disorders characterised by sudden periods of elevated and low mood.
- *Dysthymia.* A chronic depressive disorder; less severe than major depression, though by definition lasts for a minimum of two years and may extend over many years.

Knowing the different types of depression provides a base from which health professionals can begin assessing a person experiencing a low mood.

Assessment of depression

There are various approaches to assessing depression in adults. Perhaps most important is that health professionals make observations and ask questions that enable them to gauge the person's mood. Ideally, this information should include details about the person's feelings, behaviours and level of functioning. Information gathering occurs over time by obtaining subjective and objective information about the person's mental health and overall wellbeing.

Table 7.2 outlines the key information to consider when assessing a person's mood, including but not limited to depression and anxiety. You can read more about the comprehensive mental health assessment in the chapter on assessment in the mental health context. The assessment of young people and women during the perinatal period is discussed in later sections of this chapter.

TABLE 7.2 Key information required when assessing mood

Facets of assessment	Key information
Subjective factors	This information includes the person's description of how they feel.
	The information can be obtained by asking the person how they feel directly or by describing how they feel on a scale of 0 to 10 (with 0 being the unhappiest and 10 being the happiest).
Objective factors	This information includes the health professional's observations of how the person feels, including a note of whether the person is: • tearful • agitated • exhibiting reduced social interaction and communication not explained by physical impairment or environment.

Physical health factors	Health professionals must note whether the person is predisposed to becoming depressed or anxious because of: • side effects or consequences of medical treatments (e.g. medication, radiotherapy), cerebral damage (e.g. following stroke, head injury) • pre-existing medical or other physical health problems.
Psychological factors	Health professionals must note the potential or actual impact of: • history of mood or other psychiatric disorder (particularly depression or anxiety) • recent significant life events (e.g. bereavement, childbirth, relationship problems).
Physical activity factors	Health professionals must note the potential or actual impact of: • physical deficits or problems as a result of illness or injury (e.g. aphasia, immobility, degree of physical dependence) • reduction of or withdrawal from physical activity or recreational pursuits.
Social factors	Health professionals must note the potential or actual impact of: • employment (e.g. role within the family unit, whether the person is the main source of family income) • housing • financial worries or concerns.
Interpersonal factors	Health professionals must note the potential or actual impact of: • input from partner/significant other, family members, friends • pre-morbid relationships (e.g. avoid making assumptions about the role of the person's partner in providing ongoing care and support; involve significant other in discussions regarding their level of input and involvement in the recovery and rehabilitation process).

Screening tools

Some health professionals will use screening tools to conduct a mental health assessment. These screening tools can assist health professionals in measuring the level of depression the person is experiencing and, as time goes by, how this improves or declines (Alavi et al., 2022). Health professionals need to find the 'best fit' tool to assess and individual's depression, and there are many validated instruments from which to choose.

There are various depression screening or assessment tools available. For example:
• Beck Depression Inventory (Beck, 1970/2006)
• Children's Depression Scale (Lang & Tisher, 1983/2004)
• Geriatric Depression Scale (Yesavage et al., 1983)
• Edinburgh Postnatal Depression Scale (Cox et al., 1987).

The American Psychological Association (2022) provides a comprehensive range of screening tools on their website, together with a comprehensive explanation.

In Australia, a commonly used instrument is the Depression Anxiety Stress Scales or 'DASS', which is a self-report instrument (i.e. the person experiencing the low mood completes it) that measures depression, anxiety and stress/tension. The DASS is valuable because it can detect depression and anxiety. This scale is in the public domain, and health professionals are encouraged to familiarise themselves with the different aspects of a person's mood that can be affected by depression.

Another useful tool is the Kessler Psychological Distress Scale-10 (K10) (Kessler et al., 2002), often used in public health services across Australia. This self-reporting instrument comprises ten items relating to the psychological distress experienced the month before completion. Each item has a five-point scale. The items broadly focus on issues of anxiety and depression. Once the person has completed the survey, the health professional can discuss their answers and explore how their mood affects their quality of life.

Interpreting the results of a screening tool requires some expertise; however, this should not preclude health professionals who work in general settings from using such tools. Most notably, simpler tools can be used to strike up a conversation about depression with a person experiencing a low mood.

Outcome measures

Screening tools can be used as outcome measures in health settings to improve quality and safety (ACSQHC, 2022). Outcome measures assess a person's current level of health. They can also measure the person's progress when utilised over time. More broadly, outcome measures — patient-reported or practitioner-reported — that are used to collect data from all those who access health services will help to:

- identify meaningful change for the person accessing a service (e.g. in wellbeing/quality of life)
- evaluate the effect of the interventions
- demonstrate the impact and value of services (e.g. to people who access them, colleagues and funders/commissioners)
- identify areas for improvement
- benchmark against other organisations/services/standards to improve health services and care (AHP Outcome Measures UK Working Group, 2019).

The Australian government established the Australian Mental Health Outcomes and Classification Network (AMHOCN) (2022) in late 2003 to work collaboratively with the Australian states, territories, and other key mental health sector stakeholders to implement routine outcome measurement in public mental health services. These outcome measures include screening tools such as the Kessler-10 (K10), a self-reporting instrument comprising ten items that measure the psychological distress a person has experienced the month before completion.

Other outcome measures used by the AMHOCN and completed by the consumer include:
- Strengths and Difficulties Questionnaire (SDQ)
- Kessler-10+ (K10+)
- Behavior and Symptom Identification Scale - 32 (BASIS-32)
- Mental Health Inventory - 38 (MHI – 38).

Outcome measures to be completed by the health professional include:
- Health of the Nation Outcome Scales - Children and Adolescents (HoNOSCA)
- Health of the Nation Outcome Scales (HoNOS)
- Health of the Nation Outcome Scales 65+ (HoNOS 65+)
- Health of the Nation Outcome Scales for Infants (HoNOSI)
- Children Global Assessment Scale
- Factors Influencing Health Status
- Life Skills Profile - 16 (LSP-16)
- Resource Utilisation Groups—Activities of Daily Living (RUG-ADL)
- Phase of Care.

Not all of these outcome measures relate to depression. However, according to the Department of Health (2015a) in Victoria, no single measurement scale offers an accurate overall picture of a person's mental health. The use of several measures can help to broaden the results and address the limitations that arise when using a single screening tool. For example, some screening tools focus on the severity of symptoms in the past two weeks without exploring the person's life skills or level of functioning.

The data collected by the AMHOCN measures the effectiveness of the mental health care being provided across Australia and allows organisations and services to identify areas of need and progress.

7.2 Anxiety

LEARNING OBJECTIVE 7.2 Discuss anxiety and its impact on people.

While depression and anxiety are often co-associated — that is, people tend to experience anxiety and depression together — this is not always the case, with many people experiencing anxiety without depression. This section focuses on anxiety, including the prevalence and experience of anxiety in Australia, the most common forms of anxiety, and how health professionals can support people with anxiety.

Prevalence of anxiety

As noted earlier in this chapter, anxiety is Australia's most common mental health issue. The Australian National Study of Mental Health and Wellbeing (ABS, 2022) reported on anxiety disorders in 2020–21, and found that almost 17 per cent of people aged 16–85 years (i.e., 3.3 million people) had experienced an anxiety disorder at some time in their life or symptoms of that disorder in the 12 months before the survey. Specifically:

* females were more likely than males to have had an anxiety disorder (21 per cent compared to just over 12 per cent)
* almost one-third of young people aged 16–24 years had an anxiety disorder, with just over 40 per cent of females this age having an anxiety disorder
* almost 45 per cent of LGBTQIA+people had an anxiety disorder
* over one-quarter of people living in one-parent family households with dependent children had an anxiety disorder
* 7 per cent of people had a social phobia disorder
* females experienced higher rates of social phobia than males (almost 10 per cent compared to just over 4 per cent).

Alongside being high prevalence, anxiety has been described as the most treatable mental health condition (Beyond Blue, 2022a). This fact enables health professionals to inspire hope in people who are embarking on their anxiety recovery journey.

Experiences of anxiety

Feelings of anxiety are a universal human experience, most likely evolved from the primitive 'fight-or-flight' response. However, anxiety can also be experienced without an apparent external threat or as a consequence of situations and events that a person finds unfamiliar or difficult (Sadock et al., 2017). Such situations can include events such as attending a health service, leading to distressing physical or **somatic** and other feelings. Table 7.3 outlines some of the common experiences of anxiety.

TABLE 7.3   Common experiences of anxiety

Autonomic symptoms	Physical symptoms	Behavioural symptoms	Psychological symptoms
Tachycardia	Tremor	Avoidance	Excessive rumination
Sweating	Muscular aches	Ritual behaviour	Indecisiveness
Dizziness	Difficulty swallowing	Distress in social situations	Irritability
Hot/cold spells	Lump in throat	Increased use of substances	Inability to relax Feeling tense Being easily startled
Frequency of micturition	Restlessness	Appearing hostile or dismissive	Poor concentration Distractibility
Diarrhoea/nausea	Fatigue	Withdrawal from social recreational pursuits	Impatience
Paraesthesia (pins and needles)	Headaches	Repetitive seeking of reassurance	Reduced sense of humour

Source: Chambers (2017); Sadock et al. (2017); RANZCP (2019a).

Risk factors for anxiety

Anxiety has various contributing factors. These include a family history of anxiety, such as a genetic predisposition or modelling by parents and/or other family members (Beyond Blue, 2022a). Other people may have personal characteristics predisposing them to anxiety (e.g. autism spectrum disorder). Those who experience ongoing stress may also develop anxiety from the high cortisol levels and other ongoing physical reactions to this stress. People with physical health issues and other mental disorders, including substance use issues, are likewise more likely to develop anxiety. These various contributing factors suggest the challenges in preventing anxiety.

Types of anxiety

According to the DSM-5 and ICD-11, there are various types of anxiety disorders based on the different experiences of anxiety with shared characteristics (APA, 2013). The most common types in Australia are generalised anxiety disorder, panic disorder and social anxiety (Beyond Blue, 2022a). Other conditions where anxiety is present include obsessive-compulsive disorder and post-traumatic stress disorder. Health professionals will also encounter acute stress reactions and health anxiety, sometimes known as hypochondriasis.

Generalised anxiety disorder

People who experience a generalised anxiety disorder (GAD) tend to worry about many things. Indeed, each day can be consumed with worry over various issues, from social engagements to financial concerns or safety issues. Such worries will often have symptoms of muscle tension, sleep disturbance, restlessness and irritability (Chambers, 2017). These behaviours are distressing for the person and concerning for family members, friends and colleagues.

For a person to be diagnosed with GAD, they must experience a heightened anxious state on most days for at least six months (Beyond Blue, 2020). Symptoms of generalised anxiety are sometimes divided into cognitive/affective, behavioural and physical symptoms.

Cognitive symptoms can include:
- constant thoughts that something bad is about to happen
- constant worry that they are not doing things correctly.

Behavioural symptoms can include:
- constantly asking questions and requiring reassurance
- perfectionism
- being argumentative, especially if trying to avoid a feared situation
- ruminating over mistakes, a change in routine, or unfamiliar places.

Physical symptoms can include:
- dry mouth and/or difficulty swallowing
- nightmares
- difficulty getting to and staying asleep
- difficulty concentrating
- muscle tension and headaches
- rapid heart rate and breathing
- sweating
- trembling
- diarrhoea
- the flare-up of another health problem or illness (e.g. dermatitis, asthma)
- sexual problems, such as not having any sexual feelings or being interested in sex APA (2013); Sadock et al. (2017); WHO (2019).

UPON REFLECTION

Experiences of generalised anxiety

The lived experience of anxiety has been described as physical, emotional and social pain. In research conducted by Woodgate et al. (2020, p. 14), one participant stated:

> I want to describe anxiety, like, this is what I'm going through, and it sucks … cause I think I can do more if anxiety wasn't there … it's … a roadblock … there's so much physical pain that I feel that's hard to describe at times, except for someone who's actually living with it.

Other participants described anxiety in terms of pain that is invisible, indeterminate, unpredictable and complex. Health professionals must recognise the levels of distress experienced by people with anxiety and take the necessary steps to support them.

Panic attacks

A panic attack occurs when a person experiences sudden, severe and uncontrollable anxiety triggered by new or previously stressful situations (Sadock et al., 2017). Particular objects, sounds, smells or other sensory stimulation can also trigger a panic attack, such as the sound of a dentist's drill or the smell of a hospital. Panic attacks are often associated with physical symptoms, such as palpitations, chest pain, tachycardia, shaking, difficulty breathing, weakness or tingling in the limbs and a fear of impending death or doom (Chambers, 2017).

While different people will report different clusters of symptoms during a panic attack, the person experiencing a panic attack often feels like they are experiencing a heart attack or serious physical problem. In this situation, it is best that the person calls the emergency services personnel or is transported to a hospital where an accurate diagnosis can be made. The person can then be provided with strategies to reduce the likelihood of further attacks and practical strategies to manage any future occurrences.

A major debilitating factor in panic disorder is the fear of future panic attacks. For example, people may avoid a variety of life or social situations for fear of the recurrence of a panic attack. Even though a person may have experienced only a few short-lived panic attacks, they may limit their whole lifestyle due to their experience.

IN PRACTICE

Panic attacks and emergency services personnel

When a person is experiencing a panic attack for the first time and/or is experiencing breathing difficulties during a panic attack, they or a family member or friend may contact the emergency services for help. Often, the person will be experiencing high levels of uncontrollable distress and feel convinced they will die. They may have palpitations, chest pain, difficulty breathing and feelings of impending doom.

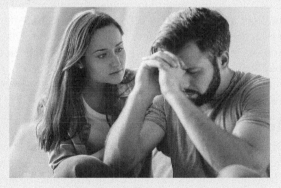

Emergency services personnel must take these symptoms seriously, including when the person has previously called for help in a similar situation. To support the person, the health professional must:

- show unconditional positive regard
- provide reassurance and information
- coach the person to manage their symptoms (e.g. slow down their breathing if hyperventilating)
- minimise stimulation
- transport the person to a hospital for a thorough assessment.

These strategies aim to assist the person in regaining control of their physical, cognitive and emotional responses.

QUESTIONS

1. What are the main differences between the signs and symptoms of a panic attack and a cardiac event?
2. How can health professionals establish trust with a person experiencing a panic attack to help them regain control of their physical, cognitive and emotional responses?

Social anxiety

A person with social anxiety fears being criticised, judged, watched, embarrassed or humiliated by others, even in everyday situations (NIMH, 2022). Social anxiety is more than shyness. Examples of such situations can include an intense fear of eating in public, being asked to answer a question in front of everyone in a classroom, being assertive at work or talking to a cashier in a shop. Social anxiety will stop some people from going to work, studying or getting on with their lives.

Health professionals will encounter people with social anxiety in their day-to-day work, including consumers, carers and colleagues. Some health professionals may also have their own social anxieties. Social anxiety can be a barrier to people asserting themselves or asking questions in health settings. When supporting people with social anxiety, it is important to offer reassurance, check that they have the information they need, and follow up to ensure they have received the services they need. Health professionals can also refer people with social anxiety for counselling or psychotherapy, including but not limited to CBT. Non-pharmacological treatments are outlined in the section that focuses on interventions for depression and anxiety.

Obsessive-compulsive disorder

People with obsessive-compulsive disorder (OCD) experience intrusive thoughts or feelings that cause anxiety. The person will try to manage the intrusive thought (consciously or unconsciously) by carrying out a particular behaviour or ritual. If the person tries to resist this behaviour, their level of anxiety will increase (Chambers, 2017). The person may or may not recognise that the rituals are excessive or inappropriate.

OCD has no specific cause, but researchers suggest genetic and environmental contributing factors (Sadock et al., 2017). A common presentation of OCD is a person who experiences intrusive thoughts about germs. They may constantly think about germs as they handle money, shake someone's hand or turn a doorknob. To relieve this anxiety, the person may develop some rituals regarding hand washing and cleaning their environment. The cleaning rituals may not always allay the anxiety, although they may be repeated frequently, performed in sequences or a predetermined number of times. These rituals can become very time-consuming and embarrassing for the person.

Some people with OCD will have concerns with checking. For example, they may have intrusive thoughts or feelings that they have left things undone, such as not turning off electrical equipment or not locking their house or car. The discomfort caused by these persistent preoccupations will lead them to develop time-consuming rituals of checking and rechecking. For example, a person may have to switch the light switches on and off six times each time they leave a room or check that the windows and doors are locked four times before leaving the house. Others may complain that they 'know' they switched the iron off, but they still have to go back and recheck to make doubly certain. The result is that the person may feel like they are 'going crazy'.

Interventions to support people with OCD are pharmacological and non-pharmacological, including CBT, antidepressant medication

Acute stress reaction

Different people will have diverse reactions to stressful events differently, including but not limited to anxiety. Most people exposed to a traumatic event will have some difficulties managing their responses. The types of events likely to cause problems for people include major stressful events such as major car accidents, serious assault, rape, torture, war and earthquake. These events and others, which place people in fear for their lives or safety, are the events that are likely to give rise to anxiety and impact the person's quality of life.

Acute stress reaction is explained in the chapter that discusses the common reactions to stressful situations. In summary, an acute stress reaction is a transient psychological or anxiety reaction that develops in response to a traumatic event. The reaction is usually self-limiting and, in most cases, does not require specific physical treatments (e.g. medication) (NHMRC, 2021). Even so, the symptoms can be severe and distressing for the person and may include:

- initial state of feeling dazed
- reduced levels of consciousness
- agitation or overactivity
- withdrawal
- dissociation
- anxiety symptoms (e.g. sweating, increased heart rate or flushing).

These symptoms can occur within a few minutes of the stressful event and usually disappear within hours or days. Some people will also experience vivid dreams about the incident or become anxious when recollecting the event.

An essential part of the care of a person experiencing an acute stress reaction includes treating the initial symptoms and providing explanations and reassurance. If symptoms of acute stress reaction persist in frequency and severity for longer than four weeks, the condition may develop into a **post-traumatic stress disorder (PTSD)**.

Post-traumatic stress disorder

Post-traumatic stress disorder or 'PTSD' is a trauma and stress-related disorder that gives rise to feelings of anxiety. Generally, the condition is diagnosed in those who have survived specific types of trauma, such as war, terrorist attacks, rape or other assault, natural disaster, refugee experiences or the sudden unexpected death of a loved one. The possibility of developing PTSD depends on the type of traumatic event experienced, with approximately 5 to 10 per cent of Australians experiencing PTSD at some point in their lives (Phoenix Australia, 2021). The ABS (2022) suggests that just under 6 per cent of people were diagnosed with PTSD in 2020-2021, including 7.6 per cent females and 3.6 per cent males.

People with PTSD experience symptoms that often significantly impact their lives. These symptoms include:
- recurrent, unwanted and distressing memories of the traumatic event
- reliving the traumatic event, including 'flashbacks'
- distressing nightmares relate to the traumatic event
- severe emotional distress, anxiety and physical reactions when something 'triggers' memories of the traumatic event
- negative changes in thinking and mood, including suicidal thoughts
- changes in physical and emotional reactions.

Treatment for PTSD includes cognitive processing therapy, exposure therapy, eye movement desensitisation and reprocessing and medications. These treatments are explained in the section that focuses on anxiety interventions.

Some health professionals may also encounter people with a diagnosis of complex PTSD or 'CPTSD'. This is a condition that includes symptoms of PTSD, along with other symptoms, such as:
- difficulty controlling emotions
- constant feelings of emptiness, hopelessness and worthlessness
- dissociative symptoms, including **depersonalisation** and **derealisation**.

Complex PTSD is most often diagnosed in people who have experienced ongoing childhood sexual abuse (Blue Knot Foundation, 2021). You can read more about complex PTSD in the chapter on the person who has self-harmed.

Health anxiety

Some people will experience anxiety about their health — for example, they may obsess over whether they have a common cold or a deadly flu virus, a headache or a brain tumour, a small problem or cancer. They may also question whether health professionals know what they are doing and if they should seek a second, third and fourth opinion.

If this type of anxiety becomes extreme, it can be diagnosed as hypochondria or hypochondriasis (Sadock et al., 2017). People with this condition have a persistent fear that they have a serious or life-threatening illness. Sometimes the person will experience symptoms that seem very real to them; however, constant testing by medical practitioners shows no abnormalities. The person does not feel reassured when they are assured there is nothing wrong and insists on further investigations, consuming many health resources.

Health professionals must not label a person with health anxiety a 'hypochondriac'. While the symptoms may not have a biological or physical cause, this does not negate the fact that the person's concerns are real and distressing to them. Alternatively, there will be times when a person's symptoms have a physical or biological cause, but health professionals have been unable to locate the source of the symptoms. Labelling will not help the person address their anxiety.

The primary treatment intervention for a person with health anxiety is a supportive relationship with the health professional. Read more about establishing clear boundaries in the chapter about people displaying challenging behaviours.

Other anxiety experiences

There are various other anxiety disorders that health professionals may encounter. These can include phobias or irrational fears that are out of proportion to the actual threat posed to the individual. For example, some people experience agoraphobia, a fear of specific places or situations. Social phobia is social anxiety taken to the extreme and can lead a person to completely avoid talking in front of others or ordering food in restaurants. Other phobias include the anxiety and feelings of panic triggered by discrete situations, such as a phobia of certain animals or creatures such as spiders (arachnophobia), flying (aviophobia), heights (acrophobia) or enclosed rooms (claustrophobia). Provided the person avoids the object, situation or event that triggers the phobia, other aspects of their life remain unaffected. In some cases, however, the avoidance behaviour becomes extreme and disabling.

IN PRACTICE

Screening and assessing for anxiety

Screening is a process for identifying the possible presence of a particular issue or condition. Assessment is a process for obtaining more detailed information, including determining the risks, coming to a diagnosis and developing specific treatment recommendations for addressing the identified issues (Department of Health, 2015b). There is a range of screening and assessment tools that health professionals can use to assess anxiety. These include the following.

- Beck Anxiety Inventory, which is completed by the person with anxiety, assesses the intensity of physical and cognitive anxiety symptoms during the past week. It comprises 21 items and scores minimal anxiety, mild anxiety, moderate anxiety and severe anxiety levels.
- Hamilton Anxiety Scale (HAM-A), which is completed by the clinician and aims to assess the severity of the symptoms of anxiety. It measures both psychic anxiety (i.e., mental agitation and psychological distress) and somatic anxiety (i.e. physical complaints related to anxiety).
- Generalised Anxiety Disorder 7 (GAD-7), completed by the person with anxiety, can be used as a screening tool and severity measure of generalised anxiety disorder.
- Panic and Agoraphobia Scale (PAS), which measures the severity of the symptoms in people with panic disorder (with or without agoraphobia). It is available in both clinician-administered and self-rating formats and contains five sub-scales: panic attacks, agoraphobic avoidance, anticipatory anxiety, disability and functional avoidance (health concerns).

You can learn more about the assessment of anxiety in the chapter that focuses on mental health assessment.

QUESTIONS

1. In what ways could health professionals use these screening and assessment tools to help the consumer?

2. How could these screening and assessment tools be misused in health settings?

Supporting people with anxiety

For health professionals working in general health contexts, it is important to remember that, for most people, anxiety is a transient feeling. People will most often respond to appropriate explanations, reassurance and sensitive communication. Only one to two people out of 10 will develop an ongoing anxiety disorder that requires further specialist input.

Generally, strategies that health professionals can use to help people who do go on to develop an issue with feelings of anxiety include:

- encouraging the person to relax, using music, breathing and relaxation exercises
- encouraging diversional activities (e.g. having a hot bath or listening to music)
- developing personal coping strategies that utilise some of the principles of formal cognitive therapy (e.g. recognising and addressing automatic negative thoughts and challenging these with more realistic alternatives)
- using short-term anxiolytic medications
- providing health advice and information that helps the person to address lifestyle issues, including:
  - achieving balance in the work, home and recreational aspects of their lives (e.g. addressing the impact of excessive work, amount of time spent at work, blurred boundaries between professional and personal life caused by 'bringing work home')

- addressing issues around the development of a healthier lifestyle (e.g. smoking, use of alcohol, exercise)
- engaging in specific strategies to manage stress (e.g. yoga, relaxation classes, aromatherapy).

If a person goes on to develop an anxiety disorder, then health professionals can assure them that anxiety is one of the most treatable mental health conditions (Beyond Blue, 2022). The interventions utilised are non-pharmacological (e.g. psychological therapies), pharmacological and brain stimulation therapies. These interventions are discussed in the section on interventions for depression and anxiety.

LIVED EXPERIENCE

Chronic pain and depression

I was in a car accident over 2 years ago. Since then, I've lived with nagging neck and back pain. It kept me awake, day and night. The doctors gave me pain medication, which made me feel doped out all the time. I just wanted my old life back, where I could think clearly, sit comfortably at work, or go hiking with the family. I even stopped enjoying sex with my husband because the pain was always there, getting in the way. Worse still, he didn't seem to understand, which upset me even more. I could see the writing on the wall — he was going to leave me. Well, I'd leave me, if I was him! The kids hated me too — how could they not? I couldn't do the things I used to do with or for them before the accident.

I started taking more and more sick days from work because I didn't want them to realise how useless I'd become. I was also feeling anxious about going outside or getting in a car. What if I had another accident? I lost energy, put on weight and felt overwhelmed by anything and everything. I started crying at nothing. It was like I'd fallen into a black hole of paralysis. Time lost its meaning.

Until one day, my husband dragged me along to the GP. I can't remember what they talked about, but the GP referred me to a pain clinic. I didn't want to go, but my husband insisted.

The health professionals at the pain clinic explained about holistic approaches to managing pain. They also asked a lot of questions about my life before and after the accident. We developed some goals. They also reduced the amount of pain medication I was on and started me on a small dose of antidepressant medication. I wasn't keen on that, I didn't want people to think I wasn't coping or there was something wrong with me in the head. But my husband seemed to think I should give it a go, and in the end, I thought, what did I have to lose? I also began talking to a dietician and a psychologist, and they suggested we bring the kids to see a family therapist. I began aqua aerobics and joined a mindfulness-based group program, where we learn how to clear our minds of obsessive thoughts, focus on the present moment and accept things for what they are.

It's been three months now. I can't say my life turned around, but I'm sleeping a little better and feeling something like hope. I have a plan to follow, people to support me, and a family keen to see me happy again. I can't help feeling that life will be good again one day.

7.3 Interventions for depression and anxiety

LEARNING OBJECTIVE 7.3 Identify the recovery-oriented interventions for adults with depression and anxiety.

This section focuses on the recovery-oriented interventions used to support adults with experiences of depression and anxiety on their recovery journey. These interventions involve non-pharmacological, pharmacological and brain stimulation therapies. Central to the success of any intervention to support people with experiences of mental illness to achieve recovery is the robust therapeutic relationship and close collaboration between the consumer and health professional (Malhi et al., 2021; Meadows et al., 2019). As explained in the chapter that looks at mental health assessment, the best recovery-oriented, therapeutic relationships involve inspiring hope and optimism, showing unconditional positive regard and kindness, clarifying expectations, empowering the person through collaborative decision-making and involving family members.

Engaging with people with depression or anxiety

Health professionals must also take a holistic or comprehensive approach when supporting a person with depression and/or anxiety. The biopsychosocial approach to care was also described in the chapter on assessment in the mental health context; it includes supporting the physical, emotional, social, sexual, spiritual, environmental and functional needs and preferences of the person. To ensure a comprehensive approach when supporting the person on their recovery journey, health professionals must work in a multidisciplinary team that includes mental health specialists.

Table 7.4 recommends the approaches to care that can be taken by members of the multidisciplinary team when supporting a person with depression and/or anxiety.

TABLE 7.4 **Approaches to care**

Approaches to care	Rationale
Take a recovery-oriented approach, highlighting to the person that recovery is possible	Maintaining hope and optimism helps the person to develop goals and be future-focused.
Include outcome measures in the initial assessment processes	Outcome measures provide a baseline against which future changes in mood can be compared
Utilise a non-judgemental approach and active listening skills when communicating with the person and their significant others	Demonstrates acceptance, value, warmth and empathy. All of these factors can have a positive therapeutic effect on the person's mood and self-esteem
Provide protected time to engage the person in a discussion regarding their current thoughts and feelings	Demonstrates acceptance and reinforces comprehensive care
Identify specific symptoms of depression and/or anxiety, including those associated with their physical illness or as a result of current treatments (e.g. side effects of medication)	Some symptoms of depression and anxiety can be a direct consequence of the underlying physical illness/injury or a side effect of medication
Identify whether there are any pre-existing or related factors contributing to apparent depressive or anxious feelings or behaviours (e.g. interpersonal difficulties, financial worries, recent bereavement)	Assists in the screening for possible anxiety or depression
If depression is suspected, then encourage and support the person in completing an appropriate screening tool	Provides a standardised baseline against which to measure changes in mood
Identify whether the person has any suicidal and/or self-harming thoughts. If self-harming or suicidal thoughts are present, complete a suicide risk screen (see the chapter that looks at caring for a person who has self-harmed)	Depression is associated with an increased risk of self-harm and suicide
Explain that depressed and anxious feelings are a common consequence of physical illness	Utilising time to discuss thoughts and feelings can assist in normalising the individual's experience
Discuss with the multidisciplinary team any concerns regarding the person's mood	This approach demonstrates effective teamwork and collaboration. Effective communication helps ensure appropriate care and can assist in the reduction of risk
Collaborating with the person and their significant others, develop the person's goals and discuss the most appropriate interventions	This approach demonstrates consumer-centred and recovery-oriented approaches.
If antidepressant medication is indicated, ensure it is administered as prescribed	This approach ensures appropriate treatment is commenced as soon as possible
Explain that antidepressant medication can take up to three weeks before demonstrating a positive therapeutic effect	Treatment adherence and collaboration are improved if the person is aware of all the facts and options regarding the use of antidepressants or other medication (see the section on psychoeducation)
Monitor the person's response to both therapeutic and side effects of any antidepressant medication prescribed	Provides valuable information about the person's response to treatment

Observe and record details of the person's verbal and non-verbal behaviour (e.g. anger, impulsivity, irritability, motor retardation, dietary and fluid intake)	Ensures that the appropriate level of care is initiated (e.g. recovery from depression is enhanced if adequate nutrition, hydration and physical activity are maintained)
If concerned about the person's mood or if deterioration continues, consider referral to a mental health consultation liaison clinician for specialist advice and assessment (see the chapter that discusses mental health service delivery)	Mental health consultation liaison clinicians can assist in treatment and care (see the chapter that discusses the approaches to mental health service delivery). Ensures specialist follow-up and onward referral are arranged, if appropriate

It is essential to highlight the following factors when supporting people with depression or anxiety. First, there is a need to ensure the safety of the person. For example, people with depression are at a higher risk of experiencing thoughts of self-harm or suicide. Identifying risk and then implementing appropriate strategies to manage specific risks are key responsibilities (see the chapter that looks at caring for a person who has self-harmed). Maintaining safety will include conducting clinical and suicidal risk assessments on an ongoing basis (see the chapter on mental health assessment) and supporting the person based on the findings of these assessments.

Second, health professionals must know that depression and anxiety can impair a person's communication ability. Common difficulties include withdrawing from routine social interaction, isolation and difficulty in expressing feelings. The ability of the health professional to demonstrate empathy, warmth and optimism will support engagement with the person.

Third, support must be provided for the physical health of people with depression. The close connection between depression and physical health was explained in a previous section of this chapter. Common physical challenges associated with depression also include:

- changes in appetite — either loss of appetite or increased food intake, unintended weight changes
- disturbed sleep — may present as either insomnia or hypersomnia (i.e. excessive sleeping)
- loss of interest in appearance — leading to difficulty in washing, dressing and maintaining personal hygiene
- increased or decreased physical activity — motor retardation may be a feature of severe depression, and increased activity, agitation and restlessness can be features of anxiety.

Health professionals must therefore take a comprehensive approach when supporting people with depression and anxiety with non-pharmacological, pharmacological and brain stimulation therapies. Comprehensive approaches will always include recommendations for people with depression and anxiety to exercise regularly, maintain a healthy diet, and ensure adequate rest and recreation.

IN PRACTICE

Tips for engaging with people experiencing depression and anxiety

Utilising the principles of active listening is critical when supporting people experiencing depression and/or anxiety. At the same time, health professionals are encouraged to adapt their interpersonal skill-set according to the needs and preferences of the person. For example:

- Avoid overt optimism when helping a person experiencing depression and/or anxiety, as this may come over as lacking authenticity.
- Avoid giving overly prescriptive advice or false reassurances. Well-meaning statements such as, 'Don't worry; everything will be all right' or 'I'm sure you are going to be just fine' are more likely to increase the person's sense of distress and disempowerment than reassure them.

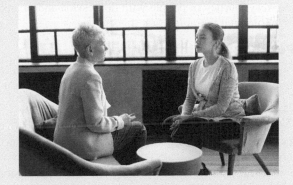

- Avoid reflecting the content and feelings of the person's conversation by making statements such as, 'You're looking exhausted today' or 'Sounds like you are feeling like you can't go on'. These kinds of statements can reinforce the person's negative emotional state.

You can also support people who lack motivation by using motivational interviewing techniques or learning to ask 'open' or 'closed' questions. Effective questioning can assist the person in identifying how they are feeling and highlight specific concerns, worries and problems that may be acting as psychological reinforcements for their negative thoughts and feelings.

Closed questions require a single-word response and help elicit or confirm factual information. Examples of closed questions include the following.
- 'Do you feel more depressed than last week?'
- 'Has your sleep pattern been disturbed?'
- 'Are you feeling suicidal?'

Although useful, such questions do not allow for exploring thoughts and feelings. Also, closed questions may impart a lack of interest if used excessively.

Open questions are a way of encouraging the person to talk. They require more than a monosyllabic response from the person being asked the question. Examples of open questions include the following.
- 'How would you describe your mood this week?'
- 'How have you been experiencing disturbed sleeping?'
- 'What are you intending to do about your suicidal thoughts?'

Open questions can create opportunities to explore what may be influencing the person's current emotional state. They may also allow the health professional to identify if the person has thoughts of self-harm or suicide, the degree of pain and discomfort, and the effect of specific treatments, such as the side effects of medication.

You can read more about therapeutic engagement, active listening and motivational interviewing in the chapters that look at mental health assessment and substance use disorders.

QUESTIONS

1. How will you know if your interpersonal skills need further development?

2. What steps can you take to develop skills in asking open and closed questions?

Non-pharmacological interventions

For mild to moderate depression, psychological therapies alone are viewed as appropriate first-line treatment, with a combination of psychosocial and pharmacological interventions recommended for moderate to severe depression (NICE, 2022). It is necessary to reiterate at this point that the choice of which interventions are best for a person with depression and/or anxiety must be made collaboratively by the person, their partner, carers or family members, and the multidisciplinary team. There is also a need to take a biopsychosocial approach, with consideration given to managing stress, ensuring appropriate sleep hygiene and enabling the uptake of healthy lifestyle changes, including regular exercise and eating well (Malhi et al., 2018).

This section briefly explains the non-pharmacological interventions commonly used to support the recovery journey of people with depression and/or anxiety. These interventions include psychosocial and psychological therapies.

Psychosocial interventions

Psychosocial interventions include psychoeducation, social or peer support groups and other services as required (e.g. housing, employment and other relevant services such as drugs and alcohol).

Psychoeducation

Psychoeducation involves providing information or education to a consumer, carer or any community member or population group about mental health concerns or services (van Erp et al., 2020). This may be information about:
- medical or other jargon that mental health professionals often use
- the symptoms affecting the person and how to manage them
- the medication they may be taking, including the side effects and how to manage them
- relevant resources or support services available in the community
- how to problem solve and develop skills to assist the person in managing their situation.

One of the benefits of psychoeducation is a reduction in stigma (Richardson & White, 2019). Also, people with an understanding of the challenges they are encountering and a knowledge of internal and external resources, including their strengths and areas of development, will feel more in control of a situation and be better able to work toward better health outcomes (Askey-Jones & Hailes, 2020).

Psychoeducation can be delivered by all health professionals, regardless of background, to individuals or groups. Facilitating psychoeducation requires the health professional to have up-to-date knowledge on accessing the information needed by the person and their carers or family. The information shared can be digital or paper-based and ideally include an understanding of the services available for people with the lived experience of mental illness. Be aware that the depressed person will have an impaired capacity to take on board and remember information due to their illness. It is, therefore, vital to repeat information for the person and their significant others.

In Australia, there is a plethora of credible online information about depression and anxiety, and the relevant services to support people with these conditions. For example, websites such as Beyond Blue, which is a high-profile national, independent, not-for-profit organisation in Australia, works to address issues associated with depression, anxiety and related substance-use disorders. Likewise, the Black Dog Institute provides information and support on mood disorders. Other online organisations and programs to support people with depression are outlined in the chapter that discusses the approaches to mental health service delivery and includes the Better Access to Mental Health Services initiative, funded by the Australian government. This program provides psychological services to people with mental ill-health at a subsidised cost.

Peer support

Peer support, including peer group support, involves people with mental health concerns meeting together to support one another with nonclinical assistance, supporting one another in their recovery journey. In recovery-oriented services, peers are sometimes employed as 'consumer consultants' or 'consumer representatives'. Some services also employ carer consultants or representatives.

Peer support, including peer support groups, can be used effectively to supplement traditional therapeutic interventions for people who are unwilling or unable to access professional support or distrust health professionals (Bernecker et al., 2020). In Australia, an example of an active and formalised peer support program is provided through Open Arms Veterans & Families Counselling, where people with the lived experience of military life and mental illness are employed to support veterans in the community who have mental health and substance misuse issues (Open Arms Veterans & Families Counselling, 2019). Peer support groups are also helpful when there are resource constraints (e.g. limited services or mental health professionals). Furthermore, subclinical symptoms and chronic stress without a mental illness often go unaddressed, despite their substantial health impact.

Other social services

Other social services that can be used effectively to support people with depression, anxiety and other mental health concerns, include housing, employment, family, education and recreation services. As explained in the chapter that looks at culturally appropriate health care, the social determinants of health mediate the health status of all people, shaping how they access resources that can support the quality of life. For example, people with lower education and employment levels have poorer mental health outcomes. It is, therefore, essential to connect people with mental health concerns with the social services that will help them. This connection is best achieved by engaging with a social worker.

UPON REFLECTION

Psychoeducation for Aboriginal and Torres Strait Islander peoples

Primary care organisations in Australia, such as Headspace, ensure that the psychoeducation they deliver is culturally sensitive and relevant to various population groups. Yarn Safe was developed for young Indigenous Australians to provide a safe place to share stories about mental health and being. Topics include stress and pressure, relationships, alcohol and drugs. You can read more about Yarn Safe at www.headspace.org.au/yarn-safe.

QUESTIONS

1. Why does psychoeducation need to be population specific?
2. What are the benefits of engaging with community members to develop appropriate psychoeducation materials?

Psychological therapies

Many different psychological therapies are used to support people with anxiety and depression. The following information describes some of these therapies. Health professionals must complete specific training and engage in ongoing supervision to deliver these interventions effectively.

Acceptance and commitment therapy

Acceptance and commitment therapy (ACT) assists the individual in accepting things that seem out of their control and committing to acting on plans or goals to improve and enrich their lives. ACT teaches the person to deal with painful thoughts, memories and feelings, and to clarify what is truly important to them. There is a focus on **mindfulness** in ACT, which teaches the person to be self-aware in the present moment, to engage fully in what they are doing and enable feelings to come and go without reaction. Recent studies suggest that ACT may be effective for various disorders, including anxiety disorders and depression (Bai et al., 2020). The benefits of internet-delivered ACT, called iACT, have also been demonstrated (Kelson et al., 2019).

Cognitive behavioural therapy

Cognitive behavioural therapy (CBT) is a talking therapy focusing on two elements shown to have a significant influence on the development and experience of depression, namely cognition (thoughts) and behaviour (actions). CBT aims to assist the person in recognising the link between negative and unhelpful thoughts (such as irrational beliefs) and the associated behaviours (Gautam et al., 2020). CBT has been evaluated positively as a treatment for depression and is a widely used intervention with a strong evidence base (Malhi et al., 2018). Internet-based CBT for depression and anxiety is available online to assist people with depression, with the intervention growing exponentially during the COVID-19 pandemic. Internet-based CBT continues to address barriers related to geographical distance, isolation, access to, and the cost of treatment, stigma and the reluctance of people to seek help (Verkleij et al., 2021).

Eye movement desensitisation and reprocessing therapy

Eye movement desensitisation and reprocessing therapy (EMDR) was developed to alleviate the distress associated with traumatic memories, including those experienced by people with PTSD. During EMDR, the person is briefly and sequentially exposed to emotionally disturbing material while simultaneously focusing on an external stimulus, such as therapist-directed lateral eye movements, hand-tapping and audio stimulation. There is clear evidence demonstrating the effectiveness of EMDR for people who have experienced traumatic events (Snoek et al., 2020).

Interpersonal psychotherapy

Interpersonal psychotherapy (IPT) is a time-limited, structured talking therapy for individuals where mental illness is associated with life events or has significantly challenged relationships and roles. The treatment goals are to reduce symptoms, alleviate interpersonal distress and assist the person in building and enhancing social supports (Durmaz & Okanli, 2021). Interpersonal psychotherapy is an effective treatment for mental illness over the longer term (Mulder et al., 2017).

Mindfulness-based interventions

These therapeutic approaches incorporate mindfulness, an Eastern meditation practice originally developed to support people in their quest for happiness and spiritual freedom (Karunamuni & Weerasekera, 2019) and have since been used to help people manage unhelpful thoughts, feelings and behaviours (Schuman-Olivier et al., 2020). Mindfulness-based interventions are often group-based and can include mindfulness-based stress reduction (MBSR) and mindfulness-based cognitive therapy (MBCT), where participants are taught practices designed to help them increase their ability to live in the present moment rather than relive, ruminate or feel stress, worry or anxiety about past events (de Sousa et al., 2021). The research evidence-base demonstrating the effectiveness of mindfulness-based interventions for depression and anxiety is substantial (Galante et al., 2021)

Problem-solving therapy

Problem-solving therapy (PST) is an effective, cognitive-behavioural intervention that focuses on training the person in adaptive problem-solving attitudes and skills (Shang et al., 2021). This training aims to help the person to identify current stressful life events and social, health or interpersonal problems; gauge the priority and impact of these problems; problem-solve them accordingly; and, with guidance from the therapist, work on strategies to implement solutions. PST also promotes adaptive attitudes and behaviours, which support the person to cope effectively with stressful life events.

Psychodynamic therapy

Psychodynamic therapy focuses on the psychosocial roots of emotional distress. This therapeutic approach uses self-reflection, self-examination, and the relationship between the person-practitioner to reflect on the relational patterns in the person's life. Psychodynamic therapy is effective for various mental health concerns, including depression and anxiety (Leichsenring et al., 2020).

Systemic family therapy

Systemic family therapy aims to work with the person and their family to explore how problems, illness, disability and disease affect them and others in everyday life. The focus of such a therapeutic approach is to view the person, their partner, carer and family as a unit functioning as a whole system. Systemic family interventions are effective for relationship issues, mood and anxiety disorders, substance use issues, psychosis and adjustment to chronic physical illness (Carr, 2019).

Complementary therapies

Many people access a range of complementary therapies to help them manage their experiences of depression and anxiety. These complementary therapies include acupuncture, aromatherapy, homeopathy, yoga, meditation and reflexology. Although many people find these therapies helpful, the empirical research evidence-base demonstrating the benefits remains a work in progress (Gray et al., 2019). For more information on complementary medicinal therapies, read the section on pharmacological interventions that discusses the value of complementary or alternative medicines.

UPON REFLECTION

Group mindfulness-based interventions

Group mindfulness-based interventions can be delivered in primary care by any health professional who has completed training in mindfulness-based interventions (Tang & Lee, 2021). This type of facilitation could be useful in light of the worldwide shortage of mental health professionals and the preferences of many consumers who are more likely to seek help from a primary care provider than a mental health specialist (Torres-Plata et al., 2019).

....

QUESTIONS

1. How likely are you to attend a group-based intervention to improve your mental health and wellbeing? Why?

2. What are the benefits and challenges of using non-mental health specialists to support people with mental health concerns?

Pharmacological interventions

As explained in the previous section, while psychological interventions are recommended as the first-line treatment for depression and/or anxiety, a combination of psychosocial and pharmacological interventions are recommended for moderate to severe depression (NICE, 2022). Malhi et al. (2021) suggest, in figure 7.1, that all pharmacological interventions aim to relieve symptoms and enable the person to resume functioning to previous levels. Psychological and psychosocial interventions can then be used to help develop the person's resilience and support their quality of life and recovery journey. This section briefly explains the pharmacological interventions commonly used to support the recovery journey of people with depression and/or anxiety.

Antidepressant medications

Antidepressant medications are used to treat depression and some anxiety disorders. There are several different types or classes of antidepressant medications. Despite extensive use, the exact mode of action of these medications is not fully understood. Some researchers suggest that levels of chemicals in the brain (neurotransmitters), such as serotonin and noradrenaline, are linked to mood and emotion, and antidepressant medications work on levels of serotonin and noradrenaline (NHS UK, 2021).

FIGURE 7.1 The spectrum of interventions

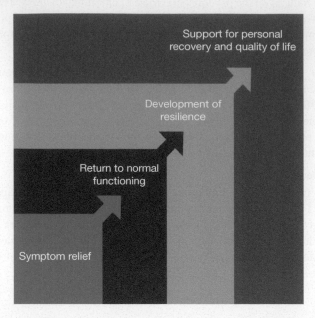

Support for personal
recovery and quality of life

Development of
resilience

Return to normal
functioning

Symptom relief

Source: Malhi et al. (2021).

Best practice guidelines suggest that antidepressant medications be prescribed only after a careful evaluation of the person's situation, including their risk of suicide, level of severity, response to psychological therapies and the existence of comorbidities (Gabriel et al., 2020). Other factors that may influence the type of antidepressant prescribed such as:

- the prescriber's experience and personal choice
- side-effect profile — groups of antidepressants have specific side-effect profiles
- the person's previous history of depression and treatment
- presence, or otherwise, of a physical illness
- safety profile of the medication in overdose — for example, it is common for people with depression to contemplate suicide; individuals who are considered to be at a high risk of suicide are generally not prescribed antidepressants with high toxicity in overdose (see the chapter that looks at caring for a person who has self-harmed)
- the consumer's preference.

Categories of antidepressant medication used in Australia are listed next, with examples using generic rather than trade names. This information has been adapted from Beyond Blue (2022b). Dosage information can be obtained from websites such as the National Health Services in the United Kingdom (NHS, 2021). Some of the side effects of the medications are listed in a later section; nevertheless health professionals are advised to refer to complete product information in a current Medical Information Management System (MIMS) or a similar resource when supporting people taking antidepressant medication.

Selective Serotonin Reuptake Inhibitors

Selective Serotonin Reuptake Inhibitors (SSRIs) are Australia's most commonly prescribed antidepressants and are often a doctor's first choice for most types of depression and anxiety. They are generally well tolerated and non-sedating. Examples of SSRIs are sertraline, citalopram, escitalopram, paroxetine, fluoxetine and fluvoxamine.

Serotonin and Noradrenalin Reuptake Inhibitors

Serotonin and Noradrenalin Reuptake Inhibitors (SNRIs) have fewer side effects than SSRIs. SNRIs are often prescribed for severe depression and are safer if a person overdoses. SNRIs include venlafaxine and desvenlafaxine.

Reversible Inhibitors of Monoamine oxidase

Reversible Inhibitors of Monoamine oxidase (RIMAs) have fewer side effects than other antidepressants and are non-sedating, but they may be less effective in treating more severe forms of depression than other antidepressants. They can be helpful for people who are experiencing anxiety or sleeping difficulties. An example of this type of antidepressant is moclobemide.

Tricyclic Antidepressants

Tricyclic Antidepressants (TCAs) are effective antidepressants but have more harmful side effects than SSRIs and are more likely to cause low blood pressure, which must be monitored carefully. Examples of TCAs are nortriptyline, clomipramine, dothiepin, imipramine and amitriptyline.

Noradrenaline-Serotonin Specific Antidepressants

Noradrenaline-Serotonin Specific Antidepressants (NaSSAs) are relatively new antidepressants and can be helpful for people with anxiety and/or depression. They are helpful for those who have trouble sleeping. In addition, these medications have fewer sexual side effects. However, they may cause weight gain. An example of the NaSSAs is mirtazapine.

Noradrenalin Reuptake Inhibitors

Noradrenalin Reuptake Inhibitors (NARIs) are designed to act selectively on one type of brain chemical — noradrenaline. They are less likely to cause sleepiness or drowsiness than some other antidepressants. However, they are more likely to make it difficult for people to sleep. They can cause increased sweating, sexual difficulties, difficulty urinating and an increased heart rate after the initial doses. An example of a NARI is reboxetine.

Monoamine Oxidase Inhibitors

Monoamine Oxidase Inhibitors (MAOIs) are prescribed only under exceptional circumstances as they require the person to have a special diet and have adverse effects. An example of an MAOI is tranyl-cypromine.

Agomelatine

Agomelatine is a synthetic analogue of melatonin and works as an atypical antidepressant by stimulating melatonin receptors. This medication has a range of side effects, and it interacts with other medicines. Side effects such as headaches and sleep disturbances are quite common. A rare side-effect is that it can affect liver function and requires regular follow-up blood tests. It is generally not recommended in people who have liver problems.

IN PRACTICE

Supporting diverse people to manage their medicines

According to the Australian Commission on Safety and Quality in Health Care (ACSQHC) (2017), culturally and linguistically diverse (CALD) groups and Aboriginal and Torres Strait Islander peoples need understandable and accessible health information that enables them to improve their knowledge, understanding and recall about their health and care, including their prescribed medicines. Such information can increase the person's feelings of empowerment, improve their ability to cope, increase satisfaction, support shared decision-making and contribute to improved health literacy. Understandable and accessible information can enable people to become partners in their health care.

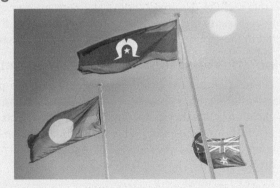

Research undertaken by the ACSQHC (2017) found that CALD and Aboriginal and Torres Strait Islander participants preferred simple, plain language information in both English and their first language. All groups sought short and visually appealing information, including culturally appropriate designs. Aboriginal and Torres Strait Islander participants also reported feelings of shame when they were unable to understand health care information. They expressed a preference for culturally sensitive in-person support and information to be provided through face-to-face discussions.

Obtaining understandable and accessible health information about medication, including the side effects, can be challenging. Visually appealing information using simple and plain language in both English and their first language is not always available. Likewise, interpreters can be difficult to access. This situation presents challenges for health professionals supporting diverse people to manage the side effects of medication prescribed for mental illness.

▶

Some solutions to these challenges include:

- NPS MedicineWise, an Australian online service that provides fact sheets on medications, written in various languages, including Arabic, simplified and traditional Chinese, Greek, Hindi, Italian, Punjabi, Spanish, Tagalog and Vietnamese. www.nps.org.au
- Pharmaceutical Society of Australia (PSA), which has produced a guide for supporting Aboriginal and Torres Strait Islander peoples with medicine management, at www.ppaonline.com.au/wp-content/uploads/2019/01/PSA-Guide-to-Providing-Pharmacy-Services.pdf
- Therapeutic Goods Administration (TGA), is an Australian Government department that provides consumer medicines information, written by the pharmaceutical company responsible for the medicine at: www.tga.gov.au/consumer-medicines-information-cmi.

Developing a comprehensive repository of visually appealing, simple and plain language information in both English and a person's first language remains a work in progress.

QUESTIONS

1. What are the main issues for diverse consumers who are unable to access information about their medications?

2. What practical steps can practitioners take to support diverse people with information about their medications?

Effectiveness of antidepressant medication

Many people, including health professionals, will suggest that antidepressants are not effective and that multinational pharmaceutical companies drive the widespread use of these medications. However, a large-scale systematic review published in the *Lancet* found that all antidepressants were more efficacious than placebo in adults with major depressive disorder, with some antidepressants demonstrating more effective than others (Cipriani et al., 2018). Antidepressants usually need to be taken for around seven to 14 days (without missing a dose) before the benefits are felt (NHS Inform, 2022).

The choice of antidepressant medication use will depend on the individual's tolerance of the side effects. The overall length of time a person needs to take an antidepressant medication will vary depending on various factors, including the severity of the depression and response to treatment. People who take antidepressant medications need to be regularly monitored. The medications should only be ceased gradually and under the supervision of a medical practitioner or other authorised prescriber. Reasons for this include the possibility of the person experiencing 'antidepressant discontinuation syndrome' if antidepressants are ceased too quickly (Gabriel & Sharma, 2017). This syndrome is explained in more detail in the section that discusses the cessation of antidepressant medication.

Side effects of antidepressant medications

It is essential that the health professional help the person taking antidepressant medication to manage the side effects they may experience. One of the main reasons people stop taking their antidepressant medication is that they cannot manage the side effects (Milan & Vasiliadis, 2020). While some side effects of medications were identified in the previous sections, many side effects will vary according to the type of antidepressant taken and individual responses to this medication. More generally, side effects may include:

- dry mouth
- urinary retention
- blurred vision
- constipation
- sedation (can interfere with driving or operating machinery)
- sleep disruption
- weight gain
- headache
- nausea
- gastrointestinal disturbance/diarrhoea
- abdominal pain
- sexual problems
- agitation
- anxiety.

The first step to helping a person manage the side effects is to identify how they affect the person's lifestyle. For example, an adolescent who is gaining weight from taking antidepressants may find it difficult to adhere to this treatment regimen in the long term. The health professional can assist the person who experiences unwanted side effects of medications by working with them to manage what is happening. This work could include referring the person to a dietitian or other allied health professional who will support the person in achieving a lifestyle change. Such assistance requires much more than the health professional simply informing the person what is required or handing them a relevant brochure. Instead, close planning or additional psychological therapy may be required to support long-term behavioural change.

Another often unspoken side effect for the health professional to consider is the sexual issues that affect many people when placed on antidepressants. As noted earlier, these issues can include low libido, difficulties achieving and maintaining an erection, orgasmic difficulties and reduced penile sensitivity. Some people feel embarrassed about discussing this topic; likewise, they may be unaware that medication can contribute to the sexual difficulties they may have experienced during an episode of depression. Health professionals must explain to the person that if this becomes an issue, it is not a permanent condition. However, unlike some other side effects of antidepressant medication, these side effects remain for the duration of treatment. It can also be helpful to suggest to the person that they discuss any sexual issues with their prescriber because there are significant differences between the different types of antidepressants and their side effects.

Generally speaking, reassuring people commencing antidepressant medication therapy is integral to treatment. A statement used by many health professionals to raise awareness of possible issues without increasing the risk of discontinuation of the pharmacological treatment could be: 'Antidepressants usually take several weeks before you start to feel the improvement. There are some side effects that you may notice early on in treatment, which will often reduce over a few weeks.' Health professionals can then go on to outline the common side effects for the class of antidepressant medication the person is taking.

Ceasing antidepressant medication

Quite often, once a person taking an antidepressant medication starts to feel their mood improving, they are keen to stop taking the medication. Some people think it is somehow shameful or a sign of weakness to be taking antidepressants. Whenever antidepressants are prescribed, treatment should be the correct therapeutic dose and should be continued under medical supervision. Health professionals could pose questions such as the following.

- 'If you were taking medication for a cardiac problem, would you stop taking it when you started to feel better?'
- 'If you were taking medication for diabetes, would you stop taking it when you started to feel better?'
- 'What are the issues if you continue on your antidepressants?'

Questions such as these can highlight misunderstandings the person may have about the antidepressants, including issues of stigma, leading to a beneficial discussion between the health professional and the person.

When discussing any medication with a person experiencing anxiety or depression, health professionals must advise them that they need to consult with the prescriber if they choose to cease the medication. There are two main reasons for this. First, ceasing antidepressant medication abruptly or a marked reduction in the dose of an antidepressant taken continuously for one month can lead to a withdrawal syndrome termed 'antidepressant discontinuation syndrome' (Gabriel & Sharma, 2017). The antidepressant discontinuation syndrome is summarised using the mnemonic FINISH: Flu-like symptoms (lethargy, fatigue, headache, achiness, sweating), Insomnia (with vivid dreams or nightmares), Nausea (sometimes vomiting), Imbalance (dizziness, vertigo, light-headedness), Sensory disturbances (burning, tingling, electric-like or shock-like sensations) and Hyperarousal (anxiety, irritability, agitation, aggression, mania, jerkiness) (Gabriel & Sharma, 2017). If a person chooses to cease antidepressant medication, the health professional may suggest increasing the frequency of monitoring the person's mood to enable an early response if the person's mood deteriorates.

Anxiolytic medications

In addition to antidepressant medication, people with depression and anxiety may also be prescribed other types of medication. In particular, people with anxiety may take **anxiolytic** or 'anti-anxiety' medications.

Medications prescribed for anxiety may include the benzodiazepines, such as alprazolam, clonazepam, diazepam (commonly known as Valium), lorazepam, midazolam, temazepam (used as a sleeping tablet) and other medications that end in the letter 'pam'. The medications are sedatives and can be ultra-short,

short- or long-acting. Unfortunately, some of these medicines are used as 'date rape' drugs, placed in a person's drink to impair judgement and make them susceptible to sexual assault. Another major issue with benzodiazepines is that they are habit-forming and often abused. If overdosed, they can lead to death. For this reason, benzodiazepines should not be widely used for the long-term treatment of anxiety.

Buspirone is not prescribed for anxiety but can be used to address symptoms of anxiety, such as sweating, a pounding heartbeat, fear, irritability, dizziness or other symptoms. Hydroxyzine was designed to treat the itching caused by an allergic reaction but can also be taken to relieve anxiety or tension. Beta-blockers were designed to control your body's fight-or-flight response and reduce its effects on your heart. They are occasionally precribed **off-label** for anxiety.

The limited number of medications designed specifically to reduce anxiety symptoms suggests why many prescribers instead use antidepressant medications. The only other pharmacological options include complementary medicines.

Complementary or alternative medicines

The terms complementary and alternative medicines refer to a range of medicines, supplements and approaches, such as herbal remedies and food supplements, including vitamin preparations and other organic and inorganic substances (e.g. omega-3 fatty acids). These substances can be purchased without the need for a prescription.

There is ongoing debate by the scientific community regarding the efficacy of these remedies in improving mental health and wellbeing; although there is some evidence to suggest St John's Wort is superior and equivalent to conventional antidepressants for the treatment of mild to moderate depression — in the short term only (Black Dog Institute, 2020; NCCIH, 2017). Interest in complementary or alternative medicine continues to grow across the western world, including Australia.

When talking to a person with depression and/or anxiety about the value of complementary or alternative therapies, health professionals can advise that:

- many people use complementary medicines or therapies to supplement medical treatment; others use the medicines and therapies alongside medical treatment. Those who use them, generally say they are helpful
- many substances or therapies labelled 'complementary', 'alternative' or 'natural' do not undergo the same safety testing as mainstream medications
- complementary therapies are not a replacement for adequate medical treatment
- consultation with an authorised prescriber must occur before using complementary or alternative medicines, including how they interact with prescribed medications (SANE, 2017).

Health professionals may also consider the interesting research on placebos, which are medicine or procedures prescribed for the psychological benefit to the person rather than for any physiological effect. According to Harvard Health (2021), scientists have found that, under the right circumstances, a placebo can be just as effective as a conventional treatment. If a person believes a treatment will work, this creates a stronger connection between the brain and body and how they work together. Placebos can work on symptoms modulated by the brain, including anxiety.

UPON REFLECTION

St John's Wort

St John's wort (*Hypericum perforatum*) is a perennial herb with a yellow flower that has been used to treat nervous conditions since ancient Greek times (Black Dog Institute, 2022). Today, it is a popular herbal remedy for mild depression.

Although some research evidence suggests that St John's Wort is superior to conventional antidepressants for the treatment of mild to moderate depression in the short term only, St. John's wort also limits the effectiveness of many prescription medicines (NCCIH, 2017). Also, combining St. John's wort and certain antidepressants can lead to a potentially life-threatening increase in a person's serotonin levels (NCCIH, 2017).

....

QUESTIONS

1. How would you begin a conversation with a person regarding this pharmacological intervention with a person who is experiencing depression?
2. What recommendations would you make about this pharmacological intervention? Why?

Brain stimulation therapies

Brain stimulation therapies are used to treat major depression, treatment-resistant depression and other serious conditions, as identified by a psychiatrist (Gouveia et al., 2020). These therapies involve activating or inhibiting the brain directly with electricity. The electricity can be given directly by electrodes implanted in the brain or noninvasively through electrodes placed on the scalp, or it can be induced by using magnetic fields applied to the head (NIMH, 2016). While these interventions are used less frequently than non-pharmacological therapies, but are nevertheless effective when provided according to clinical practice guidelines based on the best research evidence. This section describes brain stimulation therapies, including the benefits and challenges of their use for people with mental illness.

Electroconvulsive therapy

Electroconvulsive therapy (ECT) is the most studied of the brain stimulation therapies (NIMH, 2016). Movies like *One Flew Over the Cuckoo's Nest* have presented the public with an ill-informed and negative perception of ECT and its effects, stigmatising this treatment unnecessarily. The intervention is an effective and safe medical treatment delivered in a hospital as an inpatient or outpatient (Malhi et al., 2018; Weiss et al., 2019).

ECT involves passing a small, pulsed electrical current to the brain sufficient to induce a seizure for therapeutic purposes and is performed under general anaesthesia (RANZCP, 2019b). Typically, ECT is administered about three times a week until the person's depression improves, which usually takes six to 12 treatments (NIMH, 2016). After that, maintenance ECT treatment may be required to reduce the chances that symptoms will return, depending on the person's needs. Maintenance ECT ranges from one session per week to one session every few months (Malhi et al., 2018). Often, a person who undergoes ECT will also be taking antidepressant or mood stabilising medications (SANE, 2021).

ECT is a most effective for people with major depressive disorders, particularly for people who have either not responded to medication or are unable to take medication (NIMH, 2016). ECT is also recommended for extremely severe or psychotic depression, especially if the person has exceptionally high levels of distress, refuses to eat or drink and/or presents a substantial suicide risk (Malhi et al., 2018).

Side effects of ECT include muscle aches, headache, confusion and memory loss (SANE, 2021). The type of memory loss varies between individuals and can be difficult to distinguish from memory loss associated with depression and some anaesthetic-induced memory loss. For most people, memory loss is temporary. However, for a small number, memory loss may last for months, or even years, depending on how many treatments they receive and the duration of treatment.

In Australia, legislation governs ECT treatment, including minimum standards and regulations around consent. This legislation is explained in more detail in the chapter that looks at the legal and ethical context of mental health care. Additionally, the RANZCP has published Professional Practice Guidelines on the administration of electroconvulsive therapy. Psychiatrists who prescribe ECT in Australia must abide by these guidelines for the administration of ECT, which state that ECT should be considered in the following circumstances.

- Only for illnesses where there is adequate evidence of effectiveness and an appropriate clinical indication, including major depression and major depression with psychotic features, major depression with melancholic features and major depression with peripartum onset.
- For other psychiatric disorders such as bipolar affective disorder (manic, mixed and depressed phases), acute and chronic treatment-resistant schizophrenia, schizoaffective disorder, catatonia, acute psychosis, puerperal psychosis and neuroleptic malignant syndrome.
- Alongside other treatments after detailed psychiatric assessment.
- For depressed patients who have not responded to adequate trials of medication and psychotherapy.
- When rapid clinical improvement is required.
- As a first-line treatment for severe depression when there is an inadequate oral intake, a high suicide risk or high levels of patient distress.
- For patients with psychotic depression, acute psychosis, catatonia, delirious mania or previous positive response to ECT (Weiss et al., 2019, p. 3).

Other criteria include people with treatment-resistive depression, especially older people who may not tolerate or respond to pharmacological interventions. Considerations such as anaesthetic risk need to be evaluated for those with cardiac or respiratory conditions.

If a person is to have ECT or they know someone who is to have ECT, and they are feeling apprehensive, health professionals should discuss the procedure with them in a matter-of-fact way, using an analogy of a pacemaker passing an electrical current through the heart to keep it beating. The difference with ECT is that instead of implanting a pacemaker-type device, ECT is performed in several sessions, often over several weeks. It is not painful during or after the procedure, aside from some people reporting headaches.

Transcranial magnetic stimulation

Transcranial magnetic stimulation (TMS) is a noninvasive intervention that uses magnetic fields to stimulate nerve cells in the brain. TMS is used when other depression treatments have failed to help improve the mood of a person with depression (Fitzgerald et al., 2022). The intervention involves placing an electromagnetic coil near the person's forehead, delivering repetitive magnetic pulses, which is why TMS is sometimes called repetitive TMS or rTMS. These magnetic pulses stimulate nerve cells in the region of the brain involved in mood control and depression. While researchers remain unclear about how TMS works, the intervention seems to ease depression symptoms and improve mood (Malhi et al., 2020).

As with ECT, if a person feels apprehensive about TMS, health professionals should discuss the intervention based on the best evidence and clinical practice guidelines. TMS is not painful and has achieved good outcomes for people with treatment-resistant depression.

UPON REFLECTION

Recovery and brain stimulation therapies

Some people may suggest that the 'last resort' notion of some brain stimulation therapies is firmly located within the medical model and incongruent with mental health recovery. Recovery-oriented approaches, in contrast, are characterised by notions of hope, optimism, self-determination and a personal journey.

However, many consumers will choose one or another of the brain stimulation therapies to keep themselves off medication or out of hospital, to live meaningful and contributing lives. In their view, brain stimulation therapies have widened their options for treatment.

....

QUESTIONS

1. What are your personal views on brain stimulation therapies?

2. What are the differences between your personal views and professional recommendations? If these differences are substantial, how will you approach the topic of brain stimulation therapies to consumers and carers asked for more information?

This section explained the various interventions that can support the recovery journey of adults with depression and/or anxiety, including non-pharmacological, pharmacological and brain stimulation therapies. One focus of the explanation was the effectiveness of these interventions, and how health professionals can support consumers in managing the side effects of their medications.

The next section focuses on perinatal mental health concerns and experiences of women, their partners and families.

7.4 Perinatal mental health issues

LEARNING OBJECTIVE 7.4 Describe how to support women and their families with perinatal mental health concerns.

Pregnancy and childbirth are significant events for a woman and her family; motherhood is viewed as bringing positive changes for a woman. But this is not always the case. Pregnancy heralds a period of rapid physical and biological change for women. Childbirth gives rise to social, emotional, relational and economic changes in the family. These changes can cause feelings of vulnerability or mental health concerns, with many women reporting feeling stressed, losing confidence and having low self-esteem (PANDA, n.d.).

About 9–21 per cent of women will experience symptoms of anxiety and/or depression during the perinatal period (McLeish & Redshaw, 2017). Partners can also experience perinatal mental health issues (Atzl et al., 2021), with about one in 10 expectant and new fathers experiencing depression, anxiety or other forms of emotional distress in the perinatal period, with these experiences also impacting the woman (PADA, n.d.). These impacts are even greater when the woman and her family experiences disadvantages, such as a low income, single parenthood, a history of abuse or domestic violence, or a history of mental illness (Palmer Molina et al., 2018; Brown et al., 2020).

The section focuses on women's mental health during the perinatal period — that is, the time from conception to 12 months after the child's birth. Topics covered are perinatal mental health promotion and illness prevention. Following this is an explanation of 'the baby blues', perinatal anxiety, perinatal depression and postnatal or puerperal psychosis. The section concludes by considering how best to support the woman, her baby, partner and family.

Perinatal mental health promotion and illness prevention

Despite the well-documented risks, mental health issues experienced in the perinatal period can often go unrecognised and untreated (Martin-Key et al., 2021). The reasons for this are complex. Some women may presume the symptoms they are experiencing are a normal part of adjusting to the changes wrought by pregnancy, childbirth and a new baby. Women with a history of mental illness may fear that reporting symptoms will result in the authorities removing their child. Another, perhaps even more concerning reason, is that many health professionals lack the awareness, skills or knowledge to identify the signs and symptoms of perinatal mental health issues (Coates & Foureur, 2019).

From 2018–19 to 2024–25, the Australian government will spend $43.9 million to support women living with or at risk of perinatal mental health issues (Department of Health, 2019). This support includes developing innovative screening programs for symptoms of mental illness, and improvements in the delivery of appropriate and accessible mental health interventions for mental health services for women and their families. The mental health services to be delivered include mental health promotion and illness prevention services to raise awareness of perinatal mental health issues in the community, and loss and bereavement peer support services for women and families after the death of a baby.

For example, the Statewide Perinatal and Infant Mental Health Program (SPIMHP) in Western Australia provides training, screening and assessment tools, and perinatal mental health promotion activities to enable health professionals to develop the skills required to support women during the perinatal period, their partners and families (King Edward Memorial Hospital, 2022). Mental health promotion and illness prevention activities provide an essential means of raising awareness for the early recognition of early warning signs of possible mental illness in the perinatal period. Such awareness and early recognition of mental health concerns will increase the possibility of implementing early intervention strategies to achieve better outcomes for all (Swami et al., 2020).

IN PRACTICE

PANDA

Perinatal Anxiety & Depression Australia or 'PANDA' supports the mental health of parents and families during pregnancy and in their first year of parenthood Australia-wide. PANDA provides the following services.

- Australia's only national helpline for individuals and their families that provides access to counselling and information to assist with perinatal anxiety and depression recovery.
- An intensive care coordination program in some states (e.g. VIC and SA).
- Training for health professionals to manage disclosure, provide appropriate referrals and facilitate ongoing support for people experiencing perinatal mental health challenges.
- A free, nationwide secondary consultation service for health professionals who need advice on supporting people with perinatal mental health challenges.
- The Community Champions Program, a national network for volunteers who support families in a positive transition to early parenthood.
- A Clinical Champions Program, a national network of health professionals working in perinatal mental health who support families during the perinatal period.
- Community education that includes volunteers sharing their stories and facilitating educational activities to raise awareness of perinatal anxiety and depression in new parent groups, playgroups and other community settings.

PANDA leverages on the lived experience of those with perinatal mental health issues to influence governments, health advocates, health care providers, employers, and the wider community to support people experiencing perinatal mental health challenges. They work toward an Australia in which stigma, shame and barriers to perinatal support no longer exist.

You can read more about the work of PANDA and the services it provides at: www.panda.org.au/about/about-panda.

▶

Types of perinatal mental health conditions

There are four main mental health conditions for women during the **perinatal period**: 'baby blues', anxiety, depression and psychosis. Each of these conditions is now explained, in turn.

'Baby blues'

The maternity 'baby blues' is a transient mood change that occurs about four days **postpartum** and affects most women generally up to five days following birth. It is a relatively mild and self-limiting condition, usually characterised by a labile (i.e. changing) mood, tearfulness, anxiety, irritability and feeling overwhelmed. The 'blues' last for two or three days and generally disappear after a few days. The treatment is supportive only, including health professionals informing new mothers that they may experience the 'baby blues' and that it is a temporary condition only.

Women and partners affected by the 'baby blues' require information and reassurance that what they are experiencing is a common and possibly hormonal reaction to an extraordinarily stressful situation. If the symptoms do not go away, the woman must discuss the situation with her health professional, as this may be a sign of developing anxiety and/or depression.

Perinatal anxiety

It is common for expecting and new parents to experience anxious feelings about the changes in their lives. People with perinatal anxiety, however, experience more sustained and more pronounced feelings. An earlier section on anxiety in adults explained that people who experience anxiety feel irritable, agitated, panicky, overwhelmed or frustrated. They can also experience social withdrawal.

According to Leach et al. (2017), one in five women report anxiety during pregnancy, and between 4–20 per cent of women experience symptoms of an anxiety disorder after giving birth. Fairbrother et al. (2016) identified anxiety disorder during the pregnancy and early postpartum periods as occurring in 15.8 and 17.1 per cent of women, respectively. These statistics suggest the prevalence is widespread.

The contributing factors for anxiety are similar to those of depression. Although anxiety is often associated with depression, it is a discrete condition with specific signs, symptoms and interventions. These signs and symptoms were described earlier in this chapter, in the section focusing on anxiety. In addition to those signs and symptoms, women who develop anxiety in the perinatal period may experience feelings ranging from persistent generalised worry to catastrophic 'what ifs' focusing on the health or wellbeing of the baby.

Perinatal depression

Perinatal depression is a broad term that incorporates both antenatal depression (experienced during pregnancy) and postnatal depression (which develops between one month and up to one year after the baby's birth). Estimates of the prevalence of **antenatal** and postnatal depression vary considerably. For example, a recent study in Italy reported the prevalence of maternal antenatal and postnatal depression at just over 6 per cent during pregnancy and just under 20 per cent in the postnatal period (Cena et al., 2021). The Royal Women's Hospital Victoria (n.d.) reports the prevalence of depression during pregnancy and in the postnatal period to be 10–15 per cent.

In high-income countries, the prevalence of prenatal depression is estimated to be 15 per cent and postnatal depression at 10 per cent, whereas in low to middle-income countries, prevalence rates are 25 per cent and 19 per cent, respectively (Fatori et al., 2020). Reasons for these differences most likely arise from factors such as the social determinants of health, referred to in the earlier section on depression in adults.

Indeed, many factors can contribute to a woman developing depression during the perinatal period. These include:

- stress during the pregnancy
- unplanned pregnancy
- unable to meet unrealistic expectations of motherhood
- a traumatic or complicated birth
- baby is sick or unsettled (Royal Women's Hospital Victoria, n.d.).

Signs and symptoms of depression during and following pregnancy are similar to those experienced by others who experience depression. These signs and symptoms were described earlier in this chapter, in the section focusing on depression. In addition, women who develop depression in the perinatal period may experience:

- preoccupation with morbid thoughts or anxiety about bad things happening to the pregnancy, their baby or their partner
- feeling disconnected from their baby, feeling that their baby is not really theirs or that they do not have a bond with their baby
- excessive feelings of guilt and/or failure that they are a 'bad mother'
- thoughts of harming themselves
- thoughts that things would be better for them or their baby if they were dead, leading to thoughts of suicide (Royal Women's Hospital Victoria, n.d.).

Early screening for perinatal depression in women can assist in raising awareness of the condition. Early screening also allows health professionals to identify at-risk women and implement early interventions if required.

UPON REFLECTION

Perinatal mental health week

In Australia, the second week of each November is Perinatal Mental Health Week. This week was established in 2005 to raise awareness about mental health issues and create opportunities for conversations about how women, their partners and families can be affected by perinatal mental health challenges and where they can find help and support (PANDA, www.panda.org.au/articles/perinatal-mental-health-week).

QUESTIONS

1. In your view, how successful are special days or weeks for raising awareness about a health issue?
2. What can you do to support the activities to raise awareness about perinatal mental health issues?

Puerperal psychosis

Puerperal, postnatal or postpartum psychosis is a psychotic episode commencing within six weeks of birth (Deas, 2017). Between one and two women per 1000 births develop puerperal psychosis. Sixty per cent of women who develop puerperal psychosis have had a previous psychotic episode (VanderKruik et al., 2017). Generally, the psychosis starts within 24 hours of birth, with symptoms becoming apparent within three days of birth and up to twelve weeks after the baby's birth (del Corral Serrano, 2019).

The psychotic features experienced by the mother are no different to psychosis generally (see the chapter that looks at caring for a person with a serious mental illness). However, most often, the content of the delusions and hallucinations in puerperal psychosis revolve around the baby and the transition to motherhood (Deas, 2017). The woman's moods can be elated but may fluctuate rapidly to depression and suicidal thoughts. There is also a markedly disturbed sleep pattern.

The symptoms of puerperal psychosis include:

- confusion and disorientation about the day and time and people
- slowed or racing thoughts
- severe physical anxiety or agitation, to the point of being unable to stay still
- variable mood, from irritability and mania to depression
- insomnia and feeling like they need less sleep or going days without sleeping
- delusions or paranoid thoughts, e.g. the hospital staff are spies or a family member is an imposter
- hallucinations or impaired sensations where the woman either hears, sees or smells things that are not present

- strange sensations that they are not themselves (depersonalisation) or others are controlling their actions and thoughts
- thoughts of and/or plans to harm themselves and their baby (Royal Women's Hospital Victoria, n.d.).

The delusions, hallucinations and confusion of psychosis can have serious, even fatal, consequences for the baby and/or mother if untreated (VanderKruik et al., 2017). For this reason, post-partum psychosis is considered a psychiatric emergency, with immediate treatment required to support the safety of the mother and baby. This treatment most often includes the hospitalisation of the mother and baby. There are mother and baby mental health units in capital cities across Australia.

A comparison of the four perinatal conditions of 'baby blues', perinatal anxiety, perinatal depression and postnatal psychosis is provided in terms of onset, severity, common duration, **incidence** and course of illness in table 7.5. This table shows that these conditions have many similarities but also some clear differences

TABLE 7.5 **Comparison of perinatal mental health challenges**

	Baby blues	Perinatal anxiety	Perinatal depression	Postnatal psychosis
Onset	3–4 days after birth	Any time before or after birth	Any time before or after birth. Peaks at 5 weeks post-birth	Within 24 hours of birth up to 12 weeks after birth
Severity	Mild	Mild to severe	Mild to severe	Severe
Common duration	1–2 days	Highly variable	Highly variable	6–9 months
Incidence	Most women	150+ per 1000 (estimations only)	100–150 per 1000 births (10–15 per cent)	1–2 per 1000 births (0.1–0.2 per cent)
Course of illness	Changeable mood and teary	As per anxiety in adults	As per depression in adults	Psychosis lasting weeks to months, followed by a depressed phase lasting weeks to months

Screening for perinatal mental health issues

Screening for perinatal and mental health issues, a poor adjustment to parenting and possible domestic violence issues involves identifying risk factors and early symptoms. Universal and routine screening of women in the antenatal period during regular health and progress checks is recommended. Such screening will enable the implementation of early intervention strategies and specialist treatment.

Screening for perinatal depression and anxiety is best undertaken using validated screening tools, such as Edinburgh Postnatal Depression Scale (EPDS) (San Martin Porter et al., 2019). The clinical practice guidelines for depression and related disorders (e.g. anxiety, bipolar disorder and puerperal psychosis) during the perinatal period, recommend the EPDS be used for universal, routine antenatal and perinatal screening for depressive symptoms (Austin, Highet & the Expert Working Group, 2017).

Screening and assessment methods for perinatal depression and anxiety must be culturally appropriate for diverse populations, including Aboriginal and Torres Strait Islander peoples, CALD groups and LGBTQIA+ people. For example, screening and assessment tools for Aboriginal and Torres Strait Islander women can include the Kimberley Mum's Mood Scale and 'Baby Coming You Ready?' (RANZCP, 2021). Other culturally appropriate screening tools can be accessed through the Centre of Perinatal Excellence, which has a range of resources to support health professionals deliver best practice services.

Centre of perinatal excellence

The Centre of Perinatal Excellence (COPE) is an Australian organisation that supports the emotional challenges of becoming a parent, and provides resources for health professionals. These resources include:

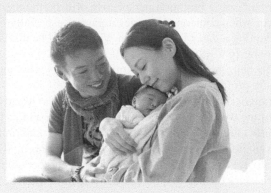

- a large range of culturally appropriate screening tools to gauge the risk of a woman developing perinatal mental health tools, including iScreening
- information (including fact sheets) on specific perinatal mental health conditions, including how to support women, partners and families to overcome the challenges involved
- online courses for health professionals on various perinatal topics
- best practice in perinatal mental health
- search facility to find local help and support for post-partum psychosis using postcode or suburb
- a list of COPE-accredited health professionals to contact for further information.

Other websites that provide information for health professionals on perinatal mental health challenges and how to support diverse woman and their families to overcome these challenges are:

- Beyond Blue Pregnancy and New Parents (www.healthyfamilies.beyondblue.org.au/pregnancy-and-new-parents)
- The Royal Women's Hospital Victoria (www.thewomens.org.au/health-information/pregnancy-and-birth/mental-health-pregnancy).

QUESTIONS

1. Which perinatal screening tool do you think is most appropriate for women in your community? Why?

2. Which of the courses offered through COPE do you think would help you in your work? In what way?

Caring for mothers with perinatal mental health issues

According to the RANZCP (2021), there are three primary considerations when a woman develops perinatal mental health issues:

- the woman's mental health
- parenting and the mother–baby relationship
- the baby's health and wellbeing.

Additionally, and across these three domains, is the need to support the woman's partner, family and key supports (Bohren et al., 2019).

Based on these considerations, specific interventions for women with anxiety, depression or psychosis during the perinatal period are similar to the treatment of all adults, as outlined in previous sections of this chapter, with the following additional considerations.

- When prescribing or administering medication for the mother, health professionals need to consider the effects of the medication on the unborn baby or the infant if the mother is breastfeeding.
- Mental health issues have the potential to affect the mother–baby relationship adversely. This situation can exacerbate the mental health issues experienced by the mother in an escalating cycle. It is vital to support the mother–baby relationship as early as possible and ensure the baby's safety.
- The baby's patterns of behaviour (e.g. difficulties in sleeping or feeding) may exacerbate the woman's symptoms, suggesting the need to ensure the woman and her partner have the skills to manage the baby appropriately.
- The transition to parenthood is as much a challenge for partners as it is for new mothers, so it is also important to screen a woman's partner for mental health issues and assist the partner in supporting the woman and baby.
- The family unit will often need assistance to function effectively. This assistance could include developing communication, coping and problem-solving skills. Individual family members may need help with specific skills, such as practical infant care and parenting skills. Partners may also need direction to obtain additional help.

Partners and other family members, such as the baby's grandparents, can provide valuable support for the mother with mental health issues and the family unit. However, before engaging with the partner and grandparents, it is crucial to understand their perspectives (Hanley & Williams, 2020). For example, although each partner's perspective will be unique, common experiences can include the changes that occur when someone becomes a parent, especially for first-time parents, and the challenges involved in becoming a carer for a woman with mental health issues (RANZCP, 2021). Both roles are stressful and require some adjustment.

To help the partner and family members who support a woman with perinatal mental health issues, health professionals can:

- obtain a release of information from the mother to allow health professionals to share important aspects of the woman's treatment with her partner and/or family
- provide psychoeducation to the partner and family about the mental health issue, including the symptoms, risks, the possibility of recurrence and strategies to support the woman
- involve the partner in a discussion about the woman's care, alternative treatment options and possible risks for the baby — the partner will most often be responsible for the baby's safety and care in addition to caring for the mother
- ascertain how the partner is coping, including discussing:
  - the importance of taking breaks and exploring ways they can take some time out for themselves
  - communication skills and coping skills, and providing options to help develop skills where needed
  - ways of strengthening relationships in the family unit, including those between the mother and partner, and parents and children
  - any parenting issues, work patterns, division of tasks at home and the organisation of other activities of daily living
- provide the partner and family with information on how to access support peer groups and specialised perinatal mental health services.

Occasionally, it may become evident that the partner or other family members are unable to provide the necessary support to the mother and baby (Bohren et al., 2019). Such situations can involve complex psychosocial issues such as family violence, alcohol and drug dependency or abuse, and trauma. Additionally, such situations require urgent discussion with the multidisciplinary team and urgent referral to specialists. In these cases, the safety of the infant and other family members under 16 must be prioritised.

Most specialised services for women and families with perinatal mental health challenges are located in the cities; however, digital perinatal mental health services are becoming more accessible for people who are isolated or live in rural and remote areas. These specialised services include midwives (until the baby is six weeks old), mental health nurses, child and family nurses, social workers, general practitioners and psychiatrists. Women who access specialised services will achieve better health outcomes (RANZCP, 2021).

7.5 Caring for children, adolescents and young people with depression or anxiety

LEARNING OBJECTIVE 7.5 Explore the issues for young people with depression or anxiety.

Mental health problems in childhood can substantially impact the wellbeing of the child and their family (AIHW, 2022a) and increase the risk of mental illness in adulthood (National Mental Health Commission [NMHC], 2021). On the other hand, there are many opportunities to support children, adolescents and their families experiencing symptoms of mental illness, including depression and anxiety. Key to this support is the delivery of mental health promotion, illness prevention and early intervention strategies (Jung & Cho, 2020).

This chapter concludes by exploring depression and anxiety in children, adolescents and young adults. The first section outlines the prevalence and types of depression and anxiety experienced by young people. Following this, risk factors for young people developing anxiety and depression and issues around the assessment are considered. Finally, the most common interventions used to support young people are discussed, including the need for health professionals to take family-focused and trauma-informed approaches.

Prevalence of depression and anxiety in young people

In Australia, one in seven children is likely to experience a mental illness, with high proportions experiencing anxiety and mood disorders such as depression. The Australian Institute of Health and Welfare (AIHW, 2022a) provides the following prevalence data about depression and anxiety in children and adolescents.

- Three of the five leading causes of the total burden of disease in children aged between 5 and 14 were mental disorders
- Anxiety disorders were the second most common disorders among children (almost 7 per cent) and the most common among girls (just over 6 per cent), with depressive disorders ranking third. Conduct disorders ranked fourth.
- Overall, almost 3 in 4 had mild disorders, 1 in 5 had moderate disorders and less than 1 in 10 had severe disorders, with the latter more common among boys (just under 10 per cent) than girls (just over 5 per cent).

Links have also been identified by the AIHW (2022a) between lower mental health outcomes in children from lower socio-economic families and families with poor functioning. These links suggest the need for health professionals to understand the risk factors for young people developing anxiety and depression, and the interventions that best support young people to achieve the best possible outcomes.

UPON REFLECTION

Socio-demographic risk factors for young people

According to the AIHW (2022a), children and adolescents from families with a lower socio-economic demographic or poor functioning are at a higher risk of developing mental health problems. For example:

- children living in families with two parents or carers were less likely to have mental disorders than children living in families with one parent or carer (12 per cent compared with 22 per cent)
- children with their original families (with two parents or carers) were less likely to have mental health disorders than children living with blended families (11 per cent compared with 21 per cent)
- mental illness was more common among children living in families with poor family functioning (34 per cent) than in families with very good family functioning (11 per cent)
- mental illness was more common among children born in Australia (14 per cent) than in children born overseas (just over eight per cent). Mental illness was also more common among children with both carers born in Australia (15 per cent) than when both carers born overseas (just over 5 per cent)
- mental illness was more common among children living in areas with the lowest socio-economic areas (19 per cent) than in those living in the highest (12 per cent).

QUESTIONS

1. What more can governments and organisations do to support young people to overcome the negative impact of some childhood experiences?
2. What more can health professionals do to support young people to overcome the negative impact of some childhood experiences?

While the various types of depression and anxiety were described in earlier sections in this chapter, there are some differences between the anxiety and depression experienced by young people and adults. For example, it is more common for adults to be diagnosed with phobias and panic disorders than young people (Raising Children Network, 2021). Also, although social anxiety is common in adolescents and young adults, it is not as common in children (Headspace, 2021). With regard to depression, diagnoses tend to be classified as mild, moderate or severe based on the number, type and severity of symptoms and the degree to which these symptoms affect day-to-day life (Schimelpfening, 2021)

Reasons for the differences between the types of anxiety and depression experienced by young people and adults are related to the young person's developmental stages. For example, children and adolescents do not process information the same way as adults. They may feel confused by the behaviours of those around them due to their stage of development. The development stage of a child affects how they think and interpret experiences, process stress or distress, grief or sadness, and express their thoughts or feelings (Cherry, 2021).

Developmental stages of children

Various theorists have explained the developmental stages of children and adolescents, including attachment, behavioural, cognitive, psychosocial, psychosexual, sociocultural and social learning theorists. These theories have been simplified by Emerging Minds (www.emergingminds.com.au), an Australian government initiative aimed at advancing infant, child and adolescent mental health.

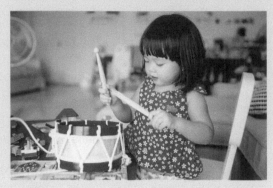

Emerging Minds provides various resources and training opportunities for parents, practitioners, organisations and researchers to support children and adolescents. In addition, Emerging Minds leads the National Workforce Centre for Child Mental Health, which is delivered in partnership with the Australian Institute of Family Studies, the Australian National University, the Parenting Research Centre and the Royal Australian College of General Practitioners.

Emerging Minds provides information about the developmental stages of children. For example:

- *0–3 years.* The major development task of infants and young children at this age is to form an attachment bond with a caregiver/s who is reliable and responsive to the child's emotional and physical needs. The child learns to trust their caregiver during this stage and also rely on their own ability to exert influence on the world. Children's attachment experiences at this stage of life are the foundation for their later social, emotional and cognitive development. A positive attachment experience is associated with consistent, reliable and responsive caregiving. Inconsistent or poor attachment is a risk factor for mental ill-health late in life (Maclean, 2020a).
- *3–5 years.* At this age, children are typically egocentric in the way they understand the world, although they are learning to interact socially and use language to connect with others. They think the world revolves around them and have genuine difficulty seeing the world from another's perspective. Children from 3–5 years have difficulty separating fact from fantasy and are likely to see themselves as causing special things to happen because of their wishful thinking. On the other hand, if something bad happens, they are likely to think they have likewise caused this. Also, they have limited understanding of concepts such as the permanence or temporary nature of events, including death. Children from 3–5 years can identify when others are sad or happy (Maclean, 2020b).
- *5–8 years.* At this age, children are beginning to be able to see things from another's perspective more reliably. They are also becoming more social and interested in others, including friendships and the world around them. Children between 5–8 years can take turns and participate in cooperative play, although these new abilities can break down under pressure. They can also use their developing language skills to interact socially, ask questions of others and more reliably distinguish between what is imaginary and what is real. They develop a sense of 'fairness' and a conscience during this time. At this age, learning difficulties and emotional regulation difficulties start to emerge, with the increase in social and learning expectations introduced by the school environment (Maclean, 2020c).
- *9–12 years.* Most children this age can reliably see things from another's perspective and, because of this, can show genuine empathy for another's experiences and feelings. They can also distinguish between fact and fantasy. Children between 9–12 years can think logically and use their verbal skills to resolve differences and solve problems. Difficulties and delays in cognitive and language abilities become more noticeable and are more likely to cause a child social distress and embarrassment. This can lead to behavioural issues, as children may be seen as the 'bad' kid rather than the 'dumb' kid.

Children at this age are also forming their self-identity and are interested in their family and cultural background. Towards the end of this stage, children develop closer relationships with friends outside of their family of origin and the influence of their peer group becomes stronger. Also, towards the end of this stage is their marked physical development. The onset of puberty can make children feel more awkward and challenge their confidence. They may begin to develop and test their emerging values, beliefs and 'identity' through arguments with parents and other significant adults (Maclean, 2020d).

Young people's experiences of depression or anxiety

The experiences of anxiety and depression in adults have been outlined in earlier sections of this chapter. Children and adults share many of the same signs and symptoms. However, the experience of anxiety and depression by children, adolescents and young adults can also be different to that of adults (Iannelli,

2021). As already noted, reasons for these differences include young people's developmental stages and possible experiences of family dysfunction, including conflict and violence, abuse and neglect, trauma and homelessness.

With regard to anxiety, children and adults both experience trouble sleeping, a lack of focus or difficulty concentrating, cold sweats, dizziness, chest pains, nausea, shortness of breath, palpitations and feelings of uneasiness, restlessness, panic or terror. Young people can also experience nightmares, sleepiness or falling asleep in school, irritability, crying and tantrums (Headspace, 2021).

Children who have ongoing anxiety or are under stress are considered at a higher risk for developing depression. It is important to note that the DSM-5 also utilises different criteria for diagnosing anxiety disorders in children versus adults. For example, children only need to show one symptom to be diagnosed with generalised anxiety disorder, whereas adults need at least three for a diagnosis (Glasofer, 2022).

Many signs and symptoms of depression in young people are similar to those experienced by adults (Orygen, 2017), described previously in this chapter. In addition, children may:

- be irritable or grumpy all the time
- not be interested in things they used to enjoy
- feel tired and exhausted a lot of the time
- interact less with friends and family
- seem unable to relax or be more lethargic than usual
- talk about feeling guilty or worthless
- have thoughts about suicide or self-harming
- complete the self-harm, such as cutting their skin or taking an overdose
- have physical symptoms, such as headaches and stomach aches
- have problems at school
- older children may misuse drugs or alcohol (NHS UK, 2020; Healthdirect, 2020).

A parent often notices changes in their child's emotions, behaviours and/or somatic (i.e. physical) symptoms. The parent may express concerns to any health professional, who must be ready to assess the situation or advise.

IN PRACTICE

Suicide in young Indigenous Australians

Suicide is the leading cause of death among all Australians aged 15–24 (AIHW, 2022b). While this is a concerning statistic, it can be in part explained by the fact that young people do not tend to die from other causes.

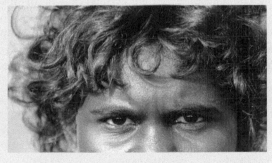

The suicide rate among young Aboriginal and Torres Strait Islander peoples is 2.6 times the rate for non-Indigenous Australians (Beyond Blue, n.d.). According to the Australian Bureau of Statistics (ABS, 2019), Indigenous Australians aged between 5–17 died at 8 deaths per 100 000 in 2018. Some researchers suggest an even higher rate, estimating that Indigenous Australian children and young people aged 5–14 were 10 to 14 times as likely, and those aged 15–24 years were 14 times as likely than non-Indigenous Australians to die by suicide (Dickson et al., 2019).

As with the suicide behaviour of Indigenous Australian adults, the suicide behaviour of young Indigenous Australians has been linked to depression. For example, two-thirds of Aboriginal and Torres Strait Islander peoples aged 15–24 experienced low to moderate levels of psychological distress in the previous month, and one-third experienced high to very high levels (AIHW, 2018).

Risk factors for young Indigenous Australians dying by suicide include:

- trauma from the effects of colonisation, such as the loss of connection to culture, Country and spirituality, which maintains social and emotional wellbeing, supports strong self-identity and provides a sense of continuity among Aboriginal and Torres Strait Islander peoples
- the effects of removal of children from their families, with the traumatic experienced involved being passed down through generations
- ongoing racial discrimination.

According to the Centre of Best Practice in Aboriginal and Torres Strait Islander Suicide Prevention (n.d.), various programs and services offered across Australia provide local, culturally appropriate strategies to identify and respond to young Indigenous Australians most at risk of suicide. These include:

- Kimberley Empowerment Healing and Leadership Program is delivered by the Kimberley Aboriginal Medical Services (KAMS) team across the Kimberley in Western Australia (www.kams.org.au/training-employment/kimberley-empowerment-healing-and-leadership-program)
- Life for Koori Kids (Redfern, Sydney NSW) provides an open network of support for families within the community, whether it be through education and training programmes, sporting activities, medical and dental support or strengthening Aboriginal cultural heritage (www.lifeforkoorikids.org.au/wp)
- GREATS Youth Services (Maningrida, NT) provides a range of community-determined programs and services for Aboriginal and Torres Strait Islander youth (www.malala.com.au/youth-services).

Read more about these and other programs at www.cbpatsisp.com.au/clearing-house/best-practice-programs-and-services/programs-for-preventing-youth-suicide.

QUESTIONS

1. What more could you do to learn about the programs and activities in your local area to support young Indigenous Australians?

2. What steps could you take to support one of the programs and activities in your local area to support young Indigenous Australians?

Assessment of children and adolescents

As with the assessment of adults, the mental health assessment of young people is linked to their risk factors. For example, most young people who present with major depressive disorder have experienced a combination of chronic illness or disability and/or ongoing psychosocial stressors, such as parental separation or family disharmony, domestic violence, physical and sexual abuse, school difficulties (e.g. bullying) or social isolation (Charles & Fazeli, 2017). Another important consideration is the young person's experience of marginalisation, including a culturally and linguistically diverse background, identifying as LGBTQIA+, experiencing homeless, living in a rural community or having a substance use problem (Orygen, 2017).

Factors to consider when assessing children and adolescents for depression or anxiety are outlined in table 7.6. These factors are divided into **predisposing factors**, which place a young person at risk of developing a problem, such as genetics, life events or temperament; **precipitating factors**, which are the specific events or triggers to the onset of the current problem; **perpetuating factors**, or those that maintain the problem once it has become established; and **protective factors** or the strengths of the young person that reduce the severity of problems and promote healthy and adaptive functioning (Racine et al., 2016)

TABLE 7.6 Factors to consider when assessing a young person for anxiety or depression

Focus of assessment	Risk factors	Triggers and perpetuating factors	Strengths	Protective
Biological	Genetic factors Physical illness Parental mental illness	Puberty Physical illness and treatments Identity issues Ethnicity	Genetic factors Physical wellbeing	Absence of comorbidity
Psychological	Behavioural approaches Cognitive style Poor emotion regulation skills Low perceived academic and social competence	Childhood trauma Poor emotion regulation skills Poor coping style Low levels of intelligence	Adaptive emotion regulation skills Problem-focused coping style Normal to high intelligence	Absence of comorbidity Sense of humour High to normal intelligence Adaptive emotion regulation skills Problem-focused coping style

| Social | Family dysfunction or family violence
Life events
Social disadvantage | Acute and chronic life events
Poor peer relationships | Positive friendship and support networks
Close relationship with one or more family members
Socially valued
Personal achievement. | Positive friendship and support networks
Close relationship with one or more family members
Socially valued
Personal achievement. |

Source: Charles and Fazeli (2017); Headspace, 2021; NICE, 2019; Orygen, 2017

According to Orygen (2017), health professionals should only assess a young person if they are competent and trained. However, all health professionals can engage positively with a young person and speak to family members to identify signs and symptoms of anxiety or depression. If the young person is at risk, health professionals can refer the young person to a general practitioner or health professional working with children and adolescents for a more comprehensive assessment.

Positive engagement is the process by which the practitioner establishes, develops and maintains connections with the person they are helping (Chowdhury, 2022). Understanding that it will take several appointments for a health professional to engage well with a young process, the following general principles can be used as a guide.

- Demonstrate unconditional positive regard, authenticity, attentiveness and an unbiased approach.
- Show respect for the young person as an autonomous individual (as appropriate to the young person's age and developmental stage).
- Actively support the young person, as appropriate to their age and developmental stage, to understand themselves and their environment.
- Simplify the therapeutic process wherever safe and possible.
- Include the young person's family, demonstrating respect, a willingness to support and a neutral (or unbiassed) stance.
- Support parents to develop their skills in communication with their child (Raising Children Network, 2022).

UPON REFLECTION

Engaging with diverse young people

Diversity in young people can mean many things, such as an Aboriginal or Torres Strait Islander background, cultural and linguistic diversity, belonging to an LGBTQIA+ population group, or diversity in experiences of trauma.

According to the Youth Affairs Council of South Australia (2016, p. 15–6), barriers to engaging diverse young people include:

- a historical distrust of people in authority
- limited literacy skills or knowledge of English
- difficulty getting parental permission to participate
- fear of being 'outed' to their parents, peers or community
- avoidance of potential discrimination such as racism and homophobia.
  Ways of overcoming these barriers include:
- the use of multiple forms of communication (in a variety of languages) to reach the widest possible audience (e.g. radio, television, social media, local and state newspapers, community groups, cultural spaces and organisations frequented by or which deliver services to young people)
- using interpreters when needed, leading up to and while the engagement is in process
- the use of inclusive and appropriate language for your target group
- being culturally sensitive, flexible and practice in a variety of ways that are tailored to the cultural and other social circumstances of young people from diverse backgrounds
- integrating the mediums that young people value into your engagement, such as online tools and music or videos, and don't forget creativity and 'doing' opportunities.

▶

QUESTIONS
1. What two or three overarching principles could guide how health professionals engage with diverse young people?
2. What are two or three overarching principles that could guide how health professionals engage with the families of diverse young people?

Common interventions for children and adolescents

The interventions used to support young people with anxiety or depression are similar to those described in earlier sections on adult interventions. However, adaptations must be made to accommodate the young person's age and developmental stage. For example, psychological therapies for young children must include play. Likewise, categories and doses of pharmacological interventions will differ according to best evidence practice, with **psychotropic medications** only prescribed to young people by specialists. Health professionals can access evidence-based guidelines that various organisations and institutions developed, such as the National Institute for Health and Care Excellence (NICE, 2019), outlining best-evidence practices when supporting young people.

For young people with mental health concerns, interventions often focus on psychoeducation and early intervention (Colizzi et al., 2020). The earlier a young person is informed and supported, the better their outcomes will be. For high-risk groups, such as children affected by violence, abuse, maltreatment or poverty, early interventions can help reduce disparities (NMHC, 2021). When supporting high-risk groups, it is also essential to consider how to approach the delivery of interventions. These approaches include trauma-informed and family-focused practice, multidisciplinary approaches and online interventions.

Trauma-informed, family-focused approaches

Trauma-informed care

Many young people have experienced trauma, including physical, psychological, emotional and sexual abuse, with these experiences increasing their risk of developing anxiety, depression and other mental illnesses (Orygen & Phoenix Australia, 2018). Supporting young people with trauma-informed care will help them feel safe and improve their health outcomes.

As explained in the chapter on mental health care in Australia, trauma-informed care is a strengths-based framework that is responsive to the impact of trauma, emphasising physical, psychological and emotional safety for both service providers and survivors; and creating opportunities for survivors to rebuild a sense of control and empowerment (Mental Health Coordinating Council, n.d.). Trauma-informed care is principles-based rather than a specific practice. Trauma-informed practice includes understanding trauma and its effects on young people, recognising the signs of trauma in young people and responding accordingly; focusing on engaging with the young person, building trust and helping them to feel safe; identifying and developing the strengths of the young person; inspiring hope and supporting recovery for the young person (Wall et al., 2016).

Trauma-informed approaches to engaging with young people must occur at the organisational, service and practitioner levels. It is also vital to use trauma-informed practices at the family-systems level to support repairing family relationships and creating new networks of caring in a young person's life (Berry Street, 2022).

Family-focused approaches

Bronfenbrenner's ecological system theory influences family-focused approaches to supporting young people (Bronfenbrenner, 1979). Bronfenbrenner's theory suggests that childhood and adolescence are a part of a larger system that includes family, community and societal influences. Children are rarely treated in isolation from their primary systems, such as their family and school, with the influences provided by these systems affecting cognitive, emotional, social and behavioural development.

Understanding the family 'system' or context and including family members when providing mental health support to children and adolescents can improve engagement with services and increase the young person's overall wellbeing (Strawa, 2022). Family-focused approaches include:
- ensuring the young person's safety
- listening to the young person regarding whom they consider 'family' and their key support network
- taking into consideration the culture and language traditions of the family

- taking a strengths-based approach
- communicating and collaborating with the family in the assessment, planning and implementation of interventions.

When first engaging with families and young people, there is a need to be clear about the roles and responsibilities of the family members and the various professionals involved, establishing rules around confidentiality (Emerging Minds, 2018). While children and most adolescents have not yet reached the age of consent, the young person needs to trust that every detail of what they say will not be immediately reported to their parents, if that is the young person's preference. Family-focused approaches will also include providing psychoeducation for family members, ensuring the family has practical, social and emotional support, coordinating care and sharing information across services, and enabling family care planning and goal setting.

UPON REFLECTION

Issues of consent with young people

According to Kang and Sanders (n.d.), in Australia, minors have the legal capacity to make their own decisions regarding their health, independently of their parents, in various situations. A practitioner must make a case-by-case assessment of whether the young person has sufficient understanding to enable fully understand the health options that are being proposed. If a child is not competent to consent to treatment, and a parent has consented to treatment on their behalf, the parent would be entitled to information about the young person's health care.

In general, if a person is under 14, the parent or guardian's consent is necessary. From around 14 years of age, dependent on:
- the state/territory of residence
- the young person's level of maturity
- the young person's understanding of the proposed treatment and its consequences
- the severity of treatment
- teenagers have the right to consent to simple health (including mental health) interventions.

From 16 years (depending on the state/territory of residence), young people have the same right to consent as adults.

....

QUESTIONS

1. What can health professionals do to improve their knowledge and understanding of the legal and ethical issues when working with young people?

2. What can health professionals do to improve their legal and ethical practice when working with young people?

Family-focused approaches to supporting young people with mental health issues lead to:
- better communication between the practitioner and the young person's family
- decreases in perceived maternal criticism
- more supportive family relationships (García-Carrión et al., 2019).

One reason for including families in assessing a young person with a mental health concern is the information they can provide to assist with the process. Another reason is to engage with them in a partnership that can empower the young person.

Family-inclusive approaches will include providing psychoeducation for family members, ensuring the family has practical, social and emotional support; coordinating care and sharing information across services; and enabling family care planning and goal setting.

Multidisciplinary approaches

Given the complex nature of youth mental health problems and disorders (especially the biopsychosocial interactions), interventions should involve various health professionals from different specialties and disciplines. For example, a young person experiencing depression and substance-use disorders may require support from a medical practitioner (prescription, and monitoring of medication and physical illness), a clinical psychologist (to conduct the individual psychotherapy), a social worker (to assist with any social issues like housing or family conflict), a drug/alcohol service (to provide specialist inpatient treatments), a youth worker (to support access to community-based services like Centrelink and recreational pursuits).

Online interventions

Given the affinity of the average young person with technology, and the level of their interactions with social media, many of the interventions developed for young people are digitally based. Online mental health services for young people include a range of early interventions, health promotion messages, telephone and virtual counselling and support services to young people. Examples of such services include:

- ReachOut (www.au.reachout.com)
- Headspace (www.headspace.org.au)
- Youth Beyond Blue (www.youthbeyondblue.com)
- Kids Helpline (www.kidshelp.com.au)
- Children of Parents with a Mental illness (www.copmi.net.au/kids-young-people).

IN PRACTICE

Cyberbullying, anxiety and depression in children

Kidshelpline (n.d.) defines bullying as an ongoing or repeated misuse of power in relationships, intending to cause deliberate psychological harm. Bullying behaviours can be verbal, physical or social. They can happen at a young person's home, with friends, in a group, on a bus or at school. Bullying behaviours can also occur online.

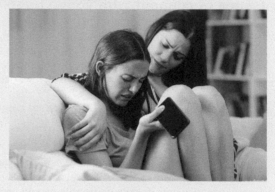

Cyberbullying occurs when someone uses the internet to be mean to a child or young person, leaving the young person to feel bad or upset (eSafety Commissioner, 2021). Some 44 per cent of Australian young people have reported negative online experiences in the last 6 months, including 15 per cent who received threats or abuse online (eSafety Commissioner, 2021).

According to Beyond Blue (2022c), young people who have been or are being bullied can behave in various ways, including:

- not wanting to go to school
- being unusually quiet or secretive
- not having many friends
- becoming more isolated — stop hanging around with friends or lose interest in school or social activities
- seeming over-sensitive or weepy
- having uncharacteristic angry outbursts
- having trouble sleeping
- complaining about having headaches, stomach aches or other physical problems
- being more unhappy or anxious than usual, especially before or after school, sport or wherever the bullying is occurring.

Bullying can lead to anxiety and depression disorders in children and also later in life, in adulthood (Winding et al., 2020). Health professionals can help families to minimise the effects of bullying by supporting them to understand the nature of bullying and why it happens, how to stand up to bullies, and the importance of building resilience. In particular, cyberbullying can be prevented by encouraging the young person or their family to:

- change the settings on the young person's devise so the messages, posts or comments from the cyberbully can't be seen
- collect evidence of the cyberbullying and report the harmful content.

Also encourage the young person to regularly contact Kidshelpline to talk about how they are feeling.

QUESTIONS

1. How can a young person be supported to understand the nature of bullying, why it happens, and how to manage it?

2. What steps can children and families take to build resilience?

SUMMARY

This chapter provided an overview of the major issues related to the care of a person with depression and/or anxiety. This included a discussion of the factors contributing to a person developing depression and anxiety. Following this was an explanation of how to assess for depression and anxiety; and the interventions that can be used to support a person with depression or anxiety, including pharmacological, non-pharmacological and brain stimulation therapies.

There was also a section on perinatal mental health and illness, focusing on experiences of 'baby blues', perinatal anxiety, perinatal depression and puerperal or postnatal psychosis and how health professionals can support the woman and baby. Supporting the mental health of the women's partner and family was then considered.

The final section of the chapter focused on depression and anxiety in young people. The discussion included the importance of implementing early intervention strategies and taking trauma-informed and family-focused approaches.

Depression and anxiety disorders are Australia's most common but treatable mental illnesses. Health professionals who can recognise these conditions in people across the lifespan can ensure that intervention and treatments are provided in a timely way.

KEY TERMS

affective disorder A mental health problem, also called a mood disorder, characterised by a consistent alteration in a person's mood that affects their thoughts, emotions and behaviours. Depression is an affective disorder.

antenatal The period before the birth of a child.

anxiolytic A treatment or approach that reduces anxiety.

baby blues A transient mood change that occurs about four days after the birth of a baby that affects most women.

closed questions Questions that require a single-word response and are useful for eliciting or confirming factual information.

contributing factors The various factors that result from interactions between the mind, body and environment and contribute to a person developing a condition.

depersonalisation A feeling of being able to observe oneself while not having control over what is happening.

derealisation Perceptual disturbance in which the world seems unreal.

dysthymia Mild to moderate depression that occurs for most of the day, more days than not, for at least two years.

hypomania A period of elevated mood which has less impact on functioning than mania.

incidence A measure of the number of new cases of a characteristic that develop in a population in a specified time period.

mania An episode of highly elevated mood which interferes significantly in day-to-day life.

mindfulness A meditation method based on Buddhist principles; the focus is achieving a state of compassionate, non-judgemental awareness in the 'here and now'.

open questions Questions that require a detailed explanation as a response.

perinatal period Generally considered to cover the time from conception to 12 months following childbirth.

perpetuating factors Factors that maintain the problem once it has become established.

postnatal The period after the birth of a child

postpartum Occurring immediately after birth.

post-traumatic stress disorder (PTSD) A diagnosed mental health condition characterised by the development of a long-lasting anxiety reaction following a traumatic or catastrophic event.

precipitating factors Specific events or triggers to the onset of the current problem.

predisposing factors Factors that place a child at risk of developing a problem, such as genetics, life events or temperament.

protective factors Strengths of the young person that reduce the severity of problems and promote healthy and adaptive functioning.

prevalence The proportion of a population who have a specific characteristic in a given time period, regardless of when they first developed the characteristic.

psychoeducation An approach that involves the provision of information to consumers and their carers or significant others regarding signs, symptoms, clinical management, Recovery planning and discharge related to mental health and mental ill-health.

psychotropic medications Medication that is prescribed to alter the mental state of a person and to treat mental illness.

sequelae The consequences of a set of circumstances, particular condition or therapeutic intervention.

somatic Relating to apparent physical symptoms.

REVIEW QUESTIONS

1 What are the main factors that contribute to a person developing depression?
2 What are the symptoms that must be present to diagnose depression?
3 What are the major contributing factors to Aboriginal and Torres Strait Islander peoples developing depression?
4 What is the prevalence of anxiety disorders in Australia?
5 How can anxiety impact the life of a person?
6 What steps can health professionals take to effectively engage with a person experiencing depression and anxiety?
7 How can psychoeducation help a person with anxiety and depression?
8 Why are psychosocial interventions necessary when supporting a person with mild to moderate depression and/or anxiety?
9 What is the most common antidepressant prescribed in Australia and what are the side effects?
10 How can health professionals help a person with a CALD background manage the side effects of antidepressant medications?
11 What are the factors that contribute to a woman developing postnatal depression?
12 Why are trauma-informed, family-focused approaches necessary when supporting young people with mental health concerns?

DISCUSSION AND DEBATE

1 Think of someone you know (of) who may have had depression. What was the hardest aspect of the experience for them? How could they have been more effectively supported?
2 Depression is more common among females than males in Australia. What are the possible reasons for this?
3 Avoidance is a common behavioural response to experiences of anxiety disorders. Discuss the consequence and impact of avoidance on the ability of a person to function in their daily life.
4 Why do many people seem keen to stop taking antidepressant medication as soon as they begin to feel better?
5 Many people view brain stimulation therapies with suspicion. What are the potential causes of and solutions for this suspicion?
6 Discuss what could be done in Australia to support new mothers at risk of developing postnatal depression in the context of limited resources and shrinking health budgets.
7 Discuss how a woman with puerperal psychosis could be supported to bond with her baby if she has negative delusions about herself or her baby. In your discussion, include the practical steps required to protect the baby.
8 What are the risk factors for developing depression for young people in rural and remote areas or from culturally and linguistically diverse locations? How can these risk factors be addressed?

PROJECT ACTIVITY

Have a look at a variety of fact sheets on credible websites that explain depression. Websites such as Beyond Blue and the Black Dog Institute are useful to begin with — both sites have clear and simple information. Once you have familiarised yourself with this information, work out how you could use this when planning or implementing care. In your considerations, you may want to think about the various consumers and carers that may present to you and reflect on how you could adapt the information according to age, cultural background and diversity.

WEBSITES

1 Beyond Blue is a national, independent, not-for-profit organisation working to address issues associated with depression, anxiety and related disorders in Australia. The website provides information about anxiety, depression and suicide to the Australian community: www.beyondblue.org.au.

2 The Black Dog Institute is an independent not-for-profit, educational, medical, research, clinical and community-oriented facility offering specialist expertise in depression, anxiety and bipolar disorder: www.blackdoginstitute.org.au.

3 Centre for Clinical Interventions (CCI) is a specialist program that conducts clinically applied psychosocial research, training and supervision for various psychological interventions. CCI offers a clinical service for adults with anxiety, mood and eating disorders. Its website contains comprehensive resources (research and clinical) for both health professionals and consumers: www.cci.health.wa.gov.au.

4 Headspace is a national initiative that provides both internet- and community-based resources for young people. This service provides information about the various issues faced by youth and provides an opportunity to locate and easily access information and appropriate support services: www.headspace.org.au.

5 Everymind deliver mental health and suicide prevention programs. Their mission is to prevent mental ill-health and suicide through world-leading programs and research with the website containing a range of resources: www.everymind.org.au.

6 Mind covers postnatal depression and other perinatal mental health problems, including causes, support and treatment options. Information for friends and family, including partners, is also provided: www.mind.org.uk/information-support/types-of-mental-health-problems/postnatal-depression-and-perinatal-mental-health/about-maternal-mental-health-problems.

7 National Institute of Mental Health (NIMH) leads research on mental disorders and the website contains a range of resources on depression (www.nimh.nih.gov/health/topics/depression#part_2256), anxiety (www.nimh.nih.gov/health/topics/anxiety-disorders) and perinatal depression (www.nimh.nih.gov/health/publications/perinatal-depression).

8 National Institute of for Health and Care Excellence (NICE) treatment and management guidelines include identifying, treating and managing depression in people aged 18 and over(www.nice.org.uk/guidance/ng222) and anxiety disorders in adults, young people and children in primary, secondary and community care (www.nice.org.uk/guidance/qs53). There guidelines cover recognising, assessing and treating mental health problems in women who are planning to have a baby, are pregnant or have had a baby or been pregnant in the past year (www.nice.org.uk/guidance/cg192).

9 ReachOut is a national site specifically designed for young people to access information on a variety of topics and available sources of help. The site also provides opportunities for young people to openly discuss their own issues in a safe and secure way: www.au.reachout.com.

REFERENCES

Alavi, M., Hunt, G., Thapa, D., & Cleary, M. (2022). Conducting systematic reviews of the quality and psychometric properties of health-related measurement instruments: Finding the right tool for the job. *Issues in Mental Health Nursing*, *43*(4), 317–322. https://doi.org/10.1080/01612840.2021.1978599

Allied Health Professions (AHP) Outcome Measures UK Working Group. (2019). *Key questions to ask when selecting outcome measures: A checklist for allied health professionals.* www.rcslt.org/wp-content/uploads/media/docs/selecting-outcome-measures.pdf

American Psychiatric Association. (2013). *Diagnostic and statistical manual of mental disorders: DSM-5* (5th ed.).

American Psychological Association. (2022). *Depression assessment instruments.* www.apa.org/depression-guideline/assessment

Askey-Jones, R., & Hailes, K. (2020). Exploring the benefits of a psychoeducation session for patients with Chronic Obstructive Pulmonary Disease (COPD) and co-morbid depression and/or anxiety. *Mental Health Practice*, *24*(4), 24–31. https://doi.org/10.7748/mhp.2020.e1435

Atzl, V., Narayan, A., Ballinger, A., Harris, W., & Lieberman, A. (2021). Maternal pregnancy wantedness and perceptions of paternal pregnancy wantedness: Associations with perinatal mental health and relationship dynamics. *Maternal & Child Health Journal, 25*(3), 450–459. https://doi.org/10.1007/s10995-020-03084-1

Austin, M.-P., Highet, N., & The Expert Working Group. (2017). *Mental health care in the perinatal period: Australian clinical practice guideline. Centre of Perinatal Excellence.* www.cope.org.au/wp-content/uploads/2017/10/Final-COPE-Perinatal-Mental-Health-Guideline.pdf

Australian Bureau of Statistics. (2018). *Mental and behavioural conditions. National Health Survey: First Results, 2017–18 (cat. no. 4364. 0.55.001).* www.abs.gov.au/statistics/health/health-conditions-and-risks/national-health-survey-first-results/latest-release

Australia Bureau of Statistics. (2019). *Causes of Death, Australia, 2019, Cat no. 3303.0, Canberra: ABS.* www.abs.gov.au/statistics/health/causes-death/causes-death-australia/2019

Australian Bureau of Statistics. (2022). *National study of mental health and wellbeing 2020–21.* www.abs.gov.au/statistics/health/mental-health/national-study-mental-health-and-wellbeing/latest-release#data-download

Australian Commission on Safety and Quality in Health Care. (2017). *Consumer health information needs and preferences: Perspective of culturally and linguistically diverse and Aboriginal and Torres Strait Islander people.* www.safetyandquality.gov.au/sites/default/files/migrated/Consumer-needs-and-preferences-Perspectives-of-culturally-and-linguistically-diverse-and-Aboriginal-and-Torres-Strait-Islanders.pdf

Australian Commission on Safety and Quality in Health Care. (2022). *Patient-reported outcome measures.* Australian Government. www.safetyandquality.gov.au/our-work/indicators-measurement-and-reporting/patient-reported-outcome-measures

Australian Institute of Health and Welfare. (2022a). *Australia's children.* Australian Government. www.aihw.gov.au/reports/children-youth/australias-children/contents/health/children-mental-illness

Australian Institute of Health and Welfare. (2022b). *Suicide & self harm monitoring. Deaths by suicide among young people.* www.aihw.gov.au/suicide-self-harm-monitoring/data/populations-age-groups/suicide-among-young-people

Australian Institute of Health and Wellbeing. (2018). *The Aboriginal and Torres Strait Islander adolescent and youth health and well-being 2018.* Australian Government. www.aihw.gov.au/reports/indigenous-australians/atsi-adolescent-youth-health-wellbeing-2018/contents/summary

Australian Mental Health Outcomes and Classification Network. (2022). *About AMHOCN.* Australian Government. www.amhocn.org/background/about-amhocn

Bai, Z., Luo, S., Zhang, L., Wu, S., & Chi, I. (2020). Acceptance and Commitment Therapy (ACT) to reduce depression: A systematic review and meta-analysis. *Journal of Affective Disorders, 260,* 728–737. https://doi.org/10.1016/j.jad.2019.09.040

Beck, A. (1970/2006). *Depression: Causes and treatment.* University of Pennsylvania Press.

Bernecker, S., Williams, J., Caporale-Berkowitz, N., Wasil, A., & Constantino, M. (2020). Nonprofessional peer support to improve mental health: Randomized trial of a scalable web-based peer counseling course. *Journal of Medical Internet Research, 22*(9), e17164. https://doi.org/10.2196/17164

Berry Street. (2022). *Therapeutic services for children, young people and families.* www.berrystreet.org.au/what-we-do/trauma-services/therapeutic-services-for-children-young-people-and-families

Beyond Blue. (n.d.). *Risk factors for suicide.* www.healthyfamilies.beyondblue.org.au/age-13/mental-health-conditions-in-young-people/suicide/risk-factors-for-suicide

Beyond Blue. (2020). *GAD. What is generalised anxiety disorder (GAD)?* www.beyondblue.org.au/the-facts/anxiety/types-of-anxiety/gad.

Beyond Blue. (2022a). *Anxiety.* www.beyondblue.org.au/the-facts/anxiety

Beyond Blue (2022b) *Medical treatments for depression.* Retrieved from: www.beyondblue.org.au/the-facts/depression/treatments-for-depression/medical-treatments-for-depression

Beyond Blue. (2022c). *Dealing with bullying.* www.healthyfamilies.beyondblue.org.au/age-6-12/raising-resilient-children/dealing-with-bullying

Black Dog Institute. (n.d.). *Facts and figures about mental health.* www.blackdoginstitute.org.au/wp-content/uploads/2020/04/1-facts_figures.pdf

Black Dog Institute. (2020). *St John's Wort as a depression treatment.* www.blackdoginstitute.org.au/wp-content/uploads/2022/06/St-Johns-Worts-treatment.pdf

Black Dog Institute. (2022). *Causes of depression.* www.blackdoginstitute.org.au/resources-support/depression/causes

Blue Knot Foundation. (2021). *Empowering recovery from complex trauma. National Centre of Excellence for Complex Trauma.* www.blueknot.org.au

Bohren, M. A., Berger, B. O., Munthe-Kaas, H., & Tunçalp, Ö. (2019, March 18). Perceptions and experiences of labour companionship: A qualitative evidence synthesis. *Cochrane Library: Cochrane Reviews, 3*(3), CD012449. https://doi.org/10.1002/14651858

Bronfenbrenner, U. (1979). *The ecology of human development: Experiments by nature and design.* Harvard University.

Brown, S., Mensah, F., Giallo, R., Woolhouse, H., Hegarty, K., Nicholson, J., & Gartland, D. (2020). Intimate partner violence and maternal mental health ten years after a first birth: An Australian prospective cohort study of first-time mothers. *Journal of Affective Disorders, 262,* 247–257. https://doi.org/10.1016/j.jad.2019.11.015

Carr, A. (2019). Couple therapy, family therapy and systemic interventions for adult-focused problems: The current evidence base. *Journal of Family Therapy, 41,* 492–536. https://doi.org/10.1111/1467-6427.12225

Cena, L., Mirabella, F., Palumbo, G., Gigantesco, A., Trainini, A., & Stefana, A. (2021). Prevalence of maternal antenatal and postnatal depression and their association with sociodemographic and socioeconomic factors: A multicentre study in Italy. *Journal of Affective Disorders, 15*(279), 217–221. https://doi.org/10.1016/j.jad.2020.09.136

Centre of Best Practice in Aboriginal and Torres Strait Islander Suicide Prevention. (n.d.). *Prevention.* www.cbpatsisp.com.au/clearing-house/best-practice-programs-and-services/programs-for-preventing-youth-suicide

Chambers, M. (Ed.). (2017). *Psychiatric and mental health nursing: The craft of caring* (3rd ed.). Hodder Arnold.

Charles, J., & Fazeli, M. (2017). Depression in children. *Australian Family Physician*, *46*(12), 901–907. www.racgp.org.au/afp/20 17/december/depression-in-children

Cherry, K. (2021). Development psychology. *Verywellmind*. www.verywellmind.com/developmental-psychology-4157180

Cho, Y., Lee, J., Kim, D., Park, J., Choi, M., Kim, H., Nam, M.-J., Lee, K.-U., Han, K., & Park, Y.-G. (2019). Factors associated with quality of life in patients with depression: A nationwide population-based study. *PloS One*, *14*(7), e0219455. https://doi.org/10.1371/journal.pone.0219455

Chowdhury, M. (2022). *What is client engagement in therapy and how to apply it?* Positive Psychology. www.positivepsychology.com/client-engagement

Cipriani, A., Furukawa, R., Salanti, G., Chaimani, A., Atkinson, L., Ogawa, Y., Leucht, S., Ruhe, H. G., Turner, E. H., Higgins, J. P. T., Egger, M., Takeshima, N., Hayasaka, Y., Imai, H., Shinohara, K., Tajika, A., Ioannidis, J. P. A., & Geddes, J. R. (2018). Comparative efficacy and acceptability of 21 antidepressant drugs for the acute treatment of adults with major depressive disorder: A systematic review and network meta-analysis. *The Lancet*, *391*(10128), 1357–1366. https://doi.org/10.1016/S0140-6736(17)32802-7

Coates, D., & Foureur, M. (2019). The role and competence of midwives in supporting women with mental health concerns during the perinatal period: A scoping review. *Health & Social Care in the Community*, *27*(4), e389–e405. https://doi.org/0.1111/hsc.12740

Colizzi, M., Lasalvia, A., & Ruggeri, M. (2020). Prevention and early intervention in youth mental health: Is it time for a multidisciplinary and trans-diagnostic model for care? *International Journal of Mental Health Systems*, *14*, 23. https://doi.org/10.1186/s13033-020-00356-9

Cox, J., Holden, J. & Sagovsky, R. (1987). Detection of postnatal depression: Development of the 10-item Edinburgh postnatal depression scale. *British Journal of Psychiatry*, *150*, 782–786

de Sousa, G., Lima-Araújo, de., G., de Araújo, D, & de Sousa, M. (2021). Brief mindfulness-based training and mindfulness trait attenuate psychological stress in university students: A randomized controlled trial. *BMC Psychology*, *9*, 21. https://doi.org/10.1186/s40359-021-00520-x

Deas, J. (2017). Puerperal psychosis: Critical analysis of a case study. *MIDIRS Midwifery Digest*, *27*(3), 339–344. www.britishjour nalofmidwifery.com/content/clinical-practice/postpartum-psychosis-and-management-a-case-study

del Corral Serrano, J. (2019). Puerperal psychosis. In M. Sáenz-Herrero (Ed.), *Psychopathology in women: Incorporating gender perspective into descriptive psychopathology* (2nd ed., pp. 581–594). Springer Nature Switzerland.

Department of Health. (2015a). *Mental health outcome measures use in Victoria*. Victoria State Government. www.health.vic.gov.au/practice-and-service-quality/mental-health-outcome-measures-used-in-victoria

Department of Health. (2015b). *Screening and assessment*. Victoria State Government. www.health.vic.gov.au/patient-care/screeni ng-and-assessment

Department of Health. (2019). *Prioritising mental health – Perinatal mental health and wellbeing program*. Australian Government. www.health.gov.au/sites/default/files/prioritising-mental-health-perinatal-mental-health-and-wellbeing-program_0.pdf

Dickson, J., Cruise, K., McCall, C., & Taylor, P. (2019). A systematic review of the antecedents and prevalence of suicide, self-harm and suicide ideation in Australian Indigenous Australian youth. *International Journal of Environmental Research and Public Health*, *16*, 3154. https://doi.org/10.3390/ijerph16173154

Durmaz, H., & Okanli, A. (2021). Effects of Interpersonal Psychotherapy (IPT) techniques and psychoeducation on self-efficacy and care burden in families of patients with schizophrenia. *American Journal of Family Therapy*, *49*(4), 373–391. https://doi.org/10.1080/01926187.2020.1820401

Emerging Minds. (2018). *Engagement. Engaging with families and children*. www.emergingminds.com.au/families/

eSafety Commissioner. (2021). *Cyber bullying*. Australian Government. www.esafety.gov.au/key-issues/cyberbullying

Fairbrother, N., Janssen, P., Antony, M., Tucker, E., & Young, A. (2016). Perinatal anxiety disorder prevalence and incidence. *Journal of Affective Disorder*, *200*, 148–155. https://doi.org/10.1016/j.jad.2015.12.082

Fatori, D., Zuccolo, P., & Polanczyk, G. (2020). A global challenge: Maternal depression and offspring mental disorders. *European Child and Adolescent Psychiatry*, *29*, 569–571. https://doi.org/10.1007/s00787-020-01556-x

Fitzgerald, P., George, M., & Pridmore, S. (2022). The evidence is in: Repetitive transcranial magnetic stimulation is an effective, safe and well-tolerated treatment for patients with major depressive disorder. *Australian & New Zealand Journal of Psychiatry*, *56*(7), 745–751. https://doi.org/10.1177/00048674211043047

Gabriel, F., de Melo, D., Fráguas, R., Leite-Santos, N., Mantovani da Silva, R. (2020). Pharmacological treatment of depression: A systematic review comparing clinical practice guideline recommendations. *PLoS ONE*, *15*(4), e0231700. https://doi.org/10.1371/journal.pone.0231700

Gabriel, M., & Sharma, V. (2017). Antidepressant discontinuation syndrome. *Canadian Medical Association Journal*, *189*(21), ee747. https://doi.org/10.1503/cmaj.160991

Galante, J., Friedrich, C., Dawson, A., Modrego-Alarcón, M., Gebbing, P., Delgado-Suárez, I., Gupta, R., Dean, L., Dalgleish, T., White, I. R., & Jones, P. B. (2021). Mindfulness-based programmes for mental health promotion in adults in nonclinical settings: A systematic review and meta-analysis of randomized controlled trials. *PLoS Medicine*, *18*(1), 1–40. https://doi.org/10.1371/journal.pmed.1003481

García-Carrión, R., Villarejo-Carballido, B., & Villardón-Gallego, L. (2019). Children and adolescents mental health: A systematic review of interaction-based interventions in schools and communities. *Frontiers in Psychology*, *10*, 918. https://doi.org/10.3389/fpsyg.2019.00918

Gautam, M., Tripathi, A., Deshmukh, D., & Gaur, M. (2020). Cognitive behavioral therapy for depression. *Indian Journal of Psychiatry*, *62*(Suppl. 2), S223–S229. https://doi.org/10.4103/psychiatry.IndianJPsychiatry_772_19

Gilbody, S., Peckham, E., Bailey, D., Arundel, C., Heron, P., Crosland, S., Fairhurst, C., Hewitt, C., Li, J., Parrott, S., Bradshaw, T., Horspool, M., Hughes, E., Hughes, T., Ker, S., Leahy, M., McCloud, T., Osborn, D., Reilly, J. . . . Vickers, C. (2019). Smoking cessation for people with severe mental illness (SCIMITAR+): A pragmatic randomised controlled trial. *The Lancet Psychiatry*, *6*(5), 379–390. https://doi.org/10.1016/S2215-0366(19)30047-1

Glasofer, D. (2022). Generalized anxiety disorder: Symptoms and DSM-5 diagnosis. *Verywell Mind*. www.verywellmind.com/dsm -5-criteria-for-generalized-anxiety-disorder-1393147

Gouveia, F., Davidson, B., Meng, Y., Gidyk, D., Rabin, J., Ng, E., Abrahao, A., Lipsman, N., Giacobbe, P., & Hamani, C. (2020). Treating post-traumatic stress disorder with neuromodulation therapies: Transcranial magnetic stimulation, transcranial direct current stimulation, and deep brain stimulation. *Neurotherapeutics*, *17*(4), 1747–1756. https://doi.org/10.1007/s13311-020-00871-0

Gray, A., Steel, A., & Adams, J. (2019). A critical integrative review of complementary medicine education research: Key issues and empirical gaps. BMC. *Complementary and Alternative Medicine*, *19*, 73. https://doi.org/10.1186/s12906-019-2466-z

Hanley, J., & Williams, M. (2020). Fathers' perinatal mental health. *British Journal of Midwifery*, *28*(2), 84–85. https://doi.org/10.12968/bjom.2020.28.2.84

Harvard Health. (2021). *The power of the placebo effect*. Harvard Health Publishing. www.health.harvard.edu/mental-health/the-power-of-the-placebo-effect

Headspace. (2021). *Understanding anxiety – For family and friends*. National Youth Mental Health Foundation. www.headspace. org.au/explore-topics/supporting-a-young-person/anxiety

Healthdirect. (2020). *Depression*. Australian Government. www.healthdirect.gov.au/depression#symptoms

Hunt, G., Malhi, G., Lai, H., & Cleary, M. (2020). Prevalence of comorbid substance use in major depressive disorder in community and clinical settings, 1990–2019: Systematic review and meta-analysis. *Journal of Affective Disorders*, *266*, 288–304. https://doi.org/10.1016/j.jad.2020.01.141

Iannelli, V. (2021). Anxiety symptoms in children. *Verywellmind*. www.verywellmind.com/anxiety-symptoms-2633863

Jung, J., & Cho, S. (2020). The effects of depression, anxiety, and parents' support on suicide ideation and attempts by gender among Korean adolescents. *Journal of Child and Family Studies*, *29*(5), 1458–1466. https://doi.org/10.1007/s10826-020-01697-2

Kang, M., & Sanders, J. (n.d). *Section 3.5. Medico-legal issues. Youth health resource kit*. NSW Health. www.health.nsw.gov.au/ kidsfamilies/youth/Documents/youth-health-resource-kit/youth-health-resource-kit-sect-3-chap-5.pdf

Karunamuni, N., & Weerasekera, R. (2019). *Theoretical foundations to guide mindfulness meditation: A path to wisdom. Current Psychology*, *38*(3), 627–646. https://doi.org/10.1007/s12144-017-9631-7

Kelson, J., Rollin, A., Ridout, B., & Campbell, A. (2019). Internet-delivered acceptance and commitment therapy for anxiety treatment: Systematic review. *Journal of Medical Internet Research*, *21*(1), e12530. https://doi.org/10.2196/12530

Kessler, R., Andrews, G., Colpe, L., Hiripi, E., Mroczek, D., Normand, S., Walters, E., & Zaslavsky, A. (2002). Short screening scales to monitor population prevalences and trends in non-specific psychological distress. *Psychological Medicine*, *32*(6), 959–976. https://doi.org/10.1017/s0033291702006074

Kidshelpline. (n.d.). *Bullying*. www.kidshelpline.com.au/teens/issues/bullying

King Edward Memorial Hospital. (2022). *Statewide Perinatal and Infant Mental Health program (SPIMHP)*. North Metropolitan Health Services, Government of Western Australia. www.kemh.health.wa.gov.au/For-Health-Professionals/SPIMHP

Krol, K., & Grossmann, T. (2018). Psychological effects of breastfeeding on children and mothers. *Bundesgesundheitsblatt Gesundheitsforschung Gesundheitsschutz*, *61*(8), 977–985. https://doi.org/10.1007/s00103-018-2769-0

Lai, H., Cleary, M., Sitharthan, T., & Hunt, G. (2015). Prevalence of comorbid substance use, anxiety and mood disorders in epidemiological surveys, 1990–2014: A systematic review and meta-analysis. *Drug and Alcohol Dependence*, *154*, 1–13. https://doi.org/10.1016/j.drugalcdep.2015.05.031

Lang, M., & Tisher, M. (1983/2004). *Children's Depression Scale (CDS)*. ACER.

Leach, S., Poyser, C., & Fairweather-Schmidt, K. (2017). Maternal perinatal anxiety: A review of prevalence and corre-lates. *Clinical. Psychologist*, *21*(1), 4–19. https://doi.org/10.1111/cp.12058

Leichsenring, F., Steinert, C., Beutel, M., Feix, L., Gündel, H., Hermann, A., Karabatsiakis, A., Knaevelsrud, C., König, H.-H., Kolassa, I. T., Kruse, J., Niemeyer, H., Nöske, F., Palmer, S., Peters, E., Reese, J.-P., Reuss, A., Salzer, S., Schade-Brittinger, C., . . . Hoyer, J. (2020). Trauma-focused psychodynamic therapy and STAIR Narrative Therapy of post-traumatic stress disorder related to childhood maltreatment: Trial protocol of a multicentre randomised controlled trial assessing psychological, neurobiological and health economic outcomes (ENHANCE. *BMJ Open*, *10*(12). https://doi.org/10.1136/bmjopen-2020-040123

Maclean, S. (2020a). Understanding child developed: Ages 0–3 years. *Emerging Minds*. www.emergingminds.com.au/resources/ understanding-child-development-ages-0-3-years

Maclean, S. (2020b). Understanding child developed: Ages 3–5 years. *Emerging Minds*. www.emergingminds.com.au/resources/ understanding-child-development-ages-3-5-years

Maclean, S. (2020c). Understanding child developed: Ages 5–8 years. *Emerging Minds*. www.emergingminds.com.au/resources/ understanding-child-development-ages-5-8-years

Maclean, S. (2020d). Understanding child developed: Ages 9–12 years. *Emerging Minds*. www.emergingminds.com.au/resources/ understanding-child-development-ages-9-12-years/#typical-development-for-children-aged-9-12-years

Malhi, G., Bell, E., Boyce, P., Bassett, D., Bryant, R., Hazell, P., Hopwood, M., Lyndon, B., Mulder, R., Porter, R., Singh, A. B., & Murray, G. (2021). The 2020 Royal Australian and New Zealand College of Psychiatrists clinical practice guidelines for mood disorders. *Australian and New Zealand Journal of Psychiatry*, *55*(1), 7–117. www.ranzcp.org/files/resources/college_ statements/clinician/cpg/mood-disorders-cpg-2020.aspx

Malhi, G., Outhred, T., Hamilton, A., Boyce, P., Bryant, R., Fitzgerald, P., Lyndon, B., Mulder, R., Murray, G., Porter, R., Singh, A., & Fritz, K. (2018). Royal Australian and New Zealand College of Psychiatrists clinical practice guidelines for mood disorders: Major depression summary. *The Medical Journal of Australia*, *208*(4), 175–180. https://doi.org/10.5694/mja17.00659

Martin-Key, N., Spadaro, B., Schei, T., & Bahn, S. (2021). Proof-of-concept support for the development and implementation of a digital assessment for perinatal mental health: Mixed methods study. *Journal of Medical Internet Research*, *23*(6), e27132. https://doi.org/10.2196/27132

McLeish, J., & Redshaw, M. (2017). Mothers' accounts of the impact on emotional wellbeing of organised peer support in pregnancy and early parenthood: A qualitative study. *BMC Pregnancy Childbirth*, *17*, 28. https://doi.org/10.1186/s12884-017-1220-0

Meadows, G., Prodan, A., Patten, S., Shawyer, F., Francis, S., Enticott, J., Rosenberg, S., Atkinson, J.-A., Fossey, E., & Kakuma, R. (2019, September). Resolving the paradox of increased mental health expenditure and stable prevalence. *Australian & New Zealand Journal of Psychiatry*, *53*(9), 844–850. https://doi.org/10.1177/0004867419857821

Mental Health Coordinating Council. (n.d.). *Trauma-Informed Care and Practice (TICP)*. www.mhcc.org.au/wp-content/uploads/2018/05/ticp_awg_position_paper__v_44_final___07_11_13-1.pdf

Mental Health Coordinating Council. (2020). *Chapter 8 Section E: Children and young people with mental health conditions*. https://mhrm.mhcc.org.au/chapters/8-people-with-mental-health-and-co-existing-conditions/8e-children-and-young-people-with-mental-health-conditions

Milan, R., & Vasiliadis, H. (2020). The association between side effects and adherence to antidepressants among primary care community-dwelling older adults. *Aging & Mental Health*, *24*(8), 1229–1236. https://doi.org/10.1080/13607863.2019.1594165

Morgan, A., Wright, J., & Reavley, N. (2021). Review of Australian initiatives to reduce stigma towards people with complex mental illness: What exists and what works? *International Journal of Mental Health Systems*, *15*(1), 10. https://doi.org/10.1186/s13033-020-00423-1

Mulder, R., Boden, J., Carter, J., Luty, S., & Joyce, P. (2017). Ten month outcome of cognitive behavioural therapy v. interpersonal psychotherapy in patients with major depression: A randomised trial of acute and maintenance psychotherapy. *Psychological Medicine*, *47*(14), 2540–2547. https://doi.org/10.1017/S0033291717001106

National Center for Complementary and Integrative Health. (2017). *St John's word and depression: In depth. National Institute of Health, US Department of Health and Human Services*. www.nccih.nih.gov/health/st-johns-wort-and-depression-in-depth

National Health and Medical Research Council. (2021). *Australian guidelines for the prevention and treatment of acute stress disorder, posttraumatic stress disorder and complex PTSD*. Australian Government. www.phoenixaustralia.org/australian-guidelines-for-ptsd

National Health Service. (2021). *Dosage – Antidepressant*. UK Government. www.nhs.uk/mental-health/talking-therapies-medicine-treatments/medicines-and-psychiatry/antidepressants/dosage

National Health Service Scotland Inform. (2022). *Antidepressants*. www.nhsinform.scot/tests-and-treatments/medicines-and-medical-aids/types-of-medicine/antidepressants

National Health Service UK. (2020). *Depression in children and young people*. www.nhs.uk/mental-health/children-and-young-adults/advice-for-parents/children-depressed-signs

National Health Service UK. (2021). *Overview – Antidepressants*. www.nhs.uk/mental-health/talking-therapies-medicine-treatments/medicines-and-psychiatry/antidepressants/overview

National Institute for Health and Care Excellence. (2019). *Depression in children and young people: Identification and management*. www.nice.org.uk/guidance/ng134

National Institute for Health and Care Excellence. (2022). *Depression in adults: Treatment and management*. www.nice.org.uk/guidance/ng222

National Institute of Mental Health. (2016). *Brain stimulation therapies*. National Institute of Health, US Department of Health and Human Services. www.nimh.nih.gov/health/topics/brain-stimulation-therapies/brain-stimulation-therapies

National Institute of Mental Health. (2021). *Chronic illness and mental health: Recognizing and treating depression*. www.nimh.nih.gov/health/publications/chronic-illness-mental-health

National Institute of Mental Health. (2022). *Social anxiety disorder: More than just shyness*. US Department of Health and Human Services. www.nimh.nih.gov/health/publications/social-anxiety-disorder-more-than-just-shyness#

National Mental Health Commission. (2021). *National Children's Mental Health and Wellbeing Strategy*. Australian Government. www.mentalhealthcommission.gov.au/getmedia/9f2d5e51-dfe0-4ac5-b06a-97dbba252e53/National-children-s-Mental-Health-and-Wellbeing-Strategy-FULL

Onycka, I., Collier Høegh, M., Nåheim Eien, E., Nwaru, B., & Melle, I. (2019). Comorbidity of physical disorders among patients with severe mental illness with and without substance use disorders: A systematic review and meta-analysis. *Journal of Dual Diagnosis*, *15*(3), 192–206. https://doi.org/10.1080/15504263.2019.1619007

Open Arms Veterans & Families Counselling. (2019). *Community and peer program*. Department of Veterans Affairs. www.openarms.gov.au/get-support/community-and-peer-program

Orygen. (2017). *Treating depression in young people: Guidance, resources and tools for assessment and management*. Orygen, The National Centre for Excellence in Youth Mental Health. www.orygen.org.au/Training/Resources/Depression/Clinical-practice-points/Treating-depression-in-yp/orygen_Clinical_practice_guide_depression_in_young?ext=

Orygen, & Phoenix Australia. (2018). *Trauma and young people: Moving towards trauma-informed services and systems. Eating depression in young people: Guidance, resources and tools for assessment and management*. Orygen, The National Centre for Excellence in Youth Mental Health & Phoenix Centre for Posttraumatic Mental Health. www.orygen.org.au/Orygen-Institute/Policy-Reports/Trauma-and-young-people-Moving-toward-trauma-info/Orygen_trauma_and_young_people_policy_report?ext=

Palmer Molina, A., Negriff, S., Monro, W., & Mennen, F. (2018). Exploring the relationships between maternal mental health symptoms and young children's functioning in a low-income, minority sample. *Journal of Child & Family Studies*, *27*(12), 3975–3985. https://doi.org/10.1007/s10826-018-1225-y

Perinatal Anxiety and Depression Australia. (n.d.). *Talking about perinatal mental health*. https://panda.org.au/articles/talking-about-perinatal-mental-health

Phoenix Australia. (2021). *Effects of trauma: PTSD*. www.phoenixaustralia.org/recovery/effects-of-trauma/ptsd

Racine, N., Riddell, R., Khan, M., Calic, M., Taddio, A., & Tablon, P. (2016). Systematic review: Predisposing, precipitating, perpetuating, and present factors predicting anticipatory distress to painful medical procedures in children. *Journal of Pediatric Psychology*, *41*(2), 159–181. https://doi.org/10.1093/jpepsy/jsv076

Raising Children Network (Australian). (2021). *Phobias, panic attacks, and post-traumatic stress in children*. The Department of Social Services, Australian Government. www.raisingchildren.net.au/toddlers/health-daily-care/mental-health/phobias-panic-attacks-pts

Raising Children Network (Australian). (2022). *Mental health assessment: Pre-teens and teenagers*. www.raisingchildren.net.au/pre-teens/mental-health-physical-health/mental-health-therapies-services/teen-mental-health-assessment

Richardson, T., & White, L. (2019). The impact of a CBT-based bipolar disorder psychoeducation group on views about diagnosis, perceived recovery, self-esteem and stigma. *Cognitive Behaviour Therapist, 12*, e43. https://doi.org/10.1017/S1754470X19000308

Rogers, C. (1951). *Client-centred therapy: Its current practice, implications and theory*. Houghton Mifflin.

Royal Australian and New Zealand College of Psychiatrists. (2019a). *Guidelines and resources for practice*. www.ranzcp.org/Resources/Statements-Guidelines.aspx

Royal Australian and New Zealand College of Psychiatrists. (2019b). Royal Australian and New Zealand College of Psychiatrists professional practice guidelines for the administration of electroconvulsive therapy. *Australian & New Zealand Journal of Psychiatry, 53*, 609–623. https://doi.org/10.1177/0004867419839139

Royal Australian and New Zealand College of Psychiatrists. (2021). *Perinatal mental health services. Position statement*. www.ranzcp.org/news-policy/policy-and-advocacy/position-statements/perinatal-mental-health-services

Royal Women's Hospital Victoria. (n.d.). *Mental health and pregnancy: Baby blues*. www.thewomens.org.au/health-information/pregnancy-and-birth/mental-health-pregnancy/baby-blues

Sadock, B., Sadock, V., & Ruiz, P. (2017). *Kaplan and Sadock's comprehensive textbook of psychiatry* (10th ed.). Wolters Kluwer.

San Martin Porter, M., Betts, K., Kisely, S., Pecoraro, G., & Alati, R. (2019). Screening for perinatal depression and predictors of underscreening: Findings of the Born in Queensland study. *The Medical Journal of Australia, 210*(1), 32–37. https://doi.org/10.5694/mja2.12030

SANE. (2017). *Complementary therapies*. www.sane.org/information-and-resources/facts-and-guides/complementary-therapies

SANE. (2021). *Electroconvulsive Therapy (ECT)*. https://www.sane.org/information-and-resources/facts-and-guides/treatments-for-mental-illness?highlight=WyJlbGVjdHJvY29udnVsc2l2ZSIsInRoZXJhcHkiLCJ0aGVyYXB5JyIsImVsZWN0cm9jb252dWxzaXZlIHRoZXJhcHkiXQ==

Schimelpfening, N. (2021). *What to know about childhood depression. Verywellmind*. www.verywellmind.com/childhood-depression-1066805

Schuman-Olivier, Z., Trombka, M., Lovas, D., Brewer, J., Vago, D., Gawande, R., Dunne, J., Lazar, S., Loucks, E., & Fulwiler, C. (2020). Mindfulness and behavior change. *Harvard Review of Psychiatry, 28*(6), 371–394. https://doi.org/10.1097/HRP.0000000000000277

Shang, P., Cao, X., You, S., Feng, X., Li, N., & Jia, Y. (2021). Problem-solving therapy for major depressive disorders in older adults: An updated systematic review and meta-analysis of randomized controlled trials. *Aging Clinical & Experimental Research, 33*(6), 1465–1475. https://doi.org/10.1007/s40520-020-01672-3

Snoek, A., Beekman, A., Dekker, J., Aarts, I., van Grootheest, G., Blankers, M., Vriend, C., van den Heuvel, O., & Thomaes, K. (2020). A randomized controlled trial comparing the clinical efficacy and cost-effectiveness of Eye Movement Desensitization and Reprocessing (EMDR) and integrated EMDR-Dialectical Behavioural Therapy (DBT) in the treatment of patients with post-traumatic stress disorder and comorbid (Sub)clinical borderline personality disorder: Study design. *BMC Psychiatry, 20*(1), 396. https://doi.org/10.1186/s12888-020-02713-x

Strawa, C. (2022). *Family-inclusive approaches when working with young people accessing mental health support*. Canberra, Australian Institute of Family Studies, Australian Government. www.aifs.gov.au/resources/short-articles/family-inclusive-approaches-when-working-young-people-accessing-mental

Swami, V., Barron, D., Smith, L., & Furnham, A. (2020). Mental health literacy of maternal and paternal postnatal (post-partum) depression in British adults. *Journal of Mental Health, 29*(2), 217–224. https://doi.org/10.1080/09638237.2019.1608932

Tang, A., & Lee, R. (2021). Effects of a group mindfulness-based cognitive programme on smartphone addictive symptoms and resilience among adolescents: Study protocol of a cluster-randomized controlled trial. *BMC Nursing, 20*, 86. https://doi.org/10.1186/s12912-021-00611-5

Torres-Platas, S.G., Escobar, S., Belliveau, C., Wu, J., Sasi, N., Fotso, J., Potes, A., Thomas, Z., Goodman, A., Looper, K., Segal, M., Berlim, M., Vasudev, A., Moscovitz, N., & Rej, S. (2019). Mindfulness-based cognitive therapy intervention for the treatment of late-life depression and anxiety symptoms in primary care: A randomized controlled trial. *Psychotherapy and Psychosomatics, 88* (4), 254–256. https://doi.org/10.1159/000501214

Tully, P., Ang, S., Lee, E., Bendig, E., Bauereiß, N., Bengel, J., & Baumeister, H. (2021). Psychological and pharmacological interventions for depression in patients with coronary artery disease. *The Cochrane Database of Systematic Reviews, 12*(12), CD008012. https://doi.org/10.1002/14651858.CD008012.pub4

van Erp, N., van Zelst, C., Delespaul, P., Wagemakers, E., van Weeghel, J., Brugmans, J., Bierbooms, J., Rabbers, G., van der Weerd, S., & Kroon, H. (2020). Positive effects of psychoeducation on mental disorders in the Netherlands. *Tijdschrift Voor Psychiatrie, 62*(6), 481–487.

VanderKruik, R., Barreix, M., Chou, D., Allen, T., Say, L., & Cohen, L. (2017). The global prevalence of post-partum psychosis: A systematic review. *BMC Psychiatry, 17*(1), 272. https://doi.org/10.1186/s12888-017-1427-7

Verkleij, M., Georgiopoulos, A., & Friedman, D. (2021). Development and evaluation of an internet-based cognitive behavioral therapy intervention for anxiety and depression in adults with cystic fibrosis (eHealth CF-CBT): An international collaboration. *Internet Interventions, 24*, 100372. https://doi.org/10.1016/j.invent.2021.100372

Wall, L., Higgins, D., & Hunter, C. (2016). *Trauma-informed care in child-family welfare services*. [Child and Family Community Australia Paper No 37]. Australian Institute of Family Studies, Australian Government. www.aifs.gov.au/cfca/publications/trauma-informed-care-child-family-welfare-services

Weiss, A., Hussain, S., Ng, B., Sarma, S., Tiller, J., Waite, S., & Loo, C. (2019). Royal Australian and New Zealand College of Psychiatrists professional practice guidelines for the administration of electroconvulsive therapy. *The Australian and New Zealand Journal of Psychiatry, 53*(7), 609–623. https://doi.org/10.1177/0004867419839139

Winding, T., Skouenborg, L., & Mortensen, V. Andersen, J. H. (2020). Is bullying in adolescence associated with the development of depressive symptoms in adulthood?: A longitudinal cohort study. *BMC Psychology, 8*, 122. https://doi.org/10.1186/s40359-020-00491

Woodgate, L., Tennent, P., Barriatge, S., & Legras, N. (2020). The lived experience of anxiety and the many facets of pain: A qualitative, arts-based approach. *Canadian Journal of Pain, 4*(3), 6–18. https://doi.org/10.1080/24740527.2020.1720501

World Health Organization. (2019). *International statistical classification of diseases and related health problems* (11th ed.). www.who.int/standards/classifications/classification-of-diseases

World Health Organization. (2021). *Depression.* www.who.int/news-room/fact-sheets/detail/depression

Yesavage, J., Brink, T., Rose, T., Lum, O., Huang, V., Adey, M., & Leirer, V. (1983). Development and validation of a geriatric depression screening scale: A preliminary report. *Journal of Psychiatric Research, 17*, 37–49.

Yokoya, S., Maeno, T., Sakamoto, N., Goto, R., & Maeno, T. (2018). Brief survey of public knowledge and stigma towards depression. *Journal of Clinical Medical Research, 10*(3), 202–209. https://doi.org/10.14740/jocmr3282w

Youth Affairs Council of South Australia. (2016). *Better together: A practice guide to effective engagement with young people.* Government of South Australia. www.yacsa.com.au/s/Better-Together-A-Practical-Guide-to-Effective-Engagement-with-Young-People.pdf

Zambrano, J., Celano, C., Januzzi, J., Massey, C., Chung, W., Millstein, R., & Huffman, J. (2020). Psychiatric and psychological interventions for depression in patients with heart disease: A scoping review. *Journal of the American Heart Association, 9*(22), e018686. https://doi.org/10.1161/JAHA.120.018686

ACKNOWLEDGEMENTS

Extract: © The Royal Women's Hospital (n.d) *Mental health and pregnancy: Baby Blues.* Retrieved August 10, 2022 from www.thewomens.org.au/health-information/pregnancy-and-birth/mental-health-pregnancy/baby-blues.

Figure 7.1: © Malhi G, et al. (2021) The 2020 Royal Australian and New Zealand College of Psychiatrists clinical practice guidelines for mood disorders. *Australian & New Zealand Journal of Psychiatry, 55* (1), 7-117.

Photo: © tommaso79 / Shutterstock.com

Photo: © Don Arnold / Getty Images

Photo: © Chinnapong / Shutterstock.com

Photo: © YAKOBCHUK VIACHESLAV / Shutterstock.com

Photo: © shurkin_son/Adobe Stock

Photo: © Brooke Ottley / Shutterstock.com

Photo: © Kei Uesugi/DigitalVision/Getty Images

Photo: © MIA Studio / Shutterstock.com

Photo: © LittlePanda29 / Shutterstock.com

Photo: © Pheelings media / Shutterstock.com

Caring for a person who has self-harmed

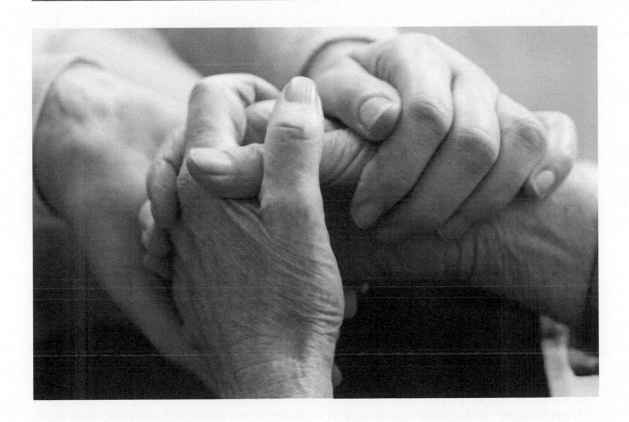

Introduction

Self-harming and suicidal behaviours are major issues for the community, government, health services and professionals across Australia. The annual Australian suicide rate, averaged from 2016 to 2020, is 3099, equating to significantly more deaths per year by suicide than by road or traffic accidents (Australian Institute of Health and Wellbeing [AIHW], 2022a; Bureau of Infrastructure, Transport and Regional Economics, 2022; Life in Mind, 2022a). Outcomes of self-harming behaviour include life-threatening injuries and accidental death (headspace, 2022b). In addition, family and friends of people who suicide or self-harm are at risk of being profoundly affected emotionally and socially (Beyond Blue, 2022a).

This chapter provides definitions for self-harm, suicide and suicidal ideation. It also outlines the incidence of self-harm and suicide in Australia, and the methods by which people choose to self-harm or suicide. The attitudes of the community and health professionals towards people who self-harm or attempt suicide are discussed, as well as how these attitudes impact health care providers. The major components of a suicide risk assessment are outlined. In addition, a description is provided of the ways in which the health professional can provide effective care and treatment to the person with self-harming behaviours, their partner or carer and family members. The chapter concludes by considering how health professionals can support a person who has been bereaved by suicide.

8.1 Definitions

LEARNING OBJECTIVE 8.1 Define deliberate self-harm, suicide and suicidal ideation.

The terms **deliberate self-harm (DSH)** or deliberate self-injury (DSI) are generic phrases used to describe a wide range of self-injurious behaviours. These behaviours can include:
- deliberately cutting the body
- scratching
- hitting
- head banging
- burning and scalding
- hair pulling
- excessive use of substances such as alcohol and illicit drugs
- self-poisoning (overdose)
- jumping from a height or in front of a moving vehicle.

Self-harming behaviours are generally defined as the intentional, direct injuring of body tissue without suicidal intent. Although people who self-harm do not necessarily have suicidal intent (headspace, 2022b), there is a very real possibility that self-harming behaviours could lead to death.

Suicide is the act of a person intentionally causing their own death, while **suicidal ideation** describes the thoughts, ideas or plans a person has about causing their own death. Suicidal behaviours are usually more lethal than self-harming behaviours and could include:
- self-poisoning (overdose)
- jumping from a height or in front of a moving vehicle
- driving a car into a tree at a high speed
- poisoning from gases and vapours (including motor vehicle exhaust)
- use of a lethal weapon
- hanging.

It is interesting to note that a number of self-harming behaviours are also suicidal behaviours. This explains why many people are confused about the difference between self-harm and suicide. The factor that differentiates the two is the motivation behind the act or behaviour.

A person who self-harms does not necessarily wish to die. Rather, people who self-harm are generally trying to express their great emotional pain. By hurting themselves, they are physically expressing what they are feeling, but cannot express in other more constructive ways. Feelings of guilt and shame can also lead some people to use DSH in order to punish themselves (Beyond Blue, 2022b).

Likewise, people who intentionally plan for or cause their own death do not necessarily want to die. Most suicide attempts occur in crisis situations; that is, they are impulsive reactions to personal crises of one form or another. A number of people who have survived suicide attempts have gone on to say their prime motivation was to escape the pain they were feeling at that time, rather than bringing about their own death. Their pain — physical or emotional — and feelings of hopelessness or helplessness were so great that they were unable to see a future for themselves. Escape from the present was the only option they could see at that moment in time. This suggests why it is important for health professionals to support a person through difficult periods or situations. Once a person has developed the skills to deal or cope with the situation and see that there are indeed other options, they can move on with hope into the future.

To clarify the difference between DSH and suicidal behaviour, it is helpful to consider self-harm as an umbrella term for three distinct but overlapping subgroups of self-injurious behaviours. These subgroups are physical self-injury, impulsive self-harm and attempted suicide. Table 8.1 provides a list of the most common forms of self-harming behaviour and their presentation.

TABLE 8.1   Common forms of self-harming behaviours and their presentation

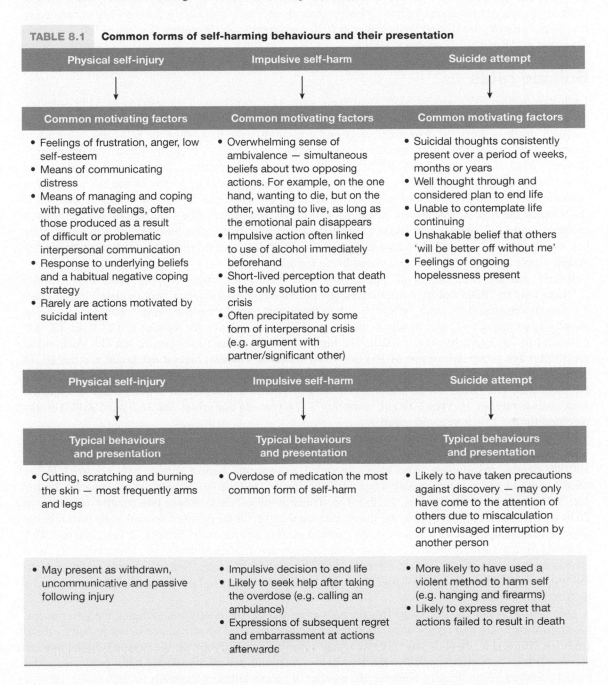

Physical self-injury	Impulsive self-harm	Suicide attempt
Common motivating factors	**Common motivating factors**	**Common motivating factors**
• Feelings of frustration, anger, low self-esteem • Means of communicating distress • Means of managing and coping with negative feelings, often those produced as a result of difficult or problematic interpersonal communication • Response to underlying beliefs and a habitual negative coping strategy • Rarely are actions motivated by suicidal intent	• Overwhelming sense of ambivalence — simultaneous beliefs about two opposing actions. For example, on the one hand, wanting to die, but on the other, wanting to live, as long as the emotional pain disappears • Impulsive action often linked to use of alcohol immediately beforehand • Short-lived perception that death is the only solution to current crisis • Often precipitated by some form of interpersonal crisis (e.g. argument with partner/significant other)	• Suicidal thoughts consistently present over a period of weeks, months or years • Well thought through and considered plan to end life • Unable to contemplate life continuing • Unshakable belief that others 'will be better off without me' • Feelings of ongoing hopelessness present
Physical self-injury	**Impulsive self-harm**	**Suicide attempt**
Typical behaviours and presentation	**Typical behaviours and presentation**	**Typical behaviours and presentation**
• Cutting, scratching and burning the skin — most frequently arms and legs	• Overdose of medication the most common form of self-harm	• Likely to have taken precautions against discovery — may only have come to the attention of others due to miscalculation or unenvisaged interruption by another person
• May present as withdrawn, uncommunicative and passive following injury	• Impulsive decision to end life • Likely to seek help after taking the overdose (e.g. calling an ambulance) • Expressions of subsequent regret and embarrassment at actions afterwards	• More likely to have used a violent method to harm self (e.g. hanging and firearms) • Likely to express regret that actions failed to result in death

It is important to remember that motivations will often overlap and individuals can present with characteristics from each subcategory. For example, a person may regularly self-harm to help them cope with stress. However, one day they may experience a particularly difficult situation, such as the breakdown of a relationship, and be unable to manage their feelings by self-harming. On impulse, they take an overdose of medication that results in their death.

8.2 Incidence of self-harming

LEARNING OBJECTIVE 8.2 Outline the incidence of self-harm and suicide in Australia.

The nature of self-harm suggests some difficulty in precisely identifying its frequency. For example, many episodes of self-harm take place in private and do not come to the attention of health professionals or other record keepers. Likewise, identifying the frequency of death by suicide presents many challenges. For example, unexplained single-vehicle road accidents may be the result of suicide; however, when there is no proof, the cause or manner of death cannot be ascertained. This is particularly relevant when considering that 55 per cent ($n = 604$) of all fatal crashes in 2020 were single-vehicle crashes (Bureau of Infrastructure, Transport and Regional Economics, 2021).

Suicide rates

Each day during 2020, almost nine Australians took their own lives. This resulted in 3139 suicides, accounting for 1.9 per cent of all deaths across the nation. In 2020, suicide was the fifteenth most common cause of death in Australia; however, injury and poisoning, including deliberate self-harm resulting in death, ranked as the third most common cause of death for Aboriginal or Torres Strait Islander peoples between 2015 and 2019 (AIHW, 2022c). Suicide is the leading cause of death for all people in the 15–44-year-old age group; however, the statistical rates change according to gender and age groups. For example, the highest proportion of male suicide deaths occur within the 20–34-year-old age group, while for females the highest rate occurs in the 45–49-year-old age group. The reporting of suicide rates in children aged 5–17 years is rare and not consistent across all jurisdictions; however, 73 per cent of child suicide deaths are in the 15–17-year-old age group. Of major concern, over one-third of all deaths for young people aged 15–24 years are attributable to suicide.

Indeed, suicide rates across all age groups were higher for males (75 per cent) than females (25 per cent) in 2020; that is, Australian males sustain death by suicide at approximately three times the rate of females. This is slightly higher than the global average male-to-female suicide ratio being slightly more than 2 to 1; specifically being 6.3 per 100 000 population for females and 13.9 per 100 000 for males in 2017 (Ritchie et al., 2020). The highest number of male age-specific suicides occurred in the 85-plus age group, with a rate of 36.2 per 100 000 deaths. The next highest age group was the 40–44 year-old group and the 50–54-year old group who both recorded 27.1 per 100 000 deaths, accounting for more than one-quarter of all male suicide deaths. This is in comparison to the lowest age-specific male suicide rates of 16.5 per 100 000, being the 70–74-year-old age group, and 16.9 per 100 000 deaths recorded for the 15–19-year-old group.

For women, the highest age-specific suicide rate occurred in the 45–49-year-old age group with 9.6 per 100 000 deaths, followed by the 25–29 and 30–34-year-old age groups, recording 8.0 and 8.2 per 100 000 deaths, respectively. The lowest recorded age-specific female suicide rate occurred in the 65–69-year-old age group recording 4.6 per 100 000 deaths, and the 70–74-year-old age range at 5.5 per 100 000 deaths (Australian [ABS], 2022a). The standardised suicide incidence rate for all Australians in 2020 was 12.1 per 100 000 deaths; the lowest rate since 2016. Of the people who took their own life, the average median age was 43.4 years old; the average median age for males being 43.6 years old and 43.1 years old for females. This is in comparison to the average age of death related to all causes, being 82 years on average, specifically, 78.9 years for males and 84.6 years for females. Suicide was the cause of death for 1.9 per cent of the population with 1.5 per cent of all male deaths and 0.5 per cent of all female deaths in 2020 (ABS, 2021).

Suicide is a preventable outcome. This suggests an important reason why communities, the government, health professionals, and family and friends who have been affected by suicide are so concerned by these statistics. Much is made of deaths on the roads in Australia — and rightly so. If a person is killed in a car accident, their death is announced on the news across Australia, and an annual road toll is published at the end of each year. Significantly, however, the number of people killed on the roads in 2020 was 1106 — a death toll more than 60 per cent lower than the number of people who died by suicide (ABS, 2021; Bureau of Infrastructure, Transport and Regional Economics, 2021). The Australian public was not made aware of this startling fact in the same way by the media.

Despite the comparable suicide rates of the past few years, it is heartening to know that since the last peak of 14.6 suicide deaths per 100 000 in 1997, the overall suicide rate has fallen, with males having a larger overall suicide reduction rate than females. The finding of a general reduction in overall suicide rates is comparable to most Western countries and should be viewed as a positive result, especially when considering that the suicide rates in the United States for the 2000–2020 period increased by 30 per cent (National Centre for Health Statistics, 2022). One reason for the Australian suicide rate reduction is the **National Suicide Prevention Strategy** and the significant fiscal resources the Commonwealth Government has committed to fund the various programs it administers. More information about the National Suicide Prevention Strategy is provided later in this chapter.

The Australian National Study of Mental Health and Wellbeing 2021

The results of the *National Study of Mental Health and Wellbeing* (ABS, 2022a) highlighted that during the period 2020–21, 16.7 per cent of Australians aged 16–85 years have, at least once in their lives, experienced some form of suicidal ideation. This is an increase from 13.3 per cent in the 2007 National Survey. The report illustrated that 7 per cent of the population in this age group had made a suicide plan, and 4.8 per cent disclosed that they had attempted suicide at least once.

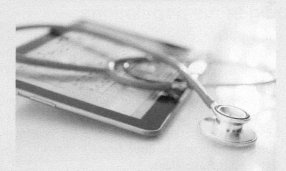

When asked what people had experienced in the 12 months prior to the survey being conducted, rather than across the life span, 3.4 per cent of the total population reported having experienced suicidal thoughts or behaviours. Females (18.7 per cent) had a higher prevalence of experiencing any suicidal thoughts or behaviours in their lifetime when compared to males (14.5 per cent).

The study also ascertained the proportion of Australians who had ever been close to someone who had taken or attempted to take their own life. Almost two in five (38.0 per cent) people aged 16–85 years had been close to someone who had taken or attempted to take their own life, while 5.9 per cent had been close to someone who had taken or attempted to take their own life in the last 12 months.

The study also collected statistics on self-harming behaviours and reported that 8.8 per cent of Australians aged 16–85 years stated that they had self-harmed at some point in their lifetime. Similarly to suicidal thoughts and behaviours, females recorded higher lifetime rates of self-harm than males (11.4 per cent versus 6.2 per cent).

Roughly one quarter (24.7 per cent) of all females aged 16–34 years had self-harmed in their lifetime, with one in fourteen (7.0 per cent) of this cohort disclosing self-harming behaviours in the last 12 months.

These alarming statistics illustrate that the overall mental health and wellbeing of Australians has declined since the last national study in 2007 (ABS, 2022a).

Rates of self-harm

The incidence of self-harm is currently measured by the number of people who present to an emergency department or other health setting and seek assistance from a health professional. Currently, there is a long-term trend of increasing hospital admissions for intentional self-harm for young women (AIHW, 2022a). During 2020–21, there were 29 910 hospital admissions for DSH. This represents roughly 25 per cent more admissions than for admissions related to injuries related to assault and homicide (AIHW, 2022b). These statistics need to be considered in the context of COVID-19 consequences, especially financial insecurity, reduced social contact and freedom-of-movement restrictions (Klenthis, 2021).

People admitted to hospitals in Australia with a primary diagnosis of intentional self-harm during the 2019–20 period accounted for 5.3 per cent of all injury hospitalisations and 24 per cent of all injury deaths in Australia (AIHW, 2022d). These admissions included people who had **attempted suicide** and those who intentionally hurt themselves but did not intend to kill themselves. It has been noted that DSH is a significant risk factor for repeated DSH and suicide (ABS, 2022a).

Other significant statistics related to DSH include the following (AIHW, 2022a).

- Females are admitted to hospital at more than double the rate of males for DSH, with a male-to-female ratio of 1 to 2.0. The incidence of DSH is higher in every age group for females up to the 75-plus age group, where the incidence for males is higher than females.
- The highest prevalence of DSH for all genders occurred in the 15–19-year-old age group bracket, at a rate of 698 instances per 100 000 population for females, with males recording 174 per 100 000 population.

- The next highest age group was 20–24-year-old with females having a higher prevalence of DSH being 363 per 100 000 as compared to 166 per 100 000 instances for males.
- The self-harm rate for females aged 0–14 increased from 41 per 100 000 population in 2019–20 to 70 in 2020–21.

There is clearly a need for ongoing research to identify the predisposing factors for these age groups at highest risk. These factors are discussed in more detail in the following sections of this chapter.

Alarmingly, there continues to be ongoing reports citing negative and pessimistic attitudes from health professionals towards people who self-harm (Gibson et al., 2019). The interventions and strategies a health professional can use to effectively care for and support people who have self-harming behaviours are outlined later in this chapter.

Indigenous populations

As noted in the chapter on delivering culturally appropriate mental health care, the suicide rate of Australia's Indigenous peoples is much higher than that of non-Indigenous Australians (AIHW, 2022c).

- Suicide accounts 6 per cent of all deaths in Aboriginal and Torres Strait Islander peoples compared to 2 per cent for non-Indigenous Australians.
- Suicide is the second leading cause of death for Indigenous males.
- Suicide is the seventh leading cause of death for Indigenous females.
- Suicide is the leading cause of death for Indigenous peoples aged 15 to 35.
- Suicide death rate is three times higher for Indigenous peoples aged 15 to 35 compared to non-Indigenous Australians.
- 40 per cent of deaths in Indigenous youth aged 5 to 17 were caused by suicide.
- 23 per cent of all suicide deaths in the 5–17 year age group were Indigenous youths.
- Intentional self-harm in youth aged 15 to 24 is five times higher in Indigenous youth compared to non-Indigenous youth in Australia (Everymind, 2022).

This trend is of great concern to health professionals, health services, governments and communities. The Australian government is committed to reducing suicide rates within Aboriginal and Torres Strait Islander communities through increased resourcing and suicide prevention activities specific to these communities. In May 2013, the Australian government released the first National Aboriginal and Torres Strait Islander Suicide Prevention Strategy, with the aim to achieve measurable improvements over a 10-year period (Department of Health, 2013). The strategy identifies six broad action areas.

1. Building strengths and capacity in Aboriginal and Torres Strait Islander communities.
2. Building strengths and resilience in individuals and families.
3. Targeted suicide prevention services.
4. Coordinating approaches to prevention.
5. Building the evidence base and disseminating information.
6. Standards and quality in suicide prevention (Department of Health, 2013).

Since 2013, ongoing strategies and policies have been developed to reduce Indigenous suicide rates, including the National Strategic Framework for Aboriginal and Torres Strait Islander Peoples Mental Health and Social and Emotional Wellbeing 2017–23 and the 2017 Fifth National Mental Health and Suicide Prevention Plan and Implementation Plan. Gayaa Dhuwi (Proud Spirit) Australia (GDPSA) was established in 2020 as the new national Indigenous social and emotional wellbeing, mental health and suicide prevention leadership body. The Australian health landscape has changed significantly in the past decade and as a consequence, the government has commissioned GDPSA to review and revise the National Aboriginal and Torres Strait Islander Suicide Prevention Strategy. This review is currently in progress, with many community consultations occurring in 2020 and 2021 (Gayaa Dhuwi (Proud Spirit) Australia, 2020).

Methods of self-harm

From a clinical perspective, injuries sustained from self-harming behaviours may be minor, moderate, serious or potentially life threatening. Self-harming behaviours include poisoning by drugs, poisoning by other methods (including alcohol, gases and vapours, and motor vehicle exhaust), hanging, strangulation and suffocation, drowning and submersion behaviours, firearm presentations, contact with sharp objects, and falls and jumping from a high place. Other less common causes include explosives, smoke/fire/flames, blunt objects, jumping or lying before a moving object, intentional crashing of a motor vehicle and other unspecified means (ABS, 2021). Globally, ingestion of pesticides, hanging and firearms are among the most common methods used (WHO, 2021).

In Australia , hanging is the most common method of suicide for both genders and it accounts for more than half of all suicide deaths. The rate of intentional hanging has been steadily increasing since the late 1980s for males and females, while other methods of suicide have decreased. In 2020, almost two-thirds (61 per cent) of male deaths by suicide and half (52 per cent) of all deaths by suicide in females were due to hanging.

Conversely, rates of suicide by use of firearms declined steeply for both males and females from 1987 and continued to decline from 1996, coinciding with the introduction of gun control restrictions and reforms.

In 2020, poisoning by substances (excluding gas) was the second most common means of suicide among females, accounting for almost a third of female deaths by suicide each year for the last decade (ABS, 2021a).

The methods by which people self-harm are significant to health professionals because they affect whether or not the person presents to a health service for assistance. For example, health professionals who work in intensive care units will often have to care for or treat a person who has deliberately taken an overdose of medication. Likewise, people who use more violent or high-impact methods, such as those that involve vehicles, weapons or hanging, may require critical care in the first instance, then long-term rehabilitative care. It is also important to identify the preferred method of the person with self-harming behaviours, as this will impact their level of risk.

UPON REFLECTION

Methods of suicide: Do we need to know?

Mindframe supports safe media reporting, portrayal and media communication about suicide, mental ill-health, alcohol and other drugs. The Australian Government supports this principle and has restricted access to specific details of annual suicide deaths to the general public. However, from a primary health care perspective, should we have access to this information?

QUESTIONS

1. Discuss how the with holding of information regarding the classification causes of suicide deaths might impact the development of suicide prevention strategies, plans and frameworks.
2. Comment on the actual and potential difficulties in the identification of potential risks given the minimisation of modes of suicide information.
3. What foreseeable issues can be anticipated concerning the restriction of access to implements, drugs, objects and so on, when the proportion of deaths occurring by these means are not known?

8.3 'Causes' of self-harming behaviour

LEARNING OBJECTIVE 8.3 Describe factors that may contribute to self-harming behaviours.

According to the Black Dog Institute (2022), the causes of suicide and self-harming behaviours are complex; contributing indicators include:
- stressful life events
- mental illness
- physical illness
- trauma
- poor living circumstances
- drug or alcohol abuse.

In short, it would seem that there is no single cause of self-harm or suicide.

Although it is important that health professionals work within a framework of person-centred care that will assess each person as an individual and according to that person's own unique set of circumstances, it can also be helpful to identify general trends. These trends are called **predisposing causes, precipitating influences** and **perpetuating factors**, which fall under the domains of social, psychological and interpersonal.

Predisposing causes are the factors that render the person liable or more prone to a particular behaviour. They are usually a part of the person's background or previous experiences and cannot be changed. For example, past childhood sexual assault is a common predisposing factor in people who self-harm (Scocco et al., 2019). Even so, the way in which the person responds to these predisposing causes can be changed or managed. Precipitating influences are the catalysts of the behaviour. They are not the underlying causes, but rather the influences or triggers that elicit or provoke the behaviour in the 'here and now'. They are difficult to predict and will often just happen; however, like predisposing causes, they can usually be managed. Finally, perpetuating factors are those that promote or support a continuation of the behaviour. These are the factors that a person has the potential to both manage or control and change.

The major predisposing, precipitating and perpetuating factors related to self-harm and suicide are listed in table 8.2. They have been categorised according to the social, psychological and interpersonal aspects of a person's life. Mental health and physical risk factors are discussed further on in this section.

TABLE 8.2   **Predisposing, precipitating and perpetuating factors relating to self-harm and suicide**

	Predisposing	Precipitating	Perpetuating
Social	Family history of self-harm and suicide Abuse as a child, particularly sexual abuse Homelessness Physical illness	Entering care Parents divorcing Bereavement Rape and sexual assault Unplanned/unwanted pregnancy Significant financial problems Lack of availability of specialist help for high-risk individuals	Being bullied Unresolved housing, employment and financial problems Ready availability of potentially lethal means of self-harm (e.g. over-the-counter analgesics)
Psychological	Family history of mental illness Reduced ability to regulate emotions Poor impulse control Low self-esteem	Mental illness (e.g. depression, psychosis) Excessive alcohol Illicit drug use	Intoxication with alcohol and/or illicit drugs Cognitive problems (e.g. negative thinking, thoughts of worthlessness, hopelessness about the future) Believing that their distress or problems are not being taken seriously by others
Interpersonal	Conflict between parents Lack of supportive, close relationship(s) Poor interpersonal problem solving	Perceived stressful situations involving others Relationship breakdown Argument/verbal conflict with partner or significant other	Unresolved conflict with parents Continuing negative experiences of care Ongoing difficulty in communicating feelings

Consideration of the different factors listed in table 8.2 can assist the health professional to understand how a person may reach the point of choosing self-harm or suicide as a way of dealing with a situation. For example, a person may belong to a family where there is a history of suicide; that is, suicide has been modelled to the person as a way of dealing with a difficult situation. This modelling predisposes the person to view suicide as an option when they feel unable to cope with a problem. The person in this example may also have poor impulse control — another factor predisposing them to behave in a certain way.

At the same time, these predisposing causes do not mean that the behaviour is inevitable. The person has choices that can enable them to manage these predisposing factors. However, to use the same example, one day the person consumes excessive amounts of alcohol. At the same time, they have an argument with their partner. These two factors precipitate a crisis that leads to self-harming behaviour. Although the person does not die on this occasion, the perpetuating factors of the excessive drinking of alcohol and ongoing relationship problems perpetuate the issues involved. This may lead the person to make an even more serious attempt to self-harm sometime in the future — a choice they may not otherwise have made if the predisposing, precipitating and perpetuating factors had been different.

It is significant that a large proportion of people who self-harm are intoxicated with alcohol or a combination of alcohol and other substances. As is noted in the chapter that looks at caring for an older person with mental illness, substance misuse has been linked to an increased risk of psychosis and depression, accidents and injuries, overdose, impaired judgement and decision making, as well as increasing levels of impulsiveness (Yang, 2017). All of these factors have been linked to suicide. At the same time, and as already noted, self-harming behaviour is also the result of a complex interplay of many different interpersonal, psychological and social factors that trigger a particular reaction. Alcohol does not always play a role in self-harming behaviour.

Perhaps what is most important to remember is that the trigger to an episode of self-harm can often be a relatively minor or insignificant incident. The challenge is to identify ways of managing the situation so that the person's reactions to the trigger can be minimised and so the self-harming behaviour is less likely to occur.

For the period 2020, the Australian Bureau of Statistics reported the following risk factor summary in a review of deaths by suicide (ABS, 2021).

- Over 90 per cent of people who died by suicide had at least one reported risk factor.
- Psychosocial risk factors were the most commonly reported risk factor.
- Both mental and behavioural disorders and psychosocial risk factors were present in over two-thirds of deaths of people who died by suicide.
- People who died by suicide had an average of three to four risk factors mentioned.

Other risk factors

The risk of suicide is higher in people who have previously attempted suicide (ABS, 2022a). Certainly, it cannot be assumed that everyone who attempts suicide will make further attempts or cause their death by suicide. Even so, prior suicidal behaviour is the single most important risk factor for completed suicide (WHO, 2021). Suicide risk assessment is discussed in more detail later in the chapter. At this point, risk is discussed as it relates to the major predisposing, precipitating and perpetuating factors, mental illness and chronic physical illness.

Mental illness

The experience of a mental illness increases the person's risk of suicide by up to seven times when compared to the general population (SANE, 2019). Bradvik (2018) reiterates previous findings of the strong association of suicide and diagnoses of:

- major depression
- psychosis
- alcohol and other substance use disorders
- borderline personality disorder
- anxiety
- eating disorders
- previous trauma.

There is a firmly established link between mental illness (in particular depression and alcohol use disorders) and suicide (WHO, 2020). Further to this, Moitra et al. (2021) conducted a systematic review covering the period 2010–19 and found that the following mental illnesses were significantly associated with suicide risk. The mental illnesses in order of prevalence are: (i) major depressive disorders, (ii) bipolar disorder, (iii) schizophrenia, (iv) anxiety disorders and (v) dysthymia. In Australia, the ABS summary of suicide data, which identified the prevalence of a diagnosed comorbid mental illness at the time of death was comparable to these findings. Mood disorder (40 per cent), acute substance use or intoxication (29 per cent), chronic substance use disorder (23 per cent) and anxiety and stress-related disorders (18 per cent) were the highest psychiatric diagnoses. Additionally, as previously mentioned, 23 per cent of deceased persons had a history of DSH (ABS, 2021). These links suggest that mental illness predisposes a person to increased suicide risk. Mental illness can also precipitate suicidal behaviour; for example, a major depressive episode or a psychotic episode could be a trigger that causes the person to react in a way they otherwise may not. Finally, mental illness may work to perpetuate certain behaviours; for example, alcohol and substance-use disorders may lead to ongoing behaviours that are risky.

Eating disorders

The American Psychiatric Association (APA) describes eating disorders as 'illnesses in which people experience severe disturbances in their eating behaviours and related thoughts and emotions. People with eating disorders typically become obsessed with food and their body weight' (APA, 2017).

The DSM-5 chapter 'Feeding and eating disorders' defines several eating disorders:
- anorexia nervosa (AN)
- bulimia nervosa (BN)
- binge eating disorder (BED)
- other specified feeding or eating disorder (OSFED)
- unspecified feeding disorder
- pica
- rumination disorder and
- avoidant/restrictive food intake disorder (ARFID).

The first five disorders are most likely to be treated in adolescence and adulthood (APA, 2013).

The DSM-5 has acknowledged BED as a separate diagnosis for the first time. It is thought that a separate category will help increase awareness of the differences between BED and the more common issue of overeating. BED is less common but much more severe than overeating and is associated with more subjective distress regarding the eating behaviour, and commonly other co-occurring psychological problems.

Eating disorders are primarily characterised by distorted or obsessive thoughts about food and a preoccupation with body shape and weight. Eating disorders are serious and potentially life threatening. The DSM-5 diagnostic criterion are listed in figure 8.1.

FIGURE 8.1 Classifying eating disorders

Anorexia nervosa (AN)
According to the DSM-5 criteria, to be diagnosed as having anorexia nervosa a person must display the following.
- Persistent restriction of energy intake leading to significantly low body weight (in context of what is minimally expected for age, sex, developmental trajectory and physical health).
- Either an intense fear of gaining weight or of becoming fat, or persistent behaviour that interferes with weight gain (even though significantly low weight).
- Disturbance in the way one's body weight or shape is experienced, undue influence of body shape and weight on self-evaluation, or persistent lack of recognition of the seriousness of the current low body weight.
  AN subtypes: restricting type; binge-eating/purging type.

Bulimia nervosa (BN)
According to the DSM-5 criteria, to be diagnosed as having bulimia nervosa a person must display the following.
- Recurrent episodes of binge eating. An episode of binge eating is characterised by both of the following.
  - Eating, in a discrete period of time (e.g. within any 2-hour period), an amount of food that is definitely larger than most people would eat during a similar period of time and under similar circumstances.
  - A sense of lack of control over eating during the episode (e.g. a feeling that one cannot stop eating or control what or how much one is eating).
- Recurrent inappropriate compensatory behaviour in order to prevent weight gain, such as self-induced vomiting, misuse of laxatives, diuretics, or other medications, fasting, or excessive exercise.
- The binge eating and inappropriate compensatory behaviours both occur, on average, at least once a week for three months.
- Self-evaluation is unduly influenced by body shape and weight.
- The disturbance does not occur exclusively during episodes of anorexia nervosa.

Binge eating disorder (BED)
According to the DSM-5 criteria, to be diagnosed as having binge eating disorder a person must display the following.
- Recurrent episodes of binge eating. An episode of binge eating is characterised by both of the following.
  - Eating, in a discrete period of time (e.g. within any 2-hour period), an amount of food that is definitely larger than most people would eat during a similar period of time and under similar circumstances.
  - A sense of lack of control over eating during the episode (e.g. a feeling that one cannot stop eating or control what or how much one is eating).

- The binge eating episodes are associated with three or more of the following.
  - Eating much more rapidly than normal.
  - Eating until feeling uncomfortably full.
  - Eating large amounts of food when not feeling physically hungry.
  - Eating alone because of feeling embarrassed by how much one is eating.
  - Feeling disgusted with oneself, depressed or very guilty afterward.
- Marked distress regarding binge eating is present.
- Binge eating occurs, on average, at least once a week for three months.
- Binge eating not associated with the recurrent use of inappropriate compensatory behaviours as in bulimia nervosa and does not occur exclusively during the course of bulimia nervosa or anorexia nervosa methods to compensate for overeating, such as self-induced vomiting.

Pica

According to the DSM-5 criteria, to be diagnosed with pica a person must display the following.
- Persistent eating of non-nutritive substances for a period of at least one month.
- The eating of non-nutritive substances is inappropriate to the developmental level of the individual.
- The eating behaviour is not part of a culturally supported or socially normative practice.
- If occurring in the presence of another mental disorder (e.g. autistic spectrum disorder), or during a medical condition (e.g. pregnancy), it is severe enough to warrant independent clinical attention.
  Note: pica often occurs with other mental health disorders associated with impaired functioning.

Rumination disorder

According to the DSM-5 criteria, to be diagnosed as having rumination disorder a person must display the following.
- Repeated regurgitation of food for a period of at least one month. Regurgitated food may be re-chewed, re-swallowed or spit out.
- The repeated regurgitation is not due to a medication condition (e.g. gastrointestinal condition).
- The behaviour does not occur exclusively in the course of anorexia nervosa, bulimia nervosa, BED or avoidant/restrictive food intake disorder.
- If occurring in the presence of another mental disorder (e.g. intellectual developmental disorder), it is severe enough to warrant independent clinical attention.

Avoidant/restrictive food intake disorder (ARFID)

According to the DSM-5 criteria, to be diagnosed as having ARFID a person must display the following.
- An eating or feeding disturbance as manifested by persistent failure to meet appropriate nutritional and/or energy needs associated with one (or more) of the following.
  1. Significant loss of weight (or failure to achieve expected weight gain or faltering growth in children).
  2. Significant nutritional deficiency.
  3. Dependence on enteral feeding or oral nutritional supplements.
  4. Marked interference with psychosocial functioning.
- The behaviour is not better explained by lack of available food or by an associated culturally sanctioned practice.
- The behaviour does not occur exclusively during the course of anorexia nervosa or bulimia nervosa, and there is no evidence of a disturbance in the way one's body weight or shape is experienced.
- The eating disturbance is not attributed to a medical condition, or better explained by another mental health disorder. When it does occur in the presence of another condition/disorder, the behaviour exceeds what is usually associated, and warrants additional clinical attention.

Other specified feeding or eating disorder (OSFED)

According to the DSM-5 criteria, to be diagnosed as having OSFED a person must present with feeding or eating behaviours that cause clinically significant distress and impairment in areas of functioning, but do not meet the full criteria for any of the other feeding and eating disorders.

A diagnosis might then be allocated that specifies a specific reason why the presentation does not meet the specifics of another disorder (e.g. bulimia nervosa — low frequency). The following are further examples for OSFED.
- Atypical anorexia nervosa: All criteria are met, except despite significant weight loss, the individual's weight is within or above the normal range.
- Binge eating disorder (of low frequency and/or limited duration): All of the criteria for BED are met, except at a lower frequency and/or for less than three months.
- Bulimia nervosa (of low frequency and/or limited duration): All of the criteria for bulimia nervosa are met, except that the binge eating and inappropriate compensatory behaviour occurs at a lower frequency and/or for less than three months.

▶

- Purging disorder: Recurrent purging behaviour to influence weight or shape in the absence of binge eating.
- Night eating syndrome: Recurrent episodes of night eating. Eating after awakening from sleep, or by excessive food consumption after the evening meal. The behaviour is not better explained by environmental influences or social norms. The behaviour causes significant distress/impairment. The behaviour is not better explained by another mental health disorder (e.g. BED).

Unspecified feeding or eating disorder (UFED)
According to the DSM-5 criteria this category applies to where behaviours cause clinically significant distress/impairment of functioning, but do not meet the full criteria of any of the feeding or eating disorder criteria. This category may be used by clinicians where a clinician chooses not to specify why criteria are not met, including presentations where there may be insufficient information to make a more specific diagnosis (e.g. in emergency room settings).

Source: Eating Disorders Victoria (2019a).

An emerging eating disorder that is yet to be included in the DSM-5 is known as orthorexia nervosa (Bratman, 1997; National Eating Disorders Association [NEDA], 2022). This disorder is when people are rigidly committed to consuming only healthy food and have an extreme list of exclusions, for example, always eliminating foods that are processed, cooked, contain sugar, salt or fat, are animal- or milk-based or non-organic. People with this disorder are likely to become fixated on food quality, nutritional value and the purity of the food that they consume. In severe cases, this preoccupation with food significantly interferes with normal activities of living and social interactions. Of great concern, there have been reports of deaths attributed to malnutrition due to a nutritional imbalance when consuming such limited food groups (NEDA, 2022). For more on orthorexia nervosa see www.nationaleatingdisorders.org/orthorexia-nervosa and www.orthorexia.com.

The Authorized Bratman Orthorexia Self-Test contains a list of questions that assists individuals to determine whether they are at risk of developing orthorexia nervosa. The self-test is available at www.orthorexia.com/the-authorized-bratman-orthorexia-self-test.

The US National Eating Disorders Association (NEDA) and the Australian National Eating Disorders Collaboration (NEDC) are both supporting active research in relation to the correlation between orthorexia nervosa and restrictive diet communities, autoimmune Paleo diet and recreational juice cleansing camps (Bóna et al., 2018; NEDA, 2022; NEDC, 2020). The Butterfly Foundation reports that:
- disordered eating is the single most important indicator of onset of an eating disorder
- extreme and unhealthy dieting practices are a major risk factor associated with developing an eating disorder
- teenagers who have moderate dieting practices are six times more likely to develop an eating disorder than those who do not diet
- the risk of developing an eating disorder is 18 times more likely for a person with extreme restrictive food intake practices (Butterfly Foundation, 2022a).

Likewise, there is concern that body dissatisfaction has a negative impact on psychological wellbeing in young Australian males, with reports that over 370 000 males are now affected by this (Butterfly Foundation, 2022b). Body dysmorphic disorder exists when a person restricts their behaviour including social commitments, due to a perceived physical flaw of some type. Muscle dysmorphia as opposed to another body part, may also be known as 'bigorexia', with the person aiming to increase muscle mass by either excessive gym exercises or with the assistance of steroids (Molloy, 2019). There is now evidence that a dysfunctional use of social media is associated with unrealistic body ideals including maladaptive physical exercise and food habits, which may increase eating disorder related symptoms (Imperatori et al., 2022).

To address this growing trend of adolescent boys displaying unhealthy thinking towards physical shape and size, the Butterfly Foundation launched RESET, the first Australian online digital body image program in 2018 (Butterfly Foundation, 2022b). Given that parents and carers are usually the first people to notice changes in eating and exercise, the Feed Your Instinct portal (www.feedyourinstinct.com.au), funded by the Victorian government, has an online Eating and Body Image Checklist for parents of children and young people. Results of the information provided can be generated into either a parent overview or a general practitioner (GP) summary.

Eating disorders are serious mental illnesses, and are associated with significant psychological distress, major physical complications and increased mortality. Additionally, self-harm is highly prevalent among young people with eating disorders (Lavis et al., 2022). The NEDC (2022a) states that people with eating disorders have significantly elevated mortality rates of up to six times higher than the general population, with the highest rates occurring in those with AN. Reasons for premature death include medical complications and suicide. Furthermore, reported suicide rates for people with eating disorders illustrate that suicide is up to 31 times more likely to occur for someone with anorexia nervosa and 7.5 times higher for someone with bulimia nervosa than in the general population (NEDC, 2022a).

The NEDC reports that approximately 4 per cent of the Australian population live with an eating disorder, with BED being the most common. The latest evidence regarding the prevalence of eating disorders among Aboriginal and Torres Strait Islander youths suggests that eating disorders and body image issues are at a similar or higher rate than non-Indigenous people (Burt et al., 2020). The NEDC further states that over 80 per cent of adults diagnosed with an eating disorder have at least one more psychiatric disorder, with the highest psychiatric comorbidities being mood disorders, anxiety disorders, post-traumatic stress disorder (PTSD) and trauma, substance misuse, personality disorders (avoidant, borderline, obsessive compulsive), sexual dysfunction and non-suicidal self injury (NEDC, 2022b). Treatments for eating disorders are diverse and include public and private specialist inpatient, specialist outpatient or routine general outpatient services. The recommended multidisciplinary approach may consist of nutritional counselling and supplementation; physical health management; psychotherapy interventions including interpersonal psychotherapy, motivational interviewing and cognitive behaviour therapy; medication and family counselling and self-help strategies as indicated. Treatment in Australia is most commonly provided in an outpatient or day-patient setting, with some people requiring medical stabilisation and weight restoration in hospital (Eating Disorders Victoria, 2022b).

Hospitalisation usually occurs when a person's body mass index (BMI) falls below 14. The BMI is a simple and common tool used to estimate a person's total percentage of body fat, and assists in determining a person's healthy weight range. Based on height and weight, the BMI helps classify people as being underweight, in a healthy weight range, overweight or obese. This tool is used for both adults and children; however, in the childhood population, care needs to be taken as the BMI in children changes significantly with age and gender, and a specific BMI sex and age chart must be used (New South Wales [NSW] Health, 2022). There are also some exceptions to the usefulness of BMI gauging body fat percentage for some groups in the population, for example, pregnant women, body builders and people with high muscle mass, older people, people with disabilities and some specific cultural groups and people who are very short or very tall (Better Health Channel, 2021).

BMI is defined as weight in kilograms divided by the square of the person's height in metres (kg/(height (m))^2). For example, the BMI calculation for a person who is 1.71-metres tall and weighs 72 kilograms is:

$$\frac{72}{(1.71 \times 1.71)} = \frac{72}{2.92} = 24.66$$

The following BMI ranges are used to determine whether a person's BMI value is considered healthy:
- < 18.5 (underweight and possibly malnourished)
- 18.5–24.9 (healthy weight range for young and middle-aged adults)
- 25.0–29.9 (overweight)
- > 30 (obese).

However, a person's general health status may be of greater significance than being mildly overweight, if they are over 70 years of age. Some research has indicated a 22–26 BMI range as acceptable for this age group (Better Health Channel, 2021).

THE BIG PICTURE

Australian Eating Disorder Research and Translation Strategy 2021–31

For the first time, Australia has a 10-year strategy that will guide critical research and transform how we treat and care for people who live with eating disorders, including bulimia and anorexia nervosa.

In September 2021, the Coalition Government launched the Australian Eating Disorder Research and Translation Strategy 2021–31. The Strategy, which has been developed under a $4 million federal grant by the InsideOut Institute, identifies the top 10 priority areas in greatest need of additional research.

▶

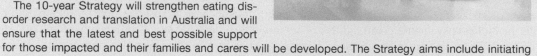

Minister for Health and Aged Care, Greg Hunt, said eating disorders were serious, complex and life-threatening mental illnesses and the Strategy provides a clear national approach to ensuring best-practice prevention, early intervention and treatment now and in the future.

It is estimated that around 1 000 000 Australians have an eating disorder. These disorders affect not only the person, but also their families and loved ones, and have one of the highest mortality rates of any psychiatric illness, with anorexia being the deadliest of all mental health conditions.

The 10-year Strategy will strengthen eating disorder research and translation in Australia and will ensure that the latest and best possible support for those impacted and their families and carers will be developed. The Strategy aims include initiating significant improvements in the wellbeing of those with an eating disorder, which will ultimately save lives.

The 10 research priorities identified in the Strategy are prevention, risk and protective factors, early identification, equity of access, treatment outcomes, individualised medicine, family support, early intervention, positive and negative treatment impacts, stigma and health promotion.

The 2021–22 Federal Budget also provided a further $26.9 million for eating disorder research and support, including $13 million to establish a National Eating Disorder Research Centre.

This Strategy builds upon the previous historic investments such as $110.7 million to provide up to 40 Medicare-subsidised psychological and 20 dietetic therapy sessions, $63 million for the establishment of a national network of residential eating disorders treatment centres, $5 million for research through the Medical Research Future Fund (MRFF), and $13.4 million for the National Eating Disorders Collaboration (NEDC).

Source: Commonwealth of Australia (2021a).

Physical illness

The suicide rate may be higher among people who experience specific ongoing disorders, for example, autism spectrum disorder (Blanchard et al., 2021), or chronic physical illnesses such as type 1 diabetes (Majidi et al., 2020). From the Australian perspective, based on 2020 suicide data analysis, the ABS found that older people had a higher proportion of chronic health conditions such as cancer, coronary heart disease and diabetes as a risk factor than younger people (ABS 2021). Furthermore, those who live with a long-term health condition (i.e., heart disease, diabetes, arthritis or asthma) are also at higher risk of developing depression and anxiety (Beyond Blue, 2022c). The 2021 Australian Census collected information for the first time regarding the health status of Australians. The survey asked about the following ten long-term groups of conditions (ABS, 2022b):

- arthritis
- asthma
- back pain
- cancer
- cardiovascular disease
- chronic obstructive pulmonary disease (COPD)
- diabetes
- kidney disease
- mental health conditions
- osteoporosis.

The key findings of the 2020–21 census were that just over three-quarters (78.6 per cent) of Australians had at least one long-term health condition, and nearly half had at least one of the ten identified chronic conditions (46.6 per cent or 11.6 million). A breakdown of these conditions reveals that mental and behavioural conditions (20.1 per cent), back problems (15.7 per cent) and arthritis (12.5 per cent) were the most common chronic conditions. Almost one in five (18.6 per cent) Australians had two or more chronic conditions, with females having slightly higher rates of physical illness compared to males.

Importantly, from the 20.1 per cent of people who account for mental and behavioural conditions, 49.5 per cent of people self-identified as also having a comorbid physical health condition (ABS, 2022b).

Therefore, health professionals who provide services to people with a chronic and/or long-term physical illness need to be aware of these risk factors and work proactively to provide appropriate support.

It is also recommended that health professionals ensure each person who presents to a health service with self-harming behaviour is assessed and treated as an individual. This will enable the health professional to reach some understanding of the person's unique reasons for engaging in the self-harming behaviour.

Person-centred care is discussed in more detail later in the chapter. Prior to this discussion, consideration is given to the attitudes of people, communities and health professionals towards people who self-harm.

The use of insulin in fatal overdoses

Insulin-induced hypoglycemia is the cause of approximately 100 000 emergency department visits per year, and severe hypoglycemia accounts for up to 10 per cent of deaths among young people with type 1 diabetes. Suicide caused by the deliberate injection of insulin has been reported for almost the entire period that insulin has been available as a hormone treatment (Rzepczyk et al., 2022). In South Australia, fatal cases of insulin overdose were reviewed over a 20-year period (2000–2019) to assess rates and characteristics of insulin-related deaths, irrespective of whether the person was insulin-dependent or not. A range of 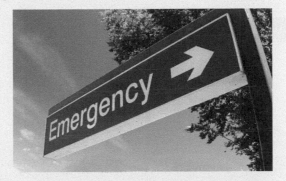 demographic and health variables were collected including age, sex, cause of death, scene findings, manner of death, decedent medical and personal histories, biochemistry, toxicology, histopathology and autopsy findings. During the period reviewed, 40 cases of insulin overdose were identified. Twenty-nine cases (72.5 per cent) were reported by the Coroner as death by suicide, with the remaining cases classified as accidental or undetermined intent.

From these 40 deaths, 22 people were known to have insulin-dependent diabetes (55 per cent), and 13 of these people (59 per cent) had a history of depression; 10 of whom had previously demonstrated suicidal ideation. The review of these deaths demonstrated that suicides using insulin among people with insulin-dependent diabetes are equally as prevalent, if not more so, than fatal accidental insulin overdoses. This can largely be attributed to people with an insulin dependence having immediate access to a potentially lethal substance (Stephenson et al., 2022).

QUESTIONS

1. When reviewing table 8.2, what practices would be useful in determining whether a person who requires insulin therapy has a predisposition to potential misuse of insulin?
2. Insulin is both a life-sustaining and potentially life-ending drug. Discuss the tension of minimising or restricting insulin access to people who have insulin-dependent diabetes, and comorbid symptoms/diagnosis of depression.
3. How could suicide prevention strategies sensitively focus on people with an insulin dependence with a history of depression, particularly for those with access to rapid-acting insulin?

8.4 Attitudes towards self-harm

LEARNING OBJECTIVE 8.4 Describe attitudes to self-harming.

The attitudes of health professionals often reflect the attitudes of the community. Many health professionals have negative attitudes or perceptions of people who self-harm because this behaviour is stigmatised by the wider community, and often viewed as 'self-destructive' or 'wrong'. At the same time, there is no doubt that providing care to a person who has self-harmed or attempted suicide can be emotionally challenging for health professionals. Self-harming behaviours can evoke strong personal feelings in people, with many of these feelings arising from the person's beliefs and values. For example, some people may perceive self-harming behaviour as a form of 'attention-seeking', which is considered invalidating and potentially dangerous (Reachout, 2022). From a clinical perspective, the health professional may think it is appropriate to distance themselves from the consumer for fear of worsening the person's symptoms (Ribeiro Coimbra

& Noakes, 2022). Alternatively, some health professionals may feel unsure about what they should say or how they should provide care to someone who has self-harmed; for example, the health professional may think that talking about the self-harming behaviour will only encourage the person to want to do it again and thus avoid the topic. Indeed, researchers have identified that health professionals consistently feel a lack of confidence when it comes to caring for the person who has self-harmed and additionally, many health professionals perceive that they have not received the education or training they need and lack the skills to care for people who have self-harmed (Rayner et al., 2019). Leddie et al. (2021) also state that training, reflective practice and self-care practices need to be adopted by nurses who provide care to adolescents who self-harm. Similarly, consumer feedback highlights that feelings of misunderstanding and not being heard, along with a perceived lack of receptiveness from health professionals towards people presenting with eating disorders, are underpinning causes of early termination of treatment (Vinchenzo et al., 2022).

UPON REFLECTION

Keeping people safe

All organisations have policies and procedures that determine how body and personal belonging searches should be conducted when a person states they are going to harm themselves. These policies and procedures are aligned with human rights legislation.

QUESTIONS

1. What search provisions and limitations are described within the policy of an organisation you have worked within or are familiar with?
2. Considering the consumer's perspective, how might you broach the issue of personal belonging searches with a consumer?
3. What legal considerations underpin your practice?

In particular, health professionals who work in the emergency context and deal on a day-to-day basis with people who are highly distressed because of accidental injury or unwanted illness or loss, often find it difficult to be non-judgemental towards people who self-harm. Rates of compassion fatigue in health care professionals working with vulnerable people range from 50 to 75 per cent, with significant consequences related to their psychological and emotional wellbeing (Amir et al., 2019). These health professionals may find themselves feeling resentful towards the person they perceive as a 'time-waster' — they may feel that if the person chose to hurt themselves, they do not deserve treatment and should be made to bear the consequences. Many of these views are also shared by the Australian public (Robinson et al., 2016, p. 24). Pintar Babič and colleagues found that nurses from non-psychotherapeutic units felt more negative emotions and less positive attitudes than those from psychotherapeutic units, when working with adolescents with self-harm behaviours (Pintar Babič et al., 2020). Indeed, Biancarelli and colleagues (2019) found that people who presented with a history of injecting drugs also experienced negative attitudes from health professionals, and experienced feelings of unfair treatment and discrimination. After reviewing 47 studies, Alshahrani (2018) found that overall, psychologists, followed by psychiatrists, were found to have the most negative attitudes of all health professionals towards those with a mental illness, with higher prevalence in younger professionals compared to older more experienced professionals.

The person who has self-harmed is often aware of these negative perceptions. Significantly, both health professionals and consumers report high levels of dissatisfaction with their experience of care when self-harm is involved (Rayner et al., 2019). This dissatisfaction, in turn, can have an impact on the consumer's willingness to receive timely and necessary treatment. Negative attitudes are also a motivating factor for people leaving a health context prematurely, before the necessary assessments, interventions or referrals have been completed. This is a significant issue in light of the fact that adolescents who self-harm carry a 100 times greater risk of death by suicide within a year compared to the general population (Burton, 2019).

In summary, the negative attitudes of health professionals towards people who have self-harmed:

- reinforce stereotypical and misinformed beliefs about the nature of self-harm and those who exhibit self-harming behaviours
- maintain a spiral of negative feelings and expectations towards people who self-harm
- reduce the ability of the health professional to view the person as an individual in need of care and treatment for their own particular health issues

- interfere with the ability of health professionals to make effective judgements regarding the assessment of risk, identification of ongoing needs and the implementation of care
- increase the likelihood of consumers feeling frustrated and dissatisfied with their care and treatment.

For these reasons, it is important that health professionals are aware of their personal values and feelings about people who self-harm and develop strategies to manage their reactions. These may include a guided practice reflection, such as that which is utilised in clinical supervision sessions and peer support groups. For example, the literature provides good evidence that positive attitudinal changes occur post suicidal behaviour training for health professionals, who identified feeling more confident and capable of managing the needs of those who self-harm (Gibson et al., 2019; Rayner et al., 2019). Negative attitudes towards consumers who self-harm will have a negative effect on both health professionals' ability to plan person-focused care and the consumer's experience of seeking help and treatment. By challenging these attitudes, the health professional will have greater ability to respond in a considered way, rather than react to the person with self-harming behaviours, and thereby support the improvement of health outcomes.

IN PRACTICE

Mitigating the development of compassion fatigue

Health care professional attitudes that are positive and non-judgemental when providing care and treatment to people who self-harm, particularly young people, will facilitate people feeling comfortable in sharing their stories in a safe environment. While clinicians have an ethical obligation to remain professional, the potential consequences of trauma (vicarious and observed) can also potentiate the vulnerability of the health care professional developing compassion fatigue, emotional exhaustion, brown-out and burnout. This spiral can have negative personal and professional consequences and can also interfere with people receiving optimal care and treatment.

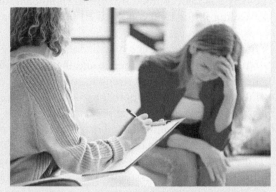

QUESTIONS

1. Thinking about your own practice, when working in high-risk areas or with people who may challenge your cultural and personal value systems in relation to self-harm behaviours, what strategies could be enacted to minimise your risk of developing compassion fatigue and burnout?
2. Compassion fatigue and burnout can negatively impact the ability to develop therapeutic alliance, empathy and compassion. What resilience and/or wellbeing training is available in your organisation to address this from occurring? What other professional training could you also proactively access?

8.5 National Suicide Prevention Strategy

LEARNING OBJECTIVE 8.5 Outline the National Suicide Prevention Strategy.

In 1999, Australia launched the National Suicide Prevention Strategy (NSPS) in response to a growing body of evidence that highlighted the risk of suicidal behaviours developing across the whole-of-life span. The NSPS provides the platform for Australia's national policy on suicide prevention with an emphasis on promotion, prevention and early intervention.

In addition to the NSPS, the National Mental Health Commission (NMHC) was established as an independent body in 2012. The NMHC reports directly to the Prime Minister and is tasked with reporting and advising on the mental health needs of the community; increasing accountability and transparency in government, non-government and private mental health and suicide prevention sectors across the country; and giving mental health reform national prominence (National Mental Health Commission, 2020). The fundamental aim of the NMHC is to support all people in Australia to achieve the best possible mental health and wellbeing, as individuals and as groups within the community from all sectors including health, education, housing, employment, human services and social support. As part of the governmental response into the NMHC *Review of mental health programs*, in November 2015 the government announced an update of the NSPS, which now includes the following.

- A systems-based regional approach to suicide prevention. This is led by Primary Health Networks (PHNs) in partnership with Local Hospital Networks, states and territories, and other local organisations through a flexible funding pool.
- National leadership and support activity. This includes whole of population activity and crisis support services.
- A renewed focus on suicide prevention in Aboriginal and Torres Strait Islander communities. This takes into account the recommendations of the Aboriginal and Torres Strait Islander Suicide Prevention Strategy.
- A joint commitment to suicide prevention by the Australian government and states and territories. This commitment was made in the context of the Fifth National Mental Health Plan to prevent suicide and ensure that effective follow-up support is given to people who have self-harmed or attempted suicide (Life in Mind, 2022b).

These objectives have a primary health care focus, with health promotion, suicide prevention and early intervention for early warning signs viewed as essential (see the chapter that discusses mental health service delivery).

The NSPS is underpinned by several significant interconnecting frameworks.

- The Living is for Everyone (LIFE) Framework (available at www.livingisforeveryone.com.au) based on six action areas:
    1. improving the evidence base and understanding of suicide prevention
    2. building individual resilience and the capacity for self-help
    3. improving community strength, resilience and capacity in suicide prevention
    4. taking a coordinated approach to suicide prevention
    5. providing targeted suicide prevention activities
    6. implementing standards and quality in suicide prevention.
- The National Aboriginal and Torres Strait Islander Suicide Prevention Strategy (available at www.in digenous.gov.au/news-and-media/postcard/national-aboriginal-and-torres-strait-islander-suicide-preve ntion-strategy). This Strategy focuses on early intervention measures and the development of strong communities through community focused and integrated approaches to suicide prevention. The strategy comprises a holistic view of mental, physical, cultural and spiritual health.
- The National LGBTI Mental Health and Suicide Prevention Strategy. The Strategy outlines effective mental health and suicide prevention strategy for the 11 per cent of the Australian population who identify as lesbian, gay, bisexual, transgender and/or intersex (LGBTI) and other sexuality, gender and bodily diverse people and communities.
- The National Mental Health and Wellbeing Pandemic Response Plan. The COVID-19 pandemic forced the rapid expansion of digital services and a seismic shift to telehealth delivery of mental health services, innovative community-based models of care, more agile coordination between primary and acute care, expanded engagement with people with lived experience, and the recognition of the importance of social and associated needs such as housing for those who are homeless.
- Australia's Long Term National Health Plan. This Plan was launched by the Department of Health in August 2019. The Plan focuses on Australian health care for a 10-year period and includes the 2030 mental health vision. The Plan also includes the inaugural Australian mental health strategy for children under 12 years of age. The Plan contains four pillars of health care covering primary care, public and private hospital preventative health, and medical research. Mental health care and suicide prevention is a key priority throughout the document (Life in Mind, 2022b).
- Prevention Compassion Care — National Mental Health and Suicide Prevention Plan. In the development of this Plan, the government recognises that 'as a country, we have faced significant challenges in recent years, enduring drought, bushfires, floods and the COVID-19 pandemic. These crises have significantly affected the mental health and wellbeing of individuals, families and communities, and continue to do so' (Commonwealth of Australia 2021a, p. 5). This national $2.3 billion plan further builds on the Coalition Government's investment in specific mental health services for Australians throughout the 2019–20 bushfires and COVID-19 pandemic periods. The National Mental Health and Suicide Prevention Plan is based on five pillars (Commonwealth of Australia, 2021a):
    1. prevention and early intervention
    2. suicide prevention
    3. treatment

4. supporting the vulnerable
5. workforce and governance.

From 1 July 2016, all PHNs across the country took responsibility for ensuring that suitable and adequate suicide prevention activities and services are in place locally, and a number of state and territories have their own suicide prevention plan, for example, the Strategic Framework for Suicide Prevention in NSW 2018–23. This framework illustrates the systems approach to suicide prevention in response to the first goal of the NSPS, which is known as 'LifeSpan'. LifeSpan is led by the Black Dog Institute and the National Health and Medical Research Centre (NHMRC) Centre for Research Excellence in Suicide Prevention. In New South Wales, LifeSpan worked collaboratively with the NSW Mental Health Commission, the NSW Department of Health, the Commonwealth Department of Health, PHNs, local health districts and a wide range of local partners in each area, to implement and deliver the nine evidence-based suicide prevention strategies across a number of trial sites, as shown in figure 8.2 (Black Dog Institute, 2022). This project was funded by a $14.5 million philanthropic grant from the Paul Ramsay Foundation, with estimates that this approach may prevent 21 per cent of suicide deaths and 30 per cent of suicide attempts if fully implemented (Black Dog Institute, 2022). The outcomes for the trial of this project are yet to be published by Black Dog Institute.

FIGURE 8.2   Nine evidence-based suicide prevention strategies

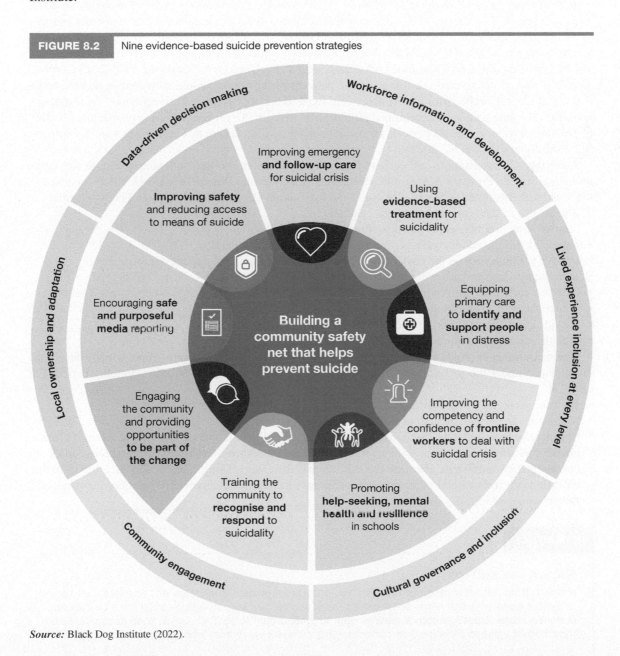

Source: Black Dog Institute (2022).

Groups 'at risk'

The NSPS provides a population-based, universal suicide prevention framework. Additionally, the NSPS targets a number of population groups that have been identified as being at particular risk of suicide (AIHW, 2022a). These include children and adolescents, veterans and Australian Defence Force personnel and Aboriginal and Torres Strait Islander peoples. Other priority populations are lesbian, gay, bisexual, transgender, queer, intersex, asexual (LGBTQIA+) and other sexually or gender diverse groups, and people from culturally and linguistically diverse (CALD) backgrounds (AIHW, 2022a). Further vulnerable groups often targeted are men, older people, people from rural and remote settings, people who are bereaved by suicide and people who have previously attempted self-harm or suicide. Finally, people at increased risk of death by suicide due to their occupation will be mentioned.

Youth

Youth suicide has increased over recent years and is the leading cause of death for young Australians aged 15–24. The proportion of deaths by suicide is relatively high among children and young people because these age groups do not tend to die from other causes. For those aged 15–17 years, 31 per cent of all deaths were due to suicide, and for those aged 18–24, suicide was the cause of 39 per cent of all deaths in 2020. Although suicide is a tragedy at any age, suicide in children generates extreme levels of distress and loss in Australian communities. In children aged 14 and below, 12 per cent of all deaths for this age group was due to suicide in 2020 (AIHW, 2022a). To obtain a demographic and clinical characteristics perspective of 10–24 year-olds who died by suicide in Australia, Hill and colleagues reviewed the 2006–2015 Coronial data. The authors uncovered the following: 41 per cent of the young people who died by suicide had a diagnosed mental health disorder; 38.4 per cent lived in areas of greater socio-economic disadvantage; one-third of young people had consumed alcohol close to death; 31 per cent of young people had a history of previous self-harm; and 28 per cent of young people who died during this period was known to misuse illicit substances (Hill et al., 2021).

A number of organisations are currently working hard to address the youth suicide rate in Australia, including Suicide Prevention Australia, ReachOut, Youth Beyond Blue, Black Dog Institute, headspace, the Australian Institute for Suicide Research and Prevention, Carers Australia, Youth Focus and Lifeline. The strategies of these organisations are generally to:

- remove structural barriers to youth wellbeing
- target risk factors and increase protective factors for suicide prevention
- involve young people in the design and implementation of youth suicide prevention programs
- increase research and access to online services
- focus on early intervention in youth mental illness
- reduce the stigma of asking for help
- provide gatekeeper training for adults
- include suicide prevention mechanisms in the school curriculum.

Again, a number of programs to promote mental health and resilience in young people initially developed or enhanced under the early phases of the NSPS have continued beyond the initial funding period. For example:

- Be You (previously KidsMatter Primary initiative) www.beyou.edu.au
- Mindspot, an online mental health and counselling service (www.mindspot.org.au) that provides cognitive behavioural therapy counselling to people with mild to moderate depression. Access is free of charge and available with or without a referral from a health professional. Health professionals are encouraged to familiarise themselves with the excellent work being done in this area by accessing the Mindspot website and other relevant websites (e.g. www.suicidepreventionaust.org/news/statsand facts).

IN PRACTICE

Reporting self-harm

Kennedy lives down the road from you and you casually know their family. Kennedy changed their name to a more gender-neutral name some months back and you are still struggling to call them by their new preferred name. Both Kennedy's parents work in professional roles: their father is an accountant and their mother works as a lawyer. Both parents are high achievers and rarely work less than 10 hours per day,

---

six days per week. Kennedy is a bright and bubbly 17-year-old and a well-liked Year 11 student at the nearby private school. Kennedy has had a part-time job for the past two years, working most weekends in a kitchen shop, which is usually where you have an informal catch-up with them.

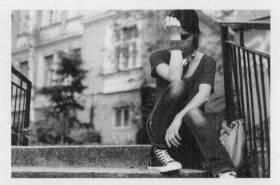

Kennedy saved enough money to purchase a small car and now drives to work and school. Some months ago, Kennedy broke up with Ryder, their boyfriend of five months. Since that time, Kennedy has found it difficult to manage their feelings, and finds it hard to concentrate at school. Kennedy's academic work has steadily declined over the past term. They are often tearful and irritable, and has begun taking regular doses of paracetamol for stress headaches. Sometimes they takes large doses of paracetamol when they don't have a headache. Kennedy hasn't bothered to tell their parents about their problems because of how busy they are.

On the way to school one day, Kennedy failed to give way to an oncoming car at a roundabout. A low-speed collision occurred, and Kennedy was transported to hospital via ambulance with an obvious fractured arm. Kennedy is overwhelmed by the noise, lights and stimulation of the hospital, and sits quietly in a corner waiting for their parents to arrive. You notice Kennedy while you are on duty and approach them. You strike up a conversation, and during this interaction you notice a large number of scratches, cut marks and scars on their arm. This is especially evident where Kennedy's jumper has been cut and pulled high above the elbow by paramedics. A few of the scars look old, but many appear to be recent wounds, and some look like they may have been significant injuries.

As a health professional, you are aware that you have a professional obligation and responsibility, underpinned by a legislative basis, to protect children and young people aged 0–18 years from any form of child abuse or neglect. You do not have to prove that abuse or neglect has occurred, only form a reasonable belief that it has occurred. Kennedy starts to cry because you're being so nice and tells you that since their boyfriend left them, they have been feeling really lousy. Kennedy also says that they're fat and ugly, their parents don't understand or have any time for them, and often feels like hurting themselves with a razor blade. That's what they usually do when feeling emotionally overwhelmed. Kennedy is called to the triage desk at that point, and you part ways. You're bothered by this conversation, and you speak to a more senior colleague, and relay the story. Your colleague suggests that perhaps you need to make a Child Protection Report.

QUESTIONS

1. What framework do you use to underpin your clinical decision about what to do in this situation?

2. What are the legal considerations that you need to factor into your decision?

3. Explain the ethical issues that need to be addressed in this situation.

4. What other options could you employ to manage this situation?

Veterans and Australian Defence Force personnel

Between 2018 and 2021, the Australian Institute of Health and Welfare (AIHW) on behalf of the Department of Veteran Affairs (DVA) collated a number of annual reports on suicide among permanent, reserve and ex-serving members of the Australian Defence Force (ADF). The reports reviewed suicide data between 2001 and 2019 related to ADF personnel who had served since 1985. The alarming results culminated in a Royal Commission being established in July 2021 to investigate Defence and veteran personnel suicide. The aim of the Royal Commission is to inquire into the systemic issues and risk factors relevant to suicide and suicide behaviours of serving and ex-serving Defence members.

Compared with the Australian population, ADF deaths by suicide rates (after adjusting for age) between 2002 and 2019 were: 51 per cent lower for male permanent ADF members; 48 per cent lower for reserve males; 24 per cent higher for ex-serving males; and 102 per cent (or 2.02 times) higher for ex-serving females. Concerningly, the suicide rate for ex-serving males who separate voluntarily is around one-third of the rate of those who separate for involuntary medical reasons (73.1 compared with 22.2 per 100 000 population per year). The Interim Report was tabled in August 2022 and highlighted preliminary observations and recommendations about these urgent and immediate issues. A final report is due in June 2024 (Commonwealth of Australia, 2022a).

Indigenous Australians

Suicide rates for Aboriginal and Torres Strait Islander peoples — in particular, youths in the 10–19-year age group — are more than four times higher than the general population (Gibson et al., 2021). From a rural and remote perspective, the Northern Territory has an alarming and disproportionately high Indigenous **suicide cluster** rate (Hanssens, 2011), and Indigenous suicide in the Kimberley region, Western Australia, is reported as being among the highest suicide rates in the world (McHugh et al., 2016). As discussed in the chapter that looks at delivering culturally appropriate mental health care, higher suicide rates in the Indigenous population are related to a number of factors. Indigenous people often live in poverty and have a lower socio-economic status; poorer levels of education and employment; reduced access to social, community and health services; higher rates of domestic violence or abuse, and alcohol and other drug abuse; and lower levels of general health. In addition, many Aboriginal and Torres Strait Islander peoples have been affected by the suicide of another family or community member, and trauma and grief issues are also ever-present within Indigenous communities. From an Indigenous Elder perspective, 'loss of cultural identity and cross cultural confusion' is a significant antecedent to youth suicide (Prince, 2018, p. 3). Similar findings related to higher deaths by suicide in areas where there are lower levels of participation in cultural and community events was also found by Gibson et al. (2021). As mentioned earlier in this chapter, in 2013 the Australian Government released the first National Aboriginal and Torres Strait Islander Suicide Prevention Strategy to address the self-harm and suicide rates of this cohort of the population (Department of Health, 2013). Further to this, the Centre for Best Practice in Aboriginal and Torres Strait Islander Suicide Prevention (CBPATSISP) and the Menzies School of Health Research have published evidence-based *Guidelines for best practice psychosocial assessment of Aboriginal and Torres Strait Islander people presenting to hospital with self-harm and suicidal thoughts* to promote enhanced outcomes for Indigenous peoples presenting with suicidal thoughts and behaviours (Leckning et al., 2019).

Yarn Safe is a national headspace initiative that was launched in 2014. Yarn Safe was the first youth-led Aboriginal and Torres Strait Islander Mental Health campaign in Australia, and aims to raise awareness of mental health issues and encourage young Aboriginal and Torres Strait Islanders to seek help at an appropriate mental health service. In the 12 months following the campaign launch, there was a dramatic 32 per cent increase in the number of young Aboriginal and Torres Strait Islander peoples accessing support at headspace centres (headspace, 2020a). Likewise, the ibobbly mobile phone app targeted at Indigenous youth is also demonstrating favourable outcomes (Tighe et al., 2017). Further issues around suicide and self-harm and the programs that are being implemented by the Indigenous communities themselves to raise the social and emotional wellbeing of Indigenous people are discussed in detail in the chapter that looks at delivering culturally appropriate mental health care.

LGBTQIA+ and other gender diverse groups

Another group often overlooked in the community, with a higher risk of suicide, are LGBTQIA+ people and other gender diverse groups (Perkins, 2019). The complex and multifaceted reasons for this identified increased risk of suicide can be largely related to the effects of negative health determinants such as barriers to gender-affirming care, gender-based victimisation, institutionalised cissexism (Zwickl et al., 2021), social marginalisation and stigma, including **homophobia**, **transphobia**, **cissexist** and **heterosexist** attitudes. More recently, **misgendering** and the incorrect us of **gender pronouns** are considered disrespectful and potentially harmful. Effects of the social marginalisation and discrimination include (Living Proud, 2017):

- exposure to discrimination
- social isolation
- family or relationship stress
- harassment, physical or sexual abuse
- substance use problems
- previous suicide attempts or DSH
- current or past mental health difficulties (notably, depressive and affective disorders).

A small number of studies have improved mental health outcomes when using identified gender minority-specific interventions, including transition-related gender-affirming care interventions (Coulter et al., 2019). Mental Health First Aid Australia has developed helpful guidelines when working with LGBTQIA+ persons who require mental health first aid. A webinar is available at the LGBTIQ+ Health Australia website: www.lgbtiqhealth.org.au/considerations_when_providing_mental_health_first_aid_to_an_lgbtiq_person.

It is difficult to establish accurate LGBTQIA+ suicide rates because, first, LGBTQIA+ people are often treated as one homogenous group in mental health and suicide research and, second, there is limited evidence regarding gender identity and sexuality collected at the time of death (additionally, each diverse subgroup is not clearly reported). This may be the result of deliberate or unintentional omission by partners, family members and friends or because questions about gender and/or sexual identity may not be asked by investigating authorities; or when they are asked, these details cannot be recorded as per the persons self-identity. Thus, it is likely that suicides for LGBTQIA+ people are under-reported. Lyons and colleagues (2019) conducted a review from 2003 to 2014 from the US National Violent Death Reporting System that discovered associations between distinct suicide groups. Intimate partner problems were found in 70 per cent of lesbian suicides, which is 6.5 times higher than non-lesbians. Lesbians also chose strangulation (35.1 per cent) and firearms (35.1 per cent) as the suicide method in contrast to 37.5 per cent of non-lesbians using poisoning to initiate death. Gay males recorded higher levels of mental illness, physical health problems and a situational crisis immediately preceding death than non-gay men. Gay males and lesbians were more likely to have a mental illness at the time of death than non-lesbians and heterosexual males.

The National LGBTI Mental Health and Suicide Prevention Strategy is a welcome acknowledgement of the uniqueness of this group; however, it is clear that further research into this situation (including subgroups), inclusive of ensuring affirming language and the developing further policy and evidence-based practice to support the needs of LGBTQIA+ members of the Australian community, is needed in order to enable social equity and inform the development of inclusive support and health services (Commonwealth of Australia, 2022b).

Culturally and linguistically diverse (CALD) people

Australia has one of the world's largest multicultural populations, with 27.6 per cent of Australians being born overseas (ABS, 2022c). Stigma driven by diverse cultural value systems can impact reporting on suicide among the migrant population, and in some cases, deaths by suicide are reported as unintentional or accidental deaths.

People from CALD communities have different risk and protective factors unique to each cultural or ethnic group. Some CALD communities are at a greater risk of suicide and poorer mental health. For example, refugees who have experienced traumatic events are at a higher risk of suicide and the asylum-seeking process can heighten the risk. People from CALD communities may also experience higher levels of psychological distress than other Australians due to having experienced traumatic events, such as war, separation from family and friends, or the migration process. Various reports in the literature have reported higher rates of mental illnesses such as PTSD, depression and anxiety amongst refugees and asylum seekers than other immigrants (Suicide Prevention Australia, 2021).

Males

In 2020, 76 per cent of people who took their own lives in Australia were male (ABS, 2021). To address and reduce the higher rate of male-versus-female suicide, specific suicide prevention programs have been developed and are aimed at providing education and support for men in high-risk age groups and high-risk occupations. For example, services targeting men in the building industry are provided through the Mates in Construction and Mates in Mining programs (www.matesinconstruction.org.au).

Many men make the decision to suicide impulsively and show few warning signs. For this reason, it is essential to respond quickly and effectively to those who seek help. Men of all ages and backgrounds can be at risk. Contributing factors include social isolation, unemployment, ill-health, old age, being part of the forensic system, work-related pressure, relationship breakdown, legal or financial problems, chronic illness or pain, suicide by a family member or close friend, substance use disorders and mental illness. Significantly, many men do not recognise symptoms of emotional distress or may prefer to try to work things out for themselves so they don't appear 'weak'. The generally lower health status of men in Australia is now receiving much deserved attention as governments target the key areas that are in need of improvement.

Older people in the community

In 2020, the highest number of age-specific suicide deaths per population for Australian men occurred in the 85-plus age group. For females, the age group recording the highest number of deaths by suicide was the 45–49-year-old group; however, in age groups above this, the 80–84-year-old group was the highest age-specific suicide deaths per population (ABS, 2021). There are a number of factors that contribute to suicide in older people, including isolation. Risk factors such as declining physical health, restricted mobility, lack of access to private transport and reduced contact with friends and family all contribute to feelings of isolation in older people (Suicide Prevention Australia, 2019). Furthermore, Conejero and colleagues (2018) report that suicide in older people is less likely to be due to a mental illness when compared to younger age groups and more likely to be related to bereavement and social isolation or physical health problems. Despite general comparative suicide rates over the past decade, men aged 80 years and over remain a high-risk group and suicide statistics for men aged over 85 years have been consistently ranking alarming high figures. There is also some concern that the rates of suicide for older men are under-reported because of stigma issues; for example, medical officers may be more likely to record a physical condition as the cause of death of older people, rather than suicide.

The needs of older people generally are often overlooked by health professionals. Older people are stigmatised and the provision of health care to older people is often viewed as somehow less important or glamorous than the provision of care to younger people. There is also a lack of choices for older people in relation to end-of-life care (Office of the Royal Commission, 2019).

People in rural and remote areas

People who live in rural and remote areas are at a higher risk of suicide than those who live in urban or metropolitan areas despite comparable diagnostic statistics (Fitzpatrick et al., 2021). This is due to economic and financial hardship, social isolation, reduced health literacy and access to health, community and support services in rural and remote areas. The regular but distressing cycles of droughts, floods, fire and cyclones that are an integral part of life in rural and remote areas are also contributing factors (Bishop et al., 2017). Finally, people in rural areas are less likely to seek help than people in urban or metropolitan areas because of perceptions of social stigma, perceived lack of confidentiality and because of the rural stoic, self-reliant nature of people living in rural areas (Royal Australian and New Zealand College of Psychiatrists, n.d.). The government has established arrangements with telecommunication service providers to ensure that crisis calls made to 1800 or 1300 numbers are free or are charged at the cost of a local call from a landline, regardless of the caller's location. For people living in a rural or remote area, this improves the affordability of contacting a telephone crisis centre in the absence of a face-to-face option, and addresses potential confidentiality issues. There are, however, significant concerns regarding the 'patchwork quilt' approach to connectivity and quality of telecommunication access and needs, including landline, web, mobile and other platform-based apps that affect accessing these types of services (Commonwealth of Australia, 2021c, p. 4). Ways and means of providing more effective care and treatment to people in rural and remote areas, including those with mental health issues, are discussed in the chapter that looks at delivering culturally appropriate mental health care.

People bereaved by suicide

Individuals and families bereaved by suicide are at higher risk of suicide themselves, irrespective of whether the deceased person was a blood relative, non-blood relative or friend. This is because people bereaved by suicide often experience a very complicated form of grief, with higher levels of prolonged grief occurring when a member of the nuclear family unexpectedly dies (Heeke et al., 2019). The sudden shock and denial of losing someone through a preventable event often generates a feeling of guilt and plays on a person's mind through unanswered questions such as 'Why?' and 'What could I have done?' The person bereaved by suicide may also experience anger, numbness, searching, self-blame, despair, shame, anxiety, depression, or a sense of rejection, or be traumatised following the discovery of the person who has taken their own life (SuicideLine Victoria, n.d.). The unique needs of people bereaved by suicide, often referred to as **suicide survivors** in the United States (Kõlves & de Leo, 2018), are identified in community prevention activities for high-risk groups. Ways of supporting the person who has been bereaved by suicide are discussed later in this chapter.

People who have self-harmed or attempted suicide

As previously stated, there is an increased suicide risk for people who have previously self-harmed when compared to those who do not self-harm (McGough et al., 2022). Nonetheless, it cannot be assumed that everyone who displays behaviours of suicidal intent will make further attempts to take their life in the future; however, it is important to acknowledge that prior suicidal behaviour is a major risk for future suicide (WHO, 2019).

Identifying those who are at risk presents some challenges. For example, self-cutting is considered common in adolescents (Hetrick et al., 2020) and is generally done in isolation (Beyond Blue, 2022b). In an English study involving 2000 general population teenagers aged 13–18 years, 75 per cent of those teenagers who admitted to cutting behaviours, cut their arms. The study found that teenagers who also cut elsewhere on their bodies presented with lower rates of wellbeing scores and were predominantly female (Morey et al., 2017). For this reason, it is important for health professionals to be aware of this risk and ensure that they talk to people who have unexplained injuries.

High-risk occupation groups

A large scoping review has been undertaken by Australian authors in an effort to identify if particular occupations pose a higher risk of suicide due to personal or occupational factors. Australian industries have unique contextual factors including workforce demographics and geographical landscape, which may additionally contribute to suicide risk among adult workers. The findings of the scoping review suggest that significant numbers of employed people in NSW are at increased risk of suicide due to their occupation. Rates among farmers, construction workers, ambulance and fire services, veterinarians, entertainers and artists, and the transport industry are particularly concerning, with elevated risk also evident in female doctors and male nurses.

A desktop study exploring Australian Coronial data conducted by the National Rural Health Alliance has highlighted that 370 farmers took their lives between 2009 and 2018. The report highlighted that farmers with certain demographic characteristics had higher suicide rates, including males, those who have separated from their spouse and middle-aged farmers. For the review period 2009–2017, the statistics illustrated that the average suicide rate in farmers was almost 59 per cent higher than non-farmers. The 2018 figures were even more tragic, revealing that this already high rate increased to 94 per cent higher than non-farmers when looking at the final year of data (Sartor, 2021).

The evidence in support of many at-risk occupations is inconsistent, and a number of studies analysed were of poor quality. Despite this, several common risk factors associated with specific employment types have been identified, including high job demands, low autonomy or control, shift work, physical danger and access to lethal means. Personal characteristics were also identified in specific occupations and may also be associated with increased risk, with socioeconomic, personality, mental health, substance use and demographic factors identified throughout the literature (Case et al., 2020). Notwithstanding the limitations of the literature evidence, health care professionals are encouraged to be mindful of these potentially high-risk occupations in relation to suicide risk and assessment processes.

Health professionals are encouraged to read more about the NSPS and about the population groups who are at risk of suicide on the Department of Health website (www1.health.gov.au/internet/publications/publishing.nsf/Content/suicide-prevention-activities-evaluation~background~national-suicide-prevention-strategy). There are also many opportunities to be involved in one or more of the programs or access information from organisations that have been developed as part of the NSPS. For example, Suicide Prevention Australia (www.suicidepreventionaust.org) provides online information about suicide, including information about the resources and supports for those who have been affected by suicide across Australia.

8.6 Assessment of risk

LEARNING OBJECTIVE 8.6 Discuss suicide risk assessment.

All people who are seen by a health professional in health services across Australia after an episode of self-harm must receive a comprehensive **suicide risk assessment** or **clinical risk assessment** from a mental health professional (Australian Commission on Safety and Quality in Health Care, 2022). A suicide risk assessment is a process by which health professionals gauge or estimate a person's immediate, medium-term and long-term risk for suicide. The assessment will include the development of interventions to ensure the person's safety, address the major issues and promote better health and wellbeing for the person.

Clinical risk assessment is a formal process by which health professionals gauge or estimate a person's short-term, medium-term and long-term risk for a variety of issues including, but not limited to, self-harm, self-neglect, aggression or violence, vulnerability/exploitation, poor adherence to treatment, child protection issues, domestic violence, homelessness, loss of income, and so on. Each or any of these factors can have an impact on a person's level of health and increase their risk of suicide and self-harm.

All health professionals are required to undertake risk assessments of consumers. The type of risk assessment undertaken will depend upon the nature of the risk that is being assessed. Adopting recommendations from national inquiries, a number of Australian states and territories have developed comprehensive training packages and guides for health professionals in light of the call by the Australian government for a 'documented system [in all states and territories] for prioritising referrals according to risk, urgency, distress, dysfunction and disability with timely advice and/or response to all those referred, at the time of assessment' (Australian Commission on Safety and Quality in Health Care, 2018, p. 35). Frustratingly, Rheinberger and colleagues reported that many emergency department staff (medical and nursing) feel that the emergency department is not conducive to providing adequate preventative care to people who present following a suicide attempt or self-harm and often defer clinical assessment, treatment and discharge decisions to colleagues with a mental health background (Rheinberger et al., 2022). There is also emerging evidence that gender-based suicide tests using blood-based biomarkers will be available to assist health care practitioners to predict those at highest suicide risk (Nimesh, 2019). It will be interesting to monitor how this research and biomarker indication affect clinical care and service delivery in future years.

The 'why' of risk assessment

Suicide and clinical risk assessments are a major component of the comprehensive biopsychosocial care that is provided to all consumers. While specialist mental health professionals will undertake a more detailed or specific risk assessment for people who have been identified as a high risk, health professionals in any setting will be required to undertake risk assessments to:
- clarify whether the person is at risk of self-harm or suicide in the short term
- identify if other people (e.g. staff or community members) are at risk of harm
- identify risk factors that will inform the person's immediate care and treatment
- ascertain whether a more detailed suicide risk assessment is indicated.

Risk assessments such as these are quite preliminary in nature and allow health professionals to identify the priorities for immediate intervention, manage any risk issues or behaviours that are being displayed at the time, and develop ongoing care.

Health professionals who work in emergency settings may also be required to undertake a suicide risk assessment because a significant number of individuals who present to a health service for assistance may not be prepared to wait or may refuse to be assessed for risk of suicide or self-harm by a mental health professional (Canberra Health Services, 2021). Reasons for leaving may include excessive waiting times, stigma, embarrassment and the negative attitudes of staff. In instances such as these, the initial or preliminary risk assessment will be used to determine whether or not the police should be notified to find the person and bring them back to the health service for treatment. Furthermore, death by suicide is associated with a recent emergency department attendance. O'Neill et al. (2019) reviewed the relationship between eating disorder presentations, hospital admission and death by suicide in 6630 medical records and, alarmingly, found that death by suicide is independently associated with eating disorder presentation and hospital admission within the previous three months. This very alarming statistic is further supported by Brenner et al. (2020), who found that approximately 1 per cent of all adults and adolescents who visit an emergency department with a self-harm injury will die by suicide within 3 months of their index visit (Brenner et al., 2020).

The 'who' of risk assessment

Many health professionals are uncertain as to whom they need to assess for risk. The most obvious answer is: if a person has expressed suicidal ideation, has attempted suicide, or has self-harmed, a suicide risk assessment is required.

Other people who may require a risk assessment are those who fall into the groups most at risk. A number of these groups have already been identified in a previous section. In addition, figure 8.3 lists the factors, situations and symptoms associated with an increased risk of suicide and self-harm. This table can be used by the health professional to help identify those people who may be in need of a risk assessment. In general, if the health professional is unsure, they are advised to go ahead with implementing the risk assessment. Even if the person is found to have a low risk, the assessment will have provided an opportunity for the health professional to engage with the person and discuss other health issues.

Individual
- Single, divorced, widowed or separated
- Access to potentially lethal means of harm/further harm (e.g. large amounts of medication, firearms)
- Physical illness — especially chronic, painful, debilitating and terminal conditions
- Family history of suicide
- Bereavement — especially loss of spouse/partner
- Occupation and job security status (Case et al., 2020)

Social
- Living alone
- Social isolation
- Prisoners and those in custody

Mental health-related
- Depression
- Psychotic illness
- Personality disorders
- Substance misuse
- History of self-harm
- Depressed thinking
- Suicidal ideas
- Suicidal plans
- Expressions of hopelessness
- Extreme variations in mood (labile mood) within relatively short periods of time ('mood swings')
- Displays of hostility and aggression
- Perceptual disturbance — particularly auditory hallucinations instructing the person to harm themselves

High-risk situations
- Recent major stress (e.g. bereavement, relationship breakdown, loss of employment, disruption to usual living arrangements)
- Recent self-harm
- Currently receiving psychiatric inpatient care — especially if on 'leave' from a mental health unit
- Recent discharge from psychiatric inpatient care — especially during the first month following discharge
- Anniversary of previously stressful or traumatic life event(s)
- Ready access to potentially lethal means

Indications of suicide risk following an episode of self-harm
- Evidence of pre-planning
- Well thought through and considered decision to choose a violent method
- Fully expects or expected to die
- Took steps to avoid discovery or intervention

Lack of appropriate ongoing care
- Consciously isolated at the time of the act
- Suicide note
- Regret at survival

The 'how' of risk assessment

Given that there continues to be no 'gold star' statistically robust and reliable way to measure self-harm and suicidality risk, it is crucial that the health professional considers how to approach risk assessments (Harmer et al., 2022; Saab et al., 2021). The decisions made will be informed by the:
- type of self-harming behaviour with which the person presents
- attitude and behaviour of the person on arrival or admission; for example, the degree of cooperativeness, level of consciousness, degree of intoxication
- information available from other sources; for example, written information brought in by the person, information from partner, friends or significant others, and access to the person's medical and general health history.

Information that will inform risk assessment can be obtained through observation, the use of questions and, as previously noted, reference to sources of written information from significant others.

Reliance on a risk assessment tool does not substitute the need for therapeutic engagement with people in order to determine a person's mental state, suicidal thoughts and emotional pain (Foster et al., 2021). When using a suicide risk assessment tool, it is necessary to consider the assessment in the context of the individual, their personal circumstances, the predisposing and precipitating factors that have led them to act or to think about acting, their current thoughts and feelings, and whether the person has any mental health issues. It is important not to avoid direct questions concerning the person's thoughts or plans regarding further self-harm. In fact, direct questioning allows the risk to be assessed and managed more effectively. In addition, the person may experience relief that previously distressing feelings can be discussed openly and honestly.

Questions the health professional may find helpful are provided here.

- What things have led up to you harming yourself?
- Have you been feeling anxious or agitated recently?
- What did you want to happen, or what did you think would happen, as a result of you harming yourself?
- Do you still have any thoughts or plans to harm yourself?
- How likely do you think you are to act on these thoughts? (It is often helpful to suggest that the person uses a 0–10 scale to rate the likelihood of further self-harm; that is, 0 = will definitely not harm myself; 10 = will definitely harm myself.)
- How do you feel now about having harmed yourself?
- Do you have anything on you right now that you could use to harm yourself with?

In addition, many health professionals make use of the variety of risk assessment tools that are available from health services across Australia or on the web.

Risk assessment tools

Currently, most states and territories have standardised assessment tools for health professionals to use across all settings. Health professionals are advised to familiarise themselves with the risk assessment policy, procedures and forms that are used in their place of work. The suicide risk assessment and clinical risk assessment tools that are available across Australia are not identical, but will almost always contain the same elements, such as those identified in figure 8.4. Like all assessment tools, these instruments are meant to provide only a gauge or estimation of the person's risk of suicide. As noted, these tools can be used by non-specialist health professionals to strike up a conversation with the person, rather than to develop a diagnosis.

Two of the most important things to note about any suicide risk assessment are, first, the process should not be undertaken by a health professional in isolation; and second, it is a dynamic process. Assessment of people at risk of suicide is a complex and demanding task. Wherever possible, health professionals need to discuss findings with the multidisciplinary team. Decisions made about the consumer must be collaborative — involving the consumer, partner or carer, and other health professionals, including a mental health specialist.

In addition, suicide risk assessments, and clinical risk assessments, are not static. Indeed, the 'change-ability' of risk status, especially in the period immediately after an experience of DSH or a suicide attempt, needs to be identified. If a person seems ambivalent and there is a level of **high changeability** in the way they present themselves to the health professional, the health professional needs to recommend reassessment (e.g. every eight hours) and closely monitor the person. Various factors will influence the person's level of risk and for this reason it is helpful to consider such an assessment in relation to the short-, medium- and long-term risk. These different levels of risk are considered in turn as follows.

Short-term risk

The most important factors in assessing a person's imminent suicide risk arise from their current personal or lived experience. Factors of concern include:

- 'at risk' mental state; for example, feelings of hopelessness, despair, agitation, shame, guilt, anger, psychosis or psychotic thought processes (see the chapter that looks at caring for a person with a serious mental illness)
- recent interpersonal crisis, especially rejection or humiliation
- recent suicide attempt
- recent major loss, trauma, or anniversary of loss or trauma
- alcohol intoxication
- drug withdrawal state
- chronic pain or illness
- financial difficulties, unemployment

- impending legal prosecution and/or child custody issues
- cultural or religious conflicts
- lack of social support network
- unwillingness to accept help
- difficulty accessing help due to language barriers and stigma for some culturally and linguistically diverse groups.

FIGURE 8.4 A risk assessment tool

Assessment categories		
1. Background history and general observations	**Yes**	**No**
• Does the person pose an *immediate* risk to self, you or others?		
• Does the person have any immediate (i.e. within the next few minutes or hours) plans to harm self or others?		
• Is the person aggressive and/or threatening?		
• Is there any suggestion or does it appear likely that the person may try to abscond?		
• Does the person have a history of self-harm?		
• Does the person have a history of mental health problems or psychiatric illness?		
If yes to any of the above, record details below:		
2. Appearance and behaviour	**Yes**	**No**
• Is the person obviously distressed, markedly anxious or highly aroused?		
• Is the person behaving inappropriately to the situation?		
• Is the person quiet and withdrawn?		
• Is the person inattentive and uncooperative?		
If yes to any of the above, record details below:		
3. Issues to be explored through brief questioning		
• Why is the person presenting now? What recent event(s) precipitated or triggered this presentation?		
• What is the person's level of social support (i.e. partner/significant other, family members, friends)?		

4. Suicide risk screen — greater number of positive responses suggests greater level of overall risk

	Yes	No	Don't know		Yes	No	Don't know
Previous self-harm	☐	☐	☐	Family history of suicide	☐	☐	☐
Previous use of violent methods	☐	☐	☐	Unemployed/retired	☐	☐	☐
Suicide plan/expressed intent	☐	☐	☐	Male gender	☐	☐	☐
Current suicidal thoughts/ideation	☐	☐	☐	Separated/widowed/divorced	☐	☐	☐
Hopelessness/helplessness	☐	☐	☐	Lack of social support	☐	☐	☐

(continued)

Assessment categories							
Depression	☐	☐	☐	Family concerned about risk	☐	☐	☐
Evidence of psychosis	☐	☐	☐	Disengaged from services	☐	☐	☐
Alcohol and/or drug misuse	☐	☐	☐	Poor adherence to psychiatric treatment	☐	☐	☐
Chronic physical illness/pain	☐	☐	☐	Access to lethal means of harm	☐	☐	☐

Management or action plan and outcomes following initial risk screen:
Describe all actions and interventions following assessment. Include details of referral to other team(s), telephone calls/advice and discharge/transfer or follow-up plans.

Researchers have proposed that suicide crisis syndrome diagnosis be adopted to reflect imminent suicide risk and cite the following five domains as essential to review: entrapment, affective disturbance, loss of cognitive control, hyperarousal and social withdrawal (Voros et al., 2021).

Collecting imminent risk factor information is best done by directly questioning the person and encouraging them to be as specific as possible about the likelihood of acting on their suicidal thoughts. Health professionals also need to be familiar with the criteria for using mental health legislation to protect the person or others from further harm. Information about mental health legislation, such as Australian state and territory Mental Health Acts, can be found in the chapter that looks at the legal and ethical context of mental health care.

Medium-term risk assessment

Some people retain suicidal thoughts, but deny any plans to act on them in the short term. These people may or may not be concurrently managing an ongoing mental illness that requires specialist mental health assessment or treatment. Some people may also describe ongoing suicidal thoughts, but, despite this, may have no plans to act on them in the short term. For a number of people, self-harm may be the culmination of a long period of distressing symptoms and difficulties. To manage and reduce the associated risks, it is important to ensure that people with medium-term risks are referred to a mental health service to receive appropriate and ongoing specialist care.

Long-term risk assessment

Statistically, all individuals who have self-harmed have an increased risk of suicide in the longer term. For a number of people, the act of self-harm is a 'one-off', an out-of-character action that they find difficult to explain and does not reflect how they are currently thinking and feeling. However, many of these individuals may also have longstanding difficulties with communication or in maintaining effective interpersonal relationships that predispose them to the risk of further self-harm or suicide in the long term. Again, to manage and reduce the associated risks, it is important to ensure people with long-term risks are referred to their general practitioner for regular monitoring or suitable community services to provide ongoing support.

UPON REFLECTION

Caring for long-term high-risk consumers

A small number of consumers are at a high risk of causing their death by suicide over a long period of time. These consumers are viewed as 'long-term high-risk' consumers. Constraining them for months, even years, under mental health legislation in an acute mental health unit is not an option. As discussed in the chapter on people displaying challenging behaviours, a large percentage of people who make repeated suicide gestures have a borderline personality disorder diagnosis.

QUESTIONS

1. When and how could you adopt the domains of the suicide crisis syndrome diagnosis into your assessment practices?

2. How would you clinically determine the importance of protective factors versus the intensity of perpetuating risk factors for people who are at long-term high risk of suicide?

3. How do you think that a person who is assessed as having a long-term high-risk of suicide could be managed in the community?

4. What long-term physical health conditions in mental health consumers significantly increase long-term suicidal risk?

5. When caring for a person who has a long-term high risk of suicide, what factors does a health professional need to be mindful of that may increase immediate risk?

8.7 Caring for the person who has self-harmed

LEARNING OBJECTIVE 8.7 Outline the care of the person who has self-harmed.

Just as the causes of self-harm and suicide are complex and multi-factorial, so is the provision of care to those with self-harming or suicidal behaviours. The decisions that are negotiated around the care and treatment provided will depend on the perceived level of risk of the person at the time of assessment, including the person's risk and protective factors, and the 'here and now' situation of the person.

In the first instance, the health professional who is providing care to a person who has self-harmed or has suicidal behaviours needs to follow a number of important steps.

- Treat any urgent complications of the self-harm to prevent or minimise the risk of future self-harm, severity of injury, disability or death.
- Undertake an initial assessment of risk as part of the comprehensive biopsychosocial assessment.
- Provide a safe environment.
- Consult with specialist mental health professionals.
- In consultation with the consumer, their partner, carer or family members and the mental health professional, develop an immediate safety management plan.
- In consultation with the consumer, their partner, carer or family members and the mental health professional, develop a Recovery plan. This may be an electronic or paper-based plan as part of the health record for the organisation. Additional options may include a digital suicide planning app for example Beyond Blue has a suicide planning app titled 'Beyond Now' that may appeal to some people (Beyond Blue, 2022d).
- Refer the person on for specialist treatment.
- Follow up and confirm that the person is receiving this specialist treatment.
- Provide suitable supportive literature to the consumer, family or carer, for example, *Finding your way back*, one of Beyond Blue *The way back* series resources (Beyond Blue, 2020a). For Aboriginal and Torres Strait Islander peoples, the specific resource is *Finding our way back* (Beyond Blue, 2020b).

Each of these steps is framed by person-centred approaches. This means that the health professional must first and foremost engage with and listen to the person, and practice empathetic communication (Foster et al., 2021). Additional suggestions that relate specifically to the person who has self-harmed are now outlined.

LIVED EXPERIENCE

This is My Brave

This is My Brave Australia is a registered charity in Australia and offers a platform for people with a mental health disorder or addiction problem to openly disclose their stories in a creative mode for the benefit of others and with the ultimate aim of reducing community stigma. Listen to Paige's story at www.thisismy brave.org/2019/03/04/paige-reitz-shares-her-story-of-recovery-from-self-harm and answer the following questions.

QUESTIONS

1. Paige stated that Recovery is 'not linear'. What implications does this have for health care workers?
2. In Paige's experience, what were the disadvantages of hospitalisation? What can you, and your service, do to mitigate this situation recurring?

▶

3. After listening to Paige's story, what can you change about your own practice to assist people who self-harm?

4. What is the underlying message of Paige's story? How can you honour her success and story in your treatment of other consumers?

Effective interpersonal communication

Many people will feel ashamed, guilty or embarrassed because they have self-harmed and it is important that health professionals are aware of this distress, accept what has happened without judgement and provide a degree of emotional support by validating the person's feelings and displaying empathy (Foster et al., 2021). This will involve the use of effective interpersonal communication. Strategies include the following.

- Adopt a non-judgemental and non-critical attitude. Overt or implied criticism usually only reinforces the person's sense of guilt and shame.
- Observe and note details of the person's emotional state and behaviour, in particular whether they are angry, impulsive, irritable, withdrawn or tearful.
- Use active listening techniques. This will assist in engaging the person in the processes of assessment and care.
- Use minimal responses. Reflecting the content and emotion of the person's story back to them will demonstrate attentive listening.
- Use open questions as a means of gaining a more detailed understanding of the person's emotional state; for example, 'How are you feeling right at this moment?', 'What would help you deal with your current difficulties?'
- Acknowledge the person's underlying distress by using empathic responses such as 'I can see you are very upset', 'You look distressed' or 'You must have found it very hard coping with these feelings of depression'.
- Avoid the use of overly reassuring or patronising statements, such as promising things that may be difficult to deliver; for example, 'Everything will be all right', 'Don't you worry; we'll sort out all your problems'.

Health professionals are also advised to stay in the present or 'here and now' with the person as much as possible, rather than going over past problems or old ground. Discussions about old problems are best left for specialist mental health professionals. On occasion, and once engagement has been achieved, the health professional may decide to make the person aware of the inconsistencies and discrepancies in their thinking, but this must be undertaken in a way that does not arouse antagonism or defensiveness.

Finally, if there comes a time when the health professional does not know what to say or how to say it, the use of empathy is always productive. Health professionals cannot 'fix' or 'cure' a person's self-harming behaviour overnight. However, by imagining what it could be like to be in the other person's shoes and sharing these thoughts with the person, the health professional will be supporting the person emotionally. It is with such support that a person can often find enough hope to move on slowly but surely into the future.

IN PRACTICE

Why do people suicide?

At times life can feel overwhelming and, to many people, numerous, stressful co-occurring problems may seem unresolvable. In these strenuous times, some people may consider suicide but won't act upon these thoughts. Others, though, sometimes feel that suicide is their only option out of a situation they deem to be hopeless. Feelings of hopelessness may be exacerbated by:

- family violence or abuse (mental, physical, sexual)
- breakdown of relationships (friends/romantic)
- poor living conditions, homelessness or poverty

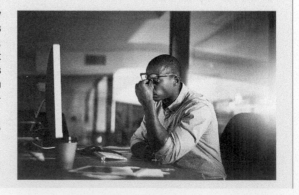

- unresolved legal problems
- lack of connectedness/no sense of belonging
- bereavement, loss and grief
- current physical or mental illness
- problems that appear to be unresolvable
- problems within the family group
- stress at school/university
- financial stressors
- work troubles or being unemployed.

DSH can at times be misinterpreted as an intention to suicide. DSH (e.g. cutting, burning) is a coping mechanism used by some people who find it difficult to process painful feelings. Most people who consider DSH don't wish to suicide.

QUESTIONS

1. How important is it to differentiate between feelings of suicide and self-harm?
2. Choose one of the situations listed that contribute to a feeling of hopelessness. What could be some predisposing, precipitating and perpetuating factors? What could be some protective factors?
3. How can you proactively predict financial, social and environmental factors that may negatively affect mental health consumers?
4. What strategies can you reasonably put in place to mitigate these identified risks?
5. Are there any additional strategies or complications to consider when an entire community group is captured within a particular event for example a natural disaster?

Managing short-term high risk

A small number of individuals may retain suicidal thoughts and plans to such an extent that they need hospitalisation. When this occurs, health professionals need to follow certain steps.

Firstly, if the person describes ongoing suicidal thoughts, health professionals need to ask the person directly if they have any means of harming themselves, such as medication or sharp objects. If this is the case, the person needs to hand these over for safe keeping while they are in the health setting. Health professionals are encouraged to refer to the policies and procedures of their workplace for guidance on the removal of personal items and/or body searches.

Observation

The person then needs to be cared for in an area that allows for easy observation and regular eye contact by health professionals. However, a balance must be struck between ensuring that health professionals know the whereabouts of the consumer to uphold their duty of care, against upholding the consumer's need for privacy. If specific risks of repetitive self-harm or suicidal behaviour have been identified, then a further assessment and updated advice from mental health professionals must be sought. If the person needs to remain in the general part of the hospital, then sedation, partial environmental confinement or one-on-one observation may need to be instigated as part of a time-limited immediate management plan. It may also be useful to refer to the relevant mental health legislation for additional measures that can be taken to ensure the safety of the person, health professionals, other staff members, consumers and the general public.

Discharge planning

Planning for discharge occurs as soon as the person has been admitted to hospital. After an episode of self-harm, discharge planning is one of the most important aspects of the person's care.

For many individuals, the act of self-harm may be a means of communicating distress relating to underlying interpersonal, family, financial, legal or social difficulties. It would not be realistic to expect to deal with all such difficulties while the person is in hospital, but these may require referral, advice and specialist assessment by other members of the multidisciplinary team or generalist community services.

If the person **absconds** or discharges themselves from hospital before a plan for future treatment has been negotiated, or before a mental health assessment has taken place, the multidisciplinary team will need to consider what actions to take to ensure that follow-up care can be arranged and is communicated to the person. Such actions will also demonstrate how the multidisciplinary team, as representatives of the health service provider, will address appropriate legal and ethical duty of care towards the person. Deciding the most appropriate action to take in such a situation will be informed by the risk assessment that was undertaken on arrival to the health service or admission to the hospital. If a person who has been assessed as having a high risk of suicide leaves the health setting without informing health professionals or against the medical officer's advice, the following actions can be taken.

1. Check the preliminary risk assessment that was undertaken and recorded in the clinical records.
2. Follow the health service's 'Missing patient/person policy'.
3. Inform the nominated next of kin, guardian or nearest relative or significant other/family member (as per your policy).
4. Inform the person's GP and other professional carers (e.g. community clinical manager or key worker), if appropriate.
5. If the preliminary risk assessment identified a high risk of suicide, health professionals must seek advice from a senior colleague about whether there is a need to inform the authorities that the person is missing. If the person was under the care provisions of mental health legislation, it is important to contact the police, health service managers and the mental health crisis assessment team (or equivalent) promptly, along with any other necessary stakeholders, as per your legislative requirements under your State or Territory Mental Health Act, and your local policy.

A person who has been hospitalised for self-harm or suicidal behaviours will be ready for discharge when they are physically well enough and when their risk of suicidality is at a level that can be managed in the community. All individuals who have self-harmed need to be assessed by a specialist mental health professional prior to discharge. They must also be referred to a community mental health specialist for follow-up after discharge. A list of key clinical tasks prior to discharge is provided here.

1. Complete all relevant documentation (e.g. risk assessment, baseline assessment tools).
2. Ensure that the person has been assessed as medically and physically well enough to leave hospital.
3. Organise a referral to mental health professionals for a comprehensive assessment.
4. Inform next of kin, guardian or relative/significant other of discharge plans.
5. Provide written information and advice to the person and next of kin, guardian or relative/significant other.
6. Inform the person's GP in writing.
7. Contact the person's clinical/case or care coordinator if the person is already known to health services.
8. Document the reason why the multidisciplinary team is discharging the person without the person being assessed by a specialist mental health professional.

While the care and treatment provided in a hospital will relate to the person's immediate level of risk, the longer term Recovery plan and specialist treatment will involve the assessment of needs related to (National Institute for Health and Care Excellence, 2022):

- skills, strengths and assets
- coping strategies
- mental health problems or disorders
- physical health problems or disorders
- social circumstances and problems
- psychosocial and occupational functioning, and vulnerabilities
- recent and current life difficulties, including personal and financial problems
- the need for psychological intervention, social care and support, occupational rehabilitation, and also drug treatment for any associated conditions
- the needs of any dependent children.

To assist with this treatment, many consumers will participate in one or more of the psychological therapies. These are now identified.

Psychological therapies

One of the major aims of the use of the psychological therapies for people with self-harming behaviours is to help the person to manage their stress and distress. It is also important to support the development of the person's ability to problem-solve. For short-term psychological therapies, the Royal Australian and New Zealand College of Psychiatrists recommends cognitive behavioural therapy (CBT), problem-solving therapy (PST) and interpersonal therapy (IPT) with CBT being reported as the superior intervention (Carter et al., 2016, p. 42).

Bahji and colleagues conducted a systematic review and network meta-analysis to determine which psychological therapies were more effective in treating and reducing self-harm and suicidal behaviours in children and adults.

Dialectical behaviour therapy (DBT) were associated with reductions in self-harm and suicidal ideation at the end of treatment, while mentalisation-based therapies were associated with decreases in self-harm and suicidal ideation (Bahji et al., 2021).

Dialectical behavioural therapies

Perhaps the most well-known psychological therapy is DBT, which has been demonstrated to be effective for women with borderline personality disorder and multiple DSH episodes (Westad et al., 2021). Favourable results using the brief therapy Attempted Suicide Short Intervention Program (ASSIP) have also been recently reported, with a clinical trial registered in Australia that will compare standard clinical approaches against standard clinical approaches combined with either brief CBT or ASSIP in the Australian context (Stapelberg et al., 2021). DBT uses cognitive and behavioural techniques to enhance interpersonal communication, develop skills to cope with emotional distress, regulate emotions and improve self-help. It is an intense and long-term form of therapy that comprises four modules: mindfulness, distress tolerance, emotion regulation and interpersonal effectiveness.

Perhaps one of the reasons DBT has been found to be so effective for people with self-harming and suicidal behaviours is that it provides them with new and more constructive ways of **self-soothing** and expressing their emotions. It also provides a means by which people are taught the skills to problem-solve and relate more effectively to others. In particular, those who self-harm often feel unable to work effectively through their problems or life experiences. The psychological therapies provide one means by which these skills can be learned.

Medication

There are no pharmacological preparations that are approved solely for the specific treatment of self-harm, but there have been reports of some randomised control trials attempting to address this issue (Witt et al., 2021). The Royal Australian and New Zealand College of Psychiatrists clinical practice guideline for the management of DSH also does not advocate the use of medication to reduce episodes of self-harm, unless clinically indicated (Carter et al., 2016).

Despite evidence which essentially does not support the use of medication, antipsychotics, antidepressants and mood stabilisers are often prescribed. This is because the person with the self-harming behaviour is looking to the authorising prescriber to 'do something' and medication is a concrete or tangible option. People with depression or psychosis may show some improvement if their DSH is related to their symptoms of mental illness. The main role of the health professional in psychopharmacological interventions is to provide the person with information about the medication and help the person to manage side effects.

The role of family and carer(s)

The NSPS has provided information for partners, carers and families on how to support the person who has self-harming behaviours. This is available through the LIFE Framework (www.livingisforeveryone.com.au), which is part of the National Suicide Prevention Initiative. Health professionals can suggest the following steps to the partner, carer or family.

- *Always take self-injury seriously* and pay particular attention if the person talks of feeling depressed, hopeless or anxious, as these feelings may also be associated with suicidal thinking.
- *Don't panic, become angry, reject the person or ignore the problem.* Don't take the self-injury personally by thinking that the person is doing it to hurt you. These reactions may increase the person's feelings of guilt and shame. Remain calm and focus on supporting the person and helping them to find better ways to cope.
- *Don't condone the self-injury.* Be non-judgemental and let the person know that you will continue to support them throughout their recovery and that you will be there for them no matter what they do.
- *Don't give ultimatums.* It can be tempting to demand that the person stop their self-injury immediately. This may drive the person away, make them feel more rejected, decrease their trust in you, and make them believe you are not listening.
- *Listen to the person* so they feel heard and supported and reassure them that the conversation will be treated confidentially.

- *Provide the support the person needs.* Self-injury is more likely to stop if the person can learn other ways to cope with their feelings and emotions, such as:
  - helping the person to find other coping strategies
  - encouraging the person to seek further help; there are many people and organisations that can help the person find better ways of coping and dealing with the issues underlying their self-injury
  - suggesting options for support (e.g. seeing their GP or other health professional) and offer to accompany the person to their appointment.
- *Do not pressure the person* into any treatment with which they are not comfortable.

Many partners or carers may feel that they do not have the skills to help or support the person who self-harms. Health professionals are able to refer or direct the partner or carer on to relevant support services that will provide them with the education and training they may need. Mental Health First Aid (2020) have developed a *Guide for care givers of people with a mental illness* and further services available are outlined in the chapter that discusses mental health service delivery.

Postvention

Postvention refers to activities and strategies undertaken after a suicide death to reduce associated trauma. Postvention Australia was launched in June 2013, and is the national association dedicated to supporting and helping people bereaved by suicide.

While the prevention of further suicide events is a role for those working in primary health care, individual health professionals also play an important role in supporting the partners, carers or families of those who die by suicide. This is because a suicide death gives rise to a complex grief in those left behind. Indeed, people left behind and bereaved by a suicide death will need ongoing and personal support. GPs can also provide targeted care and support to people who are bereaved or affected by a suspected suicide (Clark et al., 2020).

Research conducted with Australian people bereaved by suicide resulted in four themes being collated based on consultative feedback (Australian Institute for Suicide Research and Prevention & Postvention Australia (2017).

1. The need for different types of support services (practical and emotional) for survivors at different stages of the bereavement process.
2. Difficulties experienced in identifying and locating appropriate support services.
3. Experiences of stigma (personal and public), insensitive attitudes and subsequent social isolation.
4. The value of connecting with others through support groups for the suicide bereaved.

Grief counselling and follow-up will generally be provided by a specialist health professional; however, all health professionals can help those affected by being aware that grieving a suicide death is a long and complex process. As already noted, people who are bereaved by suicide may have unanswered questions that will never be answered. They may also experience anger or a sense of rejection or be traumatised following the discovery of the person who has taken their own life. In addition, there is still some stigma associated with death by suicide in Australian society, and the person left behind must learn to deal with this. This can be a long and tortuous journey for the person, and the effective health professional will understand this and demonstrate empathy regardless of the amount of time that has passed since the suicide (Government of South Australia, 2019).

IN PRACTICE

How many people are impacted by a suicide death?

It is generally accepted that approximately five immediate family members are intimately and directly affected by a suicide death. In addition, on average around 15 extended family members, 20 friends and 20 class or workmates may be affected. Of course, these numbers vary depending on the age, characteristics and the closeness of the relationship with the person who has died by suicide. A continuum of suicide 'survivorship' has been suggested by Cerel et al. (2014). This continuum covers (Australian Institute for Suicide Research and Prevention & Postvention Australia, 2017):

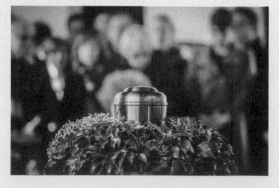

- *exposed* — everyone who knew or identified with the deceased
- *affected* — those who are experiencing significant psychological stress
- *short-term bereaved* — everyone who has grief-related reactions
- *long-term bereaved* — those who have to face extensive grief reactions over a longer period.

....

QUESTIONS

1. How does this continuum assist or distract you when considering those potentially bereaved by suicide?

2. Using the formula, calculate the amount of family, friends, class and work mates who are considered 'exposed' for every death by suicide. Multiply your answer by the annual suicide statistic. Discuss the widespread consequences of people bereaved by suicide when there are limited resources available to meet their needs.

The NSPS has funded each state and territory to provide an information and support pack for those who have been bereaved by suicide and other sudden death. It is recommended that health professionals obtain the information pack relevant to their location for ready access to provide to those in need in a timely way. Additionally, there are specific population-targeted postvention packages available for secondary schools (Department of Education and Training Victoria, 2022) and those recommended for Indigenous peoples by the Indigenous Suicide Postvention Service (Thirrili, 2019). Information on postvention is also available through Lifeline, via its website or by phoning 13 11 14. The Suicide Call Back Service (SCBS), the Salvation Army National Hope Line and the Standby Response Service are all nation-wide 24-hour telephone counselling services that also offer immediate online support for families, friends and communities who have been bereaved by suicide.

SUMMARY

People will often attend a health service after they have self-harmed, yet many health professionals find it challenging to maintain a positive approach to their assessment and the care they provide. To develop professional confidence and skills in this area, it is necessary for health professionals to become aware of the reasons people engage in self-harming behaviour, and actively participate in ongoing training and clinical supervision to minimise compassion fatigue and burnout.

This chapter focused on the ways the health professional can provide care to the person who self-harms. The chapter commenced by explaining the difference between self-harm and suicide, and the incidence of suicide and rate of DSH are discussed. Methods people use to self-harm are identified, as well as the predisposing, precipitating and perpetuating contributors and risk factors. The effects of the attitudes of health professionals towards the person who has self-harmed are also considered. This is followed by an overview of the NSPS and the major population groups in Australia that have a higher risk of suicide.

The chapter then moves on to explain risk assessment, including the 'why', 'when' and 'how' of risk assessment. A suicide risk assessment tool is provided and the major principles of negotiating and implementing care and treatment to the person with self-harming behaviours are considered. The role of partners or carers is summarised. Finally, the concept of postvention is described, including a description of how health professionals can support those who are bereaved by suicide. Further information about carers and the role they play in supporting consumers is provided in the chapter on caring for a person with a serious mental illness.

KEY TERMS

abscond When a person leaves or does not return to a health service setting without informing health professionals, when leaving is against a medical officer's advice or in breach of a legal order.

attempted suicide An action that involves a person endeavouring to intentionally cause their own death, but death does not result.

clinical risk assessment The formal process by which health professionals gauge or estimate risk for a person in relation to factors such as self-harm, self-neglect, violence or aggression, vulnerability, limited engagement with treatment and homelessness.

cissexist Showing or feeling discrimination or prejudice against transgender people.

deliberate self-harm (DSH) The intentional injuring of body tissue without suicidal intent.

dialectical behavioural therapy (DBT) A type of cognitive and behavioural therapy used with positive outcomes for people with a borderline personality disorder and self-harming behaviours.

gender pronouns How a person publicly expresses their gender identity through the use of a pronoun. Pronouns can be gender-specific or gender-neutral and can include the traditional he or she, as well as gender-neutral pronouns such as they, their, ze and hir. See also *misgendering*.

heterosexist Showing or feeling discrimination or prejudice against homosexuals on the assumption that heterosexuality is the normal sexual orientation.

high changeability A state of being that is demonstrated by a person who is quite ambivalent about suicide or self-harm.

homophobia An individual's or society's misunderstanding or negative beliefs that exist toward same-sex attracted people. It can range from the use of offensive language to bullying, abuse and physical violence and can include systemic barriers, such as being denied housing or being fired from their employment due to a person's sexual orientation.

misgendering Occurs when a person is described or addressed using language that does not match their gender identity. This can include the incorrect use of pronouns (she/he/they), familial titles (dad, sister, uncle, niece) and, at times, other words that traditionally have gendered applications (pretty, handsome, etc.). See also *gender pronouns*.

National Suicide Prevention Strategy This Strategy provides the platform for Australia's national policy on suicide prevention with an emphasis on promotion, prevention and early intervention for mental health.

perpetuating factors The factors that prolong or support the continuation of a behaviour.

postvention Activities and strategies undertaken after a death by suicide to reduce associated trauma, such as providing bereavement support and advocacy to prevent contagion suicides and suicide clusters.

precipitating influences The influences or triggers that elicit or provoke a behaviour in the present or 'here and now'.

predisposing causes Factors that render the person liable or more prone to the behaviour.

self-soothing The processes or internal resources used by an individual to lower their personal stress and distress level.

suicidal ideation The thought, ideas or plans of a person about causing their own death.

suicide cluster A number of suicides that are proximal but not usually simultaneous and grouped by association in a community.

suicide risk assessment The formal process by which a health professional gauges or estimates a person's short-term, medium-term and long-term risk for suicide.

suicide survivor Someone who experiences a high level of self-perceived psychological, physical and/or social distress for a considerable length of time after exposure to the suicide of another person.

suicide The act of a person intentionally causing their own death.

transphobia An individual's or society's misunderstanding, fear, ignorance of or prejudice against transgender people.

REVIEW QUESTIONS

1 What are the differences between self-harm, suicide and suicidal ideation?
2 Outline what is meant by the terms 'predisposing causes', 'precipitating influences' and 'perpetuating factors' of suicide.
3 Name at least six risk factors for suicide.
4 What are the defining characteristics of eating disorders? List the five most common types of eating disorder.
5 Describe the link between mental illness, physical illness and suicide.
6 Describe the main objectives of the NSPS, including the main action areas of the National Aboriginal and Torres Strait Islander Suicide Prevention Strategy.
7 Identify the key strategies that support the population groups in Australia that are most vulnerable to suicide.
8 List the high-risk occupation groups in Australia that are most vulnerable to suicide.
9 List the essential components of a suicide risk assessment.
10 What are the key factors for effective interpersonal communication when speaking with a person who has self-harmed or is a suicide survivor?
11 What is dialectical behavioural therapy?
12 What are the key points to remember about 'postvention'?

DISCUSSION AND DEBATE

1 Many people will be familiar with situations that potentially exacerbate feelings of 'hopelessness'. Discuss which comes first: the feeling of hopelessness resulting in a spiral of social and personal problems, or, a socially and personally challenged life that is the catalyst for feelings of hopelessness.
2 List three personal considerations from your background that might consciously or unconsciously limit your ability to care for people in a non-judgemental way.
3 Discuss whether talking about suicide with people will increase or decrease the risk of a person considering suicide, or acting upon suicidal thoughts.
4 How might important ethical considerations guide and assist your interactions when working with people who may self-harm?
5 Self-harming behaviours may be initially noticed in a primary health setting. Is the primary health or tertiary health sector the most appropriate setting for managing non-suicidal acts of self-harm? Explain your answer.
6 What behaviours constitute self-harm in the younger population? For example, do you consider risk-taking behaviours such as unprotected sex, self-cutting, self-inflicted cigarette and match burns, body piercings, eating disorders, alcohol use, dangerous driving and tattoos as self-harm, or just typical younger generation behaviour? Discuss your reasons using a clinical, legal and ethical framework.

7 Discuss whether social media contributes to either perpetuating or reducing self-harm rates in adolescents and young people. Provide evidence for your responses.

8 Consider large-scale disasters, such as flood, bushfire or cyclone. What is the best way to engage with known vulnerable groups within our communities in times of crisis? For example, people who are deaf, children, older residents and those from a culturally and linguistically diverse background? The MHFA Fact sheets might be useful for this activity and can be found at www.mhfa.com.au/mental-health-first-aid-guidelines.

PROJECT ACTIVITY

1 Read the Suicide Prevention Australia Turning points: Imagine a world without suicide white paper. Based on the content of the paper, draft a social media campaign highlighting suicide preventive actions for your local community. Include details of the content, the format, which social media platforms and types of media you will use, how it will be promoted across social media platforms, budget, audience and so on. In order to ensure a co-designed and evidenced-based campaign, which community stakeholders would you invite to participate?

2 Review the LGBTIQA+ Dictionary. What terms are unfamiliar? How can you insert these terms into your practice? Discuss the pros and cons of using these specific terms (i) regularly in professional language and (ii) only during the assessment process.

WEBSITES

1 Open Arms is a government service addressing the experiences of sadness, distress or anger that Department of Veterans Affairs (DVA) personnel may encounter after deployment. Open Arms can help veterans, Australian Defence Force (ADF) personnel and family members identify the symptoms of not coping. Open Arms can provide treatment options and resources to ADF personnel, including the Operation Life online platform and the Operation Life app. Open Arms also has clinical resources for health professionals who may be treating members of the veteran and defence community: www.openarms.gov.au.

2 The Bereaved by Suicide Centre for Intense Therapy provides advice on how to talk to children affected by the suicide of a loved one, using an age-appropriate suicide resource kit to facilitate the conversation. The Red Chocolate Elephants tool consists of a DVD and book which can help guide clinicians through a confusing and distressing time for children: www.bereavedbysuicide.com.au/red-chocolate-elephants.html.

3 The Butterfly Foundation is a non-government organisation that represents all people affected by eating disorders, including individuals, their families and friends. As a leading national voice in supporting these people's needs, the Butterfly Foundation highlights the realities of seeking treatment for Recovery, and advocates for improved services from both government and independent sources: www.thebutterflyfoundation.org.au.

4 The Centre for Rural and Remote Mental Health is based in Orange. It is a major rural initiative of the University of Newcastle, Faculty of Health and the NSW Department of Health. The Centre aims to bring quality education and research programs to all rural areas of New South Wales through effective partnerships. It also seeks to improve the mental health of rural and remote communities through academic leadership, collaboration and achievements in research, education, service development and information services: www.crrmh.com.au.

5 Conversations Matter is an online resource managed by the Hunter Institute of Mental Health, New South Wales. The site provides information and fact sheets for both health professionals and members of the public, in relation to understanding, preventing and responding to suicidal behaviours from a talking/understanding perspective, rather than a treatment or intervention perspective: www.conversationsmatter.com.au.

6 headspace provides mental and health wellbeing support, information and services to young people and their families across Australia: www.headspace.org.au.

7 Kids Help Line is a free, private and confidential, telephone and online counselling service specifically for young people aged between 5 and 25 years in Australia: www.kidshelpline.com.au or ph 1800 55 18 00

8 LGBTI National Health Alliance knowledge hub is a useful site where a number of webinars are available explaining sexuality and gender diversity issues in Australia: www.lgbtihealth.org.au.

9 Lifeline is a national charity that provides all Australians experiencing a personal crisis with access to 24-hour crisis support and suicide prevention services. Lifeline provides education and counselling on a large range of topics including suicidal thoughts or attempts, personal crisis, anxiety, depression, loneliness, abuse and trauma, stresses from work, family or society, and self-help information for friends and family: www.lifeline.org.au.

10 The Living is for Everyone (LIFE) website is a world-class suicide and self-harm prevention resource. Dedicated to providing the best available evidence and resources to guide activities aimed at reducing the rate at which people take their lives in Australia. The LIFE website is designed for people across the community who are involved in suicide and self-harm prevention activities: www.livingisforever yone.com.au.

11 MensLine Australia is a professional telephone and online support and information service for Australian men. Services are available 24 hours a day: ph 1300 78 99 78 or www.mensline.org.au.

12 The Embrace Multicultural Mental Health (Embrace Project) is run by Mental Health Australia and funded by the Australian government Department of Health, to provide a national focus for advice and support to providers and governments on mental health and suicide prevention for people from culturally and linguistically diverse (CALD) backgrounds. Additionally, the Embrace Project can provide education, training and resources to health provider services. Translated mental health information for consumers is available in excess of 30 languages: www.embracementalhealth.org.au.

13 Mindframe provides access to up-to-date, evidence-based information to support the reporting, portrayal and communication about suicide and mental illness: www.mindframe.org.au.

14 Postvention Australia is the National Association for the bereaved by suicide website. The website contains resources and information for people bereaved by suicide and helpful information for those who are supporting family and friends bereaved by suicide. There is specific information on grief, and Indigenous grief and loss issues: www.postventionaustralia.org.

15 QLife is Australia's first nationally oriented counselling and referral service for people who are lesbian, gay, bisexual, trans and/or intersex (LGBTI). QLife provides nation wide, early intervention, peer-supported telephone and web-based services to people of all ages across the full breadth of people's bodies, genders, relationships, sexualities and lived experiences. This service is available between 3 pm and midnight every day. QLife is a safe place to talk about mental health, relationships, isolation, coming out and a whole host of other concerns: www.qlife.org.au.

16 The Royal Australian and New Zealand College of Psychiatrist's Consumer and Carer Clinical Practice Guidelines are provided free of charge and are a valuable resource to support consumers and their carers, families and friends in learning more about mental illness and the treatments that are available: www.ranzcp.org/Publications/Guidelines-and-resources-for-practice.aspx.

17 OzHelp is a leading suicide prevention organisation that works with the government, blue collar workplaces, corporate partners and the community to provide mental health and wellbeing support and training services to hard-to-reach industries that are most at risk of suicide. These industries include building and construction, transport and logistics, mining and agriculture: www.ozhelp. org.au.

18 The Suicide Call Back Service (SCBS) is a 24-hour, nationwide service that provides immediate telephone counselling and support in a crisis to people 15 years and over, and is especially suited to people who are geographically or emotionally isolated. Services are provided to individuals who are suicidal, are caring for someone who is suicidal, people bereaved by suicide, and health professionals supporting people affected by suicide. The SCBS can additionally provide up to six further telephone counselling sessions with the same counsellor scheduled to suit consumer preferences: www.suicidec allbackservice.org.au.

19 Suicide Prevention Australia is a not-for-profit, non-government organisation working as a public health advocate in suicide prevention. It is the only national umbrella body active in suicide prevention throughout Australia: www.suicidepreventionaust.org.

REFERENCES

Alshahrani, W. (2018). A literature review of healthcare professionals' attitudes towards patients with mental illness. *Journal of Medical Research and Health Education, 2*(1), 5.

American Psychiatric Association. (2017). *Help with eating disorders.* www.psychiatry.org/patients-families/eating-disorders

American Psychiatric Association. (2013). *Diagnostic and statistical manual of mental disorders:. DSM-5.*

Amir, K., Betty, A., & Kenneth., A. (2019). Emotional intelligence as predictor of compassion fatigue among mental health practitioners. *Open Access Library Journal, 6*, 1–10. www.scirp.org/journal/paperinformation.aspx?paperid=92498

Australian Bureau of Statistics. (2021). *Causes of death, Australia 2020.* www.abs.gov.au/statistics/health/causes-death/causes-death-australia/2020#intentional-self-harm-deaths-suicide-in-australia

Australian Bureau of Statistics. (2022a). *Australian national study of mental health and wellbeing: Summary of results.* www.abs.gov.au/statistics/health/mental-health/national-study-mental-health-and-wellbeing/latest-release

Australian Bureau of Statistics. (2022b). *Australian national study of mental health and wellbeing. Health conditions prevalence: Key findings on selected long-term health conditions and prevalence in Australia.* www.abs.gov.au/statistics/health/health-conditions-and-risks/health-conditions-prevalence/latest-release

Australian Bureau of Statistics. (2022c). *Cultural diversity: Census.* www.abs.gov.au/statistics/people/people-and-communities/cultural-diversity-census/2021

Australian Commission on Safety and Quality in Health Care. (2018). *Map of the national safety and quality health service standards (second edition) with the National Standards for Mental Health Services.*

Australian Commission on Safety and Quality in Health Care. (2022). *Action 5.31. Predicting, preventing and managing self-harm and suicide.* www.safetyandquality.gov.au/standards/nsqhs-standards/comprehensive-care-standard/minimising-patient-harm/action-531.

Australian Institute of Health and Wellbeing. (2022a). *Suicide and self-harm monitoring.* www.aihw.gov.au/suicide-self-harm-monitoring/summary

Australian Institute of Health and Wellbeing. (2022b). *Injury in Australia: Assault and homicide.* www.aihw.gov.au/reports/injury/assault-and-homicide

Australian Institute of Health and Wellbeing. (2022c). *National Indigenous Australians Agency. Aboriginal and torres strait islander health performance framework. 1.23 Leading causes of Mortality.* www.indigenoushpf.gov.au/measures/1-23-leading-causes-mortality#findings.

Australian Institute of Health and Wellbeing. (2022d). *Injury in Australia: Intentional self-harm and suicide.* www.aihw.gov.au/reports/injury/intentional-self-harm-and-suicide

Australian Institute for Suicide Research and Prevention & Postvention Australia. (2017). *Postvention Australia Guidelines: A resource for organisations and individuals providing services to people bereaved by suicide.* Australian Institute for Suicide Research and Prevention.

Bahji, A., Pierce, M., Wong, J., Roberge, J. N., Ortega, I., & Patten, S. (2021). Comparative efficacy and acceptability of psychotherapies for self-harm and suicidal behaviour among children and adolescents: A systematic review and network meta-analysis. *Journal of the American Association (JAMA) Network Open, 4*(4), e216614. https://jamanetwork.com/journals/jamanetworkopen/fullarticle/2778571

Better Health Channel. (2021). *Body Mass Index (BMI).* Department of Health & Human Services, State Government of Victoria. www.betterhealth.vic.gov.au/health/healthyliving/body-mass-index).

Beyond Blue. (2022a). *Looking after yourself.* www.beyondblue.org.au/the-facts/supporting-someone/looking-after-yourself

Beyond Blue. (2022b). *Self-harm and self-injury.* www.beyondblue.org.au/the-facts/suicide-prevention/feeling-suicidal/self-harm-and-self-injury.

Beyond Blue. (2022c). *Serious health events and chronic illness.* www.beyondblue.org.au/who-does-it-affect/men/what-causes-anxiety-and-depression-in-men/serious-health-events-and-chronic-illness

Beyond Blue. (2022d). Beyond now. Suicide safety planning (app). www.beyondblue.org.au/get-support/beyondnow-suicide-safety-planning.

Beyond Blue. (2020a). *Finding your way back. A resource for people who have attempted suicide.* www.beyondblue.org.au/the-facts/suicide-prevention/after-a-suicide-attempt/the-way-back-support-service

Beyond Blue. (2020b). *Finding our way back. A resource specifically for Aboriginal and Torres Strait Islander people after a suicide attempt.* www.beyondblue.org.au/the-facts/suicide-prevention/after-a-suicide-attempt/the-way-back-support-service

Biancarelli, D. L., Biello, K. B., Childs, E., Drainoni, M., Salhaney, P., Edeza, A., Mimiaga, M. J., Saitz, R., & Bazzi, A. R. (2019). Strategies used by people who inject drugs to avoid stigma in healthcare settings. *Drug and Alcohol Dependence, 198,* 80–86.

Bishop, L., Ransom, A., Laverty, M., & Gale, L. (2017). *Mental health in remote and rural communities.* Royal Flying Doctor Service of Australia.

Black Dog Institute. (2022). *Research: Centres and collaboration. LifeSpan Trials.* www.blackdoginstitute.org.au/research-centres/lifespan-trials

Blanchard, A., Chihuri, S., DiGuiseppi, C. G., & Li, G. (2021). Psychiatry risk of self-harm in children and adults with autism spectrum disorder a systematic review and meta-analysis. *JAMA Network Open, 4*(10).www.jamanetworkopen.com/journals/jamanetworkopen/fullarticle/2785235

Bóna, E., Forgács, A., & Túry, F. (2018). Potential relationship between juice cleanse diets and eating disorders. A qualitative pilot study. *Orvosi Hetilap, 159*(28), 1153–1157.

Brådvik, L. (2018). Suicide risk and mental disorders. *International Journal of Environmental Research and Public Health, 15*(9), 2028.

Bratman, S. (1997). Health food junkie. *Yoga Journal, 136,* 42–50.

Brenner, J. M., Marco, C. A., Kluesner, N. H., Schears, R. M., & Martin, D. R. (2020). Assessing psychiatric safety in suicidal emergency department patients. *Journal of the American College of Emergency Physicians Open, 1*,1, 30–37. https://doi.org/10.1002/emp2.12017

Bureau of Infrastructure, Transport and Regional Economics. (2021). *Road Trauma Australia 2020 Statistical summary.* www.bitre.gov.au/sites/default/files/documents/road_trauma_australia_2020_statistical_summary.pdf

Bureau of Infrastructure, Transport and Regional Economics. (2022). *Road Trauma Australia: Annual Summaries.* BITRE, Canberra ACT. www.bitre.gov.au/publications/ongoing/road_deaths_australia_annual_summaries

Burt, A., Mitchison, D., Dale, E., Bussey, K., Trompeter, N., Lonergan, A., & Hay, P. (2020). Prevalence, features and health impacts of eating disorders amongst First-Australian Yiramarang (adolescents) and in comparison with other Australian adolescents. *Journal of Eating Disorders, 8*, 10. https://doi.org/10.1186/s40337-020-0286-7

Burton, M. (2019). Suicide and self-harm: Vulnerable children and young people. *Practice Nursing, 30*(5). https://doi.org/10.12968/pnur.2019.30.5.218

Butterfly Foundation. (2022a). *Risks and warning signs.* www.butterfly.org.au/eating-disorders/risks-and-warning-signs

Butterfly Foundation. (2022b). *RESET: A conversation about boys' body image.* www.butterfly.org.au/get-involved/campaigns/reset

Canberra Health Services. (2021). *Canberra hospital services procedure: Emergency Department and Mental Health Interface. 21/418*

Carter, G., Page, A., Large, M., Hetrick, S., Milner, A. J., Bendit, N., Walton, C., Draper, B., Hazell, P., Fortune, S., Burns, J., Patton, G., Lawrence, M., Dadd, L., Robinson, J., & Christensen, H. (2016). Royal Australian and New Zealand College of Psychiatrists clinical practice guideline for the management of deliberate self-harm. *Australian and New Zealand Journal of Psychiatry, 50*(10), 939–1000.

Case, R., Alabakis, J., Bowles, K.-A., & Smith, K. (2020). *High-risk occupations—Suicide: An evidence check rapid review brokered by the Sax Institute for the NSW Ministry of Health.* www.saxinstitute.org.au/wp-content/uploads/20.10_Evidence-Check_Suicide-prevention-in-high-risk-occupations.pdf

Cerel, J., McIntosh, J. L., Neimeyer, R. A., Maple, M., & Marshall, D. (2014). The continuum of "survivorship": Definitional issues in the aftermath of suicide. *Suicide and Life-Threatening Behaviour, 44*, 591–600. https://doi.org/10.1111/sltb.12093

Clark, S., Smith, N., Griesbach, A., Rivers, D., & Kuliwaba, A. (2020). Supporting general practitioners and practice staff after a patient suicide: A proposal for the development of a guideline for general practice. *Australian Journal of General Practice, 49*(5), 261–266. www1.racgp.org.au/ajgp/2020/may/supporting-general-practitioners-and-practice-staf

Commonwealth of Australia. (2021a, September 21). *New Strategy and Research Centre to Support Australians with Eating Disorders.* Department of Health and Aged Care. [Media release]. www.health.gov.au/ministers/the-hon-greg-hunt-mp/media/new-strategy-and-research-centre-to-support-australians-with-eating-disorders

Commonwealth of Australia. (2021b). *Prevention compassion care. National Mental Health and Suicide Prevention Plan.* www.health.gov.au/resources/publications/the-australian-governments-national-mental-health-and-suicide-prevention-plan

Commonwealth of Australia. (2021c). *2021 Regional Telecommunications Review. A step change in demand.* www.rtirc.gov.au

Commonwealth of Australia. (2022a). *Royal Commission into Defence and Veteran suicide.* https://defenceveteransuicide.royalcommission.gov.au

Commonwealth of Australia. (2022b). *LGBTQIA+ Glossary of common terms. CFCA Resource sheet. Child Family Community Australia.* Australian Institute of Family Studies. www.aifs.gov.au/sites/default/files/publication-documents/22-02_rs_lgbtiqa_glossary_of_common_terms_0.pdf

Conejero, I., Olié, E., &, Courtet, P., & Calati, R. (2018). Suicide in older adults: Current perspectives. *Clinical Interventions in Aging, 13*, 691–699.

Coulter, R. W. S., Egan, J. E., Kinsky, S., Friedman, M. R., Eckstrand, K. L., Frankeberger, J., Folb, B. L., Mair, C., Markovic, N., Silvestre, A., Stall, R., & Miller, E. (2019). Mental health, drug, and violence interventions for sexual/gender minorities: A systematic review. *Paediatrics, 144*(3), e20183367.

Department of Education and Training Victoria. (2022). *Policy and advisory library. School operations. Suicide response (Postvention).* www2.education.vic.gov.au/pal/suicide-response-postvention/policy

Department of Health. (2013). *National aboriginal and Torres Strait Islander suicide prevention strategy. Aboriginal and Torres Strait Islander suicide: Origins, trends and incidence.* Australian Government. www.health.gov.au/sites/default/files/documents/2021/05/national-aboriginal-and-torres-strait-islander-suicide-prevention-strategy.pdf

Department of Health and Aging. (2007). Living is For Everyone. Fact Sheet 16. *Suicide Prevention in Indigenous Communities.* Australian Government. https://earlytraumagrief.anu.edu.au/files/Suicide-prevention-in-Indigenous-communities.pdf

Eating Disorders Victoria. (2019a). *Classifying eating disorders — DSM-5.* www.eatingdisorders.org.au/eating-disorders/what-is-an-eating-disorder/classifying-eating-disorders/dsm-5

Eating Disorders Victoria. (2022b). *Treatment options for eating disorders. Eating Disorders Foundation of Victoria.* www.eatingdisorders.org.au/my-eating-disorder-recovery-journey/eating-disorder-treatment-for-adults

Everymind. (2022). *Life in mind. About suicide. Suicide prevention for Aboriginal and Torres Strait Islander communities. What we know about suicide for Aboriginal and Torres Strait Islander peoples.* www.lifeinmind.org.au/about-suicide/aboriginal-and-torres-strait-islander-communities/what-we-know-about-suicide-for-aboriginal-and-torres-strait-islander-peoples

Fitzpatrick, S. J., Handley, T., Powell, N., Read, D., Inder, K. J., Perkins, D., & Brew, B. K. (2021). Suicide in rural Australia: A retrospective study of mental health problems, health-seeking and service utilisation. *PLoS One, 16*(7), e0245271. https://doi.org/10.1371/journal.pone.0245271

Foster, A., Alderman, M., Safin, D., Aponte, X., McCoy, K., Caughey, M., & Galynker, I. (2021). Teaching suicide risk assessment: Spotlight on the therapeutic relationship. *Academic Psychiatry, 45*, 257–261. https://doi.org/10.1007/s40596-021-01421-2

Gayaa Dhuwi (Proud Spirit) Australia. (2020). *Suicide prevention strategy renewal. The Final consultation of the dDraft national aboriginal and torres strait Islander suicide prevention strategy.* https://www.gayaadhuwi.org.au/home/suicide-prevention-strategy-renewal/

Gibson, M., Stuart, J., Leske, S., Ward, R., & Tanton, R. (2021). Suicide rates for young Aboriginal and Torres Strait Islander people: The influence of community level cultural connectedness. *Medical Journal of Australia*, *214*(11), 514–518. https://doi.org/10.5694/mja2.51084

Gibson, R., Carson, J., & Houghton, T. (2019). Stigma towards non-suicidal self-harm: Evaluating a brief educational intervention. *British Journal of Nursing*, *28*(5), 307–312.

Hanssens, L. (2011). "Suicide (echo) clusters" — Are they socially determined, the result of a pre-existing vulnerability in Indigenous communities in the Northern Territory and how can we contain cluster suicides? *Aboriginal and Islander Health Worker Journal*, *5*(1), 14–23.

Harmer, B., Lee, S., Duong, T. V. H., & Saadabadi, A. (2022). Suicidal ideation. *StatPearls* [*Internet*]. StatPearls Publishing. PMID: 33351435 www.pubmed.ncbi.nlm.nih.gov/33351435

headspace. (2020a). *The Yarn Safe story*. www.headspace.org.au/yarn-safe/the-yarn-safe-story

headspace. (2022b). *What you need to know about self-harm*. www.headspace.org.au/explore-topics/for-young-people/self-harm

Heeke, C., Kampisiou, C., Niemeyer, H., & Knaevelsrud, C. (2019). A systematic review and meta-analysis of correlates of prolonged grief disorder in adults exposed to violent loss. *European Journal of Psychotraumatology*, *10*(1), 1583524.

Hetrick, S. E., Subasinghe, A., Anglin, K., Hart, L., Morgan, A., & Robinson, J. (2020). Understanding the needs of young people who engage in self-harm: A qualitative investigation. *Frontiers in Psychology*, *10*, 2916. https://doi.org/10.3389/fpsyg.2019.02916

Hill, N. T., Witt, K., Rajaram, G., McGorry, P. D., & Robinson, J. (2021). Suicide by young Australians, 2006-2015: A cross-sectional analysis of national coronial data. *Medical Journal of Australia*, *214*(3), 133–139. https://doi.org/10.5694/mja2.50876 PMID: 33236400

Imperatori, C., Panno, A., Carbone, G. A., Corazza, O., Taddei, I., Bernabei, L., Massullo, C., Prevete, E., Tarsitani, L., Pasquini, M., Farina, B., Biondi, M., & Bersani, F. S. (2022). The association between social media addiction and eating disturbances is mediated by muscle dysmorphia-related symptoms: A cross-sectional study in a sample of young adults. *Eating and Weight Disorders - Studies on Anorexia, Bulimia and Obesity*, *27*(3), 1131–1140. https://doi.org/10.1007/s40519-021-01232-2

Klenthis, A. (2021). *Lockdowns due to COVID-19 and the mental health consequences for the Australian general population: An integrative literature review and narrative synthesis*. https://doi.org/10.13140/RG.2.2.22751.18082

Kõlves, K., & de Leo, D. (2018). Suicide bereavement: Piloting a longitudinal study in Australia. *British Medical Journal Open*, *8*, e019504.

Lavis, A., McNeil, S., Bould, H., Winston, A., Reid, K., Easter, C. L., Pendrous, R., & Michail, M. (2022). *Self-Harm in Eating Disorders (SHINE): a mixed-methods exploratory study*. *British Medical Journal Open*, e065065. https://doi.org/10.1136/bmjopen-2022-065065

Leckning, B., Ringbauer, A., Robinson, G., Carey, T. A., Hirvonen, T., & Armstrong, G. (2019). *Guidelines for best practice psychosocial assessment of Aboriginal and Torres Strait Islander people presenting to hospital with self-harm and suicidal thoughts*. Menzies School of Health Research. www.menzies.edu.au/icms_docs/310034_The_BestPrAxIS_study.pdf

Leddie, G., Fox, C., & Simmonds, S. (2021). Nurses' experiences of working in the community with adolescents who self-harm: A qualitative exploration. *Journal of Psychiatric and Mental Health Nursing*. *29*(5), 744–754. https://doi.org/10.1111/jpm.12806

Life in Mind. (2022a). *Australian Bureau of Statistics Causes of death data*. Everymind. www.lifeinmind.org.au/about-suicide/suicide-data/suicide-facts-and-stats-2

Life in Mind. (2022b). *Policy and Strategy. National suicide prevention strategies in Australia*. Everymind. www.lifeinmind.org.au/policies/national-policy

Living Proud. (2017). *LGBTI people and suicide risk. LGBTI Community Services of WA*. www.livingproud.org.au/risk.

Lyons, B. H., Walters, M. L., Jack, S. P. D., Petrosky, E., Blair, J. M., & Ivey-Stephenson, A. Z. (2019). Suicides among lesbian and gay males individuals: Findings from the national violent death reporting system. *American Journal of Preventive Medicine*, *56*(4), 512–521.

Majidi, S., O'Donnell, H. K., Stanek, K., Youngkin, E., Gomer, T., & Driscoll, K. A. (2020). Suicide risk assessment in youth and young adults with type 1 diabetes. *Diabetes Care*, *43*(2), 343–348. https://doi.org/10.2337/dc19-0831

McGough, S., Wynaden, D., Ngune, I., Janerka, C., Hasking, P., & Rees, C. (2022). Emergency nurses' perceptions of the health care system and how it impacts provision of care to people who self-harm. *Collegian*, *29*(1), 38–43. https://doi.org/10.1016/j.colegn.2021.04.004

McHugh, C., Campbell, A., Chapman, M., & Balaratnasingam, S. (2016). Increasing indigenous self-harm and suicide in the Kimberley: An audit of the 2005–2014 data. *Medical Journal of Australia*, *205*(1), 33.

Mental Health First Aid (MHFA) (International). (2020). *A guide for care givers of people with a mental illness*. MHFA Australia. www.mhfa.com.au/sites/default/files/guide_for_caregivers_of_people_with_mental_illness_-_may_2020.pdf

Moitra, M., Santomauro, D., Degenhardt, L., Collins, P. Y., Whiteford, H., Vos, T., & Ferrari, A. (2021). Estimating the risk of suicide associated with mental disorders: A systematic review and meta-regression analysis. *Journal of Psychiatric Research*, *137*, 242–249. https://doi.org/10.1016/j.jpsychires.2021.02.053 ISSN 0022-3956

Molloy, S. (2019). *The risky obsession with building the perfect muscular body snaring Aussie men. News.com.au*.

Morey, Y., Mellon, D., Dailami, N., Verne, J., & Tapp, A. (2017). Adolescent self-harm in the community: An update on prevalence using a self-report survey of adolescents aged 13–18 in England. *Journal of Public Health*, *39*(1), 58–64.

National Centre for Health Statistics. (2022). *Suicide mortality in the United States, 2000–2020*. www.nchstats.com/2022/03/03/suicide-mortality-in-the-united-states-2000-2020

National Eating Disorders Association. (2022). *Orthorexia nervosa*. www.nationaleatingdisorders.org/learn/by-eating-disorder/other/orthorexia

National Eating Disorders Collaboration. (2020). *Other specified feeding or eating disorders*. www.nedc.com.au/eating-disorders/eating-disorders-explained/types/other-specified-feeding-or-eating-disorders

National Eating Disorders Collaboration. (2022a). *What is an eating disorder*. www.nedc.com.au/eating-disorders/eating-disorders-explained/the-facts/whats-an-eating-disorder

National Eating Disorders Collaboration. (2022b). *Eating disorders in Australia*. www.nedc.com.au/eating-disorders/eating-disorders-explained/the-facts/eating-disorders-in-australia.

National Institute for Health and Care Excellence (UK). (2022). *Self-harm in over 8s: Long-term management*. Clinical guidelines [133]. www.nice.org.uk/guidance/cg133/resources/selfharm-in-over-8s-longterm-management-pdf-35109508689349

National Mental Health Commission. (2020). *About*. www.mentalhealthcommission.gov.au/About

New South Wales (NSW) Health. (2022). *Healthy kids for professionals*. Assess. Healthy eating Actively living. www.pro.healthykids.nsw.gov.au/assess

Nimesh, A. (2019). Can suicide risk be detected in the blood? *Specialty Medical Dialogues*. www.speciality.medicaldialogues.in/can-suicide-risk-be-detected-in-the-blood.

Office of the Royal Commission. (2019). *Royal Commission into aged care quality and safety. A history of aged care reviews* Background paper 8. Commonwealth of Australia. www.agedcare.royalcommission.gov.au/publications/Documents/background-paper-8.pdf

O'Neill, S., Graham, B., & Ennis, E. (2019). Emergency department and hospital care prior to suicide: A population based case control study. *Journal of Affective Disorders, 249*, 366–370.

Perkins, M. (2019). *High LGBTI suicide rate 'unacceptable': Mental health commissioner. The Age*. www.theage.com.au/national/victoria/high-LGBTQIA-suicide-rate-unacceptable-mental-health-commissioner-20190717-p5282r.html

Pintar Babič, M., Bregar, B., & Drobnič Radobuljac, M. (2020). The attitudes and feelings of mental health nurses towards adolescents and young adults with nonsuicidal self-injuring behaviors. *Child and Adolescent Psychiatry Mental Health, 14*, 37. https://doi.org/10.1186/s13034-020-00343-5

Prince, J. (2018). *Stories from community. How suicide rates fell in two Indigenous communities*. Healing Foundation.

Rayner, G., Blackburn, J., Edward, K., Stephenson, J., & Ousey, K. (2019). Emergency department nurse's attitudes towards patients who self-harm: A meta-analysis. *International Journal of Mental health Nursing, 28*(1), 40–53. https://doi.org/10.1111/inm.12550

Reachout. (2022). *Is self-harm linked to attentions seeking*? www.schools.au.reachout.com/articles/self-harm-attention-seeking.

Rheinberger, D., Wang, J., McGillivray, L., Shand, F., Torok, M., Maple, M., & Wayland, S. (2022). Understanding emergency department healthcare professionals' perspectives of caring for individuals in suicidal crisis: A qualitative study. *Frontiers in Psychiatry, 13*, 918135. https://doi.org/10.3389/fpsyt.2022.918135

Ribeiro Coimbra, L. R., & Noakes, A. (2022). A systematic review into healthcare professionals' attitudes towards self-harm in children and young people and its impact on care provision. *Journal of Child Health Care, 26*(2), 290–306. https://doi.org/10.1177/13674935211014405 PMID: 33929264

Ritchie, H., Roser, M., & Ortiz-Ospina, E. (2020). *Suicide. Our world in data*. www.ourworldindata.org/suicide#suicide-by-gender.

Robinson, J., McCutcheon, L., Browne, V., & Witt, K. (2016). *Looking the other way: Young people and self-harm*. Orygen, The National Centre of Excellence in Youth Mental Health.

Royal Australian and New Zealand College of Psychiatrists. (n.d.). *Mental health in rural areas*. www.ranzcp.org/practice-education/rural-psychiatry/mental-health-in-rural-areas.

Rzepczyk, S., Dolinska-Kaczmarek, K., Uruska, A., & Czeslaw, Z. (2022). The other face of insulin- overdose and its effects. *Toxics, 10*(3), 123. https://doi.org/10.3390/toxics10030123

Saab, M. M., Murphy, M., Meehan, E., Dillon, C. B., O'Connell, S., Hegarty, J., Heffernan, S., Greaney, S., Kilty, C., Goodwin, J., Hartigan, I., O'Brien, M., Chambers, D., Twomey, U., & O'Donovan, A. (2021). Suicide and self-harm risk assessment: A systematic review of prospective research. *Archives of Suicide Research*. https://doi.org/10.1080/13811118.2021.1938321

SANE. (2019). *Suicidal behaviour. www.sane.org/information-stories/facts-and-guides/suicidal-behaviour*.

Sartor, L. (2021). *Farmer suicides: Exploring ten years of Coronial data (2009–2018)*. National Rural Health Alliance. www.ruralhealth.org.au/news/first-national-study-farmer-suicide-rates-using-coronial-data#:~:text=National%20Rural%20Health%20Alliance%20Policy,were%20370%20farmer%20suicides%20reported

Scocco, P., Macis, A., Ferrari, C., Bava, M., Bianconi, G., & Bulgari, V. (2019). Self-harm behaviour and externally-directed aggression in psychiatric outpatients: A multicentre, prospective study (viormed-2 study). *Scientific Reports, 9*, 17857.

Stapelberg, N. J. C., Bowman, C., Woerwag-Mehta, S., Walker, S., Davies, A., Hughes, I., Michel, K., Pisani, A. R., Van Engelen, H., Delos, M., Hageman, T., Fullerton-Smith, K., Krishnaiah, R., McDowell, S., Cameron, A., Scales, T. L., Dillon, C., Gigante, T., Heddle, C. … Turner, K. (2021). A lived experience co-designed study protocol for a randomised control trial: the Attempted Suicide Short Intervention Program (ASSIP) or Brief Cognitive Behavioural Therapy as additional interventions after a suicide attempt compared to a standard Suicide Prevention Pathway (SPP). *Trials, 22*(1), 723. https://doi.org/10.1186/s13063-021-05658-y

Stephenson, L., van den Heuvel, C., Humphries, M., & Byard, R. W. (2022, August 9). *Characteristics of fatal insulin overdoses. Forensic Science, Medicine and Patholgy*. https://doi.org/10.1007/s12024-022-00511-3 Epub ahead of print. PMID: 35943711. https://doi.org/10.1007/s12024-022-00511-3

SuicideLine Victoria. (n.d.). *Have you been bereaved by suicide?* www.suicideline.org.au/resource/have-you-been-bereaved-by-suicide

Suicide Prevention Australia. (2019). *Turning points: Imagine a world without suicide*. www.suicidepreventionaust.org/turning-points-imagine-a-world-without-suicide

Suicide Prevention Australia. (2021). *Fact sheet: Suicidality among culturally and linguistically diverse communities. CALD suicide prevention fact sheet*. www.suicidepreventionaust.org/wp-content/uploads/2021/06/CALD-Suicide-Prevention-Fact-Sheet.pdf

Thirrili. (2019). *Postvention support*. National Indigenous Australians Agency. Australian Government. https://thirrili.com.au/postvention-support

Tighe, J., Shand, F., Ridani, R., Mackinnon, A., De La Mata, N., & Christensen, H. (2017). Ibobbly mobile health intervention for suicide prevention in Australian Indigenous youth: A pilot randomised controlled trial. *British Medical Journal Open, 7*(1), e013518.

Vinchenzo, C., Lawrence, V., & McCombie, C. (2022). Patient perspectives on premature termination of eating disorder treatment: A systematic review and qualitative synthesis. *Journal of Eating Disorders*, *10*(1), 39. https://doi.org/10.1186/s40337-022-00568-z

Voros, V., Tenyi, T., Nagy, A., Fekete, S., & Osvath, P. (2021). Crisis concept re-loaded?—The recently described suicide-specific syndromes may help to better understand suicidal behaviour and assess imminent suicide risk more effectively. *Frontiers of Psychiatry*, *12*, 598923. https://doi.org/10.3389/fpsyt.2021.598923

Westad, Y. A. S., Hagen, K., Jonsbu, E., & Solem, S. (2021). Cessation of deliberate self-harm behaviour in patients with borderline personality traits treated with outpatient dialectical behaviour therapy. *Frontiers in Psychology*, *12*, 578230. https://doi.org/10.3389/fpsyg.2021.578230

Witt, K. G., Hetrick, S. E., Rajaram, G., Hazell, P., Taylor Salisbury, T. L., Townsend, E., & Hawton, K. (2021). Pharmacological interventions for self-harm in adults. *Cochrane Database of Systematic Reviews*, *1*. https://doi.org/10.1002/14651858.CD013669.pub2

World Health Organization. (2019). *Suicide*. www.who.int/news-room/fact-sheets/detail/suicide

World Health Organization. (2020). *Suicide prevention*. www.who.int/health-topics/suicide#tab=tab–2

World Health Organisation. (2021). *Suicide. Key facts*. www.who.int/news-room/fact-sheets/detail/suicide

Yang, Z. (2017). Alcohol related psychosis. *Medscape*. https://emedicine.medscape.com/article/289848-overview

Zwickl, S., Wong, A. F. Q., Dowers, E., Leemaqz, S. Y., Bertherton, I., Cook, T., Zajac, J. D., Yip, P. S. F., & Cheung, A. S. (2021). Correction to: Factors associated with suicide attempts among Australian transgender adults. *BMC Psychiatry*, *21*(1), 551. https://doi.org/10.1186/s12888-021-03491-w

---

ACKNOWLEDGEMENTS

Photo: © Jenny Sturm / Shutterstock.com

Photo: © Jamie Grill / Getty Images

Photo: © Tero Vesalainen / Shutterstock.com

Photo: © ymgerman / Shutterstock.com

Photo: © New Africa / Shutterstock.com

Photo: © martin-dm / E+ / Getty Images

Photo: © PeopleImages / E+ / Getty Images

Photo: © Anze Furlan / Shutterstock.com

Extract: © Commonwealth of Australia. (2021a). New strategy and research centre to support Australians with eating disorders. Minister: Department of Health and Aged Care. Media Release. 21 September 2021. www.health.gov.au/ministers/the-hon-greg-hunt-mp/media/new-strategy-and-research-centre-to-support-australians-with-eating-disorders.

Caring for a person with a serious mental illness

LEARNING OBJECTIVES

This chapter will:

9.1 explain the term 'serious mental illness' in the context of mental health Recovery

9.2 explore experiences of serious mental illness

9.3 describe the Recovery-oriented interventions for people with serious mental illness

9.4 investigate the connections between physical and mental health in people with a serious mental illness

9.5 clarify the role of carers in supporting people with a serious mental illness.

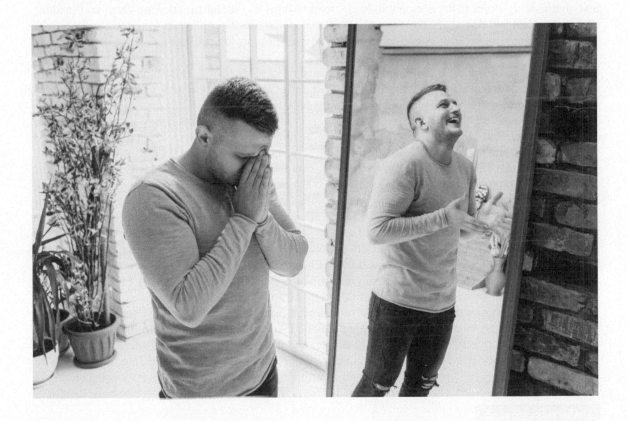

Introduction

All health professionals, regardless of background or specialty area, will encounter a person with a serious mental illness at some point in their careers. Paramedics may be required to transport a person with serious mental illness who is experiencing a cardiac event; Aboriginal and Torres Strait Islander mental health workers may be asked to support an Indigenous Australian with a serious mental illness who is being treated off country; nurses working in hospitals or primary health care settings will care for people with serious mental illness and comorbid physical health issues; counsellors may be use psychosocial therapy to support a person with a serious mental illness. This chapter supports all health professionals in providing effective care to a person with a serious mental illness.

The chapter begins by explaining the term 'serious mental illness' in the context of Recovery-oriented care. Following this is a description of the mental illnesses regarded as serious in Australia: schizophrenia, bipolar disorder, major depression and schizoaffective disorder. Also provided is an overview of the psychosocial and pharmacological interventions used to support people with serious mental illness. The importance of treating the physical health of people with serious mental illness is highlighted, with the chapter concluding by discussing the key role of carers in supporting people with serious mental illness on their Recovery journey.

9.1 Serious mental illness and Recovery

LEARNING OBJECTIVE 9.1 Explain the term 'serious mental illness' in the context of mental health Recovery.

The term 'serious mental illness' or 'severe mental illness' is generally understood to refer to mental, behavioural or emotional disorders that substantially interfere with or limit one or more major life activities and significantly impacts the person's lifestyle, relationships and **social functioning** (National Institute of Mental Health [NIMH], 2022b). A serious mental illness usually follows a long-term course, with fluctuating symptom severity. A person must be aged over 18 years to be diagnosed with a serious mental illness.

The mental illnesses most commonly defined as serious are schizophrenia, bipolar disorder, major depressive disorder and schizoaffective disorder (Whitley et al., 2015). Other serious mental illnesses can include substance use disorder and some personality disorders.

Whether or not a mental illness is classified as serious will depend on the nature and severity of the symptoms experienced by the person, the duration of the illness, and the extent to which illness has affected the person's life and ability to function independently.

In Australia, some 5 per pent or approximately 800 000 people have a serious mental illness, with around 500 000 having an episodic mental illness and 300 000 a persistent mental illness (Australian Institute of Health and Welfare [AIHW], 2022c). Many people with a serious mental illness also have issues with their physical health, which adds to the overall disease burden. For example, people with serious mental illness have a lower life expectancy of between 10 and 36 years than the general population, with most dying prematurely from a comorbid physical health condition (Royal Australian and New Zealand College of Psychiatrists [RANZCP], 2016). The annual cost of health care, welfare and lost productivity for people with serious mental illness and comorbid physical illness is estimated to be $15 billion, ballooning to over $45 billion when substance use disorders are added to the mix (RANZCP, 2016).

Such statistics suggest the need for focused attention on caring for a person with a serious mental illness. While the support provided to a person with a serious mental illness has many similarities to the care given to people whose mental illness is less debilitating, there are additional considerations for health professionals providinng care. Understanding these additional considerations will ensure the person with serious mental illness can live a meaningful and contributing life and achieve the best possible outcomes.

UPON REFLECTION

Deficit or strengths approaches to serious mental illness

Serious mental illness is defined according to the functional impairment experienced by the person and the limitations or impacts on the person's lifestyle, relationships and social functioning. This approach, however, is based on the person's deficits rather than their strengths and is often aligned to the medical

---

model. Unfortunately, the deficit model also underpins the funding models that drive Australia's health and disability systems (e.g. Medicare and the National Disability Insurance Scheme).

In contrast, strengths-based approaches work with the person's abilities, rather than disabilities. Strengths-based approaches aim to determine what a person can or could do and support them to live meaningful and contributing lives. An example of a strengths-based approach is the Recovery-oriented mental health service.

....

QUESTIONS

1. What are the benefits and challenges of the deficit approach to supporting people with serious mental illness?

2. What are the benefits and challenges of Recovery-oriented approaches to supporting people with serious mental illness?

3. How can the tension between these two approaches be resolved?

Recovery from serious mental illness

Following the de-institutionalisation of psychiatric facilities that occurred worldwide in the 1960s–80s, many people with serious mental illness found themselves homeless, unemployed and without social support (Whitley et al., 2015). This situation increased the levels of stigma and vulnerability they experienced.

The concept of mental health Recovery emerged in response to the injustices experienced by people with serious mental illness, including the overemphasis on psychiatric treatment through medication and under-emphasis on psychosocial support. As outlined in the chapter on mental health care in Australia, mental health Recovery includes notions of personal journey or development in the life domains important to the person. The consumer is positioned as the expert in their own lived experience of mental illness who collaborates or works in partnership with health professionals to make choices about the health care and social support they receive (De Ruysscher et al., 2019).

Recovery-oriented approaches to delivering mental health care are less about an absence of symptoms or illness and more about enabling people with mental illness to move beyond the negative consequences of their health condition (Elsegood et al., 2018). Recovery-oriented approaches include supporting the person to accept that they may continue to experience symptoms of mental illness and to move towards a future framed by hope, optimism, individual strengths, wellness, collaboration and community engagement, empowerment, agency and personal growth.

Recovery-oriented approaches also require health professionals to move from the role of 'expert' and 'authority' to that of a 'life coach' or 'trainer' (Petros & Solomon, 2021). Recovery-oriented practice for health professionals could include:

* providing the person with information about the symptoms they are experiencing, interventions or treatment options, stress management, coping strategies, and how to recognise and respond to the early warning signs of relapse
* encouraging the person to develop achievable goals for the future and supporting them to achieve a way of life that is meaningful to them
* enabling the person to gain a sense of control over their lives by actively participating as a member of their community
* accessing and maximising the benefits of support networks, such as other health professionals, practitioners or services, partners and carers, family members, friends or community programs
* supporting the person to build resilience and overcome the discrimination, community ignorance and **self-stigma** associated with serious mental illness.

There is strong evidence that people with serious mental illness can live autonomous, contributing and satisfying lives in the community (Jørgensen & Rendtorff, 2018). Health professionals play a key role in supporting the Recovery journey of people with serious mental illness in various ways. This role, and the interventions used, are described in the following sections of this chapter.

Digital Opportunities for Outcomes in Recovery Services (DOORS)

Digital health technologies provide an important means by which mental health consumers can access care and support (Hoffman et al., 2020). For example, the Black Dog Institute in Australia provides a list of digital apps and online technologies to help people with mental illness to monitor and self-manage their symptoms, connect with care and predict relapse (Black Dog Institute, 2022a).

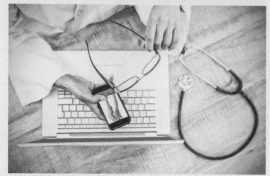

While many people with a serious mental illness own a smartphone, few have been offered the opportunity to learn how to fully utilise the digital health technologies that are now available to support them.

The DOORS project was framed by self-determination theory and built on the therapeutic alliance already developed between practitioners and people with a serious mental illness. A hands-on and interactive training program was developed to engage participants, training them to use digital health technologies on their smartphones and to teach others how to use them (Hoffman et al., 2020). The program targeted three main components.

1. *Competence.* Participants developed skills in using smartphones, and assessing and selecting the safe digital health tools that best suited their needs.
2. *Autonomy.* Participants learned how to use digital health tools to help them achieve their goals. For example, smartphone step counters and exercise apps helped patients meet goals for physical activity; an important approach to reducing symptoms.
3. *Relatedness.* Participants were encouraged to share with and learn about digital health tools and strategies and work with health professionals.

Outcomes of this project for people with serious mental illness who participated in the program included improved equity of access to suitable health technologies, and knowledge and skills related to technology use in health care (Hoffman et al., 2020).

QUESTIONS

1. How is teaching people with serious mental illness about digital technologies and self-managing their symptoms consistent with a Recovery-oriented approach to mental health care?
2. How can participation in the DOORS program challenge the stigma often associated with people with serious mental illness?

9.2 Experiences of serious mental illness

LEARNING OBJECTIVE 9.2 Explore experiences of serious mental illness.

This section explores various experiences of serious mental illness, with a focus on schizophrenia, bipolar disorder and schizoaffective disorder. Information about major depression was described in the chapter on depression, anxiety and perinatal mental health care, and substance use issues are the focus of a later chapter. In this section, consideration is given to the prevalence of and contributing factors to the experiences of schizophrenia, bipolar disorder and schizoaffective disorder. Descriptions are also provided of the lived experiences of these conditions, including signs and symptoms. The principles by which health professionals effectively care for people with serious mental illness are then identified, with interventions and treatment options examined in more depth later in this chapter.

Psychosis

Psychosis is not a serious mental illness on its own; however, people with serious mental illness will often experience psychosis as one of the symptoms. People with psychosis are said to have 'lost touch with reality', unable to distinguish what is real from what is a creation of their mind, perceptions or senses. The symptoms of psychosis include hallucinations, affecting the person's perceptions of sound, sight, smell, taste and touch; delusions, affecting the person's thinking; and marked changes in feelings and behaviours.

There are various types of psychotic disorders, including:

- single-episode or first-episode psychosis, comprising symptoms of psychosis that are sometimes triggered by a stressful event and last for a short time only (e.g. from hours to days)
- drug-induced psychosis, caused by drugs such as alcohol, speed, marijuana, ecstasy or magic mushrooms. The symptoms usually only last until the effects of the drugs wear off (e.g. hours or days). However, sometimes a drug-induced psychosis will trigger ongoing psychosis and schizophrenia
- organic psychosis, the result of a head injury, illness or infection that has affected the brain
- schizophrenia, comprising various persistent or chronic psychotic symptoms
- bipolar disorder, marked by extreme moods (either very high or very low) that can sometimes involve psychotic symptoms
- psychotic depression, involving depression that can be so intense that it causes psychotic symptoms
- schizoaffective disorder, involving a mix of extreme moods and psychotic symptoms (National Alliance on Mental Illness [NAMI], 2022b).

The time prior to a person developing symptoms of psychosis is called the **prodrome** or prodromal phase. During the prodromal phase, the person (most often a young person) will experience changes in the way they feel, think and behave that are sometimes difficult to identify due to either their gradual onset or subtle presentation. Indeed, prodromal symptoms are usually identified retrospectively after the person has developed a more pronounced symptom set or diagnosed mental illness; the symptoms are experienced as something that is 'not quite right' (Ohwovoriole, 2022). The phase is also called 'psychosis risk syndrome' or the 'early warning signs', which are described in more detail in the chapter that looks at mental health service delivery.

It is important to note that early warning signs are not a definite marker of the onset of a serious mental illness. Identifying the early warning signs will enable early treatment and improve health outcomes for the person experiencing the event (McGorry, 2015).

UPON REFLECTION

Early intervention for young people with psychosis

Orygen, the National Centre of Excellence in Youth Mental Health, Australia, is a high-profile not-for-profit Australian organisation conducting research and providing advocacy and education on youth mental illness. Orygen is a strong advocate of early intervention strategies for young people who experience the early signs of mental illness and operates the Early Psychosis Prevention and Intervention Centre (FPPIC), which provides a range of services options and treatment goals for young people (Orygen, 2017).

Orygen (2022) argues that early intervention approaches enable young people with symptoms of mental illness to be treated with greater care and respect, be exposed to a hopeful and optimistic culture, have their family included and supported, prioritise finding and maintaining work, and experience less stigma and trauma related to their treatment. According to Orygen (2022), although early intervention strategies may initially cost more, they deliver a greater return on investment. Psychotic illnesses can be delayed or prevented, people with psychosis can return to work and enjoy good vocational and social outcomes, and some people with psychosis can manage their mental health with little or no medication.

QUESTIONS

1. If the prodromal period of psychosis is recognised retrospectively, how else can young people who would benefit from early intervention strategies be identified?
2. How important are education, employment and social support in the recovery journey of people who experience psychosis? Justify your answer.

Schizophrenia

Although descriptions of psychotic behaviour date back to early written history, schizophrenia was not described until the late 1800s by Emil Kraepelin (1856–1926) and Eugen Bleuler (1857–1939). Kraepelin described the syndrome as a dementia praecox or decline in functioning with an early onset; Bleuler coined the name 'schizophrenia'. The term was derived from two Greek words meaning 'to split' and 'mind' — a derivative that most likely contributes to the common misunderstanding that schizophrenia relates to split personality. Schizophrenia is not a split personality; rather, it more closely resembles a split between a dream state and reality. A person diagnosed with schizophrenia will experience episodes of psychosis, including disturbances in perceptions, thinking, emotions and behaviours. It is important to note that the term 'schizophrenic' is no longer used to describe a person diagnosed with schizophrenia due to its pejorative connotations. The power of language and the need for health professionals to use inclusive and de-stigmatising language is explained in the chapter focusing on mental health care in Australia.

Prevalence and burden of disease

Schizophrenia is a relatively rare condition that occurs in about 1 per cent of the population worldwide, with 1.5 per cent of Australians diagnosed with the condition; and two-thirds of people experiencing their first episode of psychosis before the age of 25 (Garvan Institute of Medical Research, 2021). Although schizophrenia is a low prevalence disorder, its relative burden of disease in both direct and indirect costs is substantial (Crespo-Facorro et al., 2021)

While the course of schizophrenia varies, 20–30 per cent of people diagnosed with schizophrenia do not experience significant impairment in the longer term. Another 20–30 per cent experience symptoms that will intermittently or otherwise cause moderate disruption to their lives. Some 40–60 per cent of people diagnosed with the illness experience severe impairment (Sadock et al., 2017).

People with schizophrenia are far more likely than the general population to die of cardiovascular disease, lung cancer, chronic obstructive pulmonary disease, influenza and pneumonia (Olfson et al., 2015). Accidental deaths accounted for more than twice as many deaths as suicide, which is also elevated in people with schizophrenia (Galletly et al., 2016). Young adults with schizophrenia have the highest suicide risk, especially those with suicidal systems and substance use (Olfson et al., 2021).

THE BIG PICTURE

Serious mental illness experienced by Indigenous Australians

According to the AIHW (2022b), an estimated 24 per cent of Aboriginal and Torres Strait Islander peoples reported having a diagnosed mental health or behavioural condition, and three in ten Indigenous adults reported 'high or very high' levels of psychological distress. Indigenous Australians also experience a high burden of disease, including **multimorbidity.**

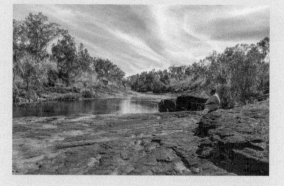

The leading five health conditions contributing to the disease burden in Indigenous Australians in 2018 were:

1. mental and substance use disorders (such as anxiety, depression and drug use)
2. injuries (such as falls, road traffic injuries and suicide)
3. cardiovascular diseases (such as coronary and rheumatic heart disease)
4. cancer and other neoplasms (such as lung and breast cancer)
5. musculoskeletal conditions (such as back pain and osteoarthritis) (AIHW, 2022c).

Accurate and generalisable estimates on rates of particular psychiatric disorders in Indigenous Australians — and indigenous peoples worldwide — are unavailable (Ogilvie et al., 2021). Therefore, the prevalence of serious mental illness in Aboriginal and Torres Strait Islander peoples is unclear.

In a study of psychiatric disorders in Indigenous Australians using hospital data, Ogilvie et al. (2021) found that:

- Indigenous Australians were overrepresented across most psychiatric disorders, particularly substance use disorders
- the over-representation of Indigenous Australians in psychiatric diagnoses begins in childhood and becomes more pronounced in adulthood
- there are important sociodemographic differences between Indigenous and non-Indigenous Australians who receive psychiatric diagnoses
- the increased likelihood of Indigenous individuals being diagnosed across all categories of psychiatric disorders except for substance use disorders disappeared after accounting for sociodemographic and other psychiatric-related variables.

The last of these points suggests the importance of the social determinants of health — that is, the conditions in which people are born, develop, live, work and grow old — in the development of mental illness, including serious mental illness. The social determinants of health are shaped by the general distribution of wealth, power and resources at global, national and local levels (Vallesi et al., 2018).

According to the AIHW (2022a), around one-third of the health gap between Indigenous and non-Indigenous Australians was due to social determinants. These determinants include:

- employment and hours worked
- highest non-school qualification
- level of schooling completed
- housing adequacy and household income.
  Just under one-fifth of the gap was due to health risk factors, such as:
- risky alcohol consumption
- high blood pressure
- overweight and obesity status
- inadequate fruit and vegetable consumption
- physical inactivity
- smoking.
  The remaining health gap of just under 50 per cent resulted from differences in access to health services and the impact of cultural and historical factors on health.

Population-based information on the prevalence of psychiatric disorders for Indigenous peoples, particularly for serious mental illness, and improving access to health services is vital for strengthening mental health policies and understanding the mental health needs of Aboriginal and Torres Strait Islander peoples (Olfson et al., 2021).

You can read more about the social determinants of health and how they influence the mental health and wellbeing of Indigenous Australians in the chapter focusing on culturally appropriate mental health care.

Development and course

The psychotic features of schizophrenia typically emerge between the late teens and mid 30s; onset prior to adolescence is rare. The peak age of onset for the first **psychotic episode** is in the early to mid 20s for males and in the late 20s for females (APA, 2013). The onset of the symptoms and episode may be abrupt; however, most people develop symptoms gradually over a period, with the severity of symptoms increasing with time (Galletly et al., 2016). The psychotic symptoms tend to diminish throughout an individual's life, with various theories postulating as to why this is so, including the possibility of connections to the reduction of dopamine observed in the normal aging process (Grunder & Cumming, 2016). No matter what the symptoms experienced, schizophrenia is often a chronic, life-long condition.

Contributing factors

The causes of schizophrenia are not well understood, with research suggesting a combination of factors related to genetics, brain structure and function, and the environment (NIMH, 2022b).

Genetic factors

Like many diseases, schizophrenia tends to run in families. It is important to note that having a family member with schizophrenia does not necessarily mean other family members will develop the condition. Studies suggest that various genes may increase a person's chances of developing schizophrenia, but there is no single gene that causes the disorder (Henriksen et al., 2017).

Brain structure

Research studies have identified that people with schizophrenia are more likely to have differences in the size of certain brain areas and connections between brain areas than those without schizophrenia (NIMH, 2022c). Some of these differences may develop before birth. This area of research remains a work in progress (Szendi et al., 2017).

Environment

A person's environment and life experiences can contribute to a person developing schizophrenia. These environmental factors can include socio-economic demographic, stress, exposure to viruses and substance use.

UPON REFLECTION

Blaming mothers for mental illness

In the 1960s and 70s, 'bad' mothers were blamed if a person developed a mental illness, in particular schizophrenia (Johnston, 2013). This blame game was recently resurrected, with the finger pointing at

▶

dysfunctional families, negative childhood experiences or childhood trauma as key contributing factors (Gaysina & Thompson, 2017). However, such views are reductionist and do not consider the wider **social determinants** of health that influence the health status of all people, including but not limited to early childhood development, disability, education, employment, gender, health services, housing, income, nutrition, social exclusion, social safety networks and race. You can read more about the social determinants of health in the chapter that looks at culturally appropriate mental health care.

QUESTIONS

1. What is the logical outcome of blaming mothers or dysfunctional families when a person develops schizophrenia?

2. What is the logical outcome of providing additional support to families when a person develops schizophrenia?

The experience of schizophrenia

There is currently no test that can diagnose schizophrenia. However, physical tests will help to exclude other conditions that may be causing the psychosis, including metabolic disorder, thyroid dysfunction, brain tumour and other possible organic causes of unexplained changes in cognition, emotions or behaviours. No single symptom is definitive for a diagnosis of schizophrenia; instead, the diagnosis is made based on a pattern of signs and symptoms together with impaired social functioning. For this reason, a diagnosis of schizophrenia takes time and is best determined by a psychiatrist. Health professionals, including GPs, who have not completed specialised education and training in the field should avoid making such a diagnosis due to the stigma attached to the condition and the potential for a misdiagnosis to cause significant distress to the person.

A useful framework for understanding schizophrenia involves separating the symptoms into **positive symptoms** and **negative symptoms**.

These are described in detail in the following sections.

Positive symptoms

The positive symptoms of schizophrenia are most often overt, observable and unusual. These positive symptoms can be understood as adding something to the person's ordinary experiences and include hallucinations, delusions and disorganised thinking.

Hallucinations can be described as false sensory perceptions or perceptual phenomena arising without any external stimulus. They include the person hearing (most common), seeing, smelling, feeling or tasting things that others do not. For many people with a serious mental illness such as schizophrenia, bipolar disorder or schizoaffective disorder, the voices will often be persecutory or critical and may command the person to behave in a certain way. Hallucinations are described according to the sensory modality, as outlined in table 9.1. When the person is relatively well, they can often recognise that these perceptions are not real and learn ways of managing or ignoring the hallucinations.

TABLE 9.1 **Examples of hallucinations**

Type of sensory disturbance	Examples of the lived experience
Auditory hallucination — hearing things that are not there (often taking the form of voices)	'I could hear someone talking to me that no one else could hear. It was outside my head, not an internal voice. It was so real.'
	'The voice kept telling me that I'm a liar and no good. It taunted and taunted me.'
	'The voice told me to kill myself.'
Visual hallucination — seeing things that are not there	'When I was unwell in hospital, I could see a young boy leaning over a small animal. I asked other people whether they could see it. They said no.'
	'I could see shadowy things at night, coming and going. I was scared.'

Tactile hallucination — feeling things that are not there	'I could feel worms crawling under my skin. I knew I could pick them out to get rid of them, so I tried and tried. I ended up in hospital when I couldn't stop picking and the wounds couldn't heal.'
Gustatory hallucination — tasting things that are not there	'I got a weird taste in my mouth. It was salty. I decided it must be blood I was tasting, but nothing would get rid of it. I tried sweet drinks and alcohol, but the taste would always come back. That lasted for about a week.'
Olfactory hallucination — smelling things that are not there	'Burning rubber was all I could smell. It stank! When I first started to smell it, I thought there was a fire, but there wasn't. The smell got stronger in my bedroom, but everyone else said there was no smell around. I even sprayed air freshener, which smelled a little better, but underneath it all, I could still smell the burning rubber.'

A **delusion** is a fixed and false belief that the person cannot be dissuaded from despite contradictory evidence. This belief is not based in the person's cultural, religious/spiritual, educational or social experience. Similarly, the belief is not shared by other members of the person's culture or religion. For example, believing that there is the possibility of life elsewhere in the universe would be in keeping with the beliefs of many other people in society, but believing that the health worker is an alien would not be in keeping with the beliefs of others and so would be classified as a delusion.

Delusions can also be bizarre or non-bizarre in nature. Bizarre delusions are completely implausible. For example, a person may believe that an alien has put a camera in their brain and is sending all their conversations back to the alien planet in preparation for the earth being invaded. There are many logical reasons why this belief is implausible. On the other hand, a non-bizarre delusion would involve a belief that, on the balance of probability, could possibly occur. For example, a person may believe their manager is constantly checking up on them for no reason.

Before deciding a belief is a delusion, health professionals must explore the person's context, life experiences and the level of the belief. For example, a person may believe their drug seller is 'out to get them'. Depending on the person's lifestyle, this may not be a paranoid delusion but rather the person's reality. Another question to ask is whether the person is obsessed with the belief. How much is the belief driving their behaviour or consuming their lives? Answers to these questions are perhaps more significant to the care and treatment provided than the content of the delusions.

Delusions can also be described in relation to their relationship with the person's mood. For example, an individual whose mood is low may become utterly convinced that a particular person or group of people hates them. However, a delusion can also be mood neutral; for example, a person may believe that people with dark hair all follow a particular football team. The different types of delusions are described in table 9.2. As with hallucinations, when the person is well, they may be able to recognise these delusions as false personal beliefs. This level of insight helps the person to challenge their thinking.

TABLE 9.2   Types of delusions

Type of delusion	Explanation and examples of delusions
Persecutory or paranoid delusions	A false belief that a person is the victim of a conspiracy, persecution or at risk of being harmed.
	The person may believe they are being spied on, poisoned or someone is out to 'get' them.
Grandiose delusions	A false belief that a person possesses special powers, talents or abilities.
	The person believes they are royalty, a film star, an entrepreneur or millionaire, or a leader in their field. The person may also believe they have been chosen to complete a particular task. Such delusions carry a risk if the task involves hurting themselves or other people.

(continued)

TABLE 9.2 *(continued)*

Type of delusion	Explanation and examples of delusions
Somatic delusions	A false belief that a person (or someone close to the person) has an illness that is not supported by medical evidence.
	Health professionals must ensure that the symptoms being reported are actually delusional. For example, most people with serious mental illness also have physical health problems.
	Somatic delusions relate more to unexplained pain or parasitic infestations.
Ideas of reference	A false belief that insignificant events have special personal significance.
	The person may believe the radio, television or computer is transmitting special messages to or for them.
Religious delusions	A false belief with religious or spiritual content.
	Health professionals must ensure that the delusions being reported are not the accepted beliefs of a religion or spiritual following.
	The person with religious delusions may be convinced that they are Jesus Christ, the prophet Muhammad or another special prophet who has returned to save the world. The person may also believe that they have been specially chosen to complete a religious or spiritual task. Such delusions carry a risk if the task involves hurting themselves or other people.

Other experiences of schizophrenia include disorganised thinking and motor behaviours. Health professionals can clearly observe this type of thinking and the behaviours it drives. For example, disorganised thinking can lead to a conversation that lacks structure and purpose. As with hallucinations and delusions, a person who can recognise their disordered thought patterns will be better able to manage their symptoms and respond to treatment.

Common speech patterns observed in people as a result of disorganised thinking include:

- *pressure of speech* — increased amount and rate of speech that is difficult to interrupt
- *thought blocking* — the person forgets what they are thinking or saying
- *circumstantial speech* — highly detailed and lengthy conversations where a simple statement would suffice
- *tangentiality* — moving from one topic to a loosely associated topic
- *'clanging'* — clang associations are a form of rhyming speech or use of words with similar sounds rather than selecting words to make logical sense
- *loose associations/derailment* — this is where a person slips from topic to topic
- *echolalia* — repeating words or phrases used by the other person in a conversation
- *neologisms* — making up new words
- *word salad* — where a person combines words in a way that does not make logical sense
- *perseveration* — where a person repeats ideas and has difficulty moving on to new ideas.

Grossly disorganised or abnormal motor behaviours are also characteristic in people with schizophrenia. Such behaviours can include anything from childlike actions (including silliness) to unpredictable agitation. Such behaviours can present barriers to a person performing and achieving activities of daily living.

Catatonic behaviour, a significant symptom within this category, presents as a marked decrease in reactivity to the environment. This behaviour may be observed as resistance to instructions (negativism); maintaining a rigid, inappropriate or bizarre posture; or a complete lack of verbal and motor responses (mutism or stupor). Catatonic behaviour can include purposeless and excessive motor activity without apparent cause. Other features include staring, grimacing and the echoing of speech.

Negative symptoms

The negative symptoms of schizophrenia are generally less evident than the positive symptoms. These symptoms involve the withdrawal or retreat of the person from social contact. Negative symptoms seem to take away from or reduce the person's common or ordinary experiences, for example, there is an absence or lack in the person's ordinary or usual experiences.

Negative symptoms of schizophrenia can be very frustrating for the person experiencing them. They can also be distressing for partners, carers and family members. Examples of the negative symptoms of schizophrenia include the following.

- *Blunted emotions.* A person's emotional responses are restricted, making them appear to be disinterested and withdrawn or lacking in emotion
- *Cognitive deficits.* These impact the person's ability to communicate; for example, the person may have difficulty concentrating and be slow to react to sensory input
- *Apathy.* The person lacks motivation or initiative and has difficulty undertaking straightforward tasks. Their movements may be slow.

IN PRACTICE

Communicating in crisis situations with people experiencing psychosis

Emergency services personnel, including paramedics, police, fire services and health professionals working in the emergency departments of hospitals, can sometimes be required to communicate with a person experiencing psychosis.

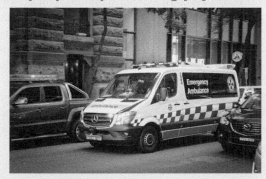

The best way to communicate with someone experiencing psychosis is to be supportive and non-judgemental (NSW Health, 2020).

People experiencing psychosis may respond to a crisis or emergency in ways that may seem bizarre, extreme or unpredictable. For example:

- they may exhibit no emotional response or appear disinterested
- disorganised thinking may lead them to be unable to respond as expected
- cognitive deficits may impact their ability to communicate what is happening or ask questions
- circumstantial speech or tangentiality may mean they are unable to describe what is happening clearly or succinctly
- paranoid delusions may lead them to think that they have caused the crisis or that someone is out to get them
- grandiose delusions may lead them to think they can help the emergency services personnel rescue the situation or 'save the day'.

A person with psychosis may also feel fearful but be unable to communicate their fears. This inability to express themselves verbally can lead the person to lash out in ways that the emergency services personnel may misinterpret. For this reason, some jurisdictions in Australia have developed programs where mental health, emergency, ambulance, and police collaborate to support people with serious mental illness who experience crisis situations. For example, the PACER (Police, Ambulance and Clinician Early Response) program in the Australian Capital Territory (ACT) has achieved inter-agency cooperation to improve outcomes for people with mental illness in need of emergency assistance (Australian Federal Police (AFP), n.d.).

According to NSW Health, when supporting a person who is experiencing psychosis, a health professional can take the following steps to improve their communication.

- Treat the person with respect.
- Listen to the way that the person explains and understands their experiences.
- Be empathetic with the person, including how they feel about their beliefs and experiences. Empathy does not mean you agree with the person; rather, it shows that you are willing to stand beside them and accept them.
- Talk clearly and use short sentences in a calm and non-threatening voice.
- Validate the person's experience of frustration or distress, as well as the positives of their experience.
- Do not argue with them about the content of their beliefs and experiences, as this will only serve to distress them all the more.
- Accept if they don't want to talk to you, but be available if they change their mind (NSW Health, 2020).

QUESTIONS

1. What is your confidence level in supporting people experiencing psychosis?

2. What steps can you take to develop your skills in supporting people experiencing psychosis?

Bipolar disorder

In the past, bipolar disorder has been referred to as 'manic depression'. The condition is now called 'bipolar affective disorder' or the 'bipolar disorder', as these terms more accurately describe the cycling of moods experienced by the person between the two poles of 'high' or elevated mood and 'low' or depressed mood.

According to Bipolar Australia (2022), bipolar disorder affects almost 3 per cent of Australians aged 16 years or older. Onset is usually before the age of 30, but can occur at any time. A person with bipolar disorder is likely to be symptom-free for most of the time and live a productive life in the community. Interestingly, some people with bipolar disorder say they would not like to be 'cured' of bipolar disorder as they view the creativity and energy generated during the hypomanic phase as a positive influence on their lives. On the other hand, other people are unequivocal in their desire to ensure the symptoms are minimised by treatment because of the destructive influence on their lives. Clearly, different people experience the symptoms of bipolar at different intensity levels and respond to these experiences in different ways.

The diagnostic criteria for bipolar disorders, as described in DSM-5, are complex (APA, 2013). There are different types of bipolar disorder, with the main types bipolar 1 and bipolar 2 disorder. In simple terms, bipolar 1 refers to people who have experienced at least one manic episode, though many will have experienced more than one episode of mania and episodes of depression. Bipolar 2 refers to people who have experienced episodes of hypomania and depression. Rapid cycling bipolar disorder describes people who cycle from elevated mood to depression at least four times in a year. This rapid cycling is more common among women than men.

Health professionals who do not work in a mental health specialty field do not need to know how to differentiate between the two types of bipolar disorder. Most important is a general understanding of the experiences of bipolar disorder and the potential impact of these experiences on a person's life.

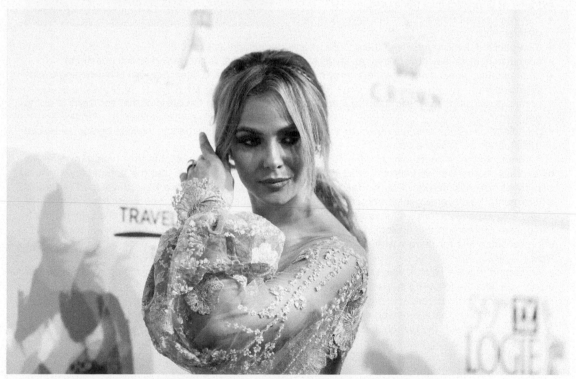

Jessica Marais is an Australian actor who has spoken openly about having bipolar disorder.

Factors contributing to bipolar disorder

Like schizophrenia, various factors contribute to the development of the bipolar disorder, including genetics, environment, substances and pregnancy.

Genetic factors

According to the Black Dog Institute (2022b), bipolar disorder is the most likely psychiatric disorder to be passed down from family, with genetic factors accounting for approximately 80 per cent of the cause.

For example, if one parent has bipolar disorder, there's a 10 per cent chance that their child will develop the illness; if both parents have bipolar disorder, the likelihood of their child developing bipolar disorder rises to 40 per cent. However, like schizophrenia, having a family member with bipolar disorder does not mean that other family members will necessarily develop the condition (NIMH, 2022a).

Environmental factors

Environmental factors contributing to the development of bipolar disorder include stress, emotional triggers and seasonal factors, with an increased chance of onset in spring (NAMI, 2022a). Reasons for the change in seasons contributing to the development of bipolar disorder have been linked to the sunshine and the pineal gland (Black Dog Institute, 2022b).

Substance use

Bipolar disorder has been linked to the use of various substances (Jergens, 2022). For example, some substances can lead to a mental state that resembles mania. These substances include cocaine, ecstasy and amphetamines, medicine for hormonal problems like prednisone or other corticosteroids, and very large amounts of caffeine. While this euphoric state is not bipolar disorder, in some circumstances, the substances may trigger the condition in vulnerable people.

Euphoric states have also been linked to antidepressant medication. For example, if the dose of antidepressant medication is too high and/or the person taking the medication is not closely monitored for symptoms of escalation, a hypomanic or manic episode may be triggered (Black Dog Institute, 2022b).

Pregnancy

Bipolar disorder can begin during pregnancy or after the birth of a baby. The experience of the symptoms of bipolar disorder may be a first episode or a continuation or relapse of the condition. Mental health issues experienced during the perinatal period are explained in detail in the chapter focusing on depression, anxiety and perinatal mental health care.

Experiences of bipolar affective disorder

As already suggested, the main experiences or symptoms of bipolar disorder are mania or hypomania, with the latter a less euphoric state than mania and depression. These two quite different experiences are explained in the following sections.

Mania

Mania refers to a period of elevated, expansive or irritable mood, high energy levels and inappropriate behaviours, which have the potential to cause major problems in relationships or the work setting. The person may also exhibit symptoms of psychosis.

A manic episode can include any number of the following symptoms:

- **grandiosity**
- decreased need for sleep
- excessive talkativeness
- racing thoughts
- distractibility and psychomotor agitation
- sexual disinhibition
- decreased ability to make sound or rational decisions
- increased focus on goal-directed activity
- disproportionate involvement in pleasurable activities.

People who experience a mania can have disjointed or distorted thinking. Hallucinations and delusions are common and often appear very real to the person. People can also experience 'mystical experiences' where they see special connections between events or other experiences. During an episode of mania, the person is at risk of behaving in an antisocial way (which may be out of character for them) or behaving in a way that may lead to serious financial, legal and relationship problems. In addition, the person may neglect their personal hygiene and physical health. In combination, these symptoms may lead to the person being hospitalised.

Hypomania is similar to mania, with symptoms that are less severe and cause less impairment for the individual. Usually, no psychotic features are evident in a hypomanic episode and the person may not require hospitalisation (APA, 2013).

In addition to mania and/or hypomania, the person with bipolar disorder will typically experience episodes of depression. The frequency or lengths of the cycles between mania and depression will depend upon the person's individual experience. However, mood-stabilising medication will often give rise to more extended periods between the highs and the lows and a decrease in the extremes of the highs and lows.

Depression, including major depression

The depression experienced in bipolar disorder has the same signs and symptoms as the depression experienced in major depressive disorder or other types of depression. Detailed information about depression, including major depression, which is classified as a serious mental illness, is described at length in the chapter focussing on depression, anxiety and perinatal mental health. This information includes details of prevalence, contributing factors, experiences and treatment. In short, people with depression find it difficult to make decisions, and they are generally uninterested in performing the tasks of everyday life or being involved in activities they once found pleasurable. Their sleep patterns may be disturbed, and they will often lose their appetite and sex drive.

Schizoaffective disorder

Another less common serious mental illness is schizoaffective disorder. This major mental illness is often incorrectly diagnosed as it involves psychotic symptoms, similar to those experienced by the person with schizophrenia, and the symptoms of a mood disorder, such as those experienced by a person with bipolar affective disorder. Schizoaffective disorder is relatively rare, with a lifetime prevalence of only 0.3 per cent, with males and females experiencing the disorder at the same rate (NAMI, 2022c). The care provided to a person with schizoaffective disorder is similar to that provided to a person with schizophrenia and bipolar disorder; that is, psychosocial and pharmacological interventions. These are described in a later section of the chapter.

Table 9.3 provides a useful grid to help health professionals differentiate between the major mental illnesses. The information provided, in turn, will enable health professionals to talk to consumers about their symptoms and how to manage these experiences.

TABLE 9.3 Symptoms seen in serious mental illness

Condition	Delusions	Hallucinations	Disorganised thinking/ behaviours	Low mood	Elevated mood
Schizophrenia	Often	Often	Often	Often	Rarely
Bipolar disorder	Sometimes	Sometimes	Sometimes	Often	Often
Major depression	Sometimes	Rarely	Rarely	Often	Not at all
Schizoaffective disorder	Often	Often	Often	Sometimes	Sometimes

LIVED EXPERIENCE

Recovery can happen!

When I was around 5 years old, my mother took me to a psychiatrist who diagnosed me with depression. She decided to ignore the diagnosis and never took me back. But my low moods didn't magically go away, and I remember my childhood as a terrible struggle with how I was feeling.

As bad as the low feelings were, even worse was the feeling that I was different, that I didn't fit in with my family. I was convinced I had some kind of intellectual disability — my siblings were brilliant academically and thrived at school; in comparison, I could hardly read, and my spelling was always wrong. As an adult, I was told this was because I had dyslexia and not because I was stupid. But as a child, then as a teenager, my only coping strategy was to skip going to school.

I left school in year nine and began working as a hairdresser. But I soon found that I couldn't follow through with that either. Everything seemed like a struggle, even work I thought I might enjoy. Completing my training was beyond me.

By that time, my moods had begun to swing from high to low. One day, I felt like I could take on the world; another day, I couldn't even get out of bed. While I was on a high, I married a man at 18. I'd only known him for three months. It could have been a disaster, but I'm still married to him, 44 years later. Without him, well, I have no idea where I'd be now.

We lost no time having babies and I loved it. The experience of birthing gave me such feelings of joy. Raising my babies likewise gave me feelings of joy. But during my last pregnancy, I suffered from a dreadful, deep depression that included delusions. I struggled to do anything, let alone care for the kids. My husband finally talked me into seeing a doctor.

It was then that I was diagnosed with bipolar disorder.

I guess the diagnosis gave us a name for my feelings, but it didn't help much otherwise. I spent years and years going in and out of acute mental health facilities with either grandiose delusions and behaviours or in the depths of despair. I felt suicidal for years and deliberately overdosed on my medication more times than I can remember — not to kill myself but to remove myself from the horrible reality of my life. While I was blessed with very good clinical support, nothing seemed to work to stop my moodiness or help me to cope. My whole miserable existence was also impacting my family.

Then, one day — and I'm not sure why, maybe it was the right time or one of those seeds that the clinicians had sown had finally taken root? — I saw another person with bipolar disorder get well. I can remember thinking, 'Man, if she can get well, so can I!'

It was like, on that day, I decided to get well. So I started to ask everyone, 'What can I do to get well' No one knew. That question began my years of discovering what makes soundness of my mind and what it means to be autonomous. I found joy in exercise, going to a gym and working, sweating, and releasing those wonderful endorphins. I experienced a complete lack of anxiety after a gym session, and I was hooked! I then tried eating healthier. I wrote a long list of what I would like to achieve, including going on a hot air balloon ride. It is incredible what writing a list did for me! Even better, while we didn't have money for hot air balloon rides and so I thought it would never happen, but a family friend owned a hot air balloon, and he offered to take me on it, and just like that, the goal was achieved.

It took me many years to get to where I am now, mentally well, working in mental health as a peer worker, and attending university. I chose to work in mental health because I knew that if I could get well, anyone could! I haven't experienced suicidal thoughts for many years now. And now that I have the gift of wellness, I am determined to help others find their road to recovery.

Recovery is unique to all; what works for me may not work for you, but there is something that will work for you. There might be some trial and error to start with, but eventually, you too can find your journey to emotional wellbeing.

Cathy Fox, Mandurah, WA.

9.3 Interventions to support the Recovery journey of people with serious mental illness

LEARNING OBJECTIVE 9.3 Describe the Recovery-oriented interventions for people with serious mental illness.

Various interventions can be used to support the recovery journey of people with serious mental illness. According to the RANZCP, people with schizophrenia are best supported with early intervention strategies, physical health and psychosocial interventions, cultural support, vocational training and pharmacological treatments (Galletly et al., 2016). People with moderate to severe bipolar disorder, are best treated with a combination of psychosocial interventions and pharmacotherapy, which has advantages in the maintenance phase (Malhi et al., 2021). This section focuses on psychosocial, including vocational interventions and pharmacological treatments. Early intervention strategies are covered in the chapter on depression, anxiety and perinatal mental health care, and cultural considerations are discussed at length in the chapter by that name. In this section, consideration is also given to how health professionals can better engage with people with serious mental illness.

The pathway of care that the consumer chooses is not always straightforward. For example, some interventions can occasionally involve involuntary treatment, where the person with a serious mental illness receives treatment against their will. Such instances can arise when the person demonstrates a lack of the capacity to make sound decisions and presents a risk to themselves or others. Such situations are complex but nevertheless require all health professionals to engage with the person actively and their family or carers to meet their goals, needs and preferences. Information about mental health legislation in Australia is provided in the chapter that looks at the legal and ethical context of mental health care.

The ethics of coercive care

Some people with serious mental illness receive treatment involuntarily. This situation occurs when the person does not understand that they have a mental illness and the symptoms they are experiencing place them or others at risk of harm.

Involuntary treatment is guided by state-level legislation, generally known as 'the mental health act'. This legislation is guided by the ethical principles of:

- upholding the human right of people with a mental illness
- facilitating choice, promoting autonomy and self-determination, and enabling shared decision making for people with a mental illness
- ensuring the use of the least restrictive care for people with a mental illness.

Many consumer advocates argue that the time has come to move away from involuntary treatment, suggesting that 'coercive care' is a contradictory notion. You can read more about this ongoing discussion and the ethics of coercive care in the chapter focussing on the legal and ethical context of mental health care.

QUESTIONS

1. How comfortable do you feel with forcing a person to receive health care, against their will?
2. What other options could there be for coercive care for people with serious mental illness who are at risk of harm to themselves or others?

Engaging with a person with serious mental illness

The principles of engaging with a person with serious mental illness are no different to engaging with other people with health problems. People with a serious mental illness have many of the same hopes, fears, needs or expectations as others. Likewise, they have relationships, day-to-day responsibilities, interests and personal issues. Similarly, each person has their own individual story to tell and Recovery journey to negotiate. Health professionals must give people with a serious mental illness the same respect and common courtesy they give others. Health professionals must also accept that it may take them a little longer to engage with the person due to the symptoms they are experiencing.

As explained in the chapter on mental health assessment, the best Recovery-oriented, therapeutic relationships involve inspiring hope and optimism in the person, showing kindness and unconditional positive regard, clarifying expectations, empowering the person through collaborative decision making, and involving family members or carers. There is also a need to take a holistic or comprehensive approach and work closely with the multidisciplinary team to meet the health needs and preferences of the person. Such approaches will include providing support for the physical health of the person. A discussion about the physical health of people with serious mental illness is provided in a later section of this chapter.

Information on the best approaches to caring for a person with mental illness is outlined in the chapter on depression, anxiety and perinatal mental health care. This information includes the need to ensure the safety of the person, particularly those who may have paranoid delusions, feel unsafe or are at risk of accidental injury, deliberate self-harm or suicide. In addition, health professionals must understand that serious mental illness can impair a person's communication ability. Common difficulties include withdrawing from routine social interactions, isolation and difficulty in expressing feelings. The ability of the health professional to demonstrate empathy, warmth and optimism will support engagement with the person using simple strategies and techniques such as:

- attending to what the person is saying or trying to communicate
- actively listening to the person
- demonstrating empathy
- validating what the person is saying is their experience (without reinforcing delusions).

Sometimes the person's delusions or behaviours may seem amusing or bizarre to the health professional. Health professionals must work hard to respond rather than react to what a person tells them or to the way the person behaves.

It can also be useful to consider why people do not engage, or disengage after the initial engagement. For example, particular populations of people with serious mental illness have historically been challenging to engage, such as young adults experiencing a first episode of psychosis, people who experience homelessness, and individuals with coexisting psychosis and substance use disorders (Dixon et al., 2016).

Indeed, comorbid substance abuse is one of the strongest factors associated with non-initiation and non-engagement in mental health treatment. Reasons for the lack of engagement or disengagement include:

- fragmentation of health care and social services, including lack of integration of services
- poor understanding of the needs for treatment
- feelings that the interventions are not working
- treatment is difficult to access
- mistrust of the health and welfare systems, and health professionals.

These barriers suggest the need for health professionals to work with managers and multi-disciplinary team members to consider how to overcome such challenges to support the individual needs of the person.

Psychosocial interventions

A person's experiences of serious mental illness will be unique to them. Consequently, health professionals cannot take a 'one-size-fits-all' approach when providing psychosocial care. For example, a person's psychosocial context includes:

- the community and physical environment in which the person lives
- their socio-economic demographic, including the level of education, and employment status
- their age, gender, sexuality, family influences, cultural background, social networks, spiritual and political beliefs
- individual emotional, cognitive and behavioural characteristics, including levels of resilience and capacity to be creative and adapt to change
- their physical health status
- their role(s) in society (e.g. 'parent', 'child', 'partner', 'carer', 'employed' or 'unemployed', 'homeless')
- their self-perception and personal needs, experiences, preferences and aspirations.

In light of the complexity of the psychosocial context of a person, there are many and varied psychosocial interventions. Broadly speaking, psychosocial interventions are non-pharmacological interventions aimed at improving symptoms, functioning, quality of life and social inclusion for people with chronic health conditions (Barbui et al., 2020). More specifically, for people with serious mental illness, psychosocial interventions can include peer support; psychological therapies, including talking therapies and psychoeducation; and social interventions that support the person with housing, occupational and vocational activities, healthy living and recreation. Also included in this section is assertive community treatment and case management, an integrated model incorporating structured clinical support and psychosocial interventions.

Peer support

Peer support, including peer group support, involves people with serious mental illness meeting together to support one another in their recovery journey (Bernecker et al., 2020). A peer is someone with whom a person shares demographic, social and/or health-related similarities. The support provided by a peer includes 'the kind of deeply felt empathy, encouragement, and assistance that people with shared experiences can offer one another within a reciprocal relationship' (Penney, 2018, p. 1).

Peers can be volunteers who work through, for example, self-help groups that combine mutuality and connection with moving forward in a common journey. As explained in the chapter on depression, anxiety and perinatal mental health care, peers are also employed in recovery-oriented services as 'consumer consultants' or 'consumer representatives'. Some services also employ carer consultants or representatives.

For people with serious mental illness, peer support is a useful intervention to improve the activation of knowledge, skills, confidence and attitudes for managing health and treatment, leading to improved quality of life, engagement with more health care practices, and treatment satisfaction symptoms (Shalaby & Agyapong, 2020). While changes have also been noted in people who engage with peer support in measures of hope, recovery and empowerment, no improvements were shown in overall symptoms (Shalaby & Agyapong, 2020).

IN PRACTICE

Peer and vocational support through Clubhouses

The original Clubhouse was started in New York towards the end of the Great Depression in the late 1940s by a group of people with serious mental illness to provide friendship and assistance to one another. Today, Clubhouses worldwide, including in Australia, provide a range of psychosocial programs ▶

to people with serious mental illness. These programs include peer support, vocational and supported employment activities, education and health promotion (Raeburn et al., 2015). In Australia, Clubhouses receive funding from the National Disability Insurance Scheme (NDIS).

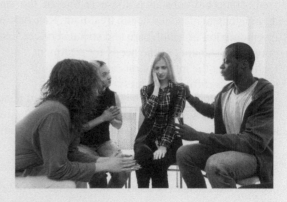

The International Standards regulate the Clubhouse model for Clubhouse Programs, including a Bill of Rights for members, a code of ethics for staff, board and administrators, and a guidelines evaluation (Clubhouse International, 2018). Participants in the Clubhouse activities are called members rather than consumers or patients. Participation is strictly voluntary, offering community experience and possibilities of participation in practical and useful activities (Fekete et al., 2021).

The essential intervention of the Clubhouse model is the work-ordered day, which provides a structure similar to that found in all workplaces. This model supports members with vocational skills they may not have previously experienced. Staff and members collaborate side by side as equals on doing tasks related to operating the Clubhouse, from cleaning bathrooms to making lunch, writing grants and planning programs. Staff or other members also provide other members with vocational employment support, education support and access to housing and entitlement. Staff do not act as service providers or care workers but rather engage members in activities and support their inclusion in the Clubhouse community (Clubhouse International, 2018).

QUESTIONS

1. Where is the closest Clubhouse to where you live? What steps could you take to visit that Clubhouse to learn more about the program?
2. What is the value of peers providing vocational support to people with serious mental illness?
3. How important is it for health professionals to know about programs such as the Clubhouse? Justify your answer.

Psychological therapies

A range of talking or psychological therapies can be used to support people with serious mental illness, including those that help to reduce or manage symptoms, prevent relapse and recurrence, restore social and psychological functioning, and support family members or carers. Depending on the needs, preferences and trajectory of the person's Recovery journey, these psychological interventions can include acceptance and commitment therapy, cognitive behavioural therapy, interpersonal therapy and complementary therapies such as massage. An explanation of these therapies is provided in the chapter focussing on depression, anxiety and perinatal mental health care.

Another important psychological therapy is psychoeducation. In its simplest form, psychoeducation involves providing information about the person's mental illness. This information provision allows the person to make decisions regarding their treatment and lifestyle based on reliable information.

While mental health specialists predominantly deliver formal, structured psychoeducation programs, all health professionals can contribute by repeating and reinforcing important health information, enabling the person to make realistic choices that will support them on their Recovery journey (Veltro et al., 2022). Psychoeducation can also be used with good effect to support carers or family members of people with serious mental illness (Qi et al., 2021)

Psychoeducation can include a range of elements in verbal and written form, including:

- Recovery planning, including goals for the future, steps required to achieve those goals, relapse prevention and self-monitoring, discussed to suit the person's readiness to consider or process information at that time (refer to 'Cycle of Change' in the chapter that looks at substance use disorders)
- information about the person's mental illness, including the symptoms of the mental illness and how these symptoms can be managed
- information about treatment options, including the management of side effects of medications
- how to build resilience and coping strategies for stress
- motivational enhancement (refer to 'motivational interviewing' in the chapter that looks at substance use disorders)

- assistance with problem solving/decision making about treatment
- family/carer education and support, including developing communication skills
- support where necessary to help the person cope with difficult and sometimes life-changing personal information (e.g. being diagnosed with a serious physical illness).

Providing psychoeducation to the person allows for tailoring information to meet individual needs, including those with impaired cognition or psychosocial functioning (Luciano et al., 2021). At the same time, there are also advantages to providing psychoeducation in a group or family setting, including enabling the person to interact with others who are grappling with similar issues. Group interventions can reduce the feelings of isolation and alienation that is often a part of the lived experience of serious mental illness (Irvine et al., 2021).

Health professionals must prepare well before facilitating psychoeducational opportunites, to increase their confidence and competence. It can also be important to have a handout containing information for the person or people to take away with them, including web addresses to reputable organisations where they can find more information. Other tips for delivering psychoeducation include:
- ask the person what they already understand about their illness
- explain information in simple terms — avoid the use of jargon; then check with people if they have understood the information
- emphasise choice and self-determination
- summarise points at the end of the discussion.

Psychoeducation has been shown to positively benefit people with serious mental illness and their carers or family members (Delibas & Erdogan 2022; Koonce Morse, 2022; Veltro et al., 2022).

Social and occupational interventions

Social workers have supported various people, including people with serious mental illness, since the late nineteenth century and, in Australia, since 1929 (Miller, 2016). Likewise, there is evidence that structured and purposeful occupational activities were delivered to white Australians on the ships bringing convicts to Australia (Cusick, 2017). While social workers and occupational therapists are not solely responsible for providing social and vocational or occupational interventions to people experiencing health problems, their roles indicate the kind of activities involved. Social and occupational interventions for people with serious mental illness can include housing support, employment opportunities, social and recreational activities, and healthy living programs.

Of particular note are the links between living meaningful and contributing lives, housing and employment, particularly for people with serious mental illness. For example, according to the Australian Housing and Urban Research Institute (AUHRI, 2021), homelessness can lead a person to experience mental health issues. Moreover, serious mental illness can:
- affect a person's ability to access and sustain tenancies
- lead to employment instability, which affects their ability to access housing
- affect a person's capacity to maintain independent living, with the support needs often fluctuating and unpredictable.

For this reason, people with serious mental illness can rely heavily on others to ensure required support is available and coordinated. Social and occupational support provides an important means of meeting these needs.

Assertive community treatment and case management

Assertive community treatment and case management is a recovery-oriented, community-based mental health care for people experiencing serious mental illness. Assertive community treatment and case management is an integrated clinical and psychosocial service often provided to people who are being treated involuntarily and require clinical monitoring and assistance to live in the community and attend appointments with professionals in clinics and hospitals (Yee et al., 2021). Assertive community treatment and case management is a less restrictive alternative to hospital or residential settings.

Assertive community treatment and case management teams are multidisciplinary, with most clinicians qualified mental health specialists. These services aim to improve the consumers' mental and physical health outcomes, enhance contact with families or support people, improve the use of community services by people with serious mental illness and reduce the reliance on hospital care (including emergency departments and acute mental health wards) by providing proactive or 'assertive' care the reduce preventable outcomes of mental illness, such as homelessness and substance abuse (Nielsen et al., 2021).

Long-term psychosocial programs

The Australian government has developed psychosocial support programs for people with severe mental illness (Department of Health & Aged Care, 2022). Commonwealth psychosocial support programs for people with severe mental illness help those who need short-term help to function daily. The program offers one-on-one and group support activities to help people with severe mental illness:

- connect with clinical care and other services they need
- build capacity in managing day-to-day activities
- strengthen social skills, friendships and relationships with family
- increase educational, vocational and training skills.

Support for people with severe mental illness is available through this program if they are not with the NDIS or a state and territory-funded service. In addition, the Australian government funds Primary Health Networks (PHNs). PHNs commission community-based organisations to run services under the Commonwealth Psychosocial Support Program. These organisations tailor their services to meet the needs of the community and clients.

QUESTIONS

1. How likely is it that people with serious mental illness will be able to build skills to live independently and contribute to their communities with short-term help?

2. How likely is that people with serious mental illness will be able to negotiate the complex layers of health and social services provided in Australia?

Pharmacological therapies

As noted previously, pharmacological treatments are a key intervention for treating schizophrenia and bipolar disorder (Galletly et al., 2016; Malhi et al., 2020). These pharmacological interventions include antipsychotic medications and mood stabilisers. Together, these drugs are called **psychotropic medications**, which are any type of medication capable of affecting the mind, emotions and behaviour. Pharmacological interventions are administered by practitioners employed by government and non-government organisations, including state-run health services and community-managed organisations. Some people with serious mental illness may also see their general practitioner (GP) regularly to monitor their pharmacological treatments in collaboration with the psychiatrist.

People with serious mental illness receiving pharmacological interventions will present to general health settings when experiencing physical health problems. For this reason, all health professionals must be aware of the types of medications used to treat people with serious mental illness, the possible side effects and drug interactions. Polypharmacy issues are addressed in the next section on the physical health of people with serious mental illness.

Antipsychotic medication

Antipsychotic medication is an effective treatment for acute and long-term management of psychotic illnesses such as schizophrenia (Galletly et al., 2016). Antipsychotic medication is also prescribed for people with bipolar disorder to control hallucinations, delusions and mania. Some prescribers recommend antipsychotic medication as **off-label** sedatives for agitation or as mood-stabilising medications

There are two broad classes of antipsychotic medication that are currently in use.

1. 'Typical', 'first generation' or older antipsychotics, which were first developed in the 1950s
2. 'Atypical', 'second generation', 'novel', or newer antipsychotics, developed from the 1970s onwards.

Of course, the so-called atypical antipsychotics are now not-so-new or novel and are more commonly used than the typical antipsychotics; even so, at this point, the names 'typical' and 'atypical' remain.

There are several possible explanations why typical and atypical antipsychotics help to reduce symptoms of psychosis. The main theory suggests they work by changing the effect of some of the chemicals in the brain: dopamine, serotonin, noradrenaline and acetylcholine. These chemicals have the effect of changing a person's emotions, mood and behaviour. Although the science behind antipsychotics continues to be debated, the outcomes achieved for people with serious mental illness who take the antipsychotic medications are mainly positive, with people previously seriously disabled now living meaningful and contributing lives.

Generally, antipsychotic medication is more effective in reducing the positive symptoms of schizophrenia and relapse rates than the negative symptoms. However, some of the more recent **atypical antipsychotic medications** are helpful in reducing negative symptoms (Cerveri et al., 2019).

Typical antipsychotics

The typical antipsychotics are generally more effective at reducing the positive symptoms of schizophrenia, such as hallucinations, delusions and disordered thinking. Even so, these medications can have a strong sedating component, and some health professionals may have experienced them being prescribed for people with dementia or substance use disorders (Hilmer et al., 2020). Examples of some typical antipsychotic medications used in Australia are:

- chlorpromazine (e.g. Largactil®)
- haloperidol (e.g. Serenace®).

One reason for the decline in the use of first-generation antipsychotic medications is the successful marketing of second-generation antipsychotic medications, which tend to have similar efficacy but better tolerability. Indeed, the first-generation antipsychotic medications are associated with a range of common and undesirable side effects, including sedation, postural hypotension and **extrapyramidal side effects (EPSEs)**. These side effects are described in more detail later in this section.

Atypical antipsychotics

Atypical antipsychotic medications are generally prescribed to people newly diagnosed with schizophrenia and appear to provide some relief from both the positive and negative symptoms of schizophrenia and reduce the cognitive decline often associated with the disorder. Atypical antipsychotic medications are thought to impact **serotonin transmission** in addition to dopamine transmission, impacting the side-effect profile of these medications. For example, although atypical antipsychotic medications are associated with a reduced risk of EPSEs compared to first-generation antipsychotics, they are more likely to be associated with **metabolic and other adverse side effects** (Hilmer et al., 2020). Examples of the more common atypical antipsychotic medications used in Australia include:

- amisulpride (e.g. Amipride®, Solian®, Sulprix®)
- aripiprazole (e.g. Abilify®)
- olanzapine (e.g. Zyprexa®)
- paliperidone (e.g. Invega®)
- quetiapine (e.g. Seroquel®)
- risperidone (e.g. Risperdal®).

These medications can be given orally or intramuscularly, with some developed for long action. Long-acting medications are often used for people with serious mental illness who are being treated involuntarily, with health professionals administering the injection. At this point in time, most of the long-acting or **depot** medications are administered fortnightly. However, since 2017, longer acting medications have become available in Australia:

- Invega Sustena® — adminstered monthly
- Invega Trinza® — adminstered 3 monthly
- Invega Hafyera® — adminstered 6 monthly.

Longer time frames between injections can help to reduce the stress and distress caused to the person receiving the injection. There is also evidence that suggests long-acting medications cause fewer side effects and physical health issues.

IN PRACTICE

Improving the safety of medication administration

In a report commissioned by the Australian Commission on Safety and Quality in Health Care (ACSQHC), Roughead et al. (2017) identified many unsafe practices when administering medications to people with mental illness. One of these unsafe practices relates to using long-acting intramuscular antipsychotics.

A coroner's investigation into the death of a person with a serious mental illness found the person's levels of zuclopenthixol to be extremely low, despite the person receiving regular treatment. The injection site primarily used for long-acting intramuscular antipsychotic received by the person was the dorsogluteal site. However, this site is known to be unpredictable in consistently achieving the optimal levels of the medication in the bloodstream, and the medication can be accidentally administered subcutaneously if the needle length is too short to reach the muscle beyond any adipose tissue. Indeed, some studies

▶

---

suggest that the dorsogluteal has a 20 per cent poorer absorption than the ventrogluteal (Rougheadet al., 2017). Moreover, using this injection site risks damaging the sciatica nerve, causing abscesses and increased pain.

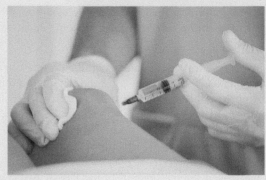

The ventrogluteal site is the more appropriate site for administering depot antipsychotic injections. The ventrogluteal site has better muscle mass and less adipose tissue. Moreover, some health services that have switched to administering long-acting intramuscular antipsychotic medication to the ventrogluteal site have reduced the prescribed doses.

There is a need for health services and health professionals to provide training on best practice administration sites and redesign depot administration charts to record the injection site used and promote rotation of injection sites. Consumers must also be involved in developing relevant and easy-to-understand information about the best administration sites for intramuscular injections.

QUESTIONS

1. How important is it that health professionals, regardless of their disciplinary background, understand the principles of medication administration? Justify your answer.

2. How can you learn more about the principles, safety features, and side effects of intramuscular medication administration?

Side effects of antipsychotic medication

All medications have the potential to induce side effects. Factors influencing the overall tolerability of medication include the seriousness of the side effects and the frequency with which they occur.

Many of the side effects of antipsychotics present challenges for people with serious mental illness, so health professionals must have detailed information on hand to assist the person. This information can be obtained from relevant pharmaceutical companies. The internet is also valuable, with government and non-government organisations providing user-friendly information.

The most common side effects of antipsychotic medication are:
- dry mouth, blurred vision, increased sweating, dizziness and/or headaches
- nausea, constipation and/or weight gain that can lead to diabetes
- movement effects (e.g. tremor, stiffness, agitation)
- sedation (e.g. causing sleepiness or low energy)
- loss of menstrual periods in women
- fluid retention
- sexual problems (SANE, 2017).

Other side effects are cardiovascular, metabolic and endocrine. A particular problem is a condition called 'metabolic syndrome'. More information about this condition is provided in the following section on the physical health of people with serious mental illness.

UPON REFLECTION

Equally Well

Australia's National Mental Health Commission published an Equally Well Consensus Statement in 2016, to improve the physical health and wellbeing of people with mental illness in Australia. According to this Statement:

> impacts of medication (both positive and negative) should be regularly assessed, and alternatives should be considered if a medication has a potential negative impact. People living with mental illness have a much higher risk of developing metabolic syndrome. Therefore anyone prescribed antipsychotic medication should be given clear and understandable verbal and written information about the medication's risks and benefits. Steps should be taken to limit side effects such as obesity, cardiovascular disease and diabetes (National Mental Health Commission, 2016, p. 18).

Extrapyramidal side effects (EPSEs)

EPSE is a broad term used to describe various movement disorders caused by antipsychotic medication. It is most often seen in young males (D'Souza & Hooten, 2022).

Most often, EPSEs result from typical antipsychotics; however, they have also been known to be caused by newer or atypical antipsychotics. Likewise, EPSEs can also occur with medically prescribed drugs that have antidopaminergic properties, such as metoclopramide (D'Souza & Hooten, 2022). The relatively common occurrence of EPSEs suggests that all health professionals need to be aware of these side effects and know how to treat them.

EPSEs can be either acute or chronic. Acute EPSEs develop within hours or days of treatment, while chronic or 'tardive syndromes' develop after a long treatment period. Sometimes EPSEs are mistaken for agitation or an underlying illness. The symptoms include involuntary muscle contraction (**dystonia**), rigidity or shaking. A list of the major EPSEs and their treatments is provided in table 9.4.

TABLE 9.4   **Extrapyramidal side effects of antipsychotic medication**

Side effect	Characterised by	Treatment
Parkinsonism	Shuffling gait, tremor, muscle stiffness, limb **cog wheeling**	Responds to dose reduction or treatment with anticholinergic medications such as benztropine or benzhexol
Dystonia	Involuntary muscular contraction	Responds to anticholinergic medication such as benztropine and dose reduction
Akathesia	The subjective or inner feeling of restlessness	Responds to dose reduction and treatment with propranolol or diazepam
Tardive dyskinesia (TD)	Involuntary movements of the mouth, lips and tongue, which may progress to the head, neck and trunk. This is most likely to be seen as a result of long-term treatment. Often irreversible	Dose reduction or treatment with anticholinergics may worsen TD. As treatment is complex, contact specialist mental health professional, ward pharmacist and local drug information service. TD has been known to affect the muscles of the respiratory and gastrointestinal systems

The most common treatment for an EPSE is an **anticholinergic** drug, such as benztropine. However, this drug is not always effective and has its own side effects. In such circumstances, the person may need to stop taking the anti-psychotic and be placed on a different medication. The role of the psychiatrist is to determine the best course of action for chronic EPSEs.

Other serious side effects

A serious side effect of antipsychotic medications is weight gain. As previously noted, weight gain is discussed in detail in the section on the physical health of people with serious mental illness.

Another far less common syndrome is neuroleptic malignant syndrome (NMS), which affects the nervous system and causes symptoms like hypertension, hypersalivation, high fever and muscle stiffness. Although the condition is serious, it is treatable if identified in time (Galletly et al., 2016).

Mood stabilisers

The term 'mood stabiliser' is often used to describe medications prescribed to help people who experience mood swings, such as those experienced by people with bipolar disorder (Malhi et al., 2021). The mood stabiliser category is not listed as a therapeutic class of medications. Instead, health professionals will only find these medications listed under classifications such as antipsychotic and anticonvulsant medications. Another common mood stabiliser is lithium carbonate or lithium citrate, which is in a different class of medications again. People who take these medications still experience changes in their moods during the day; these medicines are used for full episodes of mania or depression that last for several days or weeks. Mood stabilisers can also reduce symptoms such as agitation, sleep problems, hallucinations and delusions, depending on the choice of medication.

Antidepressant medications are not classed as mood stabilisers, even though they are used to treat depression. Reasons for this include their different mode of action than mood stabilisers. The more common mood stabilisers are:

- carbamazepine (e.g. Tegretol®, Teril®)(this medication is also an anticonvulsant)
- lamotrigine (e.g. Elmendos®, Lamictal®, Lamidus®, Lamogine®) (this medication is also an an anticonvulsant)
- lithium carbonate (e.g. Lithicarb®, Quilonum SR®)
- olanzapine (e.g. Zyprexa®)(this medication is also an antipsychotic)
- quetiapine (e.g. Seroquel®)(this medication is also an antipsychotic)
- sodium valproate (e.g. Epili®, Valprease®, Valpro®, Valproate Winthrop®)(this medication is also an anticonvulsant).

Like all medications, mood-stabilising medications have various side effects. The side effects of antipsychotic medications have already been described. The side effects of the anticonvulsants or, as they are also known, antiepileptic medication include nausea, weight gain, fatigue, headache, decreased sexual desire and tremors. There are also warnings against taking sodium valproate during pregnancy, during the higher risk of congenital abnormalities and learning disabilities.

Lithium carbonate

Health professionals working in any area of health or aged care will encounter people who have been prescribed lithium carbonate. This medication has been around for many years and was first used to treat mania in the late 1800s. An Australian psychiatrist, John Cade, who survived a Changi prisoner-of-war camp, is credited with discovering the mood-stabilising effects of lithium carbonate in the 1940s. Today, lithium carbonate remains the first-line treatment and is often given in conjunction with antipsychotic medication if the person has psychotic features to their symptoms.

An important fact to remember about pharmacological treatment that includes lithium is that it is the serum concentration rather than the dose of lithium that will determine effective treatment (Hedya et al., 2022). The oral dose required to maintain a therapeutic serum concentration of around 0.90 mmol/L will vary between individuals. Lithium has a narrow therapeutic index, and an optimal serum lithium concentration needs to be maintained. Outside of this range, a lower level will be ineffective and may lead to relapse.

The person with the mood disorder, family members and health professionals must remember that toxicity can occur if the level rises above the therapeutic range, while concentrations over 2.00 mmol/L can be potentially fatal. For this reason, blood tests for lithium levels need to be checked after the person has been taking a regular dose of the medication for 5–7 days. Blood must be taken 12 hours following the last dose of lithium to test for lithium levels. If levels are above 1.5 mmol/L, the authorised prescriber must be consulted before administering the next dose.

Risk factors for developing lithium toxicity are conditions that lead to sodium depletion, for example, diarrhoea, vomiting and excessive sweating (Hedya et al., 2022). Medication that reduces renal excretion of lithium, such as thiazide diuretics and certain non-steroidal anti-inflammatory drugs, can also lead to toxicity.

A baseline serum lithium level must be taken if a person taking lithium is admitted to a hospital for a physical illness. The signs and symptoms of acute lithium toxicity are:

- nausea, diarrhoea, vomiting
- severe tremor, **ataxia**, slurred speech, irregular jerky movements, **Parkinsonian** movements, muscular twitching, seizures
- impaired concentration, drowsiness, disorientation.

With medical approval, treatment must be discontinued and serum lithium, urea and electrolytes monitored. Providing adequate salt and fluids, including saline infusions, will reduce toxicity. Caution is also needed when prescribing lithium to individuals with renal failure, heart failure, recent myocardial infarction, electrolyte imbalance, pregnant women and older people.

Side effects of clozapine

Clozapine (Clopine®, Clozaril®, CloSyn®) is an atypical antipsychotic medication that has been shown to have superior efficacy in helping people to overcome treatment-resistant schizophrenia (Correll et al., 2022). Treatment resistance is a term used to describe the situation when a person does not respond positively or significantly to treatment. This definition reflects the viewpoint of people with this illness, their family members and mental health professionals. Although clozapine has been shown to provide effective treatment in many cases, this medication can induce very serious side effects for some people, such as **agranulocytosis**, **cardiomyopathy** and **neutropenia**, which could precipitate a medical emergency.

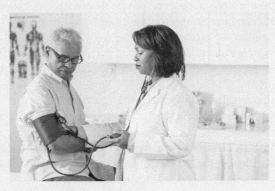

There are stringent procedures for monitoring people prescribed clozapine involving blood tests and physical observations. Clozapine cannot simply be discontinued or restarted at previous doses. Its use is also contraindicated in a variety of medical conditions. People treated with clozapine in Australia must be registered with and monitored through a standardised system called the Clozapine Patient Monitoring System (or equivalent), which involves pre-treatment medical screening followed by weekly to monthly blood tests.

QUESTIONS

1. Discuss the importance of all health professionals understanding clozapine and its potentially harmful side effect profile.
2. What strategies do health professionals need to adopt to ensure they adequately monitor a person on clozapine? Include how to obtain collateral information if this was required.
3. Benefit versus the risk of a particular treatment is not always easy to evaluate. Consider the benefits and disadvantages of clozapine treatment and discuss these findings from the symptom, physical, financial, social, ethical and Recovery perspectives.

9.4 The physical health of people with serious mental illness

LEARNING OBJECTIVE 9.4 Investigate the connections between physical and mental health in people with a serious mental illness.

People with a serious illness are more likely to develop physical illnesses, leading to a mortality rate that is 2.2 times more than the general population (AIHW, 2022d). This statistic translates to a 10–20 year reduction in life expectancy (World Health Organisation [WHO], 2018). Around 60 per cent of people with serious mental illness have a comorbid physical health condition, with these physical illnesses occurring at a younger age than in the general population (Launders et al., 2022).

The most common chronic physical illnesses in people with serious mental illness are obesity, diabetes, hypertension and chronic obstructive pulmonary disease (O'Neill, 2021). There is also a strong association between the use of alcohol, tobacco and/or illicit drugs and mental illness, which markedly increase risk factors and incidence of cancer, cirrhosis and cardiovascular disease (AIHW, 2022d).

The physical conditions of people with serious mental illness tend to be under-recognised and under-treated (Mitchell & Hill, 2020). Outcomes of this lack of recognition and treatment include higher levels of disability, reduced participation in the workforce, increased poverty and welfare dependency, and premature death (RANZCP, 2015).

Factors contributing to poorer physical health

There are various reasons why a person with a serious mental illness is more likely than the general population to develop physical health problems. Key factors arise from the social determinants of health, which were mentioned earlier on in this chapter. According to the RANZCP (2015, p. 15) and the AIHW (2022d), other contributing factors include:

- greater exposure to the known risk factors for physical diseases such as socio-economic status, smoking, poor nutrition, reduced physical activity and higher sedentary behaviour
- reduced access to and quality of health care due to financial barriers, stigma and discrimination among health care providers
- systemic issues in health care delivery, especially the separation of mental and physical health services, and a lack of clarity about who is responsible for monitoring the physical health of people with serious mental illness
- impacts from polypharmacy, prescribing practices and adverse effects of psychotropic medication, particularly their contribution to metabolic syndrome, obesity, cardiovascular disease and type 2 diabetes
- lack of capability among both generalist and specialist health care staff to deal with complex comorbidities — mental health staff may lack skills, training and confidence to treat physical conditions and vice versa for physical health teams.

Of particular note are the issues arising from weight gain, substance use and polypharmacy. These three issues are now considered, in turn.

Weight gain

Weight gain can lead to obesity in people with serious mental illness. In turn, obesity can give rise to various conditions, including diabetes, musculoskeletal disorders, cardiovascular disease and a poorer self-concept (Holt, 2019). People with serious mental illness are disproportionately affected by weight gain and obesity, with the overall prevalence some two to three times higher than that of the general population (Afzal et al., 2021).

There are various reasons why people with serious mental illness tend to gain weight. These include:

- side effects of psychotropic medication
- poor nutrition, including the individual's tendency to eat when stressed
- reduced physical activity
- higher sedentary behaviour
- disease-specific factors such as altered neuro-endocrine functioning (Afzal et al., 2021; Barnard-Kelly et al., 2022).

The complexity of these causes or contributing factors suggests that helping people with serious mental illness to manage their weight is not a straightforward process. Interventions must be multifaceted and include lifestyle changes, psychological and other therapy, medication and bariatric surgery. Health professionals must also monitor the person for conditions such as metabolic syndrome.

Metabolic syndrome

Metabolic syndrome is a collection of conditions that often occur together and increase the risk of heart disease, stroke and type 2 diabetes. According to Mazereel et al. (2020), metabolic abnormalities are most common in people taking antipsychotic medication. Antidepressants and mood stabilisers seem to have less impact, although the effects vary greatly with different medications and individual factors. The use of high dosages and/or multiple medications seems to be associated with more harmful metabolic consequences.

It is vital that health professionals screen for metabolic syndrome in people with serious mental illness so that integrated physical and mental health programs to address these risk factors through lifestyle and other changes are implemented as soon as possible.

Substance misuse

Substance use issues in people with serious mental illness include licit and illicit substances, including alcohol consumption and use of alcohol, cannabis, opioids and amphetamines. For example, lifetime alcohol use disorders may affect up to 20 per cent of people with schizophrenia, and between 24 and 35 per cent of people with bipolar disorders (Das-Munchi et al., 2020). As already noted, comorbid serious mental illness and substance use disorder markedly increase risk factors and incidence of cancer, cirrhosis and cardiovascular disease (AIHW, 2022d), with Indigenous Australians rating higher again (RANZCP, 2015).

Perhaps one of the most concerning substance used by people with serious mental illness are their use of tobacco, which is more prevalent in people with serious mental illness, who often start smoking earlier and more heavily than the general population (Das-Munchi et al., 2020). Smoking can reduce the effectiveness of some antipsychotic medications (WHO, 2018). Also, smoking is known to lead to increased rates of cardiovascular and lung disease, and cancer (O'Donoghue, 2021).

The use of tobacco is a modifiable behaviour. However, people with serious mental illness who smoke are less likely to receive advice on the harmful effects of smoking and the benefits of smoking cessation (WHO, 2018). Of concern is that smoking is often seen as more acceptable for people with a serious mental illness by those who regard it as 'their only pleasure' or as a coping mechanism. The stigma associated with mental illness may also lead health professionals to believe that people with a serious mental illness do not have the capacity to stop smoking or that the value of their lives is somehow less than that of other people. Such viewpoints suggest it is not as important to promote good strategies for maintaining good health.

In contrast, smoking cessation programs for people with serious mental illness have been conducted worldwide with positive outcomes, in both inpatient and community settings (Hawes et al., 2021; Lappin et al., 2020). Health professionals enable measurable improvements in the health outcomes of people with serious mental illness by actively supporting these programs.

Polypharmacy

Polypharmacy results from the prescribing of numerous medications for comorbid health conditions or multimorbidity (Carmona-Huerta et al., 2019). When a person consumes multiple medications, there is a high probability that these medications' **pharmacokinetic** and **pharmacodynamic** properties will affect one another.

For people with serious mental illness, polypharmacy issues can include two or more psychotropic medications, including antipsychotics, mood stabilisers, antidepressants, anxiolytics and medications used to treat physical health problems, with multiple interactions and side effects that can be counterproductive for the person and their health.

It is important to note that not all polypharmacy has negative consequences. For example, some people with serious mental illness can benefit from psychotropic polypharmacy (Lin, 2020). In many cases, however, there is a need for health professionals to flag possible polypharmacy issues with senior practitioners for further investigation, particularly if the person has been hospitalised for physical health conditions (Carmona-Huerta et al., 2019).

Also of concern is the use of over-the-counter medications and alternative or herbal medicines and their interactions with prescribed medications. Likewise, concurrent substance use can impact prescribed medications' pharmacokinetic and pharmacodynamic properties. Health professionals are advised to carefully consider all medications used by a person with a serious mental illness, and consider how the interactions may impact the person physically, mentally and socially.

THE BIG PICTURE

World Health Organization supporting improvements in the physical health of people with serious mental illness

The World Health Organization (WHO) published their guidelines for the Management of Physical Health Conditions in Adults With Severe Mental Disorders in 2018. These guidelines were published in response to the ever-rising global burden of disease due to increases in mental illness, particularly in low-to-middle income countries, and the concerning statistics around the morbidity and mortality rates of people with serious mental illness, worldwide.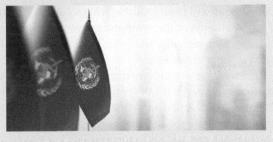

Of particular concern to WHO is the lack of equitable access to comprehensive health services for most people with serious mental illness, including promotion and prevention, screening, and treatment. This lack of equitable access explains why the aim of the guidelines for the Management of Physical Health Conditions in Adults With Severe Mental Disorders is:

To improve the management of physical health conditions in adults with serious mental illness and support the reduction of individual health behaviours constituting risk factors for these illnesses, to decrease morbidity and premature mortality amongst people with serious mental illness (WHO, 2018, p. 4).

▶

The recommendations of the Management of Physical Health Conditions in Adults With Severe Mental Disorders guidelines relate to:

- tobacco cessation
- weight management
- substance use disorders
- cardiovascular risk and disease
- diabetes mellitus
- HIV/AIDS
- other infectious diseases (e.g. tuberculosis, hepatitis B/C).

WHO acknowledges that some of the treatment recommendations for the general population require adaptation for people with serious mental illness. For example, the benefits and risks of pharmacological interventions need to be balanced against the potential side effects and drug interactions commonly used for serious mental illness. People with serious mental illness often experience impairment in functioning, making it difficult for them to take the initiative to access health care, keep appointments or take medications for physical health conditions as prescribed. For this reason, non-pharmacological interventions must be tailored according to the cognitive, motivational and sociocultural needs of people with serious mental illnesses.

The outcomes to be achieved by WHO include people with serious mental illness being offered at least the same level of treatment for physical health conditions and their risk factors as the general population.

Caring for the person with comorbid mental and physical health conditions

There will be occasions when a person with serious mental illness requires support from the emergency services for a physical health condition. Such crises could result from cardiovascular disease, diabetes, infections, substance use or other issues. Likewise, people with serious mental illness will present to various health services settings, including hospitals, community health centres and primary health services, for help with their physical health issues.

Caring for a person with a serious mental illness and physical health problem is no different to caring for any other person with a physical health problem, with a few additional considerations. These considerations include supporting someone who may be exhibiting symptoms of serious mental illness, managing psychotropic medication, reassessing their mental state, if required and the need for intersectoral collaboration and integrated care.

Supporting a person exhibiting signs of serious mental illness

People with serious mental illness do not exhibit signs of that illness all the time. Indeed, if the person's symptoms are well managed with non-pharmacological or pharmacological interventions, the health professional may not even be aware that the person has a serious mental illness.

On the other hand, if the person exhibits signs or symptoms of their serious mental illness, the health professional will need to know what to do to help the person. In particular, the **florid positive symptoms** of schizophrenia or the symptoms of mania will affect the person's thinking and behaviour, which, in turn, will affect the person's ability to cooperate with health professionals who are providing care and treatment for a physical condition.

Receiving health care and treatment for a physical condition is a stressful event for all people. The health service context can seem formal and daunting to anyone seeking help and leaves the person feeling disempowered. A person with a serious mental illness will feel doubly disempowered because of the stigma attached to their mental illness. They may also find it more difficult than others to tolerate and cope with sudden and unfamiliar events, giving rise to reactions that can increase their symptoms of mental illness.

It is important, then, for health professionals to work hard to engage to develop a rapport with the person with a serious mental illness. Such a connection can realise the following benefits.

- The health professional can gain an accurate picture of the person's health issues through the acquisition of comprehensive and accurate clinical information, leading to the effective application of appropriately matched treatment.
- The person is less likely to feel distressed, fearful, anxious and uncertain, and express this through behaviours that are difficult to manage in a health environment.

- The person is more likely to be satisfied with their care and accept the interventions that are being offered by health professionals.
- The person is more likely to adhere to the treatment that is being provided for their physical and mental health issues.

The principles for engaging a person with a serious mental illness were outlined earlier in this chapter.

In addition, when a person is experiencing the positive symptoms of schizophrenia or mania, it is best to provide them with a low-stimulus environment with little noise and low levels of activity and interruption. Health professionals are advised to speak slowly and calmly, and frequently check that what they say is clear. If a person shares the content of their delusional ideas with a health professional, it is best to neither agree with the content nor try to persuade the person that they are mistaken. Instead, health professionals can respond empathically by saying, for example, 'It must be hard for you when you believe these things and other people don't' or 'Although I do not share the same belief, I believe that these thoughts must be distressing for you'. If the person asks the health professional outright if they agree, the health professional may respond by saying, for example, 'I don't see it the same way you do, but I can see that this is very real for you'.

Health professionals will also find it helpful to establish boundaries or practise limit setting with the person experiencing hypomania or mania. Most often, people with these symptoms cannot set their own limits and, once they have commenced treatment, will usually appreciate being guided by a health professional. A person who has experienced symptoms of mania will sometimes look back at their behaviour when they were unwell and feel embarrassed or have great regrets. Such situations suggest the importance of health professionals talking to the person about limit setting and negotiating the rules and consequences together. An authoritarian approach must be avoided as it will increase the person's level of irritability and is not consistent with the consumer-centred, person-focused approaches outlined in the chapter on assessment in the mental health context.

Other suggestions for working with a person with a serious mental illness who is exhibiting acute or florid symptoms are outlined in table 9.5.

TABLE 9.5   **Tips for working with a person experiencing acute symptoms**

Intervention	Rationale
Maintain your own safety and the safety of the person who is acutely unwell.	A person who is acutely unwell may behave in ways that are out of character for them — particularly if they are experiencing psychotic phenomena or are suicidal.
Ensure evaluation of mental state as part of health professional's assessment.	Provides a baseline against which to assess improvement or deterioration.
Use non-judgemental and non-critical responses; offer reassurance and demonstrate acceptance.	Reduces the stress associated with alterations in thinking and perception.
Maintain regular social contact — do not avoid the person or isolate them.	Isolating and avoiding the person is likely to increase feelings of anxiety and suspicion.
Use clear straightforward language (e.g. avoid jargon, approach unhurriedly, maintain eye contact and open posture). Avoid overt criticism and negative comments; be accepting of bizarre conversations.	Ensures that communication is clear and unambiguous. Reduces the likelihood of the person displaying apparently uncooperative or 'difficult' behaviours.
Reassure the person that they are safe and of your non-harmful intent.	This can act to reduce suspicious thoughts and anxious feelings.
Maintain accurate records of the person's verbal and non-verbal behaviour (e.g. angry, hallucinating, impulsive, irritable, withdrawn, dietary and fluid intake).	Enables any improvements or deterioration in symptomology to be monitored and evaluated. Ensures that physical health needs are met.
If the person is disturbed or agitated, refrain from unnecessary actions or procedures.	These may increase feelings of anxiety and suspicious thoughts.
If possible and practicable, involve the person's partner/carer/significant other in the assessment and delivery of care.	This can provide reassurance and consistency in care delivery and helps maintain a vital link to the person's usual routine.

Negative symptoms of schizophrenia and depression can also have a profound but less dramatic impact how health care is provided to people with a physical illness. When working with a person experience the negative symptoms of schizophrenia, health professionals must find a balance between maintaining a positive therapeutic approach and accepting that less than optimal adherence to treatment may be the norm. People with negative symptoms may not always keep appointments or retain a full understanding of their health needs despite being provided with relevant information.

Specific negative symptoms require targeted interpersonal responses; for example, problems with concentration can be addressed by checking the person's understanding. Other helpful strategies for working with people who have negative symptoms of schizophrenia and depression include:
- offering reminders, or setting up a system of reminders or schedules
- involving carers and family members when providing health advice and education, wherever possible
- making appointments later in the day to allow for the sedating side effects of the previous evening's antipsychotic medication to wear off
- providing written information to reinforce verbal advice.

Health professionals must show patience and a willingness to work with the person, regardless of the difficulties.

'Who has the time?'

Health professionals are often poorly resourced and pushed for time. This situation makes it difficult to engage with a person who is experiencing symptoms of serious mental illness. Engaging with the person will take more time than the health professional ordinarily spends with a consumer. Even so, the time spent initially with a person with schizophrenia will improve health outcomes for the individual in the long run.

A lack of engagement with the person with a serious mental illness early in the treatment process will reduce clinical understanding and treatment adherence and may lead to poorer health outcomes. It is necessary to ensure that the person is given adequate time to express their needs, even though this can be challenging in a busy clinical environment. If adequate attention is not given to these issues, it is likely that the person will not fully understand the care and treatment being offered. Complications and further difficulties may then ensue, which will prove even more costly in terms of time.

Supporting a person taking psychotropic medication

If a person with a serious mental illness attends a hospital or health service to be treated for a physical health condition, the person must continue to take the prescribed psychotropic medication. While this suggestion may seem obvious, complexities can arise if the person is prescribed a long-acting anti-psychotic medication by intramuscular injection. There is a need to ascertain the frequency and details of when the medication is next due. If clarification is required, gain the person's consent, then contact the person's carer or case manager in the community mental health team, GP or a practice nurse or community support workers.

It is also essential to observe for interactions between the psychotropic medications and all other medicines prescribed for the physical health condition. It is the role of all health professionals to ask questions about side effects and adverse reactions, especially if the person's symptoms of mental illness are affecting their cognitive function.

Re-assessment of mental illness

If the person with a serious mental illness also has a physical illness and is receiving treatment for that physical illness, there may be times when an additional mental health assessment is necessary. Such situations are likely to arise if the physical symptoms or treatments exacerbate the psychotic symptoms.

As explained in the chapter that looks at mental health services delivery, some health services can access mental health consultation liaison services to assist with this assessment; other health services will not have that option. For example, many rural and remote areas do not have any kind of specialist mental health services. Alternatively, in an emergency, practitioners may be required to assess the person to help the team manage the situation. In such cases, a mental health assessment, including a mental state examination and a risk assessment, must be conducted to determine the person's immediate risk and needs.

Details of how to undertake a mental health assessment are provided in the chapter on mental health assessment in the mental health context.

An essential part of this process would be ensuring that the care and treatment provided for the physical health problem is compatible with the treatment already received for the serious mental illness. In particular, it is important to consider interactions between medications.

Intersectoral collaboration

Intersectoral collaboration refers to the collective actions involving more than one service, organisation or agency, performing different roles for a common purpose (Diminic et al., 2015). For people with serious mental illness, such collaboration will include generic public health services (including acute and community services), primary health services, and community services organisations (including profit and not-for-profit services) that the NDIS often fund. Some health professionals refer to this kind of teamwork as multidisciplinary collaboration; however, there is a tendency for this term to include health professionals only. Intersectoral collaboration is more relevant for people with serious mental illness as they are often supported by various community services for accommodation, daily care, employment, healthy living and so on. Such collaboration is crucial to ensure optimal aftercare and follow-up arrangements before discharge to enable the best possible outcomes for the person (Isaacs, 2022). The collaboration must also involve working closely with carers. The role of carers in supporting people with serious mental illness is explained in the next section.

UPON REFLECTION

Recovery 'coaches' through the NDIS

People with serious mental illness can access support through the NDIS. The allocation of funds operates on a deficit model because it depends on the level of psychosocial disability and its impact on the person. Nevertheless, the NDIS (2022) describes the model used as 'Recovery-oriented'. Funds enable the person with a serious mental illness to buy in services such as a 'Recovery coach' to support people with serious mental illness to live full and contributing lives.

QUESTIONS

1. What is the logical outcome of funding people according to their level of disability?
2. How can the tension be resolved between the deficit model of funding and Recovery-oriented services that guides the operations of the NDIS?
3. How can health professionals work with 'Recovery coaches' of people with mental illness who also have a physical health condition?

9.5 Carers

LEARNING OBJECTIVE 9.5 Clarify the role of carers in supporting people with a serious mental illness.

People with mental illness supported by family or carers achieve better outcomes than those with no or limited family or carer support (Javed & Herrman, 2017). A carer is a person who, through a family relationship or other relationship, provides unpaid support to a person who has a disability, mental illness, chronic condition, terminal illness, an alcohol or other drug issue, or who is frail aged (Carers Australia, 2022). Carers are sometimes known as 'informal' carers to differentiate them from paid carers.

A primary carer is someone who provides the most informal support to a family member or friend undertaking tasks such as:

- planning collaboratively with the care recipient to identify their goals, skills and strengths
- providing emotional and crisis support
- assisting with personal care, cooking and shopping
- providing transport
- preparing notes, reports and other required documentation for appointments
- attending appointments
- coordinating, communicating and collaborating with multiple service providers (Diminic et al., 2017, p. 4).

In addition to taking care of the everyday needs of the person in need of care, carers also act as advocates, ensuring their family member is receiving the best possible and most appropriate care.

Carers make up nearly 11 per cent of Australia's population. Nearly 900 000 are primary carers, with one-third of these providing 40 hours or more of unpaid care per week (Carers Australia, 2022). The average age of the primary carer is 54 years, with one in 11 carers under 25. Seven out of 10 carers are women (Carers Australia, 2022).

The Australian government recognises the role of carers by providing a range of supports, services and financial assistance (Department of Social Services, 2021).

However, despite this recognition, there is sometimes a difference between policy and practice, leaving many carers feeling that their work goes unrecognised by health professionals.

There are various reasons for this lack of recognition. One reason is the privacy laws that guide how health professionals communicate with carers, with many practitioners uncertain of what they can and can't say to a carer with or without the person's consent. The pressure of workloads and institutional cultures can mean that carers and their needs are sometimes sidelined. There has also been a lack of clarity about the carer's role for professionals and carers alike. The following section outlines some of the responsibilities of carers and the burden this places on them.

Carer burden

Caregiver burden is the level of multifaceted strain the caregiver perceives from caring for a family member and/or loved one over time (Liu et al., 2020). Many carers express feelings of stress, frustration, anger and resentment, fatigue and being overwhelmed (Bademli et al., 2017). Carers are more likely to be affected by carer burden if they have insufficient financial resources, multiple responsibilities, and limited options for socialising or participating in social activities (Mulud & McCarthy, 2017). The consequences of carer burden are subjective and objective and include a decreased capacity to provide care, lower quality of life, and physical and mental health deterioration (Liu et al., 2020).

Understanding the challenges carers face can be enhanced by comparing the roles of health professionals.

Table 9.6 outlines the similarities and differences between these roles. One of the most important differences is the preparation or training each receives to undertake their role.

TABLE 9.6 **Comparison of role of carers and health professionals**

Activities	Carers	Health professionals
Choice	Carers have little choice in taking on the role Cannot exit role when they need a break	Health professionals choose to enter and leave the health workforce at any time
Preparation for role	Occurs after carers have taken on the role	Occurs before
Training	Limited and self-directed	Extensive formal education before starting Course of study determined by professional bodies Ongoing education once in the role
Supervision	None	Part of ongoing quality assurance
Relationship with person with mental health issues	Personal relationship, with less emotional distance separating them Different basis for negotiating May be pre-existing Long term	Professional–client relationship Starts after the person becomes ill May be transitory
Hours and breaks	Can be 24 hours a day, seven days a week with no breaks	Determined by work hours
Formal status in health care team	No formal status	Formal status defined by the profession Workplace codes and policies
Number of 'consumers'	One	Many

To help support carers and reduce the burden they can experience, health professionals must understand that carers have varying levels of resilience to undertake their role, and knowledge and skills to provide the support needed. Generally, carers have not been prepared or educated for their role of carer, unlike health professionals who spend many years receiving an education and supervision in practice. For this reason, carers may not recognise if or when a situation is deteriorating. Likewise, they may be unable to communicate what is happening with the consumer to the health professional.

Carers need training and support to undertake what is often expected of them. Health professionals are key stakeholders in helping carers to identify their needs. Health professionals are also in a key position to identify where the carer may find relevant training and support appropriate to their needs.

Another critical difference between carers and health professionals is that carers can be 'on duty' 24 hours a day, seven days a week. The carer does not receive a break, unlike health professionals, who go home after eight hours at work, have weekends or a few days off, and annual leave. There is a need, then, for health professionals to talk to carers about fatigue and how they are managing their personal needs. This conversation must include identifying options for regular respite.

Providing information

Alongside training and support, carers also need information to do their job (Bademli et al., 2017). Such information may relate to the illness and symptoms their loved one is experiencing, the different treatment options available, what to do in a crisis and the services available to support them.

Caregivers' knowledge and skills change over time (Lui et al., 2020). For example, at the beginning of their caring journey, carers do not necessarily know what is important or unimportant. Questions a carer may have or the information they need at the start of their care journey differ as time passes. Therefore, when meeting a carer, it is necessary to assess what they know, what they don't know — and what they don't know they don't know. For example, some carers report that they do not know what they do not know and so cannot ask the right questions. Health professionals can support carers in understanding what they can expect in the future and may need to know.

Carers often take on the caring role or contact health professionals in times of high stress. Such situations impede the carer's ability to absorb the information the health professional provides them or to develop skills the health professionals may be trying to teach them. Carers nevertheless need the same information that health professionals need to provide safe and effective care to a person with a serious mental illness. This information could include clinical knowledge regarding assessment, risk, and Recovery planning. It could also include practical information about employment, tasks at home, socialising and so on. Health professionals must ask whether carers access support and information when needed. Organisations such as Mental Health Carers Australia can offer support and information to people who care for a person with a serious mental illness.

IN PRACTICE

Mental Health Carers Australia

Mental Health Carers Australia is the only national advocacy group concerned with the wellbeing and promotion of the needs of families and carers supporting someone with mental illness (Mental Health Carers Australia, 2019). Mental Health Carers Australia was instituted as a national voice for families and carers, influencing systemic change in government policy and service provider practice to improve the family and carer experience of the mental health system.

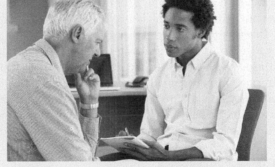

While people who support or care for a person with serious mental illness share common issues and experiences with carers of people with other conditions, they can also experience unique factors. For example, challenges faced by all carers include the:

- nature of the caring role, including the high levels of stress that can impact adversely on the carer's physical, psychological, emotional, social, financial, vocational and other aspects of their life
- lack of recognition from health professionals of the important role they play in caring for consumers
- lack of information received from health professionals and other services providers.

Carers of people with serious mental illness must also negotiate the complex and confusing systems and structural barriers comprising public mental health services. These barriers include the structural barriers that can impede carers' inclusion in decision making about the treatment provided to their family members, and the issues related to building and maintaining active partnerships with health professionals and other services providers in settings often characterised by an ongoing turnover of staff.

Mental Health Carers Australia are there to help carers of people with serious mental illness to overcome some of these barriers. Find out more about Mental Health Carers Australia at www.mentalhealthcarersaustralia.org.au.

▶

Information sharing

Carers need information to help them provide safe and effective care for a person with a serious mental illness. While carers may not have a 'health professional' status and are not paid for their role, they have many responsibilities. Carers are also a valuable resource for health professionals when undertaking an assessment or supporting a person in the long term. Indeed, carers spend more time with the person with a mental illness than the health professional, so they are often more able to report how the consumer is feeling or behaving. A carer may share information with the health professional without breaching laws or codes of conduct. Significantly, the carer often has more time or opportunity than the health professional to influence the consumer and the Recovery process. Effective health professionals will work closely with carers to facilitate positive outcomes.

Many health professionals are concerned about how much information they can give a carer and whether they are breaching confidentiality. Health professionals often make presumptions and refuse to pass on any information whatsoever to the carer. Often this presumption is nothing more than exactly that; the health professional makes the decision without checking. It is always worth discovering whether the person with a serious mental illness is happy for their information to be shared with the carer. Obtaining consent includes discussing the advantages and disadvantages of limiting the flow of information. Such a discussion can save much time and distress for all concerned.

Mental health legislation across Australia is continually being reviewed in relation to the role of the carer and their rights. Carers now have more rights to receive information about the person's condition and make treatment decisions. It is important to note that there is no law preventing a carer from speaking to a health professional about their family member, nor is there a law preventing a health professional from speaking to the carer. General information can be shared between the carer and health professional. However, if a person with a serious mental illness has identified their personal information as confidential, then this information cannot be disclosed during these conversations.

One way to address the issues of providing information to carers is for the health professional to arrange for a group or family meeting where the multidisciplinary team, consumer and carer meet to talk about all aspects of care with the consumer present. This approach enables a clear and transparent flow of information between all stakeholders at a time when they are all present and can discuss the issues. A carer may be unaware of the range of information available to them. They may also be unaware that they have gaps in their knowledge. The health professional has a role to play in identifying these issues and providing assistance, rather than waiting to be asked.

SUMMARY

This chapter provided an overview of the care and support given to people with serious mental illness on their journey of Recovery. The term 'serious mental illness' was defined as a mental illness significantly affecting a person's lifestyle, relationships and social functioning. The examples of schizophrenia, bipolar affective disorder, major depression and schizoaffective disorder were discussed, including the experiences of these mental illnesses and the interventions that can be provided to support people with these serious mental illnesses. Detailed information about the psychosocial and pharmacological interventions utilised to support people with serious mental illness, including pharmacological interventions' side effects, were also examined.

The chapter went on to investigate the connections between the physical and mental health of people with serious mental illness, who have a mortality rate much higher than the general population. Around 60 per cent of people have comorbid mental illness and physical health conditions. Reasons for this were discussed, together with how health professionals can better support the physical health of people with serious mental illness.

The chapter concluded by explaining the critical role of family or informal carers in supporting people with serious mental illness. The need for health professionals to work with family or carers was highlighted, including exchanging information about the serious mental illness. The experience of carer burden was also discussed, with health professionals encouraged to provide carers with the support they need to enable the person with serious mental illness to achieve Recovery.

KEY TERMS

agranulocytosis Medically serious condition relating to low levels of white blood cells.

anticholinergic An action that inhibits the effects of the neurohormone acetylcholine or inhibits its cholinergic neuroeffects.

ataxia Difficulty with coordination, leading to people becoming unsteady on their feet.

atypical antipsychotic medications The newer generation of antipsychotic medications that treat psychosis.

cardiomyopathy Deterioration of the myocardium or heart muscle.

cog wheeling Muscular tension in limbs that gives way in small jerks when the limb is extended or flexed.

delusion A fixed and false belief that the person cannot be dissuaded from despite contradictory evidence.

depot Medication that is given by intramuscular injection and absorbed over a period of weeks (please note zuclopenthixol acetate is a shorter acting depot with its effect peaking at 48–72 hours).

dystonia Symptoms that include prolonged and unintentional muscular contractions of the voluntary or involuntary muscles.

extrapyramidal side effects (EPSEs) Physical symptoms sometimes associated with antipsychotic medications, including tremor, dystonia, slurred speech and akathisia.

florid positive symptoms Positive symptoms of schizophrenia that are pronounced or in their fully developed form.

grandiosity Overvalued sense of self — often related to elevated mood state in bipolar disorder.

hallucination False sensory perceptions or perceptual phenomena arising without any external stimulus.

hypomania A period of elevated mood which has less impact on functioning than mania.

intersectoral collaboration Collective actions involving more than one service, organisation or agency, performing different roles for a common purpose.

mania An episode of highly elevated mood which interferes significantly in day-to-day life.

metabolic syndrome Related to a set of risk factors associated with heart disease and diabetes; symptoms include central obesity, insulin resistance, high blood pressure and high lipids.

multimorbidity The presence of two or more chronic conditions in a person at the same time. Multimorbidity is a slightly different from 'comorbidity', which refers to additional conditions (comorbidities) experienced by a person who has a specific condition of interest.

negative symptoms Psychotic symptoms that seem to be a deficit of ordinary thinking processes — where there is an absence or lack in the person's experience.

neutropenia Low levels of neutrophils — a subtype of white blood cells.

off-label Refers to when a drug is prescribed for an indication, a route of administration, or a patient group that is not included in the approved product information document for that drug. Prescribing off label is often unavoidable and very common.

pharmacodynamic The physiological action of a drug on the body.

pharmacokinetic The absorption, metabolism, distribution and elimination of a drug.

polypharmacy The concurrent use of multiple medications by a person; these medications often interact in a way that is problematic for the person.

positive symptoms Psychotic symptoms that seem to be excesses or distortions of ordinary thinking processes — where phenomena are added to the person's experience.

prodrome A symptom, or group of symptoms, that appears shortly before the development of an illness; most often indicates the period before the appearance of the first symptoms of schizophrenia.

psychosis A state of being in which a person loses touch with reality and experiences hallucinations, delusions or disorganised thinking.

psychotropic medication Any type of medication capable of affecting the mind, emotions and behaviour.

psychotic episode A temporary event in which a person experiences symptoms of psychosis.

self-stigma When people with mental health issues view themselves in a negative light, giving rise to low self-worth, feelings of shame and a negative self-image.

serotonin transmission Serotonin is a neurotransmitter associated with mood, sleep cycle, learning, memory, appetite and muscle contraction; antidepressant medications are the best-known medications that modulate serotonin transmission at the synapse.

social determinants of health The social factors that determine the health status of all people, including (but not limited to) early childhood development, disability, education, employment, gender, health services, housing, income, nutrition, social exclusion, social safety networks and race.

social functioning The ability of a person to interact in a group or as part of society.

tardive dyskinesia (TD) Symptoms that include repetitive, involuntary, purposeless movements, such as grimacing, tongue protrusion, lip smacking, puckering and pursing of the lips, and rapid eye blinking.

REVIEW QUESTIONS

1 What is the difference between a mental illness and a serious mental illness?
2 How has mental health Recovery been described for individuals with a severe mental illness?
3 What are the four mental health conditions most commonly regarded as 'serious' in Australia?
4 Describe the positive and negative symptoms of schizophrenia.
5 What are five types of hallucinations a person might experience?
6 Describe the essential features of a delusion.
7 What is the difference between mania and hypomania?
8 Explain the need for psychosocial support for those experiencing serious mental illness.
9 What is the role and value of a peer worker?
10 What are some common side effects of antipsychotic medications?
11 List the factors that contribute to poor physical health in an individual with severe mental illness.
12 Describe why it is essential, when possible, to involve carers in the treatment of a person with a serious mental illness. What benefits may the individual gain from such an approach?

DISCUSSION AND DEBATE

1 Would you consider it relevant to have a knowledge of serious mental illness if you worked in an environment other than a mental health service? Give your reasons and rationale.
2 What are your fears about supporting a person with serious mental illness? How can these fears be overcome?
3 How does stigma influence Recovery for a person with a serious mental illness and what does it mean for a person who is seeking to achieve Recovery?
4 Discuss the steps needed to engage with a person with a serious mental illness, and how these steps may differ to those taken when working with the general population.
5 How would you manage a conversation with a person with a serious mental illness who tells you that they have the power to get inside your head and make you do whatever they want?

6 Why is it important for a person with a serious mental illness to have stable housing and social support?

7 Pharmacological interventions are an important component of the treatment interventions used to support people with serious mental illness. Who should have knowledge of these pharmacological treatments, and what sort of information should they be given?

8 Discuss why people with mental illness who have the support of family or informal carers achieve better outcomes than those who don't.

PROJECT ACTIVITY

Metabolic syndrome is a collection of conditions that often occur together and increase the person's risk of diabetes, stroke and heart disease. The main components of metabolic syndrome are obesity, high blood pressure, high blood triglycerides, low levels of HDL cholesterol and insulin resistance. Metabolic abnormalities are most common in people who are taking antipsychotic medication.

All health professionals must be aware of the risks related to metabolic syndrome, particularly for people with serious mental illness.

1 What policies and/or procedures does the workplace have in relation to the monitoring of symptoms of metabolic syndrome?

2 What is your role in preventing, monitoring and reducing contributing risks of metabolic syndrome?

3 What additional education or training do you require to effectively support people with serious mental illness who may be at risk of metabolic syndrome? What steps could you take to obtain this education or training?

WEBSITES

1 Clubhouse International is a non-profit organization that helps start and grow Clubhouses globally, including in Australia, where people with serious mental illness can go to get their lives back. Clubhouse International aims to create community and drive growth in mental illness recovery: https://clubhouse-intl.org.

2 SMI Adviser is a clinical support system for mental illness. It aims to transform care for people who have serious mental illness so they can live their best lives. SMI Adviser is supported by the American Psychiatric Associate and the Substance Abuse and Mental Health Services Administration (SAMHSA): www.smiadviser.org.

3 The Black Dog Institute is an Australian not-for-profit educational, research, clinical and community-oriented facility offering specialist expertise in depression and bipolar disorder: www.blackdoginstitute.org.au.

4 The Mental Health Carers Australia (MHCA) is the only national advocacy group solely concerned with the well-being and promotion of the needs of families and carers supporting someone with mental illness. The mission of this community organisation is to be the national voice for families and carers to enable the best possible life: www.mentalhealthcarersaustralia.org.au.

5 The Mental Illness Fellowship of Australia Inc is a non-government, not-for-profit, grassroots, self-help, support and advocacy organisation dedicated to helping people with serious mental illness, their families and friends: www.mifa.org.au.

6 SANE Australia is a national charity working for a better life for people affected by mental illness through campaigning, education and research: www.sane.org.

REFERENCES

Afzal, M., Siddiqi, N., Ahmad, B., Afsheen, N., Aslam, F., Ali, A., Ayesha, R., Bryant, M., Holt, R., Khalid, H., Ishaq, K., Koly, K. N., Rajan, S., Saba, J., Tirbhowan, N., & Zavala1, G. A. (2021). Prevalence of overweight and obesity in people with severe mental illness: Systematic review and meta-analysis. *Frontiers in Endocrinology*, *12*, 769309. https://doi.org/10.3389/fendo.2021.769309

American Psychiatric Association. (2013). *Diagnostic and statistical manual of mental disorders: DSM-5*.

Australian Federal Police. (n.d.). *ACT Policing: PACFA and the mental health, emergency, ambulance and police collaboration*. www.police.act.gov.au/about-us/programs-and-partners/pacer-and-mental-health-emergency-ambulance-and-police-collaboration

Australian Housing and Urban Research Institute. (2021). *Mental health and housing*. www.ahuri.edu.au/analysis/policy-analysis/mental-health-and-housing

Australian Institute of Health and Welfare. (2022a). *Determinants of health for Indigenous Australians*. Australian Government. www.aihw.gov.au/reports/australias-health/social-determinants-and-indigenous-health

Australian Institute of Health and Welfare. (2022b). *Indigenous health and wellbeing*. Australian Government. www.aihw.gov.au/reports/australias-health/indigenous-health-and-wellbeing

Australian Institute of Health and Welfare. (2022c). *Mental health services in Australia*. Australian Government. www.aihw.gov.au/reports/mental-health-services/mental-health-services-in-australia/report-contents/prevalance-impact-and-burden

Australian Institute of Health and Welfare. (2022d). *Physical health of people with mental illness*. www.aihw.gov.au/reports/mental-health-services/physical-health-of-people-with-mental-illness

Bademli, K., Lök, N., & Kılıc, A. (2017). Relationship between caregiving burden and anger level in primary caregivers of individuals with chronic mental illness. *Archives of Psychiatric Nursing, 31*(3), 263–268. https://doi.org/10.1016/j.apnu.2016.12.001

Barbui, C., Purgato, M., Abdulmalik, J., Acarturk, C., Eaton, J., Gastaldon, C., Gureje, O., Hanlon, C., Jordans, M., Lund, C., Nosè, M., Ostuzzi, G., Papola, D., Tedeschi, F., Tol, W., Turrini, G., Patel, V., & Thornicroft, G. (2020). Efficacy of psychosocial interventions for mental health outcomes in low-income and middle-income countries: An umbrella review. *Lancet Psychiatry, 7*(2), 162–172. https://doi.org/10.1016/S2215-0366(19)30511-5

Barnard-Kelly, K., Whicher, C., Price, H., Phiri, P., Rathod, S., Asher, C., Peveler, R. C., & Holt, R. I. G. (2022). Liraglutide and the management of overweight and obesity in people with severe mental illness: Qualitative sub-study. *BMC Psychiatry, 22*(1), 21. https://doi.org/10.1186/s12888-021-03666-5

Bernecker, S., Williams, J., Caporale-Berkowitz, N., Wasil, A., & Constantino, M. (2020). Nonprofessional peer support to improve mental health: Randomized trial of a scalable web-based peer counseling course. *Journal of Medical Internet Research, 22*(9), e17164. https://doi.org/10.2196/17164

Bipolar Australia. (2022). *What is bipolar? Bipolar Australia: Recovering together*. www.bipolaraustralia.org.au/bipolar-information

Black Dog Institute. (2022b). *Bipolar disorder causes*. www.blackdoginstitute.org.au/resources-support/bipolar-disorder/causes

Black Dog Institute. (2022a). *Digital tools & apps*. www.blackdoginstitute.org.au/resources-support/digital-tools-apps

Carers Australia. (2022). *Who is a carer?* www.carersaustralia.com.au/about-carers/who-is-a-carer.

Carmona-Huerta, J., Castiello-de Obeso, S., Ramírez-Palomino, J., Duran-Gutiérrez, R., Cardona-Muller, D., Grover-Paez, F., Fernández-Dorantes, P., & Medina-Dávalos, R. (2019). Polypharmacy in a hospitalized psychiatric population: Risk estimation and damage quantification. *BMC Psychiatry, 19*, 78. https://doi.org/10.1186/s12888-019-2056-0

Cerveri, G., Gesi, C., & Mencacci, C. (2019). Pharmacological treatment of negative symptoms in schizophrenia: Update and proposal of a clinical algorithm. *Neuropsychiatrist Disease and Treatment, 15*, 1525–1535. https://doi.org/10.2147/NDT.S201726

Clubhouse International. (2018). *International standards for clubhouse programs*. www.clubhouse-intl.org/resources/quality-standards

Correll, C., Agid, O., Crespo-Facorro, B., de Bartolomeis, A., Fagiolini, A., Seppälä, N., & Howes, O. (2022). A guideline and checklist for initiating and managing clozapine treatment in patients with treatment-resistant schizophrenia. *CNS Drugs, 36*(7), 659–679. https://doi.org/10.1007/s40263-022-00946-w

Crespo-Facorro, B., Such, P., Nylander, A., Madera, J., Resemann, H., Worthington, E., O'Connor, M., Drane, E., & Steeves, S. (2021). The burden of disease in early schizophrenia – A systematic literature review. *Current Medical Research and Opinion, 37*(1), 109–121. https://doi.org/10.1080/03007995.2020.1841618

Cusick, A. (2017). History of Australian occupational therapy. In T. Broan, H. Bourke-Taylor, S. Isbel, & R. Cordier (Eds.), *Occupational therapy in Australia: Professional and practice issues* (pp. 27–48). Routledge.

Das-Munshi, J., Semrau, M., Barbui, C., Chowdhary, N., Gronholm, P., Kolappa, K., Krupchanka, D., Dua, T., & Thornicroft, G. (2020). Gaps and challenges: WHO treatment recommendations for tobacco cessation and management of substance use disorders in people with severe mental illness. *BMC Psychiatry, 20*(1), 237. https://doi.org/10.1186/s12888-020-02623-y

Delibas, D., & Erdogan, E. (2022). Effects of a psychoeducation program on disease burden, depression, and anxiety levels in relatives of psychotic patients in a community mental health center. *Perspectives in Psychiatric Care, 58*(3), 940–945. https://doi.org/10.1111/ppc.12880

Department of Health & Aged Care. (2022). *Commonwealth psychosocial support programs for people with severe mental illness, Canberra, Australian Government*. www.health.gov.au/initiatives-and-programs/commonwealth-psychosocial-support-programs-for-people-with-severe-mental-illness

Department of Social Services. (2021). *Supporting Carers*. Australian Government. www.dss.gov.au/disability-and-carers/carers

De Ruysscher, C., Tomlinson, P., Vanheule, S., & Vandevelde, S. (2019). Questioning the professionalization of recovery: A collaborative exploration of a recovery process. *Disability & Society, 34*(5), 797–818.

Diminic, S., Carstensen, G., Harris, M., Reavley, N., Pirkis, J., Meurk, C., Wong, I., Bassilios, B., & Whiteford, H. A. (2015). Intersectoral policy for severe and persistent mental illness: Review of approaches in a sample of high-income countries. *Global Mental Health, 2*, e18. https://doi.org/10.1017/gmh.2015.16

Diminic, S., Hielscher, E., Yi Lee, Y., Harris, M., Schess, J., Kealton, J., & Whiteford, H. (2017). The economic value of informal mental health caring in Australia. *Mind Australia*. www.mindaustralia.org.au/sites/default/files/Mind_value_of_informal_caring_full_report.pdf

Dixon, L., Holoshitz, Y., & Nossel, I. (2016). Treatment engagement of individuals experiencing mental illness: Review and update. *World Psychiatry, 15*(1), 13–20. http://dx.doi.org/10.1002/wps.20306

D'Souza, R., & Hooten, W. (2022). Extrapyramidal Symptoms. *StatPearls*. www.ncbi.nlm.nih.gov/books/NBK534115

Elsegood, K ., Anderson, L., & Newton, R. (2018). Introducing the recovery inspiration group: Promoting hope for recovery with inspirational recovery stories. *Advances in Dual Diagnosis, 11*(4), 137–146.

Fekete, O., Langeland, E., Larsen, T., Davidson, L., & Kinn, L. (2021). Recovery at the Clubhouse: Challenge, responsibility and growing into a role. *International Journal of Qualitative Studies in Health and Wellbeing*, *16*(1), 1938957. https://doi.org/10.1080/17482631.2021.1938957

Galletly, C., Castle, D., Dark, F., Humberstone, V., Jablensky, A., Killackey, E., Kulkarni, J., McGorry, P., Nielssen, O., & Tran, N. (2016). *Schizophrenia and Related Disorders: Clinical practice guidelines an associated resources*. Royal Australian and New Zealand College of Psychiatrists (RANZCP) www.ranzcp.org/practice-education/guidelines-and-resources-for-practice/schizophrenia-cpg-and-associated-resources

Garvan Institute of Medical Research. (2021). *Schizophrenia. St Vincent's Health Australia and UNSW*. www.garvan.org.au/research/diseases/schizophrenia

Gaysina, D., & Thompson, E. (2017). Are your parents to blame for your psychological problems? *The Conversation*. www.theconversation.com/are-your-parents-to-blame-for-your-psychological-problems-81203

Grunder, G., & Cumming, P. (2016). The dopamine hypothesis of schizophrenia. In T. Abel & T. Nickl-Jockschat (Eds.), *The neurobiology of schizophrenia* (pp. 109–124). Elsevier. https://doi.org/10.1016/C2014-0-00423-6

Hawes, M., Roth, K., & Cabassa, L. (2021). Systematic review of psychosocial smoking cessation interventions for people with serious mental illness. *Journal of Dual Diagnosis*, *17*(3), 216–235. https://doi.org/10.1080/15504263.2021.1944712

Hedya, S., Avula, A., & Swoboda, H. (2022). Lithium toxicity. *StatPearls*. www.ncbi.nlm.nih.gov/books/NBK499992

Henriksen, M., Nordgaard, J., & Jansson, L. (2017). Genetics of schizophrenia: Overview of methods, findings and limitations. *Frontiers in Human Neuroscience*, *11*, 322. https://doi.org/10.3389/fnhum.2017.00322

Hilmer, S., Raymond, J., Gnjidic, D., Reeve, E., Kalisch, L., & Wu, H. (2020). *Use of antipsychotic medicines a literature review*. Australian Commission on Safety and Quality in Health Care. www.safetyandquality.gov.au/sites/default/files/2020-08/use_of_antipsychotic_medicines_-_a_literature_review_2020.pdf

Hoffman, L., Wisniewski, H., Hays, R., Henson, P., Vaidym, A., Hendel, V., Keshavan, M., & Torous, J. (2020). Digital Opportunities for Outcomes in Recovery Services (DOORS): A pragmatic hands-on group approach toward increasing digital health and smartphone competencies, autonomy, relatedness, and alliance for those with serious mental illness. *Journal of Psychiatric Practice*, *26*(2), 80–88. https://doi.org/10.1097/PRA.0000000000000450

Holt, R. (2019). The management of obesity in people with severe mental illness: An unresolved conundrum. *Psychotherapy and Psychosomatics*, *88*, 327–332. https://doi.org/10.1159/000503835

Irvine, A., Rawlinson, C., Bor, W., & Hoehn, E. (2021). Evaluation of a collaborative group intervention for mothers with moderate to severe perinatal mental illness and their infants in Australia. *Infant Mental Health Journal*, *42*(4), 560–572. https://doi.org/10.1002/imhj.21922

Isaacs, A. (2022). Care coordination as a collaborative element of recovery oriented services for persons with severe mental illness. *Australasian Psychiatry*, *30*(1), 110–112. https://doi.org/10.1177/10398562211037331

Javed, A., & Herrman, H. (2017). Involving patients, carers and families: An international perspective on emerging priorities. *BJPsych International*, *14*(1), 1–4. https://doi.org/10.1192/s2056474000001550

Jergens, J. (2022). *Understanding bipolar disorder. Addiction Center, Recovery Worldwide*. www.addictioncenter.com/addiction/bipolar-disorder

Johnston, J. (2013). The ghost of the schizophrenogenic mother. *Virtual Mentor*, *15*(9), 801–805. https://doi.org/10.1001/virtualmentor.2013.15.9.oped1-1309

Jørgensen, K., & Rendtorff, J. (2018). Patient participation in mental health care — Perspectives of healthcare professionals: An integrative review. *Scandinavian Journal of Caring Sciences*, *32*(2), 490–501.

Koonce Morse, W. L., Mankowski, S., & Harrold, S. A. (2022). Utilization of an innovative psychoeducational group for veterans with severe mental illness: A program evaluation of a quality improvement initiative. *Journal of the American Psychiatric Nurses Association*, *28*(3), 249–257. https://doi.org/10.1177/1078390320970637

Lappin, J., Thomas, D., Curtis, J., Blowfield, S., Gatsi, M., Marr, G., & Courtney, R. (2020). Targeted intervention to reduce smoking among people with severe mental illness: Implementation of a smoking cessation intervention in an inpatient mental health setting. *Medicina*, *56*(4), 204. https://doi.org/10.3390/medicina56040204

Launders, N., Hayes, J., Price, G., & Osborn, D. (2022). Clustering of physical health multimorbidity in people with severe mental illness: An accumulated prevalence analysis of United Kingdom primary care data. *PLoS Medicine*, *19*(4), 1–23. https://doi.org/10.1371/journal.pmed.1003976

Lin, S. (2020). Antipsychotic polypharmacy: A dirty little secret or a fashion? *International Journal of Neuropsychopharmacology*, *23*(2), 125–131. https://doi.org/10.1093/ijnp/pyz068

Liu, Z., Heffernan, C., & Tan, J. (2020). Caregiver burden: A concept analysis. *International Journal of Nursing Science*, *7*(4), 438–445. https://doi.org/10.1016/j.ijnss.2020.07.012

Luciano, M., Sampogna, G., Amore, M. Andriola., I, Calcagno., P, Carmassi., C., Del Vecchio, V, Dell'Osso, L., Di Lorenzo, G., Di Lorenzo, G., & Gelao, B. (2021). How to improve the physical health of people with severe mental illness? A multicentric randomized controlled trial on the efficacy of a lifestyle group intervention. *European Psychiatry*, *64*(1), e72. http://dx.doi.org/10.1192/j.eurpsy.2021.2253

Malhi, G., Bell, E., Boyce, P., Bassett, D., Bryant, R., Hazell, P, Hopwood, M., Lyndon, B., Mulder, R., Porter, R., Singh, A. B., & Murray, G. (2021). The 2020 Royal Australian and New Zealand College of Psychiatrists Clinical Practice Guidelines for Mood Disorders. *Australian & New Zealand Journal of Psychiatry*, *55*(1), 7–117. www.ranzcp.org/files/resources/college_statements/clinician/cpg/mood-disorders-cpg-2020.aspx

Mazereel, V., Detraux, J., Vancampfort, D., van Winkel, R., & De Hert, M. (2020). Impact of psychotropic medication effects on obesity and the metabolic syndrome in people with serious mental illness. *Frontiers in Endocrinology*, *11*, 573479. https://doi.org/10.3389/fendo.2020.573479

McGorry, P. (2015). Early intervention in psychosis: Obvious, effective, overdue. *Journal of Nervous Mental Disorders*, *203*(5), 310–318. https://doi.org/10.1097/NMD.0000000000000284

Mental Health Carers Australia. (2019). *What is a mental health carers?* www.mentalhealthcarersaustralia.org.au.

Miller, J. (2016). The people and the time: Founding of the Australian Association of Social Workers in 1946. *Social Work Focus*, *1*(1), 9–15. www.aasw.asn.au/document/item/8836

Mitchell, A., & Hill, B. (2020). Physical health assessment for people with a severe mental illness. *British Journal of Nursing*, *29*(10), 553–556. https://doi.org/10.12968/bjon.2020.29.10.553

Mulud, Z.A., & McCarthy, G. (2017). Caregiver burden among caregivers of individuals with severe mental illness: Testing the moderation and mediation models of resilience. *Archives of Psychiatric Nursing*, *31*(1), 24–30. https://doi.org/10.1016/j.apnu.2016.07.019

National Alliance on Mental Illness. (2022a). *Bipolar disorder*. www.nami.org/About-Mental-Illness/Mental-Health-Conditions/Bipolar-Disorder

National Alliance on Mental Illness. (2022b). *Psychosis*. www.nami.org/About-Mental-Illness/Mental-Health-Conditions/Psychosis

National Alliance on Mental Illness. (2022c). *Schizoaffective disorder*. www.nami.org/About-Mental-Illness/Mental-Health-Conditions/Schizoaffective-Disorder

National Disability Insurance Scheme. (2022). *Mental health and the NDIS*. www.ndis.gov.au/understanding/how-ndis-works/mental-health-and-ndis

National Institute of Mental Health. (2022a). *Bipolar disorder*. US Department of Health and Human Services. www.nimh.nih.gov/health/publications/bipolar-disorder

National Institute of Mental Health. (2022b). *Mental illness*. US Department of Health and Human Services. www.nimh.nih.gov/health/statistics/mental-illness

National Institute of Mental Health. (2022c). *Schizophrenia*. US Department of Health and Human Services. www.nimh.nih.gov/health/statistics/mental-illness

National Mental Health Commission. (2016). *Equally well consensus statement: Improving the physical health and wellbeing of people living with mental illness in Australia*. www.equallywell.org.au/wp-content/uploads/2018/12/Equally-Well-National-Consensus-Booklet-47537.pdf

Nielsen, C., Hjorthøj, C., Nordentoft, M., & Christensen, U. (2021). A qualitative study on the implementation of flexible assertive community treatment - An integrated community-based treatment model for patients with severe mental illness. *International Journal of Integrated Care*, *21*(2), 13. https://doi.org/10.5334/ijic.5540

New South Wales (NSW) Health. (2020). *How can I communicate with someone experiencing a psychosis?* www.health.nsw.gov.au/mentalhealth/psychosocial/strategies/Pages/communicating-psychosis.aspx

O'Donoghue, B. (2021). Addressing physical health in mental illness: The urgent need to translate evidence-based interventions into routine clinical practice. *Irish Journal of Psychological Medicine*, *38*(1), 1–5. https://doi.org/10.1017/ipm.2021.4

Ogilvie, J., Tzoumakis, S., Allard, T., Thomspon, C., Kisely, S., & Stewart, A. (2021). Prevalence of psychiatric disorders for Indigenous Australians: A population-based birth cohort study. *Epidemiology and Psychiatric Sciences*, *30*, e21. https://doi.org/10.1017/S204579602100010X

Ohwovoriole, T. (2022). *What is the prodromal phase in schizophrenia? Verywellmind*. www.verywellmind.com/the-prodromal-phase-in-schizophrenia-5203945

Olfson, M., Gerhard, T., Huang, C., Crystal, S., & Stroup, T. (2015). Premature mortality among adults with schizophrenia in the United States. *JAMA Psychiatry*, *72*(12), 1172–1181. https://doi.org/10.1001/jamapsychiatry.2015.1737

Olfson, M., Stroup, T., Huang, C., Wall, M., Crystal, S., & Gerhard, T. (2021). Suicide risk in medicare patients with schizophrenia across the life span. *JAMA Psychiatry*, *78*(8), 876–885. https://doi.org/10.1001/jamapsychiatry.2021.0841

O'Neill, E. (2021). Relationships between physical health and employment among people with serious mental illness. *Social Work Research*, *45*(1), 30–42. https://doi.org/10.1093/swr/svaa025

Orygen. (2017). *Early Psychosis: first episode psychosis*. www.orygen.org.au/Research/Research-Areas/First-Episode-Psychosis

Orygen. (2022). *News and events: Early intervention for psychosis: Why does it matter?* www.orygen.org.au/About/News-And-Events/2022/Early-intervention-for-psychosis-why-does-it-matte

Penney, D. (2018). *Defining "peer support": Implications for policy, practice, and research. Advocates for Human Potential*. www.ahpnet.com/AHPNet/media/AHPNetMediaLibrary/White%20Papers/DPenney_Defining_peer_support_2018_Final.pdf

Petros, R., & Solomon. (2021, March). How adults with serious mental illness learn and use wellness recovery action plan's recovery framework. *Qualitative Health Research*, *31*(4), 631–642. https://doi.org/10.1177/1049732320975729

Qi, L., Zhou, Y., Wang, R., Wang, Y., Liu, Y., & Zeng, L. (2021). Perceived quality of primary healthcare services and its association with institutional trust among caregivers of persons diagnosed with a severe mental illness in China. *Journal of Psychiatric and Mental Health Nursing*, *28*(3), 394–408. https://doi.org/10.1111/jpm.12687

Raeburn, T., Schmied, B., Hungerford, C., & Cleary, M. (2015). Self-determination theory: A framework for Clubhouse psychiatric rehabilitation research. *Issues in Mental Health Nursing*, *36*(2), 145–151. https://doi.org/10.3109/01612840.2014.927544

Roughead, L., Procter, N., Westaway, K., Sluggett, J., & Alderman, C. (2017). *Medication Safety in Mental Health. Australian Commission on Safety and Quality in Health Care*. www.safetyandquality.gov.au/sites/default/files/migrated/Medication-Safety-in-Mental-Health-final-report-2017.pdf

Royal Australian and New Zealand College of Psychiatrists. (2016). *The economic cost of serious mental illness and comorbidities in Australia and New Zealand*. https://vuir.vu.edu.au/31128/1/RANZCP-Serious-Mental-Illness.pdf

Royal Australian and New Zealand College of Psychiatrists. (2015). *Physical health*. https://www.ranzcp.org/clinical-guidelines-publications/clinical-guidelines-publications-library/physical-health

Sadock, B., Sadock, V., & Ruiz, P. (2017). *Kaplan and Sadock's comprehensive textbook of psychiatry* (10th ed.). Wolters Kluwer.

SANE. (2017). *Antipsychotic medication*. www.sane.org/information-and-resources/facts-and-guides/antipsychotic-medication

Shalaby, R., & Agyapong, V. (2020). Peer support in mental health: Literature review. *JMIR Mental Health*, *7*(6), e15572. https://doi.org/10.2196/15572

Szendi, I., Szabó, N., Domján, N., Tamás Kincses, Z., Palkó, A., Vécsei, L., & Racsmány, M. (2017). A new division of schizophrenia revealed expanded bilateral brain structural abnormalities of the association cortices. *Frontiers in Psychiatry*, *8*, 127. https://doi.org/10.3389/fpsyt.2017.00127

Vallesi, S., Wood, L., Dimer, L., & Zada, M. (2018). "In their own voice." Incorporating underlying social determinants into Aboriginal health promotion programs. *International Journal of Environmental Research and Public Health*, *15*(7), 1514. https://doi.org/10.3390/ijerph15071514

Veltro, F., Latte, G., Pontarelli, I., Pontarelli, C., Nicchiniello, I., & Zappone, L. (2022). Long term outcome study of a salutogenic psychoeducational recovery oriented intervention (Inte.G.R.O.) in severe mental illness patients. *BMC Psychiatry*, *22*, 240. http://dx.doi.org/10.1186/s12888-022-03887-2

Whitley, R., Palmer, V., & Gunn, J. (2015). Recovery from severe mental illness. *Canadian Medical Association Journal*, *187*(13), 951–952. https://doi.org/10.1503/cmaj.141558

World Health Organization. (2018). *Management of physical health conditions in adults with severe mental disorders*. www.who.int/publications/i/item/978-92-4-155038-3

Yee, M., Espiridon, E., Oladunjoye, A., Millsaps, U., Harvey, N., & Vora, A. (2021). The use of clozapine in the serious mental illness patients enrolled in an assertive community treatment program. *Cureus*, *13*(5), e15238. https://doi.org/10.7759/cureus.15238

ACKNOWLEDGEMENTS

Photo: © Sotnikov Misha / Shutterstock.com
Photo: © vectorfusionart / Shutterstock.com
Photo: © Philip Schubert / Shutterstock.com
Photo: © arliftatoz2205 - stock.adobe.com
Photo: © Ryan Pierse / Getty Images
Photo: © Prostock-studio / Shutterstock.com
Photo: © Elena Vasilchenko / Shutterstock.com
Photo: © TVP Inc / DigitalVision / Getty Images
Photo: © BUTENKOV ALEKSEI / Shutterstock.com
Photo: © monkeybusinessimages / iStock / Getty Images

Substance use disorders

This chapter will:

10.1 outline the difference between substance use and misuse

10.2 describe the attitudes of health professionals and the community to substance use and misuse

10.3 consider health promotion and harm minimisation approaches

10.4 describe the categories of substances — stimulants, depressants and hallucinogens

10.5 examine issues related to substance use disorders

10.6 explore common substances misused

10.7 outline screening and assessment for substance use issues and disorders

10.8 explain the issues facing family members of a person with a substance misuse issue

10.9 explain how care is provided to people with a substance use disorder, including the use of motivational interviewing and brief interventions

10.10 describe how the stress–vulnerability model can explain how substance use and other factors interact with a person's biological vulnerability to developing a mental illness.

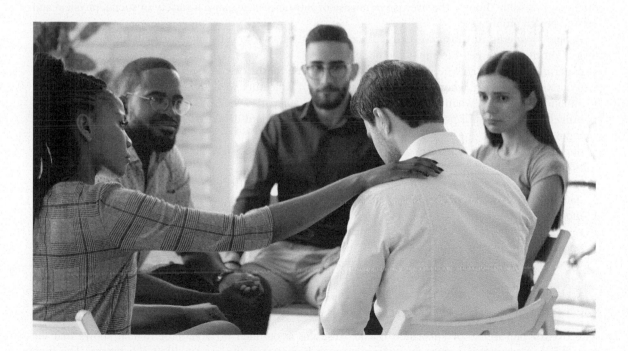

Introduction

In Australia, the use of native tobacco was widespread and alcohol was consumed in a small number of Indigenous communities before European colonisation. Following British settlement, the introduction of rum had detrimental effects on Indigenous communities and dominated the early years of the predominately White male colony (Ritter et al., 2017). Throughout history, people have most often used substances for pleasure; however, substance use also has the potential to have a negative impact on a variety of social, physical, psychological, legal and financial issues.

The focus of this chapter is substance use and misuse and its effects on a person's mental, physical and social wellbeing. The chapter begins with a definition of the difference between use and misuse, followed by a summary of the prevalence of substance use in Australia and its effects. This is followed by a description of the harm minimisation approach taken by health services across Australia when assisting people with substance use problems. There is an explanation of the screening and assessment tools that are available to assist health professionals in identifying the extent of the person's substance use, and a discussion of the most common issues related to substance withdrawal. Treatment options that can be used when caring for the person with a substance use problem are outlined, together with the health professional's role in promoting good health and encouraging personal change. The chapter concludes by outlining the transtheoretical model or 'Cycle of Change', the core principles of motivational interviewing and the stress–vulnerability model.

10.1 Substance use and substance misuse

LEARNING OBJECTIVE 10.1 Outline the difference between substance use and misuse.

There are many different terms used by health professionals working with people who use and/or misuse substances. In this chapter, the term **substance** refers to psychoactive compounds such as alcohol, caffeine, nicotine or other drugs that are used by people to achieve certain effects. The terms 'substance misuse' and 'substance dependence' relate to the continued use of a substance despite negative consequences, often leading to various substance use disorders that will be discussed in greater detail in a later section of this chapter. It is important to distinguish between **substance use** and **substance misuse** before proceeding in this chapter to ensure that the distinctions can be made in assessment and treatment.

The majority of people who do use substances are able to do so without significant adverse consequences. For some though, the overuse or misuse of substances can cause a variety of social, physical and mental health problems.

People's patterns of substance use will vary from substance to substance and will often change over time. Common patterns of use may include:

- experimental use (e.g. when a teenager tries a cigarette for the first time)
- recreational use (e.g. when a person drinks a glass of wine after work to help them to relax)
- situational use (e.g. when a person smokes cannabis at a party when it is offered to them)
- bingeing (e.g. when a person drinks more than four standard drinks of alcohol on occasion but not regularly)
- dependent use (e.g. when a person repeatedly prioritises their substance use over other activities in their life, possibly as a result of psychological or physical yearning)
- intoxication (e.g. when a person experiences the psychoactive effects of a substance; often described as getting tipsy/drunk/stoned/tripping, and so on. Disinhibition and altered mental state and reaction times increase risks of harm)
- regular excessive use (problems arising from using substances regularly and excessively over a sustained period of time. The use does not allow for the body to recover completely from the last time they used. The consequences include physical or medical consequences, e.g. disease of the liver, brain damage or cancer).

Prevalence of substance use

The overall prevalence of substance use in Australia is outlined in table 10.1, which shows that the use of legal substances across the nation is much higher than the use of illicit substances. The high frequency of use of alcohol and tobacco contributes to their association with high morbidity and mortality in Australia. The most commonly used illicit substance was cannabis, with just over 10 per cent of respondents reporting that they had used cannabis in the 12 months preceding the survey. It should be noted that population surveys, such as the National Drug Strategy Household Survey rely on self-report of substance use behaviour, which is prone to bias. Sampling bias is also impossible to eliminate, affecting the generalisability of findings relating to Indigenous communities and other populations. Also, note that caffeine use is not reported here.

TABLE 10.1	12-month prevalence of substance use in the Australian population aged 14 years and older (2019)
Substance	**%**
Alcohol	76.6
Tobacco	14.0
Cannabis	11.6
Prescribed analgesics	2.7
Cocaine	4.2
Ecstasy	3.0
Meth/amphetamine	1.3
Hallucinogens	1.6
Inhalants	1.4
Ketamine	0.9
New and emerging psychoactive substances	0.1
Heroin	<0.1
GHB	0.1

Source: Australian Institute of Health and Welfare (AIHW, 2020).

Over 40 per cent of people in Australia have smoked, drunk alcohol at risky levels or used illicit substances within a 12-month period. However, trends related to smoking rates show a significant reduction in tobacco use over recent years (as noted in figure 10.1).

FIGURE 10.1	Recent substance use trends excluding alcohol in Australia: people aged over 15 years

Source: AIHW (2020).

Patterns of substance use vary among communities, so sometimes it may appear that results from national surveys are at odds with sensational news stories reporting on 'drug epidemics sweeping the nation'. Geographic and demographic factors are associated with patterns of substance use: in rural and remote locations, the rates of amphetamine use, cigarette smoking and risky alcohol use are twice as high as rates in metropolitan areas. Twenty per cent of Australians with a mental illness smoke daily compared to less than 10 per cent among people without a mental illness. They are also more than twice as likely to have used meth and to have used pharmaceuticals for non-medical purposes, such as amphetamines (AIHW, 2020).

Indigenous Australians have higher rates of smoking than non-Indigenous Australians, though smoking rates in Indigenous populations are falling significantly. There is an increase in the proportion of Aboriginal and Torres Strait Islander peoples abstaining or drinking within the The National Health and Medical Research Council (NHMRC) guidelines (AIHW, 2020). Illicit substance use is more common among people who identify as being homosexual or bisexual (AIHW, 2020).

Around 7.5 per cent of Australians aged 14 years or older may meet the criteria for alcohol dependence, with an additional 22 per cent drinking at harmful levels (based on the 2009 Australian alcohol guidelines which were current at the time the survey was conducted). Males and people aged over 70 are at higher risk.

Twenty-one per cent of respondents, equating to around 4.5 million Australians, experienced an alcohol-related 'incident', such as verbal or physical abuse or were put in fear in the 12-month reporting period (AIHW, 2020).

Adverse effects of substance use

There are a number of health risks associated with substance use. Some health risks are associated with the substance itself, while other risks are associated with lifestyle, route of administration and increased risk of injury while intoxicated. There is an increased risk of physical, psychological, social, financial and legal issues.

Substances that are widely used may, of course, affect more individuals, while the very nature of other substances or the route of administration may affect a higher proportion of people who choose to use them.

Alcohol was the attributable cause of death for 6512 people in Australia in 2018, while illicit substance use accounted for 2855 deaths during the same period. Tobacco use was the attributable cause of death for 20 482 Australians (AIHW, 2021).

Many people experience adverse effects associated with tobacco use and excessive alcohol use. Smoking accounts for nearly 9 per cent of Australia's total burden of disease and injury, making it the leading preventable cause of morbidity and mortality (AIHW, 2021). The main adverse effects of tobacco use include cancer, and respiratory and cardiovascular diseases. Vaping, which is increasing in popularity in many countries, has an unknown profile in terms of health consequences (Rehan et al., 2018). The effects of excessive alcohol consumption include injury (see the chapter that discusses people displaying challenging behaviours), mental disorders, cancer, and cardiovascular, neurological and gastrointestinal disorders (AIHW, 2021).

In terms of personal health costs, the **disability-adjusted life years (DALYs)** attributable to substance use in Australia in 2018 were tobacco use: >430 000 DALY, alcohol >220 000 DALY and illicit substance use >149 000 (AIHW, 2021).

There are obvious pleasurable effects associated with using substances, as well as potential long-term harms. Given the preventable nature of substance use disorders, the role of the health professional extends beyond treating the immediate health sequelae of problematic substance use and extends into a health promotion and harm prevention focus.

Attitudes to substance use

In Australia, there are mixed attitudes towards the use of substances. Most people will drink tea or coffee without considering the fact that they are using a substance. Indeed, it is quite acceptable to 'use' caffeine in our culture.

Likewise, some sectors of the Australian community laud the use of alcohol — alcohol forms the centrepiece of many social interactions and features prominently in advertisements at major sporting events. This is despite the cost to taxpayers through the health budget, at an estimated $66 billion, with $18 billion attributed to tangible costs (e.g. labour and health costs) and $48 billion to intangible costs, such as morbidity and mortality related loss of productivity and quality of life (Whetton et al., 2021).

A large proportion of the community (65 per cent) supported a proposal to introduce health warnings on alcohol containers, while less than 10 per cent of people were opposed to the proposal (AIHW, 2020).

On the other hand, attitudes to the use of nicotine have changed over time, with legislation in states and territories across Australia now banning smoking in public buildings and spaces, restaurants and hotels. Smoke-free health campuses have also been implemented nationwide, with health services actively discouraging nicotine use by staff and service users alike. Prisons, too, are becoming smoke-free, with bans implemented in a number of jurisdictions in recent years (Puljević and Segan, 2019). While around 11 per cent of Australians continue to smoke regularly, attitudes towards people who use nicotine in Australia are ambivalent as social norms slowly swing away from acceptance (AIHW, 2020).

Community attitudes to the use of many **illicit substances** generally remain negative. The use and distribution of a number of newer stimulants, depressants and hallucinogens have been outlawed in Australia. This legislation was instituted to minimise the risk of harm to the physical, mental, emotional and social wellbeing of the population that the misuse of these substances can cause. Changing views around the acceptance of cannabis use are reflected in changes in patterns of use in the community (Chan et al., 2021). Prescribed opioid medications may have received increased attention in recent years including in relation to multi-billion-dollar lawsuits filed against big pharma for their role in contributing to opioid-related harm in different jurisdictions.

UPON REFLECTION

The legal status of substances

Many substances cause harm, including some legal substances. Some of these consequences are predictable, others are not. The legal status of a substance can play a role in reducing or increasing various harms associated with a substance.

QUESTIONS

1. If tobacco was made illegal in this country, what might some negative and positive consequences be?

2. If cannabis were to be legalised in this country, what might some negative and positive consequences be?

3. What impact did prohibition laws have on alcohol-related issues in the United States when they were introduced in 1920?

Substance use and stigma

Stigma is the term used to describe society's negative and stereotypical attitudes towards people who are perceived as different (see the chapter on mental health care in Australia for information about stigma in the mental health context). Stigma may be based on many factors, including gender, race, religion, sexual orientation, mental health and substance use problems. Stigma labels some people or groups as less worthy of respect than others. People with a substance use disorder are often stigmatised in the community, while people with comorbid substance use and mental health issues are further stigmatised. This situation has a profound impact on people's lives, leading to feelings of low self-worth (self-stigma) and the avoidance of contact with mainstream society and health professionals. With regard to people who use substances, research in the United Kingdom identified the following issues.

- The street policing of problem drug users can be publicly humiliating and add to feelings of injustice, alienation and stigmatisation. For recovering users, the continued labelling of them as drug users makes change extremely difficult.
- Attending a drug and alcohol program can increase stigmatisation with some people feeling that the very act of seeking treatment serves to cement an 'addict' or 'junkie' identity, leading to further rejection from family and friends.
- The supervised consumption of methadone in pharmacies provides a context where a person's problems are made public, with many feeling stigmatised by the attitudes of pharmacy staff and other customers (United Kingdom Policy Drug Commission, 2010).

Across the Western world, there is much work to be done to change attitudes. People with substance use issues have a health problem, not a personality deficit or criminal tendencies. They must be provided with fair and equitable care and treatment.

The Australian Injecting and Illicit Drug Users League (AIVL) and the NSW Users and AIDS Association (NUAA) are two Australian peer organisations working to reduce discriminatory behaviour and attitudes towards people who use illicit substances.

10.2 Attitudes of health professionals

LEARNING OBJECTIVE 10.2 Describe the attitudes of health professionals and the community to substance use and misuse.

The human condition assumes that everyone has personal values, beliefs and opinions. These are developed over many years of education, exposure and experience.

As a health professional, these values will be challenged at times and will change over time. This is particularly true in relation to the attitudes towards those who have substance use issues. On a personal level, the health professional may have individual beliefs that some substance use behaviour is 'bad' or that the person lacks 'will power'. The health professional may believe that the client has chosen to use the substance, so the problems they have are their own fault and they do not deserve treatment. Health professionals are encouraged to reflect upon their personal attitudes, values and judgements towards the choices and lifestyles of the people they are helping and consider how they affect the attitudes they display and the treatment they provide. In public health settings, substance use should be viewed as a health issue, not a moral issue.

On a professional level, many health professionals may think that the assessment and treatment of drug and alcohol issues lie outside of their scope of practise. For this reason, they lack confidence in their ability to treat the person who has a substance use issue or they do not believe that any interventions will make a difference (National Centre for Education and Training on Addiction, 2006). Further, there may be specific organisational mandates that limit a health professional's capacity to provide a more holistic approach to the treatment of persons with substance use issues. This is often referred to in practice as gatekeeping; for example, busy mental health services may reject referrals on the basis that the person has substance misuse issues and, as such, would be better treated in a drug and alcohol setting. This is also true for some specialist drug and alcohol services that reject referrals on the basis that the referred person has mental health issues and, as such, would be better treated in a mental health setting.

It is essential that all health professionals view the person who has substance use issues from a health perspective rather than a moralistic or legalistic perspective. It is also crucial that all health professionals develop a level of confidence in providing care to people with substance use issues. The health professional will most certainly encounter a person who uses substances in the course of their work. Health professionals who are not confident in what they do are less likely to inspire confidence in the person seeking assistance.

More broadly, discrimination and our prejudices play a role in perpetuating stigma in the wider community. Health professionals can play a role in bringing about social change by challenging their own prejudices (see the chapter on assessment in the mental health context). The first step to overcoming prejudice and building confidence for health professionals is to proactively seek out training (van Boekel et al., 2013). It is also important that health professionals are familiar with local policies and procedures related to substance use, and the availability of local support services.

Substance use disorders are health issues that require intervention in the same way as any other health issue. Effective health professionals will place their personal values to one side when providing health care and respond in a professional manner with evidence-based interventions rather than community attitudes or personal perceptions.

Language use

The use of labels and pejorative language reinforces the shame, guilt and embarrassment that challenge people with substance use issues and may prevent them from accessing treatment (Volkow et al., 2021). For example, 'junkie' and 'addict' are pejorative terms that connote social decay. As a result, a person is less likely to seek help from a health professional who uses such language. Likewise, the descriptor 'drug seeker' is a negative label often imposed by health professionals upon a person requesting assistance to manage physical symptoms after ceasing to use a substance. This label often gives rise to health professionals and their respective service environments (e.g. emergency departments) generally treating the person punitively. Pejorative language is more likely to be used when the person with the problem is not present. One way to encourage staff to use less pejorative language is to speak as though the person you are speaking about is present in the room. Similarly, write each note in someone's file as though you expect they will be reading it.

There is a range of strategies that health professionals and health services can employ to challenge negative community attitudes towards people with substance use disorders. These strategies include:

- becoming more active in challenging inaccurate or sensationalised media reporting of substance use issues
- encouraging iconic public figures to talk openly about their recovery from substance use and dependence
- participating in training to develop skills and confidence in assisting people with health issues arising from substance use
- providing education and information to service users about substance use issues
- not sharing or supporting social media content that is discriminatory or pejorative.

It is important to note that partners and families/carers will likewise struggle with the stigma associated with substance use. Health services and community organisations across Australia now provide excellent resources, including pamphlets, information sessions on substance use and support groups for families and carers. Information is also readily available on the Internet through a range of government and non-government sources. There is more detailed information about the kind of support available for partners and families of people with substance use issues in later sections of this chapter.

The following points are useful to remember when providing information to partners, family members or friends of people with a substance use problem.

- Substance dependence is a physical condition with behavioural implications. For this reason, people will sometimes use substances to control uncomfortable physical withdrawal symptoms.
- When someone is substance dependent, their ability to connect their substance use and the negative consequences is often impaired.
- These factors do not abrogate the person from being responsible — just as the person with diabetes needs to make difficult lifestyle changes to manage their disorder, so too does a person who is dependent on a substance.
- Managing substance dependence is not just a matter of 'will power'. While a desire to change is an important factor in changing behaviour, the person may also need assistance to manage different aspects of their behaviour change.
- Partners, family members or friends may love the person without condoning their challenging behaviours. 'Trust the person — not the addiction.'

Perhaps the most important thing for the health professional to remember is to be non-judgemental and willing to listen. Anyone who presents with substance-related issues may have experienced trauma, but this history may not be immediately obvious. Some minority populations have experienced high rates of exposure to trauma and discrimination (Oakley et al., 2021), including, but not limited to refugees, other immigrants, LGBTQIA+ and Indigenous populations. All clinicians should be routinely delivering trauma-informed care and minimising the chance of re-traumatisation.

When working with Indigenous and culturally diverse individuals, it is appropriate to include Indigenous health team members, multicultural workers and interpreters as needed. Also, make a point of familiarising yourself with important cultural issues relating to people who access your service.

Comorbidities

There is overwhelming evidence that the rates of substance use issues are much higher in people with mental health problems and, likewise, that the incidence of mental health problems is significantly higher in people seeking treatment for substance use issues (Marel et al., 2016). In clinical practice, it is often found that a high proportion of people seeking assistance for substance misuse concurrently experience psychological distress. **Comorbidity** is a broad term that indicates the presence of two or more health conditions, illnesses or disorders. In this chapter, 'comorbidity' refers to the coexistence of a mental illness and an alcohol or drug problem. Health professionals need to be aware that a range of terms are used within health services that for the most part mean the same thing. For example, the terms 'dual-diagnosis' and 'co-occurring disorders' are sometimes used interchangeably with comorbidity.

People with comorbid mental health and substance use disorders comprise a heterogeneous grouping. This can refer to people of any age or gender who have a range of different mental health disorders with differing degrees of acuity and chronicity combined with a similarly diverse array of substance-related issues pertaining to different substances and differing levels of severity that may pose problems of intoxication, withdrawal and dependence. For each disorder, there may be different levels of awareness or insight, differing levels of motivation for treatment and functional capacity.

In Australia, people who report recent substance use have significantly higher rates of psychological distress than those not using substances (Australian Institute of Health & Welfare, 2019). People who use substances every day have a 60 per cent chance of having experienced a mental health issue in the previous 12 months, and these rates are likely to be higher for people who seek alcohol and other drug (AOD) treatment (Deady et al., 2013; Marel et al., 2016). These mental health problems include but are not limited to:

- major depression
- schizophrenia
- bipolar disorder
- obsessive-compulsive disorder
- anxiety
- post-traumatic stress disorder.

On the other hand, 45–55 per cent of people with a mental health problem have a substance use disorder (National Institute on Drug Abuse, 2010). Reasons for this include:

- 'self-medication' to manage the symptoms of mental illness
- 'self-medication' to manage side effects of psychotropics
- lower levels of coping or capacity to deal with stress
- boredom
- loneliness.

There have been many discussions about which issue tends to occur first — the substance use or the mental health problem (Degenhardt et al., 2018). Likewise, there have been many discussions about which is the 'primary' disorder — the mental health problem or the substance use issues (NSW Health, 2009). Determining the answer to this discussion is interesting; however, health professionals are strongly encouraged to ensure that their focus is on the person they are helping. For non-prescribing health professionals, the treatment would usually be the same no matter which disorder emerged first. When screening and assessing clients with comorbid disorders, it is useful to consider how a client perceives his or her symptoms and motivation to receive treatment for both disorders (substance misuse and mental illness). Please refer to the Integrated Motivational Assessment Tool (IMAT) (Clancy & Terry, 2007) in the 'Understanding motivation' section of this chapter. It is vital that health professionals stay with the 'here and now' experience of the person, identify their particular needs and provide options for them so they can make informed lifestyle choices.

It is also crucial for health professionals to acknowledge the importance of addressing comorbidity issues with an **integrated treatment** approach. Many people with comorbid mental health and substance use issues report being pushed from the mental health service to the drug and alcohol service and back again, with health professionals from both services suggesting that the responsibility for providing care and treatment lies with the other. Developing evidence to support integrated approaches of treatment for comorbid conditions is complicated and results in a paucity of high-quality evidence. What is clear though, is that referring people between services leads to poor outcomes. For this reason, all health professionals should give due consideration to the person first and foremost, and which service they 'belong' to second. This is often referred to as the 'no wrong door policy' within service policy; essentially, all persons are assessed at their first access point and not just 'turned away' because they do not have the 'primary' condition required for entry. This is person-centred care at its best.

Most states in Australia have developed guidelines for the management of people with coexisting mental health and substance use disorders. Each of these guidelines emphasises the importance of ensuring that the person does not fall between the gaps thatwhich exist between services. Synthesising information for consumers reduces the likelihood that they will receive conflicting information by accessing multiple services and possibly receive conflicting information from different services.

Comorbidity is a key contributing factor associated with poor engagement and retention in treatment and, most likely, relapse (NSW Health, 2009). Also, people with comorbid issues are viewed as 'complex' by health service providers and may be rejected for entry into particular programs (e.g. accommodation support) because of this label. This demonstrates the level of need — and stigma — with which people with comorbid issues struggle. All health professionals have a duty of care to assist people with comorbid issues, regardless of so-called complexity.

IN PRACTICE

Resources for people accessing services

Finding accurate, up-to-date resources for consumers with substance related issues can be a challenge.

Your Room (www.yourroom.health.nsw.gov.au) is a NSW government online resource for people who wish to find information about substances of abuse. The information is approved by health experts and the site contains a range of resources. Each piece of provided information has been checked for accuracy and applicability in the Australian context and includes:

- information about drugs
- links to resources including mobile apps
- games
- links to support services
- information for families
- information for Aboriginal peoples.

QUESTIONS

1. What would increase the likelihood of you recommending a resource such as Your Room to people you work with in a clinical setting?
2. What strategies can you use to increase the likelihood of someone using a website you recommend?
3. What are the advantages and disadvantages of providing information in different formats (e.g. written, verbal or online)?

10.3 Health promotion and disease prevention

LEARNING OBJECTIVE 10.3 Consider health promotion and harm minimisation approaches.

Health promotion programs have the ability to change health behaviours at a population level (Thompson, 2015). In Australia, current health promotion strategies are tackling the community's beliefs about health and illness. A number of primary health care initiatives related to substance use issues have been rolled out across Australia. These form part of the National Drug Strategy (NDS), which is a cooperative venture between the federal and state/territory governments and the non-government sector. The NDS aims to improve health, social and economic outcomes for Australians by preventing the uptake of harmful drug use and reducing the harmful effects of licit and illicit drugs in the community.

The *National Drug Strategy 2017–2026* details Australia's national commitment and strategies to achieve harm minimisation as well as measurement indicators to monitor progress.

Health professionals with an interest in public health strategies are encouraged to visit the NDS website (www.health.gov.au/resources/collections/national-drug-strategy) to obtain more information about ongoing developments.

Harm minimisation

In the Australian health system, the approach taken in relation to the care and treatment of people with substance use issues is **harm minimisation** (Department of Health, 2017a). This concept acknowledges that substance use will continue in the community and the work of health services and health professionals is to assist to reduce the harm associated with substance use for individuals and also for the community as a whole.

Adopting a harm minimisation approach does not preclude abstinence-based interventions (Department of Health, 2017a). In fact, if the health professional were to view harm minimisation interventions on a continuum, abstinence-based interventions would be placed at one extreme end of the continuum; that is, the ultimate form of harm minimisation. However, if the health professional were to adopt an abstinence-based approach only, then people who are not prepared to consider abstinence would not be offered help at all. This means that no harm minimisation would be achieved. For this reason, the Australian health system offers a range of interventions, with an acceptance that many people will choose to continue to use substances.

Since the NDS began in 1985, harm minimisation has been its overarching approach. This encompasses the three equally important pillars of demand reduction, supply reduction and harm reduction (shown in figure 10.2) being applied together in a balanced way.

FIGURE 10.2 The three pillars of harm minimisation

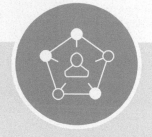
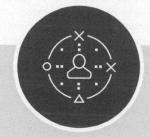

Demand reduction	Supply reduction	Harm reduction
Preventing the uptake and/or delaying the onset of use of alcohol, tobacco and other drugs; reducing the misuse of alcohol, tobacco and other drugs in the community; and supporting people to recover from dependence through evidence-informed treatment.	Preventing, stopping, disrupting or otherwise reducing the production and supply of illegal drugs; and controlling, managing and/or regulating the availability of legal drugs.	Reducing the adverse health, social and economic consequences of the use of drugs, for the user, their families and the wider community.

Source: Department of Health (2017a).

It is important to reiterate that accepting a person and their choice does not imply that health professionals, health services or even governments condone that person's choice. Rather, such acceptance acknowledges that people will make a choice. This is one of the basic ethical principles upon which Australian society stands.

10.4 Categories of substances

LEARNING OBJECTIVE 10.4 Describe the categories of substances — stimulants, depressants and hallucinogens.

As already noted, the use of substances in Australia, including **psychoactive substances**, is not uncommon. Several models can be used to categorise them. The simplest way to understand the psychoactive effects of substances is to divide them into three major categories based on their effect on the

central nervous system (CNS) during intoxication. These three categories are stimulants, depressants and hallucinogens. Each of these categories is now described in turn.

Stimulants

During intoxication, stimulants speed up neurochemical activity in some areas of the brain. Stimulants also have a level of peripheral sympathomimetic action, which produces mild tachycardia, hypertension and tachypnoea. Substances classed as stimulants include amphetamine-type substances, cocaine, caffeine and nicotine. Ecstasy (methylenedioxymethamphetamine [MDMA]) is a stimulant that possesses some hallucinogenic qualities.

People use stimulants for a variety of reasons, including:
- a sense of euphoria and wellbeing
- boost in energy levels
- wakefulness and self-confidence
- improved physical and cognitive performance
- reduced appetite.

Once a person has developed a **tolerance** for a substance or becomes **physically dependent** or **psychologically dependent** on that substance, the dependence itself — including withdrawal avoidance — will contribute to a person's continued substance use (Volkow et al., 2016).

Depressants

The major defining quality of a substance that is a CNS depressant is the slowing down of neurochemical activity. This affects cognitive processing, impairs coordination and induces sedation. In larger doses, CNS depressants may cause respiratory depression.

Substances classed as depressants include alcohol, benzodiazepines, fantasy (gamma hydroxybutyrate or GHB), inhalants and opioids. Cannabis (delta-9-tetrahydrocannabinol, or Δ9 THC) is a depressant with some mild hallucinogenic properties.

People often use depressants such as alcohol to socialise and relax. Opioids are also commonly used for their pain-relieving qualities, making them useful for treating short-term pain.

Hallucinogens

Hallucinogens alter the perceptions of the user. This alteration may affect the senses (visual, auditory, kinaesthetic, olfactory or gustatory), awareness of the passage of time and gating (the ability to dismiss extraneous stimuli). Out-of-body experiences may also be reported. Substances classed as hallucinogens include LSD (lysergic acid diethylamide) trips, mushrooms (psilocybin), Special-K (ketamine), angel dust (phencyclidine, or PCP) and datura (scopolamine). Cannabis and ecstasy may also have some hallucinogenic properties.

A summary of these three categories of substances and the different types of substances that fall into these categories is provided in table 10.2. As already noted, not everyone who uses substances will develop a substance use disorder. Instead some people use substances recreationally, with no issues, for many years. Substance use disorders are described in the next section.

TABLE 10.2   Types of substances

Depressants	Stimulants	Hallucinogens
Alcohol	(Meth)amphetamines (including mimetics, e.g. cathinones and phenthylamines)	Ketamine
Inhalants	Cocaine	LSD (acid)
Opioids	Nicotine	Magic mushrooms
Benzodiazepines	MDMA/ecstasy (including mimetics, e.g. aminoindanes and piperazines)	Cannabis (in larger doses)
GHB	Caffeine	Datura
Cannabis (including synthetic cannabinoids)		Tryptamines (e.g. NBOMe)

10.5 Substance use disorders

LEARNING OBJECTIVE 10.5 Examine issues related to substance use disorders.

Defining a substance use problem is challenging, especially since the identifiable line between use and misuse is not always apparent to the health professional or the consumer. For some people, the amount of substances they use may be the problem, while others will experience problems even though they use small amounts of substances infrequently. For this reason, the *Diagnostic and Statistical Manual of Mental Disorders*, 5th edition (DSM-5) (APA, 2013, p. 483) defines a substance use disorder as 'a cluster of cognitive, behavioural, and physiological symptoms indicating that the individual continues using the substance despite significant substance-related problems'.

As defined by the DSM-5, substance use disorders can be characterised as a change or alteration in brain chemistry whereby symptoms and impacts may continue well beyond detoxification or withdrawal. The following are the criteria groupings for recognising a substance use disorder (APA, 2013, p. 481).

- Impaired control
  - Consumption of the substance in larger amounts or over a longer period than was originally intended.
  - A persistent desire to cut down or regulate substance use and may report multiple unsuccessful efforts to decrease or discontinue use.
  - Large amounts of time spent obtaining the substance, using or recovering from a substance; in more severe substance use disorders, all daily activities may centre around the substance.
  - Craving as seen by an intense desire or urge for the drug.
- Social impairment
  - Recurrent use — may result in a failure to fulfil major role obligations at work, school or home.
  - Continued use despite having persistent or recurrent social or interpersonal problems.
  - Withdrawal from, or reduction of, important social, recreational or occupational activities.
- Risky use
  - Recurrent use of the substance in situations considered hazardous.
  - Continued use of the substance despite knowledge of having a persistent or recurrent physical or psychological problem.
- Pharmacological criteria
  - Tolerance as seen by a markedly increased level of use to achieve the desired effect or a reduced effect of the substance when usual dose levels are used.
  - Withdrawal symptoms (when there is a cessation or reduction in regular use of a substance).

Substance-induced disorders

The DSM-5 (APA, 2013) also distinguishes between problems directly associated with patterns of substance use (substance use disorders) and secondary mental health issues that develop as a result of substance use (substance-induced disorders). The classification of substance-induced disorders includes intoxication, withdrawal and other substance/medication-induced mental disorders (e.g. substance-induced psychosis, substance-induced depressive disorder).

The essential features of substance-induced disorders are:

1. the development of a reversible substance-specific syndrome due to the recent ingestion of a substance
2. clinically significant problematic behavioural or psychological changes associated with intoxication (e.g. belligerence, mood lability, impaired judgement) that are attributable to the physiological effects of the substance on the CNS and develop during or shortly after use of the substance
3. the symptoms that are not attributable to another medical condition and are not better explained by another mental disorder.

Acute intoxication

Acute intoxication occurs after the use of psychoactive substances and results in altered consciousness, **impaired cognition**, altered perception and out-of-character behaviour (e.g. disinhibition) or changes to other psycho-physiological functions and responses. It is the outcome of the acute pharmacological effects of the use of substances. It resolves in time with complete recovery, except where specific complications have arisen; e.g. trauma or inhalation of vomit.

Substance withdrawal

Substance **withdrawal** is a group of symptoms that occur following sudden cessation or reduction of the substance after persistent use. The onset, course and symptoms of the withdrawal are time-limited and related to the type and dosage of the substance. It is important that health professionals are aware of the symptoms of withdrawal across the range of substances that are most commonly used. Withdrawal from most substances is an unpleasant experience, but generally will not require hospitalisation (although the withdrawal may begin to manifest itself while the person is admitted to hospital for another condition). Severe alcohol, benzodiazepine or GHB withdrawal, on the other hand, can be quite dangerous and hospitalisation may be required. Severe opioid withdrawal, while not life threatening, is such an uncomfortable experience that many people will choose to undertake their detoxification in a specialised detoxification facility. Cessation of many other substances, including stimulants, hallucinogens, cannabis and solvents, can be undertaken without significant physical complications (NSW Ministry of Health, 2021).

This section has provided general information about each substance use disorder a person may experience. In the next sections, more specific information is provided about the substances that are used most often in Australian society, their effects, and the major disorders that a person who uses substances can experience. It is also acknowledged that substances other than those listed in this chapter are used. Health professionals who require more detail are encouraged to seek out a specialised text.

Substance or medication-induced mental disorders

A range of mental and neurocognitive disorders may arise as a result of exposure to substances of abuse and some medications. These may include psychotic, mood, anxiety and other disorders. These substance-induced disorders usually ameliorate within a month after cessation of the substance, but some conditions persist much longer. Clinicians interested in exploring these disorders in more detail are encouraged to access the DSM-5, the chapter on substance-related disorders.

Reward pathways

An exciting field of neuropsychiatric research involves the study of the mesolimbic dopaminergic pathway, otherwise known as the **reward pathway**. This pathway has its roots deep in brain structures of the ventral tegmental area, through the nucleus accumbens and connecting to the prefrontal cortex (as shown in figure 10.3). The role of the reward pathway is to reinforce behaviours to ensure the survival of individuals and species, including humankind. When a person or animal engages in behaviors, such as eating, drinking, having sex and nurturing their offspring, they receive a small burst of dopamine along this pathway that is related to the activity. This gives rise to feelings of wellbeing, and increases the person's likelihood of repeating the behaviour. Likewise, when a person uses substances, these substances provide a large boost in dopamine along this 'reward pathway'. Eventually, after prolonged substance use, the pathway becomes desensitised, resulting in diminished pleasure from non-drug activities. The net result is that the nucleus accumbens reconfigures a person's priorities so that using a substance becomes more salient than socialising, eating, drinking and sex (Koob & Volkow, 2010).

| FIGURE 10.3 | The brain's reward pathway |

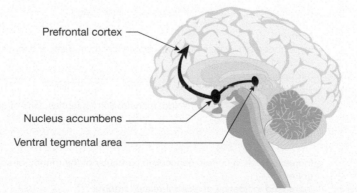

Prefrontal cortex

Nucleus accumbens

Ventral tegmental area

The US Surgeon General has confirmed three stages of addiction related to the impact on the brain: binge intoxication, withdrawal/negative affect and preoccupation/anticipation. The three stages are associated with executive function deficits, increased stress, reduced pleasure and increased salience of the substance (US Department of Health and Human Services Office of the Surgeon General, 2016). This understanding of brain adaptation contributes to the view of serious addiction as a disease of the brain.

10.6 Commonly misused substances

LEARNING OBJECTIVE 10.6 Explore common substances misused.

As outlined earlier in this chapter, substance use is quite common in Australia. Substance use issues are more prevalent among people who present to health services for treatment of other disorders. Therefore, it is important for all health professionals to have a basic understanding of the major issues relating to commonly misused substances. The following section outlines some basic information on a range of substances that clinicians may encounter in health care settings.

Alcohol

The use of alcohol by Australians is widespread. According to the 2019 National Drug Strategy Household Survey, the number of people drinking in Australia remained largely unchanged, more than three-quarters of Australians over the age of 14 having consumed a full serve of alcohol during the preceding year, though the number of people drinking at risky levels has fallen (AIHW, 2020).

Virtually every system in the human body can be damaged by alcohol (see table 10.3). Individuals who use excessive amounts of alcohol are also at an increased risk of psychological problems, including impaired judgement and decision making, as well as increased levels of impulsiveness. For a small proportion of drinkers, this can lead to antisocial and disinhibited behaviour, such as engaging in violent or criminal activity.

TABLE 10.3   **The health and medical complications of excessive alcohol use**

Body system	Complication
Gastrointestinal	Cirrhosis of liver, hepatitis Gastritis Pancreatitis Gastrointestinal haemorrhage Malnutrition, weight loss, malabsorption
Cardiovascular	Cardiac arrhythmias Cardiomyopathy Hypertension — often difficult to treat
Neurological	Blackouts Seizures Peripheral neuropathy Acute confusional states Head injuries Long-term brain damage Depression
Respiratory	Pneumonia — inhalation of vomit while intoxicated
Reproductive	*Men* Hypogonadism — loss of libido, impotence, loss of secondary sexual characteristics, enlarged breasts in males Infertility *Women* Hypogonadism — loss of libido, menstrual irregularities, loss of secondary sexual characteristics
Musculoskeletal	Gout
Other	Increased risk of certain cancers, in particular of the mouth, oesophagus, liver and colon Increased incidence of alcohol-related trauma Increased risk of self-harm and suicide

Safer drinking levels

As noted, alcohol is a CNS depressant. Ethanol or ethyl alcohol is the active, intoxicating ingredient in all alcoholic beverages, including beer, wine and spirits. In small doses, people report feeling relaxed with mild euphoria after consuming alcohol. At larger doses, people become disinhibited and report poor concentration and coordination. A healthy person metabolises alcohol at the rate of around one standard drink per hour. It is important to note that gender, physical build and health will influence an individual's blood alcohol levels after consuming alcohol. Women generally have a lower blood volume than men, so will tend to record a higher blood alcohol level than males who have consumed the same amount of alcohol.

The National Health and Medical Research Council (NHMRC) (2020) released comprehensive guidelines on ways to reduce harm associated with alcohol consumption. To understand these guidelines, there is a need to understand the concept of the Australian 'standard drink'. This concept was developed to help drinkers monitor their alcohol consumption and help simplify communication about the amounts of alcohol that it is safe to drink.

In Australia, a 'standard drink' refers to a drink containing 10 grams of alcohol, and equates to:

- schooner of light beer (425 mL)
- 'middy' or 'pot' of full strength beer (285 mL)
- small glass of wine or sparkling wine (100 mL) (note that some red wines have a higher alcohol content)
- glass of fortified wine (60 mL)
- nip of spirits (30 mL).

These drink sizes are illustrated in figure 10.4.

| FIGURE 10.4 | What is a standard drink? |

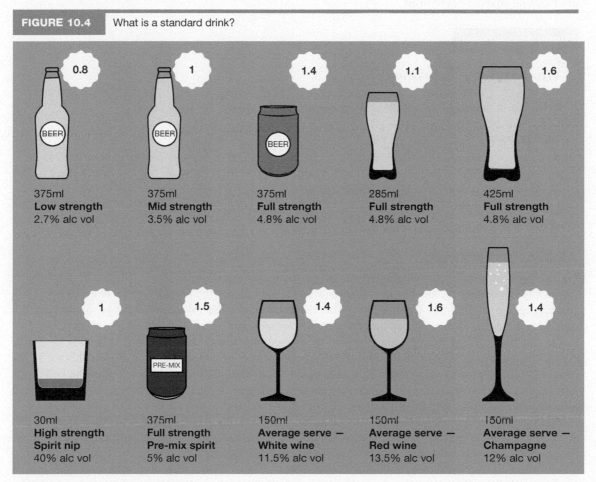

Source: NSW Ministry of Health (2018).

According to the NHMRC (2020) guidelines for healthy men and women:

- *Guideline 1:* To reduce the risk of harm from alcohol-related disease or injury, healthy men and women should drink no more than 10 standard drinks a week and no more than 4 standard drinks on any one day. The less you drink, the lower your risk of harm from alcohol.
- *Guideline 2:* To reduce the risk of injury and other harms to health, children and people under 18 years of age should not drink alcohol.
- *Guideline 3*: To prevent harm from alcohol to their unborn child, women who are pregnant or planning a pregnancy should not drink alcohol.

For women who are breastfeeding, not drinking alcohol is safest for their baby.

The full current version of the guidelines can be found on the NHMRC website at www.nhmrc.gov.au.

The physiological and pharmacokinetic effects of alcohol are influenced by factors, such as gender, body weight and the rate and amount of alcohol consumed. To reach the same blood level concentration, a greater amount of alcohol will generally be required by a heavier person than someone of lower body weight. There is little difference in associated risk for men and women at lower levels of drinking; at increased levels of consumption; however, women place themselves at significantly higher risk than men of alcohol-related disease. Men, on the other hand, have a greater incidence of alcohol-related injuries. The highest risk group for alcohol-related injuries are individuals aged 15–24 years. This is primarily due to traffic accidents where alcohol is involved.

For people under the age of 18, the NHMRC (2020) guidelines advise that the safest option is not to drink alcohol at all. This is especially important for people under 15. Women who are pregnant or breastfeeding are likewise advised not to drink.

UPON REFLECTION

What is 'safe' drinking?

The NHMRC (2020) has set guidelines to reduce the risks of drinking; however, they clearly state that there is no level of drinking alcohol that can be guaranteed to be completely safe.

QUESTIONS

1. Do you feel that there are 'safe levels' of alcohol consumption? Can these guidelines be applied to all Australians? Explain your reasons.
2. Other than the safe drinking guidelines set by the NRMRC, how else can we encourage people to drink at less harmful levels?

Alcohol withdrawal

One complication of excessive alcohol use over time is the risk of withdrawal. When a person who is physically dependent on alcohol ceases their drinking or reduces their intake, there is a risk they will experience the symptoms of withdrawal. The cessation of the use of alcohol may be unplanned, for example, if the person has been admitted to hospital for treatment of an acute illness or injury.

The Australian *Guidelines for the treatment of alcohol problems* (Haber et al., 2021) include evidence-based information to support health professionals in managing people at risk of alcohol withdrawal. The onset of alcohol withdrawal symptoms is most likely to occur in the first 6–24 hours after the last drink, although drinkers with a heavy dependence may experience symptoms of withdrawal when their blood alcohol level indicates they have consumed alcohol more recently.

The use of an alcohol withdrawal scale, such as the Clinical Institute Withdrawal Assessment for Alcohol (CIWA-Ar) scale, is the most reliable way to monitor the severity and progression of withdrawal symptoms. Severe, untreated alcohol withdrawal is a life-threatening condition.

Early identification of the possibility of withdrawal is the key to providing effective care. Health professionals are advised not to rule out the risk of alcohol withdrawal simply by the appearance of the person. While social stigma and stereotypes may suggest a person who is withdrawing from alcohol has a particular appearance, in reality any person who consumes alcohol regularly may experience symptoms of withdrawal. For this reason, a routine and comprehensive substance use history should be obtained from all people.

The information may be obtained by self-report, collateral sources of information and clinical examination.

Indicators of risk of alcohol withdrawal include:
- alcohol consumption pattern of eight or more standard drinks per day (higher consumption is associated with greater risk)
- history of withdrawal symptoms, such as tremor, nausea or anxiety, on awakening that are relieved by consuming alcohol
- past history of severe withdrawal including seizures or delirium tremens
- comorbid biomedical conditions including epilepsy, liver disease, infection, head injury, pain malnutrition
- comorbid mental health issues such as anxiety, depression or psychosis
- other substance use.

By identifying those at risk early, the heath professional may provide early interventions and strategies that have been demonstrated to improve health outcomes.

Complications of withdrawal

Most people will experience mild symptoms when withdrawing from alcohol. The following early symptoms of alcohol withdrawal are classified as 'minor'.
- Coarse tremor of the hands, tongue or eyelids
- Nausea, abdominal discomfort and loss of appetite
- Paroxysmal sweats
- Tachycardia
- Insomnia
- Irritability

If unaddressed, however, these symptoms can develop into more serious or 'moderate' symptoms, such as:
- disorientation
- confusion
- perceptual disturbance (most commonly visual hallucinations), 'seeing things', possibly insects or spiders
- marked tachycardia
- profuse sweating and flushed appearance.

If these symptoms are left untreated, withdrawal can progress to very serious **delirium tremens** (DTs) and other complications of alcohol withdrawal.

These complications are related to the CNS being in a state of hyper-excitement. There are three main complications of withdrawal that health professionals must observe or monitor. These include:
1. *seizures* — these generally occur 6–48 hours after the last drink
2. *delirium* — the DTs are characterised by confusion, disorientation, psychomotor agitation, seizure, coma and eventual death
3. *hallucinations* — these perceptual disturbances may be visual, tactile or auditory and may be accompanied by paranoid ideation and/or abnormal effects, such as anxiety, agitation or **dysphoria**.

Such complications can be life threatening and the health professional must treat the situation as a medical emergency.

Individuals with a history of seizures should be reviewed and considered for inpatient treatment during initial withdrawal from alcohol, as seizures can become so severe that they warrant urgent medical treatment. As already noted, untreated acute alcohol withdrawal can be fatal.

Providing care

The care provided to a person who is withdrawing from alcohol will depend upon the specific symptoms the person is experiencing.

Mild withdrawal (including people with a CIWA-Ar score of <10) in people with low indicators of risk can be managed with supportive care in a destimulating environment. Most people in this state of mild withdrawal will not require medication to help to deal with the symptoms. Care provision would address the following.
- The ideal environment is quiet and calm, and lighting needs to be clear but not too bright.
- Health professionals are best to communicate in a quiet, reassuring and confident manner.
- Provide frequent reassurance and reorient the person to their environment as needed.
- Offer the person fluids and monitor their hydration.

- Continue to monitor using the CIWA-Ar or similar standardised withdrawal scale.
- For people who experience moderate withdrawal (CIWA-Ar >10), diazepam may be prescribed early in the withdrawal process according to local protocols. Although treatment protocols will vary, it is uncommon for diazepam to be prescribed for more than 2 to 6 days.
- Symptom relief may also include medications such as paracetamol for headaches, metoclopramide or prochlorperazine for nausea or vomiting and possibly loperamide for diarrhoea (NCETA Consortium, 2004).

Health professionals need to ensure that they provide this care with a non-judgemental attitude and encourage the person as much as possible.

Acute alcohol withdrawal

The following list offers some suggestions for the health professional who is providing care and treatment options for acute alcohol withdrawal. These suggestions are similar to those provided for mild withdrawal symptoms, but also involve a much closer monitoring of the person for signs of physical deterioration.

- Maintain a non-judgemental attitude — avoid implied or overt criticism.
- Speak with a calm, reassuring, quiet and unhurried voice.
- Use clear, straightforward communication strategies (e.g. avoid complex instructions and maintain eye contact).
- Ensure that the person is easily observed.
- Monitor vital signs closely — blood pressure, pulse, temperature and respiration.
- Ensure adequate hydration — may require intravenous fluids.
- Monitor effects and side effects of medication used to manage withdrawal.
- If appropriate, involve the person's family, partner or significant other in the planning and delivery of care.
- Manage the person in an area with good lighting and appropriate environmental cues (e.g. clocks that work, a calendar and natural light).

It is also important the health professional observes for the signs and symptoms of Wernicke's encephalopathy and Korsakoff's syndrome, which are described in the following.

Wernicke's encephalopathy and Korsakoff's syndrome

There are two conditions that can result in brain damage as a consequence of a lack of vitamin B1 (thiamine): **Wernicke's encephalopathy** and Korsakoff's syndrome. Heavy drinkers undergoing alcohol withdrawal need to be treated with **thiamine**. This is because people who are dependent upon alcohol are often deficient in nutrients, which can cause severe complications during alcohol withdrawal. Of particular importance are thiamine and folic acid. The thiamine deficiency can trigger the development of Wernicke's encephalopathy.

Vitamin B1 is an essential nutrient required by all tissues within the body, including the brain (Gupta et al., 2012). A reduction in the availability of thiamine to the brains of individuals who are chronic consumers of alcohol can result in brain damage or even death.

Wernicke's encephalopathy is a short-term but severe condition, while Korsakoff's syndrome is a more debilitating long-term condition. Wernicke's encephalopathy causes damage to the lower parts of the brain, namely the thalamus and hypothalamus, and is completely reversible with treatment. Korsakoff's syndrome, also known as Korsakoff's psychosis, affects areas of the brain associated with memory. There is only a 20 per cent recovery rate among individuals with Korsakoff's syndrome (Thomson et al., 2012).

Symptoms of Wernicke's encephalopathy

Wernicke's encephalopathy can seriously complicate the alcohol withdrawal process and is characterised by:

- *confusion* — global memory impairment
- *ataxia* — most notably a wide gait
- *vision changes* — abnormal eye movement, most notably nystagmus.

It is important to note that not all people will exhibit all three of these signs and symptoms. Indeed, health professionals working with people with alcohol-use disorders need to be aware that Wernicke's encephalopathy may be present even if the person presents with only one or two of the symptoms (Lough, 2012). Providing care to these individuals may be challenging for health professionals; the person may present as intoxicated, dishevelled, malodorous or abusive. However, if left untreated, Wernicke's encephalopathy may progress to Korsakoff's psychosis, which can result in permanent cognitive damage (Lough, 2012; Thomson et al., 2012).

Caring for the person with Wernicke's encephalopathy

Wernicke's encephalopathy can be prevented in heavy alcohol users by providing balanced nutritional intake and the early routine use of thiamine in all people who present for treatment. The condition responds rapidly to large doses of thiamine, which is known to be useful in preventing the progression to Korsakoff's syndrome. All people presenting with alcohol withdrawal should routinely receive thiamine as per local treatment protocols. Initially, thiamine should be given intramuscularly or intravenously (Lough, 2012; Thomson et al., 2012). Thiamine should be administered before giving glucose to malnourished people (Sinha et al., 2019).

Symptoms of Korsakoff's syndrome

Korsakoff's syndrome is a preventable memory disorder that can emerge (though not always) as a result of Wernicke's encephalopathy. The main symptom — memory loss — results from damage to the areas of the brain associated with memory. Symptoms include:

- inability to form new memories
- difficulty gaining new information and skills
- memory impairment, which can be severe
- fabrication of stories (confabulation)
- seeing or hearing things that are not really there (hallucinations).

People with Korsakoff's syndrome may also exhibit a change in personality. They may demonstrate a lack of interest and concern for people and things around them or they may become overly talkative and repetitive in their behaviour. Their sense of responsibility may diminish and they will have difficulty initiating good behaviour (Thomson et al., 2012).

This section outlined the major issues related to the use of alcohol. These include the signs and symptoms experienced by people who are withdrawing from alcohol and the importance of health professionals monitoring these signs and symptoms. Acute alcohol withdrawal is a potentially life-threatening condition and it is important that all health professionals are aware of the best-evidence care required to support a person through this difficult time. The next section outlines the major issues related to the use of amphetamines.

Amphetamines

Amphetamines are widely used illicit substances in Australia (see figure 10.1). Amphetamines are CNS stimulants that stimulate dopaminergic, serotonergic and noradrenergic activity, giving the user a euphoric sense of wellbeing and confidence. In intoxication, a person also has increased physical and cognitive performance, increased talkativeness, heightened sexuality, teeth grinding, as well as reduced appetite and need for sleep (Paulus & Stewart, 2020). Most street amphetamines available in Australia are methamphetamine-based. Four types of methamphetamine are broadly available:

1. *crystal* — looks like crushed ice (smoked, snorted, swallowed or injected)
2. *powder* — looks like white or coloured powder (injected, snorted or swallowed)
3. *pills* — look like prescription pills (swallowed)
4. *base* — looks like gluggy paste (smoked, snorted, swallowed or injected).

Trends in the use of methamphetamine and amphetamine use in Australia show a reduction in recent methamphetamine use by young people. Crystal methamphetamine is most commonly used form of the drug (AIHW, 2020).

The physical signs of intoxication from stimulants include pupil dilation, tachycardia, hypertension, increased respiratory rate and increased body temperature. If the level of ingestion is high, seizures and cardiovascular collapse can occur. The use of amphetamines is associated with a range of physical and psychological problems.

The route of administration contributes to some of the physiological risks for people who use amphetamines. For people who inject, there are risks of bloodborne viruses, abscesses, infected injection sites and emboli related to the injection of undissolved contaminants. People who snort amphetamines risk damaging the mucosa and surrounding tissues of the nose (e.g. damage to the septum). For people who smoke amphetamines, there are risks of irritation to the airways leading to sore throat, blood in the sputum and exacerbation of asthma in those who are susceptible. People who swallow amphetamines have fewer identifiable risks related to the mode of administration, although the delay in intoxication may lead people to increase their dose. People who choose 'shelving' or 'shafting', which involves placing the substance in the anus or the vagina, may irritate the mucosa (NCETA Consortium, 2004).

Other physical effects of using amphetamines include, but are not limited to:

- severe hypertension, which can lead to cerebrovascular and cardiovascular accidents, seizures, coma and death
- psychological sequelae, including dysphoria, depression, delirium, psychosis, anxiety, sleep disorders and sexual dysfunction (Rincon, 2012).

When health professionals are working with pregnant women who are using amphetamines (or other substances), they need to refer to their state's relevant clinical guidelines (Centre for Population Health, 2014). If your state has not implemented guidelines, refer to the *National clinical guidelines for the management of drug use during pregnancy, birth and the early development years of the newborn* (Bell & Ali, 2006), which are available online. There are numerous clinical guidelines available in Australia pertaining to methamphetamine use disorder in different settings (Roche et al., 2019). Clinical guidelines can be found at:

- National guidelines: www.health.gov.au/resources/pregnancy-care-guidelines/part-c-lifestyle-considerations/substance-use
- New South Wales guidelines: www1.health.nsw.gov.au/pds/ActivePDSDocuments/GL2014_022.pdf
- Queensland guidelines: www.health.qld.gov.au/__data/assets/pdf_file/0023/140738/g-psumat.pdf
- Victoria clinical guidance: www.bettersafercare.vic.gov.au/resources/clinical-guidance/maternity-and-newborn/substance-use-during-pregnancy-care-of-the-mother-and-newborn
- South Australia guidelines: www.sahealth.sa.gov.au/wps/wcm/connect/public+content/sa+health+internet/resources/policies/substance+use+in+pregnancy+-+sa+perinatal+practice+guidelines.

Benzodiazepines

Benzodiazepines are also known as tranquillisers, sometimes referred to as 'benzos'. They are most often prescribed by doctors to relieve stress and anxiety, relax muscles and help a person to sleep. Benzodiazepines are CNS depressants — they work by slowing down the activity of the CNS. There are many benzodiazepines on the market and a list is provided in table 10.4. Benzodiazepines possess variable but significant addiction potential.

TABLE 10.4 Common benzodiazepines used in Australia

Generic name	Common trade names
Alprazolam	Xanax®, Kalma®, Alprax®
Bromazepam	Lexotan®
Clobazam	Frisium®
Clonazepam	Rivotril®, Paxam®
Diazepam	Valium®, Ducene®, Valpam®, Antenex®, Ranzepam®
Flunitrazepam	Hypnodorm® — previously Rohypnol®
Lorazepam	Ativan®
Midazolam	Hypnovel®
Nitrazepam	Mogadon®, Alodorm®
Oxazepam	Serepax®, Murelax®, Alepam®
Temazepam	Normison®, Temaze®, Temtabs®, Euhypnos®
Triazolam	Halcion®
Zolpidem	Stilnox®, Dormizol®, Somidem®, Stildem®, Zolpibell® — (a 'Z drug'. A hypnotic with similarities to benzodiazepines)
Zopiclone	Imovane®, Imoclone®, Imrest®, (a 'Z drug'. A hypnotic with similarities to benzodiazepines)

Risks associated with benzodiazepine use include overdose, either alone or in combination with other substances, especially other CNS depressants, including alcohol and opioids. Complications with overdose include respiratory depression. Benzodiazepine overdose alone is often not life threatening. The risk of developing benzodiazepine dependence is increased when benzodiazepines are used for periods exceeding one month, particularly at high doses and benzodiazepines with a shorter **half-life**. The risk of dependence continues to increase with the duration of treatment, even at low doses. While there is significant individual variability, it is estimated that about a third of people who have been taking benzodiazepines over a long period will have significant difficulties reducing their dose or stopping. For this reason, benzodiazepines are viewed as highly addictive.

The delay of onset of benzodiazepine withdrawal will vary considerably depending on the half-life of the benzodiazepine used and may commence one to ten days or more after the last dose. The withdrawal syndrome varies greatly and may include symptoms that resemble alcohol withdrawal, including anxiety, dysphoria, irritability, insomnia, nightmares, sweating, memory impairment, hallucinations, hypertension, tachycardia, psychosis, tremors and seizures (Therapeutic Guidelines Limited, 2013).

As with alcohol withdrawal, severe untreated withdrawal from benzodiazepines can be life threatening. People withdrawing from benzodiazepines will require a medical review to assess the need for inpatient treatment and the process of withdrawal supervised by a treating team.

Cannabis

Cannabis is the most widely used illicit drug in Australia, although legislation exists that allows for the use of medicinal cannabis (Commonwealth of Australia, 2016).

Cannabis is commonly available in three forms — **marijuana**, hashish and hash oil. Community attitudes to the use of cannabis are changing in many countries, which is reflected in legislation changes in a number of jurisdictions. It is clear that cannabis use, as with all substances, comes with some risks, but community attitudes are leaning towards individuals choosing whether or not they wish to take the risk, rather than imposing criminal penalties.

Epidemiological studies have concluded that cannabis use is associated with a number of negative outcomes, including risk of dependence, increased risk of psychosis and cognitive deficits and with increased risk of motor vehicle accidents (Hall, 2015) and lung disorders (Schwartz, 2018). Synthetic cannabinoids have also been sold in Australia under a range of brand names including Kronic and Spice. The cannabis that is commonly smoked in Australia comes from the plant *Cannabis sativa*. Over 480 compounds have been isolated in cannabis, including over 100 **cannabinoids**. The main cannabinoid responsible for the cannabis 'high' is known as delta-9-tetrahydrocannabinol or THC. The subjective perception of cannabis intoxication may continue for three to five hours following use.

The psychoactive effects of cannabis are difficult to classify. Cannabis can possess some CNS depressant qualities and, in higher doses, has some hallucinogenic properties. These properties distort perception of time, distance and some sensory input.

It is important to note that a positive urine drug screen result for cannabis does not necessarily indicate *recent* use. This is because cannabis metabolites are stored in fat cells; chronic cannabis users may continue to show positive urine screen results for around six weeks after cessation.

In intoxication, people may become talkative or introspective. Many people refer to increased hunger (the 'munchies') after using cannabis. External signs of intoxication may include bloodshot eyes and changes in behaviour as previously described.

Cannabis and mental health

The longer-term effects of cannabis use on the mental health of a person have been debated in the literature over many years (Testai et al., 2022), but the synthesis of information is now pointing towards the view that cannabis causes psychosis and schizophrenia in vulnerable individuals (Lynch et al., 2012). Cannabis use is also associated with depression and suicidality, but the evidence is not always consistent (Halladay et al., 2020). Heavy cannabis use is associated with anxiety disorders, but it is not clear whether a true causal relationship exists (Shalit & Lev-Ran, 2020). Smoking cannabis can lead to mild cognitive impairments, reduced sperm count, respiratory diseases, such as chronic bronchitis, and the development of several cancers (NCETA Consortium, 2004). The risk of cancer is exacerbated by the common practice of combining tobacco (spin) with cannabis prior to smoking.

The safety of cannabis use in pregnancy has not been established (Gerardin et al., 2011) though the use of cannabis during pregnancy is associated with increased odds of moderate to severe nausea (Metz et al., 2022), low birth weight and NICU admission (Joseph-Lemon et al., 2022). Evidence is also accumulating that prenatal exposure to cannabis may lead to enduring cognitive and emotional problems for offspring (Testai et al., 2022).

Breastfeeding mothers are advised not to use cannabis as it is passed through the breast milk to the baby.

Cannabis withdrawal

Cannabis withdrawal syndrome is usually a mildly uncomfortable experience for people. Gorelick and colleagues (2012) evaluated the diagnostic criteria in the DSM-5 relating to the symptoms of cannabis withdrawal:

- irritability, anger and aggression
- anxiety
- reduced appetite
- restlessness
- sleep disturbance including unusual dreams
- dysphoria/depressed mood.
   Physical symptoms that occur less frequently can include:
- chills
- tremor
- stomach pain or discomfort
- night sweats.

Cannabis withdrawal is a self-limiting syndrome. Health professionals can provide reassurance to people that these symptoms tend to last for only one or two weeks. Assisting people in managing individual symptoms may be beneficial.

Not using cannabis at all is best, particularly for young people where the risk of harm is greatest. For people who choose to continue to use cannabis, it is important to offer harm minimisation information, such as the following.

- Where possible, avoid using large amounts or high-potency cannabis.
- Cannabis affects reaction times; avoid driving, operating machinery or risky behaviours while intoxicated.
- Smoking cannabis introduces an additional risk of harm when compared to ingesting or vaping.
- For people who smoke cannabis, avoid mixing it with tobacco as it increases the risk of cancer and reinforces dependence.
- Avoid smoking from a bong that isn't cleaned regularly.
- Avoid smoking cannabis from an aluminium foil cone.
- Avoid smoking cannabis from a bong that uses a garden hose or other plastic for the stem that holds the cone because toxins may be released when plastic is heated.
- Avoid smoking a cone in one large 'hit' and holding it in; this doesn't increase the blood level of THC, but it does increase the risk of harm by allowing tars and other chemicals contact with deeper parts of the lungs for longer periods.
- For people who are heavily dependent on cannabis, avoid using cannabis during the day and have some cannabis-free days; this may allow the person to re-instate some other activities.
- Synthetic cannabis use is associated with a risk of harm and should be avoided.

Medicinal cannabis

The legal status of cannabis for recreational and medicinal purposes is undergoing significant change in many jurisdictions. Some news reports of cannabis treatments for a range of disorders have been misleading due to lack of detail and context. Clinicians, researchers and consumers have expressed a range of opinions and quote diverse sources of evidence in support of and in opposition to the use of **medicinal cannabis** for various disorders (O'Brien, 2019). Several cannabinoid preparations (CBD and/or THC extracts, cannabis sativa, nabilone and dronabinol) have been studied in relation to treating a number of disorders (Campbell et al., 2019). The Australian Therapeutic Goods Administration (TGA) describes medicinal cannabis as experimental (with the exception of nabiximols for spasticity in multiple sclerosis and cannabidiol for seizures associated with specific conditions) and are not registered medicines in Australia.

Approval for the prescription of cannabinoids can be provided to any registered medical doctor by the TGA under the Special Access Scheme for conditions including refractory paediatric epilepsy, neuropathic pain and spasticity from neurological conditions (www.tga.gov.au/news/blog/introduction-medicinal-cannabis-regulation-australia).

For most conditions, more research is required in order to establish the comparative efficacy and safety of cannabinoids in comparison with other treatments (Abrams, 2018; Stockings et al., 2018).

Cocaine

Cocaine is a potent CNS stimulant. Derived from the coca plant, most cocaine originates from South America. For this reason, cocaine is a relatively expensive substance in Australia, so is less commonly used. It has a shorter duration of 'high' than other potent psychostimulants. Cocaine powder is snorted or sometimes injected, while freebase or 'crack' cocaine is smoked. In large doses, cocaine can cause myriad unwanted effects, including agitation, anxiety, psychosis, aggression, delirium, convulsions, dizziness, angina, respiratory failure, elevated blood pressure, stroke, hyperthermia and myocardial infarction (NCETA Consortium, 2004).

Ecstasy

Ecstasy (3,4-methylenedioxymethamphetamine) or MDMA is also known as 'E', 'eccies' or Molly. It is a 'designer' methamphetamine with both stimulant and hallucinogenic properties. It is an empathogen. An estimated 2.5 per cent of the Australian population aged over 13 years reported using ecstasy in 2016, with people in their 20s more likely to report using ecstasy than other age groups. Ecstasy is used by many people infrequently — once or twice per year (AIHW, 2017).

Ecstasy is usually sold in tablet form. Historically, many tablets sold as ecstasy contained little or no MDMA, though purity appears to be increasing. Swallowing pills remained the most common form of ecstasy use (Peacock et al., 2019). Long-term use of MDMA can contribute to problems, such as depression, insomnia, headaches, teeth grinding and hyperthermia. Furthermore, the risk of **hyponatraemia** following MDMA use is heightened when people consume excessive quantities of water.

People need to be informed of the recommendation to drink water regularly if using MDMA, but not in excess of 500 mL/hr. People who choose to use MDMA also need to be warned of the potentially fatal risk of serotonin syndrome associated with using large amounts of MDMA or using other serotonergic substances and medicines (e.g. antidepressants and tramadol) (Makunts et al., 2022). Interest is developing around research into the therapeutic uses of MDMA in conjunction with psychotherapy in the treatment of **post-traumatic stress disorder (PTSD)**. Results from the small number of controlled studies conducted to date are promising and research continues (Smith et al., 2022).

Hallucinogens and GHB

As already noted, hallucinogens typically distort a person's perceptions. Types of hallucinogens include:
- psychedelics
  - lysergic acid diethylamide (LSD, acid), a potent hallucinogen with intoxicating effects lasting 8–12 hours
  - magic mushrooms (gold tops, mushies) containing psilocybin infused into a 'tea'. Dosing is variable and psychedelic effects continue for four hours
  - mescaline (peyote) and synthetic mimetics have similar effects to LSD
  - DMT — a short-acting, plant-based psychedelic more commonly available as a synthesised mimetic
- delirients — datura (angels' trumpet) flower chopped and infused into a 'tea'. Contains chemicals including atropine and scopolamine
- dissociatives
  - ketamine (Special-K) dissociative anaesthetic properties
  - gamma hydroxybutyrate (GHB, fantasy, liquid ecstasy, GBH) dissociative anaesthetic properties
  - phencyclidine (PCP, angel dust) has dissociative anaesthetic properties (also used as pesticide and disinfectant)
  - nitrous oxide (laughing gas, 'nangs').

Intoxication with a hallucinogenic drug is usually characterised by mild signs of autonomic arousal, such as tachycardia and pupillary dilation. Protecting the person from harm and 'talking them down' is usually sufficient when providing care to the intoxicated person. Dependence is not common with hallucinogenic drugs. While tolerance to the psychotropic effect of hallucinogens does occur, no withdrawal syndrome is reported (APA, 2013). Ketamine has been studied as a treatment for post-traumatic stress disorder both alone and as an adjunctive treatment along with psychotherapy. So far, there is insufficient evidence to confidently recommend ketamine as a treatment for PTSD, but research continues (Varker et al., 2021).

Opiates and opioids

Although the term opiate is often used interchangeably with **opioid**, the term **opiate** actually denotes the natural alkaloids found in the resin of the opium poppy. This group of drugs includes opium, morphine, heroin and codeine. In contrast, an opioid is a chemical that works by binding to opioid receptors, which are found principally in the CNS, peripheral nervous system and the gastrointestinal tract. The receptors in these systems mediate both the beneficial effects and the side effects of opioids.

Opioids are sometimes referred to as narcotics (though the term narcotic is sometimes used as a general term to describe illegal substances of abuse). They are a group of drugs that are used legally and very effectively as analgesics to relieve pain. They are also used illicitly for the relaxing or 'good' feeling they give the user. Pethidine and methadone are examples of synthetic compounds that work in a similar way as morphine on opioid receptors. Other opiates, such as morphine, heroin and codeine, come in a variety of forms, including powder, capsules, tablets, syrups, solutions and suppositories.

Dependence on prescribed narcotics has recently developed into a serious public health issue (Bolliger & Stevens, 2019). As already noted, in the health care setting, it is important that professionals view any substance use as a health issue and provide appropriate interventions to reduce harm to the individual and the community.

Heroin

Heroin is processed from the same raw gum opium that can produce morphine, codeine or thebaine; it is a product of morphine. Heroin is known on the streets as 'hammer', 'harry', 'H', 'junk', 'gear' and 'smack'. It can be a white or brownish powder with a bitter taste that is usually dissolved in water and then injected. Most street preparations of heroin are diluted or 'cut' with other substances such as sugar or quinine. Heroin can be injected, snorted, smoked, eaten or dissolved in a drink. Health professionals may also hear those who use heroin talk about the equipment they need. The most common is a needle and syringe — also known as a 'fit'.

The risks of using heroin include:

- high risk of addiction
- mood swings
- depression
- menstrual irregularity and infertility in women
- loss of sex drive in men
- anxiety disorders
- chronic constipation
- infection at the site of injections
- HIV and hepatitis infections through needle sharing
- non-fatal overdose
- death from overdose (Rastegar & Walley, 2013).

People who use heroin will begin to withdraw 8–12 hours after their last dose. The symptoms of acute withdrawal can last for five days, while cravings may continue considerably longer. Symptoms include sweating, dilated pupils, goose bumps, nausea, cramps and cravings (see table 10.5). Withdrawal from heroin can be painful and very difficult for the person to manage, but it is not life threatening. Strategies for supporting the person who is withdrawing from an opiate are outlined in the next section.

TABLE 10.5 **Opioid withdrawal symptoms**

Subjective symptoms	Objective signs
Drug craving	Dilated pupils
Abdominal discomfort and cramps	Sweating
Nausea	Tremor
Aching muscles and joints	Diarrhoea
Appetite loss	Rhinorrhea (runny nose)
Hot and cold flushes	Vomiting

Fatigue	Tachycardia (increased heart rate)
Restlessness	Hypertension
Irritability	Frequent yawning
Low mood	Lacrimation (tears) Sneezing Pyrexia (high temperature)

Prescription opioids

In recent years, there has been increasing discussion about people who have developed dependencies on medications that have been prescribed for pain by authorised health professionals (e.g. Lustman et al., 2011). This discussion has encompassed the deaths of a number of celebrities, including the artist Prince, from accidental overdoses of prescription medications. Sales of oxycodone exceeded US$35 billion between 1996 and 2017. Multi-billion-dollar class action lawsuits in the United States have been instigated by people who claim to have developed a dependence on these opioid analgesics (Allman, 2019).

As noted, narcotics are a group of drugs that can be legally prescribed and are effective analgesics to relieve pain. Chronic pain can be debilitating as it is pain that persists over a long period of time, often unrelentingly. Examples of chronic pain include headache, lower back pain, cancer pain, arthritis pain, inflammatory bowel disease, neurogenic pain resulting from damage to the peripheral nerves or CNS and psychogenic pain, which has no identifiable cause. PRN (as needed) use of narcotics by people with chronic pain can provide much-needed relief and improve their quality of life.

Some individuals who become dependent on opioids will go from health professional to health professional, complaining of pain and requesting more medication as the severity of their dependence increases. Pejorative terms, such as 'doctor shopping' and 'drug seeking' are unhelpful and unprofessional. These terms contribute to self-stigma and reduce the likelihood an individual will seek appropriate treatment for their substance use disorder and associated tolerance issues.

It is recommended that health professionals monitor for behaviours that may suggest such a dependency, while also ensuring that they do not react punitively. It is important to remember that prescription drug dependencies are the same as other substance dependencies and the person needs to be treated without judgement. Providing information about the health risks, including accidental death from **polypharmacy** issues or overdose, can also be provided.

Caring for the person with an opioid dependence

Providing acute pain relief (e.g. following trauma or surgery) for people who have an existing dependence on opioids is complex and consultation with pain management experts is recommended. As with regular alcohol consumption, the sudden cessation of an illicit opiate by a person may occur for a number of reasons, including unexpected hospital admission. Although opiate withdrawal is not a life-threatening or particularly hazardous process, it can nevertheless be an extremely distressing experience for the person. As a result, there is a need to minimise the impact of withdrawal and provide substitute alternatives to illicit narcotics. Taking a proactive approach to the provision of care and treatment options for the person with a dependence will:

- prevent the experience of unpleasant withdrawal symptoms
- increase the likelihood of establishing the person's participation in care and treatment interventions; if the person is pre-occupied and concerned about withdrawal symptoms, they are less likely to collaborate
- reduce the personal, health and social risks associated with the use of illicit drugs; for instance, quantities of opiates used are controlled, the need for the person to engage in antisocial or potentially criminal behaviour is avoided
- provide opportunities for harm reduction and physical and mental health promotion.

Methadone has historically been the medication of choice for the short-term care and treatment provided to people who are experiencing opiate withdrawal.

Methadone

Methadone is an opioid agonist that is used as an opiate substitute. It has a long half-life, ranging from 14 to 72 hours, and does not provide the 'rush' that heroin gives. It is itself addictive and can be lethal in overdose or when taken in combination with other opiates, benzodiazepines or alcohol. Methadone is one of several medications prescribed in the community as a substitute for heroin or other opiates to reduce the harm associated with the use of illicit opiates.

Methadone usually comes in syrup form, but it is also available in tablet form (Physeptone®) as an **analgesic**. For individuals to be prescribed methadone, they must meet the criteria for dependence, which are outlined in the National Guidelines for Medication-assisted Treatment of Opioid Dependence (Gowing et al., 2014). There are strict controls governing the prescribing of methadone, and the prescriber must be authorised.

Treatment with methadone and other opioid replacement therapies has a number of benefits. First, it gives the person some stability in their lives; they are no longer driven by their dependence and can be sure their needs will be met. As methadone is an oral preparation, there is no risk of the person acquiring a bloodborne disease or condition, such as HIV/AIDS or hepatitis C as well as a reduced risk of a person who already has a bloodborne virus from spreading the infection to others. It is low cost for the person, which reduces the crime associated with continued use of heroin. Perhaps best of all, the methadone program provides an opportunity for the health professional to monitor the person for health issues each time the person picks up their dose.

Only a small proportion of those who are prescribed methadone in a maintenance program go on to reduce the dose completely. Methadone provides an excellent means by which the social issues that are associated with opioid dependence or addiction can be managed.

Other medications that can be prescribed for care and treatment of opioid dependence include:
- buprenorphine (Subutex® sublingual tablets) (Bivudal® and Sublocade® depot preparations)
- buprenorphine/naloxone combination (Suboxone® sublingual film).

Buprenorphine is described here in more detail.

Buprenorphine

Buprenorphine is another maintenance replacement drug that acts to halt the symptoms of opioid withdrawal. It comes in a tablet form and is dissolved under the tongue. Many people prefer buprenorphine over methadone as it provides them with more freedom. This is because buprenorphine may be taken every two to three days, rather than daily. However, other people dislike buprenorphine for subjective reasons, including the taste, and so prefer methadone.

Buprenorphine is a partial agonist/antagonist, giving it the additional benefit that it is safer than methadone in overdose. As such, it has a lower risk of death by accident or suicide. A long-acting depot formulation of buprenorphine has been released in Australia for the management of opioid dependence. The preparation is administered weekly or monthly by subcutaneous injection.

Buprenorphine is also available in combination with naloxone as a sublingual film. The addition of naloxone reduces the likelihood that the medication will be diverted (passed on to others to use). The naloxone is not absorbed sublingually, but if injected, would precipitate a rapid and powerful opioid withdrawal. Thus, the combination preparation increases the likelihood that the medication will be taken as prescribed.

When a person is dependent on opioids and seeks admission to a hospital, there is an immediate requirement to review the person's need for care and treatment for withdrawal. This will include reviewing their need for substitute opioids. Where a person who has been admitted to hospital is engaged in a treatment program, protocols must be followed to ascertain information from the prescriber about the person's medication, usual dose, time of last dose and takeaway doses dispensed. It is also important that the usual dosing agency is contacted and given information about dosing during the hospital stay. This communication is usually undertaken by the AOD team, medical officer or nurse practitioner (NCETA Consortium, 2004).

Naltrexone

Naltrexone is an opioid receptor antagonist used primarily in the management of alcohol and opioid dependence, particularly post-withdrawal, to increase the likelihood of sustained abstinence. It comes in the form of a tablet and works by blocking the opioid receptors in the brain and, therefore, blocking the effects of substances like heroin and other opioids. It can be prescribed to assist people to maintain abstinence from opioids following detoxification by preventing a 'high' from using heroin. There is a danger of naltrexone precipitating a severe opioid withdrawal if the individual has not been abstinent prior to dosing. It does not stop a person wanting to use, although it may reduce the cravings. Naltrexone is not addictive. In the past, there were media reports on naltrexone, often describing it as a 'miracle cure' for heroin dependence. However, most health professionals agree that the success of naltrexone treatment depends on multiple factors, including the person's particular situation, their level of commitment to change, and the involvement of a treatment team of multidisciplinary professionals.

Pain management

As already noted, people who experience chronic pain are prescribed narcotics to help them to manage that pain. Chronic pain is a debilitating condition and opioids provide an important means by which sufferers are able to participate meaningfully in life. Pain management is an important consideration for people who are dependent on opioids. Where available, a pain team needs to be consulted in conjunction with the drug and alcohol treatment team, as they will have developed a tolerance to the analgesic effects of opioids and may require significantly higher doses or combinations of analgesic medication to achieve adequate pain relief. The pain management plan needs to consider the future reduction and cessation of analgesic medication. It is vital that analgesia is not withheld from people because they are dependent on the medication, unless a decision is made by the multidisciplinary team due to immediate medical risks. It is also important to remember that if opioid analgesia is administered in inadequate amounts, or withdrawn too early, it can exacerbate behaviour that some health professionals may describe as 'drug seeking'.

Opioid withdrawal

As described in table 10.5, the symptoms of opioid withdrawal can be very unpleasant. However, they are rarely life threatening, except in cases of severe comorbid physical illness. Opioid withdrawal in pregnant women also places the foetus at risk and the neonate is likewise at risk of opioid withdrawal.

It is important that health professionals across Australia refer to local guidelines to review the recommended supportive therapies to manage symptoms of opioid withdrawal. Consultation with a drug and alcohol specialist is also recommended.

Tobacco

Nicotine, the addictive component of tobacco, is a mild CNS stimulant. Cigarettes, which contain tobacco, contain upward of 4000 chemicals, many of which are known to cause harm. Cigarettes contain at least 72 chemicals known to be harmful to humans (Morgan et al., 2017).

Of all the substances discussed in this chapter, tobacco will kill more people than any other (Australian Bureau of Statistics, 2012). Smoking contributes to one in every eight deaths in Australia (AIHW, 2018). The people who are still smoking today, despite years of public health campaigns educating people on the health risks associated with cigarettes, are arguably among the most heavily dependent substance users. A number of these people will have made several previous attempts to stop and it is important for health professionals to inform people that there are new options available that have demonstrated effectiveness.

In Australia, the national Quitline (13 78 48) provides excellent support and resources to help people to develop a plan and decide on a nicotine replacement.

Other options include those below; combined interventions are more successful than one intervention alone:

- nicotine replacement therapy (NRT), which is available over the counter in various forms, including patches, gum, inhalers, spray and lozenges (including mini-lozenges)
- online resources such as QuitCoach (www.quitcoach.org.au), My Quit Buddy app (www.health.gov.au/resources/apps-and-tools/my-quitbuddy-app).
- bupropion (Zyban®), which is available from a general practitioner by prescription (this is a medication that reduces the urge to smoke)
- varenicline tartrate (Champix®), which reduces the urge to smoke and also reduces the enjoyment the person experiences from smoking if a lapse occurs
- e-cigarettes containing nicotine (prescription required).

As with any harmful substance use, it is important to raise the issue with a non-judgemental approach (NSW Ministry of Health, 2021).

This section provided information about the different types of substances, licit and illicit, that are available in Australia. This includes a description of the effects of these substances and also the signs and symptoms a person may experience when they withdraw from those substances. In the next section, health professionals are informed about how they can conduct an assessment of a person's substance use. This includes an explanation of the different types of screening tools available.

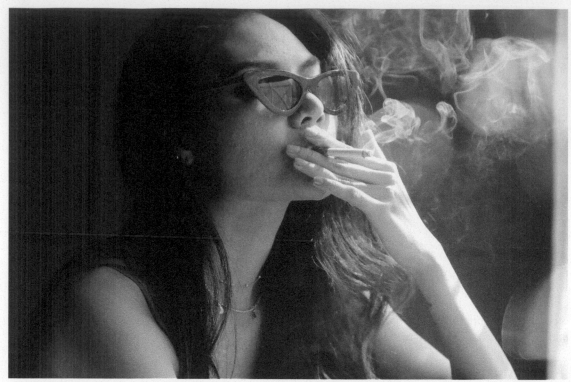

Of all the substances discussed in this chapter, tobacco will kill more people than any other.

Australia's plain packaging legislation is world first

Data modelling predicts that over a quarter of a million Australians will die from cancers directly attributable to smoking between 2020 and 2044 (Luo et al., 2022). Government agencies have implemented a number of public health campaigns to reduce smoking. Figure 10.5 illustrates the timing of the introduction of some major tobacco initiatives in relation to annual cigarette consumption in Australia.

The *Tobacco Plain Packaging Act 2011* requires that all tobacco products sold in Australia are in plain packaging. The legislation bans the use of logos, brand imagery, symbols, other images, colours and promotional text on tobacco product packaging. The packaging must be a standard drab dark brown colour in a matte finish. The only thing on the packs to distinguish one brand from another will be the brand and product name in a standard colour, position, font size and style. Cigarette packets are also required to display large health warnings.

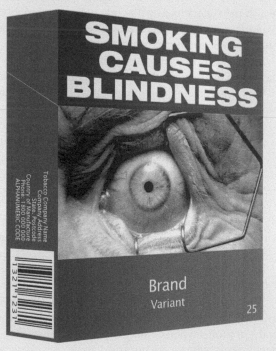

The plain packaging legislation aims to:

- reduce the attractiveness and appeal of tobacco products to consumers, particularly young people
- increase the noticeability and effectiveness of mandated health warnings
- reduce the ability of the retail packaging of tobacco products to mislead consumers about the harmful effects of smoking or using tobacco products.

These plain packaging laws will contribute to the Australian government's comprehensive package of efforts to reduce smoking rates as agreed by the Council of Australian Governments (COAG) in 2008. Figure 10.5 illustrates the timing of the introduction of some major tobacco initiatives in relation to annual cigarette consumption in Australia.

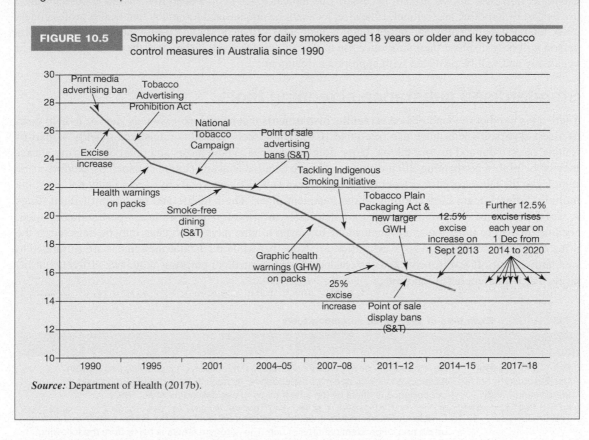

FIGURE 10.5 Smoking prevalence rates for daily smokers aged 18 years or older and key tobacco control measures in Australia since 1990

Source: Department of Health (2017b).

10.7 Assessment of substance use

LEARNING OBJECTIVE 10.7 Outline screening and assessment for substance use issues and disorders.

People can present to any health professional for help with a substance use problem; for instance, when they are intoxicated (e.g. in an emergency department) or experiencing symptoms of acute withdrawal. In circumstances such as these, it is important that the health professional undertake the following.

- Conduct an accurate and comprehensive assessment, including a substance use history.
  - Complete a full medical screen for physical health problems.
  - Conduct a risk assessment and, if indicated, a mental state exam.
- Provide short-term interventions to stabilise the presentation.
- Discuss ongoing issues related to substance use with the person.
- Assess the person's motivation and problem severity.
- Make a referral to an appropriate drug and alcohol service.

The majority of people with alcohol and drug-related problems, however, will present to health professionals for reasons that may not appear to be directly connected to their underlying alcohol or drug problem, for example, a mental illness, heart disease or trauma.

It is important for the health professional to recognise the condition and provide appropriate care and treatment. Indeed, it is recommended that all people are screened or assessed for their substance use, with a more in-depth assessment conducted as required. The rationale for this approach is that it will increase the likelihood of the identification of underlying substance use problems and will benefit the consumer by ensuring that:

- the care and treatment required for withdrawal or maintenance can be instigated; e.g. the prompt implementation of treatment for symptoms of withdrawal
- the appropriate care and treatment are provided, increasing the likelihood of the person participating and cooperating in the care and treatment for their comorbid health issue

- opportunities for health promotion and harm reduction interventions can be provided
- the person may be helped to gain insight into their behaviour and consequences and make informed choices regarding seeking further help to change their lifestyle.

As noted previously, a health professional may think a person does not 'look' like they have a substance use issue; however, 'looks' are not necessarily an indicator. All people need to be asked about substance use as part of a routine assessment. Likewise, it cannot be emphasised too much that health professionals must demonstrate empathy and adopt a non-judgemental attitude and non-confrontational approach. The person will only disclose their substance use to a health professional if they feel they will not be viewed negatively and will be provided with appropriate treatment.

Standardised substance screening tools

There are a number of standardised **screening instruments** that health professionals can use to help them to assess a person's substance use (see table 10.6). These tools can be administered quickly as part of routine assessment and history taking. Urine drug screens can aid diagnosis and point of care 'dip sticks' may be helpful in confirming illicit drug use. A more detailed analysis can be obtained by sending urine samples to the laboratory for screening. However, results will take several days and so may not assist the multidisciplinary team in developing initial treatment plans. The half-life and excretion of illicit drugs is variable; for instance, amphetamines are detectable in urine for up to 48 hours post-administration; cocaine for two to three days; and methadone for seven to nine days. Marijuana may be detected in the urine of heavy smokers up to six weeks after use. Note that while medical urine screens are calibrated to standardised cut-off levels, urine screens conducted for non-medical purposes may have different cut-off levels that will affect detection times.

TABLE 10.6   **Examples of substance screening tools**

Tool	Use
The AUDIT (Alcohol Use Disorders Identification Test)	Developed for use in primary care settings. It focuses on identifying people with hazardous drinking and mild dependence. Its sensitivity at picking up on mild dependence is offset by the time it takes to use (Saunders et al., 1993).
The CAGE	Simple and quick to use. It identifies dependent level use, but is less sensitive at picking up on non-dependent patterns of use. The acronym CAGE is taken from the following four questions asked to screen for alcohol-related problems. 1. Have you ever felt that you should Cut down on your drinking? 2. Have people Annoyed you by criticising your drinking? 3. Have you ever felt Guilty about your drinking? 4. Have you ever had a drink first thing in the morning to steady your nerves or get rid of a hangover (Eye-opener)?
The ASSIST	The drug quiz ASSIST (Alcohol, smoking and substance involvement screening test) is promoted by the World Health Organization for use in primary care settings to guide brief screening for a range of substances. The tool is available online at https://apps.who.int/iris/handle/10665/44320 and includes some guides for brief intervention.
The DAST (Drug Abuse Screening Test)	This test specifically does not include alcohol use. It is a 20-question self-test, also available online, that helps a person to become more aware of their patterns of substance use. However, the language in the DAST uses terms such as 'abuse', with which some respondents may be uncomfortable.
Severity of Dependence Scale (SDS)	The SDS was devised to provide a short, easily administered scale that can be used to measure the degree of dependence experienced by users of different types of drugs. The SDS contains five items, all of which are explicitly concerned with psychological components of dependence. These items are specifically concerned with impaired control over drug taking and with preoccupation and anxieties about drug use.

Source: Adapted from Babor et al. (2007); Humeniuk et al. (2018).

The interpretation of urine screen results, particularly for cannabis, can be a complex issue. Consulting a drug and alcohol specialist to assist in interpreting results is recommended where possible.

Once the health professional has identified that a substance use issue is likely, a more comprehensive alcohol or drug history needs to be obtained, as this will help identify whether the person may benefit from a specialist assessment and referral. Most health services in Australia utilise standardised substance assessment forms that begin by asking questions about legal substances, such as tobacco, alcohol and prescribed medications. These forms will generally come with instructions so that all health professionals are able to provide them to a client. Many health services in Australia have established **drug and alcohol consultation liaison** services. These services are similar to the mental health consultation liaison services that are described at length in the chapter that looks at mental health service delivery. They provide a means by which health professionals can access specialist drug and alcohol workers to assist them in providing care and treatment to people with a substance use issue.

Assessment of alcohol and drug use

Alcohol and drug use history taking includes comprehensive assessments that cover the substance use, general health, mental health and risk of the patient. Alcohol and drug history taking is part of a comprehensive assessment, which will include a general medical exam, mental state exam, and a thorough risk assessment.

Health professionals must ensure that they document this information in the clinical records for future reference. The information can also be used to correlate improvement or deterioration in the client's symptoms as time goes by. If the health professional is using specific screening tools, they are to be completed only as an accompaniment to the clinical interview and medical exam. The key elements of a detailed substance use history include:

- substance of choice (e.g. which substance does the person primarily seek/crave; what happens when this substance is not available)
- amounts used
- when did the person last use (including amount used; also question historical information like frequency and duration)
- route of administration (e.g. oral, smoked, nasal, intravenous) or in the case of alcohol, number of standard drinks per day
- previous experience of substance withdrawal, in particular, whether the person has any history of seizures or delirium tremens
- signs of any symptoms of dependence or withdrawal
- reasons for use (e.g. recreational, to cope, peer group pressure)
- trigger for use (e.g. any particular event or situation including emotional states that may trigger the urge for use)
- periods of abstinence (if there have been times when the person has not used, include reasons why this period began/ended)
- any specific behavioural changes associated with use (e.g. criminal, suicidal, sexual, accidental)
- potential for suicide, homicide or accidental injury
- social situation — effects of substance on specific issues (e.g. childcare, employment, driving, work/school, relationships and recreation)
- present or past contact with specialist treatment services
- the presence of behaviours associated with increased risk (e.g. sharing of needles, intoxication).

Referrals

When health professionals make a referral to a specialist drug and alcohol service, it is essential that the health professional goes on to support the person through the process of referral. This includes providing them with information about the service they are being referred to, ascertaining their preferred point of access to the service and personally assisting with the transfer of care, for example, helping to make the initial appointment, clarifying any questions the person may have and providing the drug and alcohol service with sufficient referral information.

It is also necessary for health professionals to follow-up with a phone call to the person around the time of their first appointment and confirm with the drug and alcohol service whether the person has attended. This is important because transitions in care from one service to another are one of the most critical points where a person can be 'lost' in the system, giving rise to negative health outcomes (Marel et al., 2016).

While a person can often be referred on to a more appropriate service for care and treatment, there will also be times when health professionals are required to provide the treatment where they are. For example, while some health services in Australia provide bed-based services that are specific to detoxification and management of withdrawal, most people will be managed in their local area, either in a general hospital bed or in the community. For this reason, there is a need for all health professionals to understand the basic principles underlying the provision of care and treatment to a person with a substance use issue.

10.8 Caring for family members

LEARNING OBJECTIVE 10.8 Explain the issues facing family members of a person with a substance misuse issue.

When substance use becomes problematic for a person, the effect on family members can be devastating. The misuse of substances in society has many implications and there is often a range of repercussions for family members, as well as the person who is using the substance. There have been times when family members were perceived by health professionals as contributing to an individual's ongoing substance misuse behaviour. This is a particularly unhelpful approach to supporting both the person and the family. Often, family members are left bewildered and at a loss to know how to best support their family member to reduce or cease their substance misuse and regain their health and wellbeing.

Health professionals need to be aware that family members are likely to be affected in different ways by the substance use issues of the person. Family members may experience a sense of shame, guilt, blame, grief, anger or hopelessness. Health professionals need to support the family by listening, addressing any issues, providing information and referring them to support services, such as Al-Anon, Centrelink or support services.

Support and education

The health professional needs to be aware that family members may require support and education to:
- manage their reactions to the use and misuse of substances by the person
- maintain their own health and wellbeing
- support the person with the substance use disorder but not the substance use behaviour (Straussner, 2012).

Sometimes, the family members are at a loss as to how to put these principles into practice. Health professionals can help by, for example, suggesting the family member refrain from giving the person cash, but rather provide them with specific items that they may need, for example, food or clothes.

Support groups such as Al-Anon and Nar-Anon Family Group play an important role in assisting families in dealing with the impact of substance misuse. It is essential that the health professional offer information to family members about how to access groups and education. The availability of programs will vary between states and territories, and health professionals are encouraged to identify those that are relevant to their local area.

There is a substantial evidence base for a number of defined family therapy approaches (US Department of Health and Human Services Office of the Surgeon General, 2016), but where specific programs are not available, family support is still helpful.

Parents and children

People with a substance use disorder may have children who are affected by the parent's substance use disorder to varying degrees. Health professionals need to be aware of these effects as well as factors that support resilience (Daley & Douaihy, 2019). Impacts may result from a parent with a substance use disorder not being physically or emotionally available for their child. The parent's cognitive capacity and functioning may also be impaired as a result of their disorder, which may place the child at risk. While the health professional must continue to demonstrate a non-judgemental attitude and support the person, there is also a need to respond to identified risk. All states and territories across Australia have child protection laws with which the health professional must comply. These laws mandate that health care workers report suspected child abuse or neglect. The criteria for mandatory reporting vary between states and territories. The Australian Institute of Family Studies maintain up-to-date criteria in different jurisdictions on their website, www.aifs.gov.au/cfca/publications/mandatory-reporting-child-abuse-and-neglect. Your state health service may also have resources to assist in decision making. Consulting with senior colleagues is often helpful, but ultimately the responsibility lies with the treating health professional.

People who develop a substance dependence may be unaware of the impact their substance use has on their children's lives.

QUESTIONS

1. What are some of these impacts?
2. How might a clinician raise a parent's consciousness about these impacts without destroying the therapeutic relationship?

Homelessness

A significant number of people with a substance use disorder may be homeless (Chamberlain & Johnson, 2011). This can cause concern for health professionals who are required to arrange follow-up appointments and possible ongoing treatment on discharge. Consideration needs to be given to involving a social worker or government services that link individuals with homeless support agencies in the local community early in treatment.

This section outlined the principles of providing care to a person with a substance use disorder, including engaging with the person and supporting them through the various stages of change in an ongoing process. The provision of care also involves supporting partners or carers, providing them with information and assistance as required. In the next section, motivational interviewing is explained. This is a therapeutic approach by which the health professional can engage with a person and influence them to think about change.

10.9 Motivation for behaviour change

LEARNING OBJECTIVE 10.9 Explain how care is provided to people with a substance use disorder, including the use of motivational interviewing and brief interventions.

Providing care for people with problems that require a significant lifestyle change can be complex. The health professional may find that their recommendations regarding lifestyle change will go unheeded by the individual to whom they are offering the advice. Identifying the ideal treatment does little to improve outcomes for the individual if they decline the treatment.

It is important to be aware of the contemporary models of change and the evidence-based strategies that increase the likelihood of the person adhering to treatment recommendations. The following section explores the Cycle of Change model and motivational interventions that will enhance the health professional's effectiveness when working with people with a range of issues.

Cycle of Change

In the past, behaviour change was viewed as a one-step process: behaviour was either instituted or stopped. However, in the late 1970s and early 1980s, Prochaska and DiClemente (1982) developed a theory of behaviour change by breaking down the process into several stages comprising definitive cognitive and behavioural shifts. The 'Cycle of Change' model describes the six discrete stages (the original model contained five) through which an individual passes when making any intentional behavioural or lifestyle change. This model is also known as the **transtheoretical model of change**.

The six stages identified are:
1. **precontemplation**
2. **contemplation**
3. **determination (or preparation)**
4. **action**
5. **maintenance**
6. **relapse** and recycling (DiClemente, 2018).

Figure 10.6 illustrates the six stages of change, including the cyclic natures of these stages. In addition, each of the stages of change will now be described in more detail.

FIGURE 10.6　Cycle of Change model

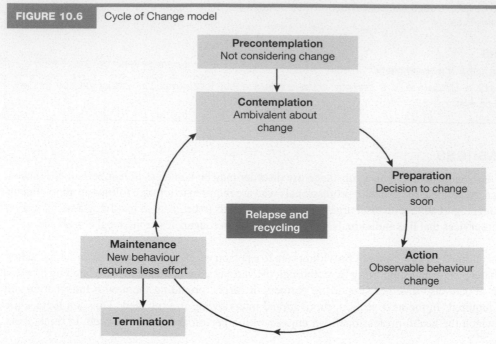

Source: DiClemente (2018).

Precontemplation stage

The hallmark of the **precontemplation** stage is that the individual is not currently considering changing their behaviour. It may be that the person does not think that their behaviour needs to change, or that the thought of changing is too difficult. The person may fail to make a connection between their behaviour and the consequences. Some precontemplators are happy with their substance use, while others have tried to change so many times before that they become resigned to continued use and feel too hopeless to change. Bear in mind, many people who are precontemplative about making a change at the moment would still prefer things to be different, for example, a smoker may desperately want a cigarette right now, but an open discussion with them may reveal that they wish they were a non-smoker. Drawing out these seemingly paradoxical feelings and discrepancies is extremely helpful in building motivation to change.

When working with a person who is precontemplative, health professionals should first work on engaging the person in a therapeutic alliance before working on strengthening the person's perceived importance of making a behaviour change, by raising the person's consciousness that there is an issue with the current behaviour. Once the person recognises the importance of the behaviour change, the health professional can help build the person's **self-efficacy** or belief that it is possible to change.

Some useful strategies to help build self-efficacy include reminding the person about other achievements they have made in the past and letting them know that many people in the same situation struggle with similar issues and manage to make changes despite the difficulties. The health professional should always be aware that the term 'precontemplator' should never be used in a pejorative way. Everyone is precontemplative about many things. For example, one might be precontemplative about ceasing coffee consumption or saving for a winter holiday in Antarctica.

Contemplation stage

In the **contemplation** stage, the person is uncomfortably ambivalent about changing their behaviour. They are seriously considering change, but they are torn between the desire to change and the difficulties of undertaking a change. Contemplators acknowledge some consequences of their behaviour.

The aim of the health professional in working with someone contemplating a health behaviour change is to increase **ambivalence**; exploring the person's reasons for change and the risks of not changing can help. It is important to continue to support an individual's self-efficacy throughout this stage. When talking with an individual who mentions the possibility of change, it is useful to explore these thoughts in more detail.

Preparation or determination stage

Working with someone who has made a decision to change their behaviour is relatively straightforward. Firstly, the health professional can assist by helping the individual strengthen their commitment to undertake the change. Provide the person with reassurance that it is quite normal to still have some doubts. The health professional can help the person plan the necessary changes that will be required, exploring which issues will be the most difficult. It is important for the health professional to use their knowledge of strategies and resources to provide a variety of options and support the person to choose the best strategies. Part of planning for a behaviour change includes identifying some strategies to deal with challenging situations before they arise.

Action stage

The **action** stage is the first point where it is possible to observe some objective behaviour change. For example, the person may have taken some small steps to change their behaviour or may have instituted a major behaviour change, such as reducing or ceasing their substance use. The early period of any behaviour change is likely to be the most difficult, so it is important to continue to offer support through this period. It can be helpful to provide affirmations for the person, such as 'You must be happy with all you've achieved so far' or 'You have really made some positive changes — you're achieving everything you said you would so far'. It is also important for the health professional to discuss which strategies have been working for the person and continue to offer a menu of options for other strategies. Some strategies can be particularly useful during the action stage, including **distraction techniques** for dealing with urges to revert to former behaviours.

Maintenance stage

In **maintenance** stage, the person recognises, after several months of behaviour change, that it requires less effort to maintain the new behaviours. This can provide the person with a sense of confidence that they have successfully made a change. In this situation, the health professional can encourage the person to remain vigilant in their efforts to avoid 'risky' situations, which might lead them back to their old behaviour patterns. It is also important to let the person know that ambivalence can creep back into their mind at any time.

Relapse and recycling

Many health professionals prefer not to label this as a 'stage of change', but it is not uncommon for people to **relapse** into their former behaviour. This may be a minor slip (lapse) or a longer-term return to former behaviour. Most people who have been successful at undertaking a difficult lifestyle behavioural change have succeeded only after making several seemingly unsuccessful attempts.

It is extremely important that the health professional avoids making any statements that could be interpreted as demoralising for the person who may have had a lapse. Another danger in this situation is to minimise the potential consequences of a lapse. The best approach is to encourage the person to learn from their experience and develop strategies to avoid the same mistakes next time.

Understanding the transtheoretical model or Cycle of Change provides health professionals with insight into how a person with a substance use issue may change their thoughts and behaviours over time. The process is ongoing and effective health professionals will support the person through the cycle as many times as it takes.

At the same time as providing support to the person, it is also important that health professionals ensure they support the partners, carers or family members of the person. Substance use issues will impact on not only the person who is using the substance, but also those with whom the person lives or is in a relationship. Partners, carers and family members play a crucial role in supporting the person and helping them to achieve change. At the same time, they also require support from the health professional. Table 10.7 describes five different precontemplator subtypes identified by DiClemente (2018). It is important to distinguish between these subtypes in order to match the most appropriate intervention to the individual.

It is important to remember that motivation fluctuates. An individual's stage of change is likely to alter based on numerous factors. The role of the health professional is to work with the person in a non-confrontational manner and attempt to build motivation.

Some rationalising precontemplators and many resigned and reluctant precontemplators will state that in a perfect world, they would prefer that their behaviour was changed. Exploring this concept can lead to an increase in ambivalence and motivation.

TABLE 10.7   Precontemplation subtypes

Type of resistance	Strategies
Revelling Those who are having too good a time to change	• Stimulate concern about the negative consequences. • Raise doubt about their illusory sense of elevated self-efficacy. • Focus on how their behaviour affects others. • Shift focus from problematic issue.
Reluctant Those who are simply unwilling to consider change	• Counter the hesitance by working through their concerns about changing. • Build confidence in their ability to change. • Use the support of individuals who have made similar changes.
Resigned Those who feel hopeless and helpless, may have a history of failed attempts and do not feel they can change	• Provide hope. • Build self-efficacy. • Share success stories of similar individuals. • Evaluate prior attempts and suggest different strategies to use.
Rebellious Those who actively resist attempts to encourage change	• Link autonomy and freedom to change. • Shift high-energy levels from rebellion to change. • Make sure they feel in charge of the change at all times. • Emphasise choice and offer options for managing their change.
Rationalising Those who rationalise why the addictive behaviour does not pose a problem; appear to have all the answers	• Continue to make a clear connection between behaviour and consequences. • Do not deride their reasons but try and work with them to your advantage. • Build confidence in their potential to change.

Source: Adapted from DiClemente (2018); Clancy and Terry (2007).

IN PRACTICE

Integrated motivational assessment tool

The simple integrated motivational assessment tool (IMAT) seen in table 10.8 was devised by Clancy and Terry (2007) to assist health professionals identify and record a client's motivation for receiving treatment interventions for both mental health and substance misuse disorders concurrently. It prompts the health professional to assess, record and subsequently focus on an issue that may be causing the greatest detriment to the client's health.

TABLE 10.8   Integrated motivational assessment tool

		Motivation regarding AOD treatment				
		Precontempla-tion	Contempla-tion	Preparation/Determination	Action	Maintenance
Motivation regarding psychiatric treatment	Precontemplation					
	Contemplation					
	Preparation/Determination					
	Action					
	Maintenance					

Source: Adapted from Clancy and Terry (2007).

We will look at a typical scenario where the IMAT may be used: Yuliya is a 24-year-old woman who is seeing a psychologist experiencing depression and is consuming 6–8 standard drinks of alcohol on a daily basis. When using this tool, a health professional would try to elicit Yuliya 's understanding of the possible contributing factors of daily alcohol consumption to her depression. For example, Yuliya may believe that due to her depression, it is useful to take antidepressant medication to deal with symptoms that she may experience (e.g. low mood); therefore, using this model, it could be argued that Yuliya is in the action phase of the transtheoretical model when considering her mental health issues. However, when questioned about her alcohol habits, Yuliya indicates that it does not affect or contribute to her depression and she has no plans to change; therefore, it can be assumed when considering her substance misuse issues that she is precontemplative. From this information, the health professional would make an assessment of the impact of Yuliya's beliefs around her drinking and mental illness and, therefore, target behaviours and motivations that may have the most detrimental effect on health. In this example, the health professional would most likely work with Yuliya with psychoeducation using a stress–vulnerability approach on the effects of alcohol and its possible contribution to exacerbating depressive symptoms. The idea being that this may possibly motivate Yuliya to shift from precontemplation to contemplation in relation to her drinking.

QUESTIONS

1. What are the advantages of recording a person's motivation to receive treatment for their mental health condition and their readiness to change their substance use disorder?
2. How would you manage a situation where another clinician in the multidisciplinary team rated the person's motivation at a lower stage than you had, on the same day?

Stages of treatment

The staged treatment model detailed by Mueser and colleagues (2003) for working with people who have comorbid mental health and substance use disorders provides a useful framework to guide health professionals as they work with complex issues. The model comprises four broad strategies for treatment that guide the clinician to provide interventions that are suited to the person's readiness to participate in treatment.

The main difference between the stage of treatment model and the Cycle of Change model is that the Cycle of Change model describes where an individual is in relation to a behaviour change, while the stages of treatment model describes interventions that a clinician or a service may implement to suit the client.

The four stages of treatment in the model are:

1. engagement
2. persuasion
3. active treatment
4. relapse prevention.

Engagement

A person who is engaged in treatment feels that the service provider has something desirable to offer. A person may be enrolled in treatment without being engaged in the treatment process. This often occurs when a person is strongly encouraged to seek treatment by a significant other. Health professionals can engage people into treatment by first making the environment as pleasant as possible, focusing on the consumer's main issues and providing practical assistance to help the person. Being friendly and not focusing on rules also helps to engage the individual.

Applying pressure on a person to cease substance use before engagement has taken place often results in treatment dropout.

Persuasion

Once engaged, the person is usually more prepared to listen to information. Motivational interviewing (MI) and psychoeducation are the strategies best suited to influencing the person to make lifestyle changes. If available, group therapy can assist in the persuasion stage.

Active treatment

People in the active treatment stage are prepared to listen to encouraging statements promoting the possibility of change. It is in the active treatment stage that people begin to make some changes. Health professionals can ensure that the person assumes control of the change by offering a range of strategies from which the person can choose.

Relapse prevention

Clients with complex issues really benefit from support in helping them expand their recovery to making the most of their life. This is likely to be more successful with some assistance from the health professional. It is important to encourage the person to try new things, take some risks and maintain some vigilance to ensure the progress that has been achieved is maintained over time (Mueser et al., 2003).

Motivational interviewing

In the past, health professionals sometimes used confrontational methods to try to convince people to change their behaviour. This is not helpful, as confrontation can be seen as pushing against the person's wishes until they relent. MI is a goal-oriented, collaborative counselling style that seeks to activate a person's intrinsic motivation to change. Miller and Rollnick (2013) suggest that the following styles and responses from health professionals have been shown to actually *increase resistance* among some clients and should be avoided.

Unhelpful strategies

* *Arguing for change*. The health professional assumes a pro-change side of the argument only.
* *Assuming the expert role*. The health professional implies that he or she knows what's best.
* *Criticising the person*. The health professional uses shaming or blaming.
* *Labelling*. The health professional needs to refrain from using pejorative and stigmatising labels when attempting to support someone in purposeful behaviour change. Terms such as 'substance abuser', 'junkie', 'druggie' and 'alcoholic' have no value or purpose in a therapeutic relationship.
* *Hurrying*. It is important not to rush people. Behaviour patterns often take years to develop, so it does not make much sense to rush things when it comes to deciding whether or not a change is required or is possible.
* *Claiming pre-eminence*. The health professional claims his/her goals and perspectives and these override those of the client (Miller & Rollnick, 2013).

At other times, health professionals have assumed that if they gave someone information about the risks associated with a behaviour, it would be enough to bring about the required health behaviour change. In reality, however, achieving change is not that easy. There are many reasons why people do or do not achieve a desired health behaviour change. Some may believe that they are unable to make a change, while others may feel that the costs — physical, psychological and/or financial — are too great. Others, again, may not place the same value on the 'need' to make a change as the health professional does. Finally, there are those who see no need to change. A lack of motivation is discussed in the next section.

Rationale for motivational interviewing

MI is a counselling strategy or 'talking therapy' that aims to increase the individual's motivation for change through the dialogue maintained between the health professional and client. MI builds on the work of Prochaska and DiClemente's 'Cycle of Change' (1982) and the underlying processes of change. It was developed by Miller and Rollnick (1991, 2002, 2013) and has since demonstrated effectiveness across a variety of clinical settings (Lundahl et al., 2013). Motivational interviewing approaches will not magically change everyone's behaviour, but even when an individual is not ready to consider change at the moment, this approach helps to minimise discord between the health professional and the person accessing treatment.

The rationale that underpins MI is simple.

* The health professional's **interpersonal style** can have an impact on a person's level of resistance towards change.
* Arguing with a person increases their resistance.
* The more a person resists an idea, the less likely they are to change.
* People who undertake a behaviour change usually experience a period of increased ambivalence just prior to change.

MI is non-confrontational and assumes equal status of the person and the health professional. While the health professional takes the guiding role, the client plays an active role in the dialogue and consequent learning. Indeed, MI emphasises an individual's right to define their own problems and choose how to deal with them. Motivation and resistance are seen as products of the interaction between the health professional and the person. If the person becomes resistive, this indicates that the health professional has been moving too fast.

The process of MI begins with engaging the person before focusing on a behaviour, evoking the person's reasons and motivation to change before helping plan the implementation of a behaviour change.

The righting reflex

An automatic response when someone makes a mistake is to gently correct the error. This is referred to as the **righting reflex**. For example, if a person makes a statement that 'amphetamines don't cause psychosis', a clinician might feel an impulse to correct the statement and say 'actually some people do experience amphetamine-induced psychosis'. While factually correct, if this correction is given immediately following the interviewee's statement, it may lead to resistance and indicate that the interviewer believes they have all the answers. In this situation, it may be better to respond with a statement that doesn't confirm the incorrect statement, but rolls with it. A response such as 'you've not noticed any problems with psychosis when you have used amphetamines' might be helpful. This can then open the door to discuss this in more detail.

Principles of MI

The main principles of MI articulated in Miller and Rollnick's early work are:
- avoid argumentation
- express empathy
- support self-efficacy
- develop discrepancy.
  These principles are described further in the following.

Avoid argumentation

Confronting or arguing with the person can be counterproductive, even though you may feel the person is denying the consequences of their substance use. Argumentation will merely increase resistance and reduce the likelihood of the person listening. The use of confrontation has been shown to increase dropout rates. The 'I know best, listen to me' attitude of the health professional can have a negative impact on attempting to engage in a therapeutic relationship with the person. Arguing can lead to an increase in resistance. Rather than trying to 'break through' the denial, it is better to work around it. Remember the decision to change is the client's decision. No-one likes being told what to do. The aim is negotiation rather than conflict. Miller & Rollnick used ⊠discord' as the preferred term to describe interactions that might previously have been labelled as argumentation or resistance.

Express empathy

The use of empathy is a key aspect of MI. This goes beyond the health professional feeling compassion, instead of relying on the health professional's ability to *express* and *articulate* empathy. Expressing empathy is critical to MI. Some examples of empathic statements are as follows.
- 'Things have been difficult for you lately.'
- 'It can be really challenging to maintain this lifestyle.'
- 'It must be hard to feel that everyone is against you.'

Empathy is different to sympathy or feeling sorry for the person. Empathy involves imagining how the person feels or perceives things. If the person believes the health professional is unable to see things from their perspective, they may feel as though they have not been listened to or understood. Therefore, they are less likely to 'open up'. However, if the person perceives empathy from a health professional, they are more likely to accept gentle challenges and questioning around lifestyle issues and substance use beliefs. Expressing empathy facilitates engagement, which is the seed of a successful therapeutic relationship.

Support self-efficacy

Self-efficacy refers to an individual's belief about whether change is possible. It is a person's belief in their ability to succeed in specific situations (Bandura, 1997). A person's sense of self-efficacy plays a key role in how a person approaches goals, tasks and challenges. Therefore, people with high self-efficacy who believe they can perform a task well are more likely to view difficult tasks as something that can be overcome or mastered, rather than avoided. It is a person's sense of control that facilitates healthy behaviour change.

A good way for the health professional to build self-efficacy is to explore changes that the person has made in the past in other areas of their life. Some individuals may have made multiple attempts in the past to change their behaviour and now feel a sense of failure. If this is the case, remind them that the majority of people who have made long-term change in their lives have usually had several unsuccessful attempts prior to succeeding, and that it is normal for this to happen. It is also useful to elicit some knowledge about a previous unsuccessful attempt, to help the person to identify what led to the last relapse and define some strategies to avoid the same result. It can also be useful to ask the person how confident they feel in being able to undertake the change using a scale of 1–10 (Miller & Rollnick, 2013).

Develop discrepancy

This principle involves the health professional gently raising a discrepancy between how the person sees their current situation and how they would like it to be. This can be achieved by exploring values and goals and the barriers to achieving them. Another strategy for developing discrepancy is to ask the person how some of their behaviours fit with the way they like to be thought of by others. Sometimes, the health professional may also notice some discrepancies in the person's history, for example, someone who has previously told the health professional that they have no problems associated with drinking, may later tell the health professional that they did something under the influence of alcohol about which they are not pleased. In this situation, the health professional might gently explore how this behaviour fits with their perception that they have no problem with drinking.

The next section provides a brief overview of microskills. When utilising MI, the health professional will apply similar skills but with a slightly different focus.

Microskills

Miller and Rollnick (2013) suggest four useful **microskills** that can be used throughout the process of MI. The following, known as the 'four OARS', have been derived from person-centred counselling.

1. **O**pen questions
2. **A**ffirming
3. **R**eflective listening
4. **S**ummarising

Open-ended questions

Open-ended questions are discussed briefly in the chapter on depression, anxiety and perinatal mental health. When using the MI strategies, health professionals will use open-ended questions to avoid a pattern of asking questions that require only short answers from the client. Open-ended questions are those that invite long answers. They could include the following.

- 'Fill me in on . . .'
- 'Tell me about . . .'
- 'What are your concerns about . . .?'
- 'Bring me up to speed on . . .'
- 'What do you think about . . .?'

Open-ended questions are used to establish an atmosphere of acceptance and trust by allowing the person to do most of the talking. They provide an opportunity to guide the person in their exploration, elicit the desired information and gain an understanding of their situation and ambivalence.

Affirming

Affirming refers to offering direct recognition of effort and statements of appreciation and understanding to the client during the interview process. Examples include the following.

- 'You took a big step in coming here today.'
- 'That's a great suggestion.'
- 'You are clearly a very strong person. Most people would struggle to cope in that situation.'

Affirmation can be important in building rapport and reinforcing open exploration. The appropriate level and frequency of affirmation within the therapeutic relationship will vary across social contexts. It is important to appropriately affirm a person's strengths and efforts. It is recommended to offer **internalising** affirmation statements (e.g. '*You* must be happy that you succeeded' rather than '*I'm* so happy you succeeded'). This provides an important means of helping the client to see the personal benefits of their changed behaviour.

Reflective listening

Reflective listening is probably one of the most important and challenging skills needed for MI. Reflective listening involves the health professional listening intently to the words and the feelings being expressed and reflecting them back to the person in the health professional's own words.

- 'You're angry with your mother.'
- 'You haven't always been like that.'
- 'And that's what worries you.'

This can be a mere substitution of the person's words, or, as the health professional gains more skill, they may make a guess at an unspoken meaning, or make an observation about how the person is feeling, or attempt the next sentence in the person's paragraph (known as continuing the paragraph). The depth of reflection increases with the level of the health professional's skilfulness. However, it is important to slightly understate what the person has said, particularly when a statement is emotionally loaded. The experts in MI aim for two to three reflections per open-ended question so that in the early stages, at least, a substantial portion of the health professional's responses are reflective listening statements. This can be quite a challenge and it can take several years to achieve this level of skill.

Summarising

Summary statements are a useful way of linking together and reinforcing the information discussed during MI. Periodic summaries also show the person that the health professional has been listening carefully and it prepares the person to elaborate further.

As noted, these communication skills are used through the process of the MI. They are a means by which the health professional can encourage the person to reflect on the issues they have raised and to continue the conversation. In the process of talking, the person will also be thinking about their situation, including their substance use and how it is impacting upon their lives. In the next section, some of the strategies related to the MI approach are outlined.

'Change talk' and 'sustain talk'

In MI, not only is it important for the interviewer not to argue for change, but also to not offer all the reasons for change.

In any conversation, a number of ideas are exchanged. If the interviewer introduces all the reasons that change would be beneficial, the only ideas left in the conversation tend to be how hard it would be to change, or reasons why a change would not be good. The role of the interviewer is to guide the conversation in such a way that they encourage the interviewee to talk about the benefits of change. This is called **change talk**. This is achieved by asking evocative questions such as 'Why would you want to change?', 'What would be different if you changed?' or 'How would you go about changing if you decided to?'

It is important to try to avoid leading the interviewee into **sustain talk**. Sustain talk involves the person talking about reasons not to change. Examples of statements that should be avoided include 'Why haven't you changed before . . .' or 'Why don't you just . . .'

The importance ruler, discussed below, provides some further strategies that lead people away from sustain talk and towards change talk.

The importance and confidence rulers

Miller and Rollnick (2013) utilise a scale from 0 to 10 to obtain the person's self-rating of how important an issue is to them to change.

If the person responds with a low number, say a one or two, the health professional can respond with something like 'You're a one out of ten, I thought you might answer a zero. I'm curious, why are you a one and not a zero (or a minus 10)?'

If the person responds with another number — such as a three or an eight — the health professional might respond with a statement such as 'So you're a three. Have a think for a minute, what would it take for you to move from a three to a four?'

This same scale and approach may be used to elicit the degree of confidence the person has in addressing the issue or their readiness to change.

Motivational interviewing and comorbidity

When using MI with people who have mental health issues as well as substance use problems, the following points need to be considered.

- When using the decisional balance (which should only be used when people are in the contemplation stage), if a person states that a substance reduces their symptoms of mental illness, resist the righting reflex to correct the response. Instead, explore this later in more detail with particular attention to the timeframe. For example, using substances may make them feel great in the short term, but may cause problems later.
- When a person begins a behaviour change, try to have as many people as possible provide the person with positive feedback (e.g. involve family and other health professionals).
- Involve the family in care as much as possible. Educate the family on the basics of non-confrontational interventions.

- Always give consistent messages, including a unified 'recommended goal'. For people with both mental health and substance use issues, abstinence is the most appropriate recommendation. It is easy to recommend abstinence while accepting an individual's decision to continue to use. This does not mean you condone continued use. In practice, this may sound like 'The experts say that if you have schizophrenia, it's best not to use amphetamines at all because of the real risk of psychosis; but if you do choose to use, then the more you use, the greater the chance of psychosis. Also, make sure that if you're injecting, that you never reuse fits'.
- Remember, abstinence may be a health professional's goal *of* treatment without being a prerequisite *for* treatment. Many people will never consider abstinence but still require support and treatment.

This section provides a brief explanation of MI, what it is, why it is used and the strategies and techniques that are used as part of the MI process. Although MI has been shown to be effective in promoting change, there will often be occasions when health professionals are unable to maintain a therapeutic relationship with the person with a substance use issue for any length of time. In such cases, brief interventions have also shown to be effective.

Brief interventions

Brief interventions present a framework for health professionals to provide standardised opportunistic interventions aimed at increasing the likelihood of behaviour change. Adopting a brief intervention focus acknowledges that the time and opportunities for health promotion and implementing behavioural change may be limited. Brief interventions have been shown to help reduce harmful substance use (Kaner et al., 2018, US Department of Health and Human Services Office of the Surgeon General, 2016). Brief interventions aim to promote moderation or harm-free substance use and involve:

- assessment and identification
- advice
- counselling with education
- promotion of self-help.

The common elements of brief intervention have been summarised by the acronym FRAMES, which provides a framework that any health professional can use to address the need for personal change. The FRAMES approach to brief intervention is depicted in figure 10.7.

FIGURE 10.7   FRAMES approach to brief intervention

Feedback	Provide feedback to the person on their assessment of the problem.
Responsibility	Advise the person that the substance use is their responsibility.
Advice	Give clear advice, both written and verbal, as to the reasons why there is a need to stop using the substance.
Menu	Help the person to identify a range ('menu') of options or choices regarding their substance-using behaviour.
Empathy	Be empathic, warm, understanding and encouraging about the person's ability to change.
Self-efficacy	Encourage and reinforce the person's ability to achieve change by being self-reliant (e.g. avoid blaming others for their problems or failure to achieve an alcohol-free or substance-free lifestyle).

Source: Adapted from Miller and Sanchez (1993).

In order to ensure that the likelihood of change is maximised, people need to receive the appropriate level of specialist help when discharged from hospital. To achieve this, health professionals need to develop contacts and links with local government and non-government specialist alcohol and drug services. Much informal support, counselling, advice and treatment is provided by these organisations, particularly 'self-help' organisations, such as Alcoholics Anonymous (AA) and Narcotics Anonymous (NA), so it is necessary to know the local contacts and means of access or referral.

Providing information

Clinicians are often in situations where they are providing treatment for people who do not wish to discuss substance use, even though it may be apparent that the individual's use of substances is an issue. This poses some ethical dilemmas for clinicians. If the clinician argues for change in substance use behaviour, it is likely to increase resistance to behaviour change; on the other hand, if the clinician does not provide objective information, the individual may never receive information related to their substance use from a health professional.

QUESTIONS

1. How can a clinician lead a discussion to address substance use issues?

2. How can discussing 'values' help raise the issue?

10.10 The stress–vulnerability model

LEARNING OBJECTIVE 10.10 Describe how the stress–vulnerability model can explain how substance use and other factors interact with a person's biological vulnerability to developing a mental illness.

Many theories have been proposed attempting to explain why some people develop symptoms of mental illness and others do not. The better we understand the causes of illness, the better equipped we are to refine treatments that work.

People's understanding of the nature of mental illness also influences the stigma associated with a diagnosis. Hence, it is important that we explain the factors that contribute to the development of mental illnesses in a way that is not only accurate, but also mindful of how the information is framed, so we don't inadvertently increase stigma within the broader community or self-stigma for people who live with mental illness.

While biological explanations of mental health aetiology have been shown to reduce people's perception of blame, they also increase non-mentally ill people's desire for social distance (Kvaale et al., 2013). Explanations of mental illness that describe mental health on a continuum and include the negative impacts of stress on 'normal' individuals are associated with less stereotyping, less social distance and less fear than biological explanations (Wiesjahn et al., 2016).

Explaining how some individuals who use substances end up with mental health problems and others do not is best approached using a simple version of the stress–vulnerability model. The stress–vulnerability model (also known as the diathesis–stress model) was proposed in a seminal article published in the late 1970s (Zubin & Spring, 1977). In their article, Zubin and Spring synthesised the dominant nature- and nurture-based theories associated with the development and course of mental illness. Each of the dominant theories of the day contributed to scientific understandings of the development of mental illness, but no theory was able to fully explain an individual's risk of developing symptoms of the illness.

The stress–vulnerability model has been refined over the 40 years since its inception (Goh & Agius, 2010; Howes & Kapur, 2009; MacKain et al., 1994; Randal et al., 2009; Rende & Plomin, 1992; Kendler, 2020; Southwick et al., 2005; Zubin & Spring, 1977). Mueser and colleagues (2003) integrated recovery concepts and substance use into the model.

The health professional may need to tailor the complexity of information provided around the stress–vulnerability model according to the individual's capacity to take the information in at the time.

At the heart of the current version of the stress–vulnerability model is our psychobiological vulnerability to develop symptoms. This vulnerability includes factors such as genetic and developmental vulnerability acquired early in life.

Stress in our lives, such as relationship problems, moving to a new house, pressure of exams or financial problems, interacts with our psychobiological vulnerability and contributes to the risk of developing symptoms of mental illness. (See the chapter on common reactions to stressful situations for more detailed information on the effects of stress.) The coping strategies we use to deal with stressors can mitigate its impact. Substance use increases the likelihood of some symptoms developing, whereas other strategies are more helpful in the long term. Some people find mediation useful as well.

Health professionals can use this simple model to explain that all of us have some degree of vulnerability to developing a range of illnesses. In fact, many illnesses run in families. These include mental illnesses, such as depression, psychosis or anxiety. This is no different to familial risk of heart disease, diabetes, some cancers and many other illnesses.

Having a higher level of vulnerability to an illness (such as a family history) does not mean that an individual will necessarily develop the illness. However, it does mean that the risk of developing the illness for that particular person is greater than for someone else in the community.

What can be helpful?

There are several factors known to interact with an individual's biological vulnerability to developing symptoms of mental illness. This concept is commonly known as the stress–vulnerability model. Figure 10.8 includes strategies that may help mitigate the effects of stressful situations and reduce a person's chance of developing symptoms. Some helpful strategies include:
- positive relationships with friends and family
- having some meaningful activities and hobbies
- learning problem-solving strategies
- learning coping skills to deal with issues or symptoms
- talking therapies, such as cognitive behavioural therapy, acceptance and commitment therapy
- healthy lifestyle activities, including exercise, healthy eating and mental stimulation, with enjoyable activities
- meditation and relaxation exercises.

FIGURE 10.8 The stress–vulnerability model

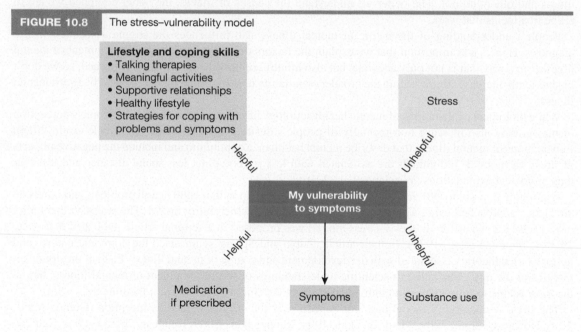

Source: Adapted from Mueser et al. (2003).

Many people find that taking medication as prescribed can also be helpful, but medication may not be for everyone. In fact, many people who have found a medication that works well for them report that it took several attempts with different medications and dosages before they found a medication that was suitable. Making sure that the prescriber is someone they can communicate with is important. Despite some of the difficulties, medication is one of the best tools we have to help manage some illnesses.

What things are unhelpful?

Stress is unhelpful and can make mental health symptoms worse. While no person can avoid stress altogether, health professionals should note that stress can increase the likelihood that a person will become unwell (Goldstein et al., 2017). For example, stress activates the hypothalamus-pituitary-adrenal (HPA) axis, which leads to an increase in cortisol released into the bloodstream, which in turn is thought to induce a decrease in the availability of neurotransmitters associated with depression, including serotonin (Keller et al., 2017).

People often use substances to manage stress. While this works for many people in the short term, using substances can also impact on a person's psychobiological vulnerability to develop symptoms of an illness. This can make a relapse of the person's mental health condition more likely.

Fauzia talks about the stress–vulnerability model

My name is Fauzia. The first time my worker showed me the stress–vulnerability model it was like a light switched on for me. She explained that depression is a physical illness that sometimes runs in families and that genes can have something to do with it.

My genes make me vulnerable to what happens around me. I get stressed when I've got problems or if I'm too bored and stress is bad for my mood. So is alcohol and weed. My worker helped me understand that smoking and drinking might make me feel better on the day, but it can make my depression worse overall. I was diagnosed with depression when I was 17. At the moment I'm doing OK, but my depression has been pretty bad at times.

My family and community are against alcohol and weed but they are slowly understanding more about my condition — especially depression. They try to help and keep me active and do things with me. Even though I know it'll help me in the long run, it's really hard to do things when I'm depressed. My worker says it's like people who start going to the gym — it's hard to begin with, but it gets easier as you get fitter.

I tried three antidepressants before I found one that I could stick with. I've got a great GP who takes time to listen to me if I've got side effects and now I know that taking it at the same time each morning helps.

People who know me know that I'm never going to stop having a few drinks or smoking weed, but I know that too much is a bad thing. Nowadays, I try to cut back when my mood is low rather than use more. Visiting my parents and my sister Aisha is good for me. Sometimes we just watch TV together or cook something. I've been trying to get into a hobby to keep busy. I've tried music and walking, but never stuck with it. I do take my mum's dog on walks, which is nice.

One thing I don't like about my medication is that I've put on weight, but it's the best out of the ones I've tried. I've spoken with my GP about it and we're keeping an eye on it and trying to watch what I eat.

Now when I do drink, I just have a couple and I don't usually smoke cones alone now, just when I'm with friends, but I don't talk about it with my family.

I'm not 'totally fixed' but I'm going OK. Learning about the things that help with depression and the things that don't has been the most practical thing for me, so I recommend that everyone should be shown the stress–vulnerability model. I wish they taught it in school.

Relapse into substance use

Many people who successfully make significant changes to their problematic substance use will relapse and resume their substance use. This can cause major problems for these individuals and their families. At times, clinicians find this behaviour difficult to comprehend. It can seem unfathomable that a person resumes their problematic substance use, particularly with the knowledge that there may be imminent life-changing consequences as a result. For example, a person may risk their health, their employment, custody of their children or gaol time when they resume their substance use. Clinicians are more likely to be required to provide care to people when they relapse, which can create an impression that every person who tries to change their substance use will relapse. Clinicians are less likely to see the individuals who have successfully made long-term changes to their substance use. Possessing an understanding of the complex and powerful biological and psychological drives that influence this behaviour can help clinicians understand some of the challenges faced by people with addiction.

QUESTIONS

1. What are the biological and psychological drives that contribute to people relapsing back into problematic substance use?
2. What can clinicians do to ensure they retain a positive and hopeful outlook for people who attempt to change their substance use?

SUMMARY

The focus of this chapter is caring for the person with a substance use disorder. The chapter provided a background to the use of substances in Australia, including prevalence rates. The majority of people in Australia use substances, from caffeine and alcohol to opioids, amphetamines or tobacco. The adverse effects of using substances are described, together with the community attitudes towards people who use substances, especially illicit substances. The work currently being undertaken across Australia as part of the National Drug Strategy is also discussed.

Following this, comorbid mental health and substance use issues are considered. People with a mental illness have a higher rate of substance use issues; likewise, people with substance use issues will often have a comorbid mental health problem. It is important that health professionals are aware of the issues involved and are ready to assist those at risk. The philosophy of harm minimisation is also considered, including the role of abstinence. Abstinence is the ultimate means of minimising harm; however, not all people will consider abstinence and they should not be excluded from care.

The different categories of substances are identified, including stimulants, depressants and hallucinogens. The major issue of alcohol misuse in Australia is also noted. It is critical that health professionals can recognise the signs and symptoms of alcohol or benzodiazepine withdrawal, as this condition is potentially life threatening. The importance of consulting local guidelines and experts to guide management of opioid withdrawal is also described.

Information about the assessment of people for substance use and misuse is provided. This includes the provision of some simple screening tools for use by health professionals. The ongoing care of people with a substance use issue is framed within person-centred approaches, with strategies such as the transtheoretical model (Cycle of Change) and stages of treatment explained. The chapter outlines the principles of motivational interviewing and brief interventions, and concludes with a simple overview of the stress–vulnerability model.

Issues related to excessive substance use are common in Australian society, and the consequences are seen frequently by health professionals in a variety of settings. Problematic substance use is a health issue and health professionals play a key role in providing care and treatment to people with a substance use disorder. The positive attitudes of health professionals are an important means by which people will be assisted to develop the motivation to change.

KEY TERMS

action A stage of change wherein a person has commenced an observable change to their behaviour.

acute intoxication The altered mental state following intake of a psychoactive substance.

ambivalence Uncertainty or indecisiveness about an issue or course of action; it can also be described as being in two minds about doing something.

analgesic Medication or drug that acts to relieve a person's pain.

cannabinoids Chemicals that interact with cannabinoid receptors in the brain.

central nervous system (CNS) The part of the nervous system that consists of the brain and spinal cord. It is one of two major divisions of the nervous system, with the peripheral nervous system lying outside of the brain and spinal cord.

change talk A person talking about desire; ability; reasons for, or need to, change a behaviour.

comorbidity The simultaneous presence of two or more health conditions, illnesses or disorders.

contemplation A stage of change wherein a person is ambivalent about a behaviour and is considering, but not yet committed to changing.

delirium tremens The 'DTs' is a complication of alcohol withdrawal involving perceptual disturbances, confusion, agitation and tremor; not to be mistaken for 'the shakes', which is a milder symptom of withdrawal.

determination (or preparation) A stage of change wherein a person has made a decision to change in the near future.

disability-adjusted life years (DALY) Standard measure of years of healthy life lost through premature death or years lived with disability (YLD).

distraction techniques A strategy used by a person to temporarily take their attention away from a strong emotion, compulsion or desire; it may involve an activity or refocusing of thoughts onto something else.

drug and alcohol consultation liaison Drug and alcohol health services that are consultative in nature and delivered by specialist drug and alcohol health professionals in a range of generalist practice settings.

dysphoria Generalised feeling of emotional discomfort.

half-life The time it takes for the body to break down or reduce the plasma concentration of a drug by half.

harm minimisation A pragmatic approach taken by health services and health professionals to reduce harm to the individual and the community.

hyponatraemia A blood electrolyte imbalance where levels of sodium are low.

illicit substances Substances that have been outlawed by governments but continue to be used illegally by people to achieve certain effects.

impaired cognition A reduced capacity to think and analyse information.

integrated treatment The synthesis of mental health and substance use treatment interventions for the consumer.

internalising A technique used by the health professional to assist the client to see the personal benefits of their changed behaviour; it replaces externalising the reasons for change.

interpersonal style Mannerisms or approaches used by a person when interacting with others, often stemming from personality and mood.

maintenance A stage of change wherein an individual has sustained a behaviour change for sufficient time to find it easier to persist.

marijuana The dried flowers and leaves of the cannabis plant; generally smoked by the user.

medicinal cannabis Products containing cannabinoids prescribed for medicinal purposes.

methadone A synthetic opioid used as a substitute for people who are dependent on, or withdrawing from, an opioid.

microskills In counselling terms, techniques that are used in the counselling situation (e.g. maintaining eye contact and using open-ended questions).

opiate A natural alkaloid found in the resin of the opium poppy. In usage refers to a drug derived from the opium poppy.

opioid A chemical that works by binding to opioid receptors, which are found principally in the central nervous system, peripheral nervous system and the gastrointestinal tract.

physically dependent When signs and symptoms with a physiological basis are experienced or manifested when a person is no longer able to use a substance or reduce their use (withdrawal).

polypharmacy The concurrent use of multiple medications by a person; these medications often interact in a way that is problematic for the person.

post-traumatic stress disorder (PTSD) A diagnosed mental health condition characterised by the development of a long-lasting anxiety reaction following a traumatic or catastrophic event.

precontemplation A stage of change wherein an individual is not currently considering changing a behaviour.

precontemplation A stage of change wherein an individual is not currently considering changing a

psychoactive substances Substances that act on the brain to alter the way a person feels, thinks or acts.

psychological dependence A strong urge, desire or attachment in relation to a substance based on the feelings aroused by the substance or the social and emotional needs it meets.

relapse A sustained resumption of former behaviours following an attempted change. Differs from a lapse which refers to a transitory slip into past behaviour.

reward pathway A system of dopamine neurons that reinforce behaviours, such as sex, eating and drinking; also implicated in substance dependence. Also called the mesolimbic pathway.

righting reflex Impulse to correct errors in others.

screening instruments Brief measures to help the health professional to identify if a person may require a more thorough assessment.

self-efficacy A person's belief about their ability or capacity to accomplish a task or achieve a goal.

substance Psychoactive material, such as alcohol, caffeine, nicotine or other drugs that are used by people to achieve certain mind-altering effects.

substance misuse The use of any substance that contributes to detrimental health effects, e.g. physical ill health or mental health problems; more likely to occur in the context of physical and/or psychological dependence.

substance use The use of any substance that does not lead to significant detrimental health effects.

sustain talk A person talking about reasons for not changing their behaviour.

thiamine A vitamin, also called vitamin B1, that is found in yeast, cereal grains, beans, nuts and meat.

tolerance When the body adapts to a substance so that increasingly larger doses are required to produce the same effect obtained earlier with smaller doses.

transtheoretical model of change The clinical name and theory behind the 'Cycle of Change' model, which describes a series of stages a person will move through when making change in their life.

Wernicke's encephalopathy A form of acute brain disorder resulting from a lack of thiamine, most commonly occurring in people with chronic alcohol dependence.

withdrawal The objective and subjective symptoms following abrupt cessation or dose reduction of a psychoactive substance after a period of continued use.

REVIEW QUESTIONS

1 What is the difference between substance use and substance misuse?
2 Describe the harm minimisation approach to substance use.
3 What are some of the adverse effects of substance use?
4 What serious complications can result from alcohol withdrawal?
5 What is meant by 'integrated' mental health and substance use health service delivery?
6 What is the difference between a stimulant, depressant and hallucinogen? Provide an example of each.
7 Outline some of the reasons that family members of people with a substance use disorder need support and education.
8 What is the HPA axis?
9 What are the six stages of the Cycle of Change?
10 What are the main principles of MI? When would you use this technique?
11 In MI, what is the 'righting reflex'?
12 How would you describe the stress–vulnerability model to discuss an individual's risk of experiencing another episode of depression?

DISCUSSION AND DEBATE

1 Discuss whether medicinal cannabis should undergo the same rigorous testing as other medications before being approved as a treatment for a condition.
2 What do you think would be the benefits and challenges of mandating people with a substance use disorder to receive treatment?
3 Think of a time you tried to change a difficult behaviour of your own. How many attempts were required to alter your behaviour? What were the challenges?
4 What substance do you think causes the most problems in Australia?
5 When a person tells you that drinking alcohol doesn't cause any harm, what are some possible ways you could respond? Consider both the evidence and how you would frame the message.
6 When a person with substance misuse issues is in treatment for only a short time and refuses to discuss substance use, what ethical dilemmas do clinicians face?
7 Opioid substitution pharmacotherapies are criticised by some for keeping a person addicted. Respond to this.
8 What are some similarities and differences between a substance addiction and a gambling problem?

PROJECT ACTIVITY

Speaking with people about problematic substance use may be challenging the first time you try. The best way to develop confidence is to practice with your peers.

Begin by reading the motivational interviewing section of this chapter. Then ask one of your peers to assume the role of a person whose alcohol consumption has caused them to lose their job, their licence and is threatening to end their relationship. Using motivational interviewing strategies, talk with them about how they feel about their alcohol use. If they mention any problems with their use, ask for more detail.

If they don't mention any negative impact of their alcohol use, ask them about their values: 'What things are important in your life?'. If the person includes anything about their relationship, their employment or anything that would require driving, ask them how they are living their life at the moment in alignment with that value and if anything might stand in the way of that in the future. Use other motivational interviewing strategies outlined in this chapter.

WEBSITES

1 Al-Anon's purpose is to help families and friends of alcoholics recover from the effects of living with someone whose drinking is a problem: www.al-anon.org.

2 Your Room is an online resource that health professionals can recommend for people to access information about alcohol and other drugs. It is a joint initiative by NSW Health and St Vincent's Alcohol and Drug Information Service: www.yourroom.health.nsw.gov.au.

3 DrugInfo Clearinghouse is a program of the Australian Drug Foundation that provides easy access to information about alcohol and other drugs, and drug prevention: www.adf.org.au.

4 Mouse Party is a website provided by the University of Utah. The site contains simple animations which illustrate the effect of substances on the brain during intoxication: https://learn.genetics.utah.edu/content/addiction/mouse.

5 The National Drug Research Institute conducts and disseminates high-quality research that contributes to the primary prevention of drug use and the reduction of drug-related harm in Australia: www.ndri.curtin.edu.au.

6 Quitnow is an Australian Government initiative that provides information and support for people who are looking to quit smoking: www.quitnow.gov.au.

7 Reachout.com provides some useful information about substances and substance use in the context of a more generalised youth mental health platform: www.au.reachout.com.

REFERENCES

Abrams, D. I. (2018). The therapeutic effects of cannabis and cannabinoids: An update from the National Academies of Sciences, Engineering and Medicine report. *European Journal of Internal Medicine, 49*, 7–11. https://doi.org/10.1016/j.ejim.2018.01.003

Allman, K. (2019). Is Australia next in line for an opioid class action? *Law Society of NSW Journal, 56*, 26–27. https://lsj.com.au/articles/is-australia-next-in-line-for-an-opioid-class-action

American Psychiatric Association. (2013). *Diagnostic and statistical manual of mental disorders* (5th ed.). APA.

Australian Bureau of Statistics. (2012). *Australian health survey: First results 2011–2012.* (cat. no. 4364.0.55.001). ABS

Australian Institute of Health and Welfare. (2021). *Australian Burden of Disease Study: Impact and causes of illness and death in Australia 2018.* Australian Burden of Disease Study series no. 23. Cat. no. BOD 29. AIHW

Australian Institute of Health and Welfare. (2022). *Illicit drug use.* www.aihw.gov.au/reports/illicit-use-of-drugs/illicit-drug-use

Australian Institute of Health and Welfare. (2018). *Impact of alcohol and illicit drug use on the burden of disease and injury in Australia: Australian Burden of Disease Study 2011.* AIHW.

Australian Institute of Health and Welfare. (2020). *National drug strategy household survey 2019.* Drug Statistics series no. 32. PHE 270. AIHW.

Babor, T. F., McRee, B. G., Kassebaum, P. A., Grimaldi, P. L., Ahmed, K., & Bray, J. (2007). Screening, brief intervention, and referral to treatment (SBIRT): Toward a public health approach to the management of substance abuse. *Substance Abuse, 28*(3), 7–30. https://doi.org/10.1300/J465v28n03_03

Bandura, A. (1997). *Self-efficacy: The exercise of control.* Freeman.

Bell, J., & Ali, R. (2006). *National clinical guidelines for the management of drug use during pregnancy, birth and the early development years of the newborn.* National Drug Strategy.

Bolliger, L., & Stevens, H. (2019). From opioid pain management to opioid crisis in the USA: How can public–private partnerships help? *Frontiers in Medicine (Lausanne), 6,* 106. https://doi.org/10.3389/fmed.2019.00106

Campbell, G., Stockings, E., & Nielsen, S. (2019). Understanding the evidence for medical cannabis and cannabis-based medicines for the treatment of chronic non cancer pain. *European Archives of Psychiatry & Clinical Neuroscience, 269,* 135–144. https://doi.org/10.1007/s00406-018-0960-9

Centre for Population Health. (2014). *NSW clinical guidelines for the management of substance use during pregnancy, birth and the postnatal period.*

Chamberlain, C., & Johnson, G. (2011). Pathways into adult homelessness. *Journal of Sociology, 49*(1), 60–77. https://doi.org/10.1177/1440783311422458

Chan, G., Chiu, V., Sun, T., Connor, J., Hall, W., & Leunig, J. (2021). Age-related trends in cannabis use in Australia. Findings from a series of large nationally representative surveys. *Addictive Behaviors, 123,* 107059. https://doi.org/10.1016/j.addbeh.2021.107059

Clancy, R., & Terry, M. (2007). *Psychiatry and substance use: an interactive resource for clinicians working with clients who have mental health and substance use problems [DVD].* NSW Health.

Commonwealth of Australia. (2016). *Narcotic Drugs Amendment Act 2016*. 7/17.

Daley, D. C., & Douaihy, A. (2019). *A family guide to coping with substance use disorders*. Oxford University Press.

Deady, M., Teesson, M., & Brady, K. T. (2013). Chapter 55. Impact of substance use on the course of serious mental disorders. In *Principles of Addiction*, *1*, 525–532. https://doi.org/10.1016/B978-0-12-398336-7.00055-3

Degenhardt, L., Saha, S., Lim, C. C., Aguilar-Gaxiola, S., Al-Hamzawi, A., Alonso, J. Andrade., H, L., Bromet, E. J., Bruffaerts, R., Caldas-de-Almeida, J. M., de Girolamo, G., Florescu, S., Gureje, O., Haro, J. M., Karam, E. G., Karam, G., Kovess-Masfety, V., Lee, S., & Lepine, J.-P. (2018). The associations between psychotic experiences and substance use and substance use disorders: Findings from the World Health Organization World Mental Health surveys. *WHO World Mental Health Survey Collaborators, Addiction*, *113*(5), 924–934.

Department of Health. (2017a). *National drug strategy 2017–2026*. Commonwealth of Australia.

Department of Health. (2017b). *Tobacco control — key facts and figures*. Australian Government. www.health.gov.au/resources/publications/tobacco-control-key-facts-and-figures

DiClemente, C. (2018). *Addiction and change: How addictions develop and addicted people recover* (2nd ed.). Guilford Press.

Ezard, N., Dunlop, A., Hall, M., Ali, R., McKetin, R., Bruno, R., Phung, N., Carr, A., White, J., Clifford, B., Liu, Z., Shanahan, M., Dolan, K., Baker, A. L., & Lintzeris, N. (2018). LiMA: A study protocol for a randomised, double-blind, placebo controlled trial of lisdexamfetamine for the treatment of methamphetamine dependence. *BMJ Open*, *8*(7), e020723. http://dx.doi.org/10.11 36/bmjopen-2017-020723

Gerardin, M., Victorri-Vigneau, C., Louvigne, C., Rivoal, M., & Jolliet, P. (2011). Management of cannabis use during pregnancy: An assessment of healthcare professionals' practices. *Pharmacoepidemiology and Drug Safety*, *20*, 464–473. https://doi.org/10.1002/pds.2095

Goh, C., & Agius, M. (2010). The stress-vulnerability model how does stress impact on mental illness at the level of the brain and what are the consequences? *Psychiatria Danubina*, *22*(2), 198–202.

Goldstein, B. L., Perlman, G., Kotov, R., Broderick, J. E., Liu, K., Ruggero, C., & Klein, D. N. (2017). Etiologic specificity of waking cortisol: Links with maternal history of depression and anxiety in adolescent girls. *Journal of Affective Disorders*, *208*, 103–109. https://doi.org/10.1016/j.jad.2016.08.079

Gorelick, D. A., Levin, K. H., Copersino, M. L., Heishman, S. J., Lui, F., Boggs, D. L., & Kelly, D. L. (2012). Diagnostic criteria for cannabis withdrawal syndrome. *Drug Alcohol Dependence*, *123*(1–3), 141–147. https://doi.org/10.1016/j.drugalcdep.2011.11.007

Gowing, L., Ali, R., Dunlop, A., Farrell, M., & Lintzeris, N. (2014). *National guidelines for medication-assisted treatment of opioid dependence*. Department of Health. www.health.gov.au/sites/default/files/national-guidelines-for-medication-assisted-treatment-of-opioid-dependence.pdf

Gupta, R. K., Yadav, S. K., Saraswat, V. A., Rangan, M., Srivastava, A., Yadav, A., Trivedi, R., Yachha, S. K., & Rathore, R. K. S. (2012). Thiamine deficiency related microstructural brain changes in acute and acute-on-chronic liver failure or non alcoholic etiology. *Clinical Nutrition*, *31*(3), 422–428. https://doi.org/10.1016/j.clnu.2011.11.018

Haber, P. S., Riordan, B. C., Winter, D. T., Barrett, L., Saunders, J., Hides, L., Gullo, M., Manning, V., Day, C. A., Bonomo, Y., Burns, L., Assan, R., Curry, K., Mooney-Somers, J., Demirkol, A., Monds, L., McDonough, M., Baillie, A. J., Clark, P. … Morley, K. C. (2021). New Australian guidelines for the treatment of alcohol problems: An overview of recommendations. *Medical Journal of Australia*, *215*(S7), S3–S32. https://doi.org/10.5694/mja2.51254

Hall, W. (2015). What has research over the past two decades revealed about the adverse health effects of recreational cannabis use? *Addiction*, *110*(1), 19–35. https://doi.org/10.1111/add.12703

Halladay, J. E., MacKillop, J., Munn, C., Jack, S. M., & Georgiades, K. (2020). Cannabis use as a risk factor for depression, anxiety, and suicidality: Epidemiological associations and implications for nurses. *Journal of Addictions Nursing*, *31*, 92–101. https://doi.org/10.1097/JAN.0000000000000334

Howes, O. D., & Kapur, S. (2009). The dopamine hypothesis of schizophrenia: Version III — The final common pathway. *Schizophrenia Bulletin*, *35*(3), 549–562. https://doi.org/10.1093/schbul/sbp006

Humeniuk, R., Newcombe, D. A. L., Dennington, V., & Ali, R. (2018). A randomised controlled trial of a brief intervention for illicit drug use linked to ASSIST screening in a primary healthcare setting: Results from the Australian component of the World Health Organization Phase III ASSIST studies. *Australian Journal of Primary Health*, *24*(2), 149–154. https://doi.org/10.1071/PY17056

Kaner, E. F. S., Beyer, F. R., Muirhead, C., Campbell, F., Pienaar, E. D., Bertholet, N., Daeppen, J. B., Saunders, J. B., & Burnand, B. (2018). Effectiveness of brief alcohol interventions in primary care populations. *Cochrane Database of Systematic Reviews*, *2018*(2), CD004148. https://doi.org/10.1002/14651858.CD004148.pub4

Keller, J., Gomez, R., Williams, G., Lembke, A., Lazzeroni, L., Murphy, G. M., Jr., & Schatzberg, A. F. (2017). HPA axis in major depression: Cortisol, clinical symptomatology and genetic variation predict cognition. *Molecular Psychiatry*, *22*(4), 527–536. https://doi.org/10.1038/mp.2016.120

Kendler, K. S. (2020). A prehistory of the diathesis-stress model: Predisposing and exciting causes of insanity in the 19th century. *The American Journal of Psychiatry*, *177*, 576–588. https://doi.org/10.1176/appi.ajp.2020.19111213

Koob, G., & Volkow, N. (2010). Neurocircuitry of addiction. *Neuropsychopharmacology*, *35*(1), 217–238. https://doi.org/10.1038/npp.2009.110

Kvaale, E. P., Gottdiener, W. H., & Haslam, N. (2013). Biogenetic explanations and stigma: A meta-analytic review of associations among laypeople. *Social Science & Medicine*, *96*, 95–103. https://doi.org/10.1016/j.socscimed.2013.07.017

Joseph-Lemon, L., Thompson, H., Verostick, L., Shizuka Oura, H., & Jolles, D. R. (2022). Outcomes of cannabis use during pregnancy within the American association of birth centers perinatal data registry 2007–2020: Opportunities within midwifery-led care. *Journal of Perinatal & Neonatal Nursing*, *36*, 264–273. https://doi.org/10.1097/JPN.0000000000000668

Lough, M. E. (2012). Wernicke's encephalopathy: Expanding the diagnostic toolbox. *Neuropsychology Review*, *22*(2), 181–187. https://doi.org/10.1007/s11065-012-9200-7

Lundahl, B., Moleni, T., Burke, B. L., Butters, R., Tollefson, D., Butler, C., & Rollnick, S. (2013). Motivational interviewing in medical care settings: A systematic review and meta-analysis of randomized controlled trials. *Patient Education & Counseling*, *93*(2), 157–168. https://doi.org/10.1016/j.pec.2013.07.012

Luo, Q., Steinberg, J., Yu, X. Q., Weber, M., Caruana, M., Yap, S., Grogan, P. B., Banks, E., O'Connell, D. L., & Canfell, K. (2022). Projections of smoking-related cancer mortality in Australia to 2044. *Journal of Epidemiology and Community Health*, *76*(9), 792–799. https://doi.org/10.1136/jech-2021-218252

Lustman, P. J., Svrakic, D. M., & Feedland, K. E. (2011). Preventing pain medication dependence. *The American Journal of Psychiatry*, *168*(10), 1118–1119. https://doi.org/10.1176/appi.ajp.2011.11060869

Lynch, M., Rabin, R., & George, T. (2012, June). The cannabis–psychosis link. *Psychiatric Times*, 35–39. www.psychiatrictimes.com/view/cannabis-psychosis-link

MacKain, S. J., Liberman, R. P., & Corrigan, P. W. (1994). Can coping and competence override stress and vulnerability in schizophrenia? In *Stress in Psychiatric Disorders* (pp. 53–82). Springer Publishing Co.

Makunts, T., Jerome, L., Abagyan, R., & de Boer, A. (2022). Reported cases of serotonin syndrome in MDMA users in FAERS Database. *Frontiers in Psychiatry*, *12*, 824288. https://doi.org/10.3389/fpsyt.2021.824288

Marel, C., Mills, K., Kingston, R., Gournay, K., Deady, M., Kay-Lambkin, F., Baker, A., & Teesson, M. (2016). Guidelines on the management of co-occurring alcohol and other drug and mental health conditions in alcohol and other drug treatment settings. In *Centre of Research Excellence in Mental Health and Substance Use* (2nd ed.). National Drug and Alcohol Research Centre, University of New South Wales.

Metz, T. D., Allshouse, A. A., McMillin, G. A., Silver, R. M., Smid, M. C., Haas, D. M., Simhan, H. N., Saade, G. R., Grobman, W. A., Parry, S., Chung, J. H., & Jarlenski, M. P. (2022). Association of cannabis use with nausea and vomiting of pregnancy. *Obstetrics & Gynecology*, *140*, 266–270. https://doi.org/10.1097/AOG.0000000000004850

Miller, W., & Rollnick, S. (2013). *Motivational interviewing: Helping people for change* (3rd ed.). Guilford Press.

Miller, W., & Rollnick, S. (2002). *Motivational interviewing: Preparing people for change* (2nd ed.). Guilford Press.

Miller, W., & Rollnick, S. (1991). *Motivational interviewing: Preparing people to change addictive behaviour*. Guilford Press.

Miller, W. R., & Sanchez, V. C. (1993). Motivating young adults for treatment and lifestyle changes. In G. Howard (Ed.), *Issues in alcohol use and misuse in young adults*. University of Notre Dame Press.

Morgan, J. C., Byron, M. J., Baig, S. A., Stepanov, I., & Brewer, N. T. (2017). How people think about the chemicals in cigarette smoke: A systematic review. *Journal of Behavioral Medicine*, *40*(4), 553–564. https://doi.org/10.1007/s10865-017-9823-5

Mueser, K., Noordsy, D., Drake, R., & Fox, L. (2003). *Integrated treatment for dual disorders: A guide to effective practice*. Guilford Press.

National Centre for Education and Training on Addiction. (2006). *Health professionals' attitudes toward licit and illicit drug users*. Flinders University.

National Health and Medical Research Council. (2020). *Australian guidelines to reduce health risks from drinking alcohol*. Commonwealth of Australia.

National Institute on Drug Abuse. (2010). *Comorbidity: Addition and other mental illnesses*. National Institutes of Health Publication (10-577110–5771).

NCETA Consortium. (2004). *Alcohol and other drugs: A handbook for health professionals*. Department of Health and Ageing.

NSW Health. (2020). *Your room. A place to get facts about alcohol and other drugs*. www.yourroom.health.nsw.gov.au/Pages/home.aspx

NSW Health. (2009). *Clinical guidelines for the care of persons with co-morbid mental illness and substance use disorders in acute care settings*. NSW.

NSW Ministry of Health. (2021). *Handbook for nurses and midwives: Responding effectively to people who use alcohol and other drugs*. NSW.

Oakley, L. D., Kuo, W., Kowalkowski, J. A., & Park, W. (2021). Meta-analysis of cultural influences in trauma exposure and PTSD prevalence rates. *Journal of Transcultural Nursing*, *32*, 412–424. https://doi.org/10.1177/1043659621993909

O'Brien, K. (2019). Medicinal cannabis: Issues of evidence. *European Journal of Integrative Medicine*, *28*, 114–120. https://doi.org/10.1016/j.eujim.2019.05.009

Paulus, M. P., & Stewart, J. L. (2020). Neurobiology, clinical presentation, and treatment of methamphetamine use disorder: A review. *JAMA Psychiatry*, *77*(9), 959–966. https://doi.org/10.1001/jamapsychiatry.2020.0246

Peacock, A., Karlsson, A., Uporova, J., Gibbs, D., Swanton, R., Kelly, G., Price, O., Bruno, R., Dietze, P., Lenton, S., Salom, C., Degenhardt, L., & Farrell, M. (2019). *Australian drug trends 2019: Key findings from the National Ecstasy and Related Drugs Reporting System (EDRS) interviews*. National Drug and Alcohol Research.

Prochaska, J., & DiClemente, C. (1982). Transtheoretical therapy: Toward a more integrative model of change. *Psychotherapy: Theory, Research, and Practice*, *19*, 276–288. https://doi.org/10.1037/h0088437

Puljević, C., & Segan, C. J. (2019). Systematic review of factors influencing smoking following release from smoke-free prisons. *Nicotine & Tobacco Research*, *21*(8), 1011–1020. https://doi.org/10.1093/ntr/nty088

Randal, P., Stewart, M. W., Proverb, D., Lampshire, D., Symes, J., & Hamer, H. (2009). 'The re-covery model' — an integrative developmental stress-vulnerability-strengths approach to mental health. *Psychosis: Psychological, Social and Integrative Approaches*, *1*(2), 122–133. https://doi.org/10.1080/17522430902948167

Rastegar, D. A., & Walley, A. Y. (2013). Preventing prescription opioid deaths. *Journal of General International Medicine*, *28*(10), 1258–1259. https://doi.org/10.1007/s11606-013-2390-8

Rehan, H. S., Maini, J., & Hungin, A. P. S. (2018). Vaping versus smoking: A quest for efficacy and safety of e-cigarette. *Current Drug Safety*, *13*(2), 92–101. https://doi.org/10.2174/1574886313666180227110556

Rende, R., & Plomin, R. (1992). Diathesis-stress models of psychopathology: A quantitative genetic perspective. *Applied and Preventive Psychology*, *1*(4), 177–182. https://doi.org/10.1016/S0962-1849(05)80123-4

Rincon, A. (2012). *Neuroscience research progress: Amphetamines — neurobiological mechanisms, pharmacology and effects*. Nova Science Publishers, Inc.

Ritter, A., King, T., & Lee, N. (2017). *Drug use in Australian society* (2nd ed.). Oxford University Press.

Roche, A. M., Ryan, K., Fischer, J., & Nicholas, R. (2019). *A review of Australian clinical guidelines for methamphetamine use disorder*. Prepared by the National Centre for Education and Training on Addiction for the National Centre for Clinical Research on Emerging Drugs.

Saunders, J. B., Aasland, O. G., & Babor, T. F. (1993). Development of the alcohol use disorders identification test (AUDIT): WHO collaborative project on early detection of persons with harmful alcohol consumption, part II. *Addiction, 88*, 791–804. https://doi.org/10.1111/j.1360-0443.1993.tb02093.x

Schwartz, D. A. (2018). Cannabis and the lung. *International Journal of Mental Health and Addiction, 16*(4), 797–800. https://doi.org/10.1007/s11469-018-9902-z

Shalit, N., & Lev-Ran, S. (2020). Does cannabis use increase anxiety disorders? A literature review. *Current Opinion in Psychiatry, 33*, 8–13. https://doi.org/10.1097/YCO.0000000000000560

Sinha, S., Kataria, A., Kolla, B. P., Thusius, N., & Loukianova, L. L. (2019). Wernicke Encephalopathy. *Clinical Pearls Mayo Clinic Proceedings, 94*(6), 1065–1072. https://doi.org/10.1016/j.mayocp.2019.02.018

Smith, K. W., Sicignano, D. J., Hernandez, A. V., & White, C. M. (2022). MDMA-Assisted Psychotherapy for treatment of posttraumatic stress disorder: A systematic review with meta-analysis. *The Journal of Clinical Pharmacology, 62*, 463–471. https://doi.org/10.1002/jcph.1995

Southwick, S. M., Vythilingam, M., & Charney, D. S. (2005). The psychobiology of depression and resilience to stress: Implications for prevention and treatment. *Annual Review of Clinical Psychology, 1*(1), 255–291.

Stockings, E., Zagic, D., Campbell, G., Weier, M., Hall, W. D., Nielsen, S., Herkes, G. K., Farrell, M., & Degenhardt, L. (2018). Evidence for cannabis and cannabinoids for epilepsy: A systematic review of controlled and observational evidence. *Journal of Neurology, Neurosurgery and Psychiatry, 89*(7), 741–753. https://doi.org/10.1136/jnnp-2017-317168

Straussner, S. L. A. (2012). Clinical treatment of substance abusers: Past, present and future. *Journal of Clinical Social Work, 40*, 127–133. https://doi.org/10.1007/s10615-012-0387-0

Therapeutic Goods Administration. (2019). *Introduction to Medicinal cannabis regulation in Australia.* www.tga.gov.au/news/blog/introduction-medicinal-cannabis-regulation-australia

Therapeutic Guidelines Limited. (2013). *Therapeutic guidelines: Psychotropic (version 7).* Therapeutic Guidelines Ltd.

Thompson, C. R. (2015). *Prevention practice and health promotion: A health care professional's guide to health, fitness, and wellness* (2nd ed.). Slack Inc.

Thomson, A. D., Guerrini, I., & Marshall, J. E. (2012). The evolution and treatment of Korsakoff's syndrome. *Neuropsychology Review, 22*(2), 81–92. https://doi.org/10.1007/s11065-012-9196-z

United Kingdom Policy Drug Commission. (2010). *Extreme social stigma holds back drug recovery.* University of York.

US Department of Health and Human Services Office of the Surgeon General. (2016). *Facing addiction in America: The surgeon general's report on alcohol, drugs, and health.* US Department of Health and Human Services.

van Boekel, L. C., Brouwers, E. P., van Weeghel, J., & Garretsen, H. F. (2013). Stigma among health professionals towards patients with substance use disorders and its consequences for healthcare delivery: A systematic review. *Drug Alcohol Dependence, 1*(131), 23–35. https://doi.org/10.1016/j.drugalcdep.2013.02.018

Varker, T., Watson, L., Gibson, K., Forbes, D., & O'Donnell, M. L. (2021). Efficacy of psychoactive drugs for the treatment of posttraumatic stress disorder: A systematic review of MDMA, Ketamine, LSD and Psilocybin. *Journal of Psychoactive Drugs, 53*(1), 85–95. https://doi.org/10.1080/02791072.2020.1817639

Volkow, N. D., Koob, G. F., & McLellan, A. T. (2016). Neurobiologic advances from the brain disease model of addiction. *New England Journal of Medicine, 374*(4), 363–371. https://doi.org/10.1056/NEJMra1511480

Volkow, N.D., Gordon, J. A., & Koob, G. F. (2021). Choosing appropriate language to reduce the stigma around mental illness and substance use disorders. *Neuropsychopharmacol, 46*, 2230–2232. https://doi.org/10.1038/s41386-021-01069-4

Whetton, S., Tait, R. J., Gilmore, W., Dey, T., Agramunt, S., Abdul Halim, S., McEntee, A., Mukhtar, A., Roche, A., Allsop, S., & Chikritzhs, T. (2021). *Examining the social and economic costs of alcohol use in Australia: 2017/18.* National Drug Research Institute, Curtin University.

Wiesjahn, M., Jung, E., Kremser, J. D., Rief, W., & Lincoln, T. M. (2016). The potential of continuum versus biogenetic beliefs in reducing stigmatization against persons with schizophrenia: An experimental study. *Journal of Behavior Therapy and Experimental Psychiatry, 50*, 231–237. https://doi.org/10.1016/j.jbtep.2015.09.007

Zubin, J., & Spring, B. (1977). Vulnerability: A new view of schizophrenia. *Journal of Abnormal Psychology, 86*(2), 103–126. https://doi.org/10.1037/0021-843X.86.2.103

ACKNOWLEDGEMENTS

Figure 10.1: © Australian Institute of Health and Welfare 2020. *National Drug Strategy Household Survey 2019.* Drug Statistics series no. 32. PHE 270. Canberra AIHW. Licensed under CC BY 4.0.

Figure 10.2: © Department of Health (2017) *National Drug Strategy 2017–2026.* Canberra: Commonwealth of Australia. Licensed under CC BY 4.0.

Figure 10.4: © NSW Ministry of Health (2018). Licensed under CC BY 4.0.

Figure 10.6: © DiClemente C. (2018). *Addiction and change: how addictions develop and addicted people recover,* 2nd Edition. New York: Guilford Press. Reproduced with permission from Carlo DiClemente.

Table 10.1: © Australian Institute of Health and Welfare 2020. *National Drug Strategy Household Survey 2019.* Drug Statistics series no. 32. PHE 270. Canberra AIHW. Licensed under CC BY 4.0.

Extract: © Your Room / NSW Health

Photo: © fizkes / Shutterstock.com

Photo: © kangwan nirach / Shutterstock.com

Photo: © Commonwealth of Australia

Caring for an older person with a mental illness

LEARNING OBJECTIVES

This chapter will:

11.1 provide an overview of caring for the older person with a mental illness

11.2 consider the notion of ageism and the impact on health outcomes for the older person

11.3 outline the major aspects of assessing the older person

11.4 clarify how to recognise depression in an older person

11.5 describe dementia from a person-centred perspective

11.6 differentiate between dementia, depression and delirium.

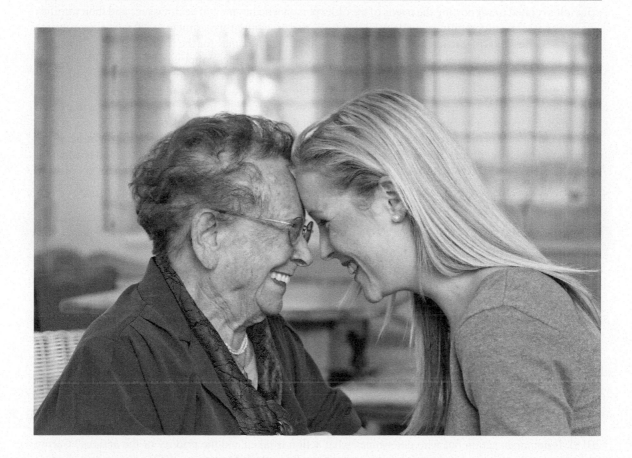

Introduction

Approximately 16 per cent of the Australian population, that is, one in six or 4.2 million people, are 65 years of age or older and 53 per cent are women (Australian Institute of Health and Welfare [AIHW], 2021). By 2066, this percentage is expected to increase to 21–23 per cent (AIHW, 2021). This trend is common to all Western nations and is a result of sustained lower birth rates, increasing life expectancy and the fact that those born shortly after the Second World War — the 'baby boomers' — are now reaching old age. The success of the Australian health system cannot be measured solely by the longevity of the population. Consideration must be given to the quality of life enjoyed by the population throughout the life span. Australian health care in the twenty-first century thus needs to focus on ensuring there are adequate resources, including the delivery of primary health care services, for its ageing population (Remm et al., 2021). The delivery of services and enhancing the quality of life of senior members of the community depends on the knowledge, skills and attitudes of those charged with supporting this group of older people.

Many older people will live a healthy and independent life regardless of the myriad health conditions that may affect them, such as arthritis, osteoporosis, cancer, stroke and vascular disease (AIHW, 2018). Although the prevalence of disability among older people has slightly decreased in the past few years, it still remains high at 49.6 per cent (ABS, 2019). For one in three people over 65 years, their lives are impacted by three or more chronic conditions (AIHW, 2018). This is especially true for those aged 85 and over, where the need for assistance with cognitive and emotional tasks is four times greater (28 per cent) than those aged 65–84 years (7 per cent) (AIHW, 2021). Anxiety and depression are high-risk issues. Likewise, dementia affects 83 people per 1000 Australians aged 65 and over and two-thirds of these people are women (AIHW, 2022). It is estimated that one in five of those with dementia will experience moderate to severe behavioural and psychiatric symptoms (Moyle et al., 2017).

These statistics suggest why supporting older people is of particular importance to governments and health services across Australia. Likewise, it is essential that health professionals are aware of the main principles related to supporting the needs of the older person who has mental health issues and their families — awareness of vulnerabilities, undertaking astute, person-centred assessment, referral to appropriate support services and treatments and follow up to evaluate the outcomes for the individual.

The focus of this chapter is the older person who is experiencing symptoms of mental illness. The chapter begins by extending the discussion around 'care' to consider the quite specific needs of older people. Notions of ageism are also discussed. Following this, approaches to the assessment of the older person are described. The importance of providing person-centred care using a biopsychosocial approach is highlighted. Assessment tools, such as the mini-mental state examination and Addenbrooke's cognitive examination are explained. The essential aspects of working with an older person with depression are described. The chapter finishes by clarifying the difference between dementia and delirium, and how health professionals can best work with older people who are experiencing symptoms of each of these conditions.

11.1 Caring for older people

LEARNING OBJECTIVE 11.1 Provide an overview of caring for the older person with a mental illness.

The meaning of 'care' and 'caring', and the principles related to the provision of care and caring, are discussed at length in the chapter on mental health care in Australia. This section extends the discussion to consider caring for the older person. This includes a reiteration of the essential nature of the relationship between the health professional and the person when providing care, and the importance of knowing the older person as an individual. In developing a person-centred relationship with an older person and ensuring an authentic focus on the person, consideration is needed about the term caring.

Notions of caring imply at least two related ideas. The first idea is that to care for another involves health professionals in a relationship with themselves as a health professional and with the person they are caring for. That is, in order to be able to form a relationship with another person and to provide care, health professionals need to be able to take care of themselves first. Essentially, they need to be able to practise what they will then preach. The second idea is that this caring relationship is an active, not a passive, engagement. While caring may be anchored in emotionality, it is not limited to it (Graffigna & Barello, 2018). It demands action but who determines what action is taken and the priority of the actions? Caring for someone can have connotations of infantalisation (Bernoth & Montayre, 2022). The attitude here is 'I am caring for you, I have the knowledge and skills to care for you and your role is to do as I say'. An example of infantalisation is when health professionals use the term 'non-compliant' when a person does not act in the way they prescribed. If we are working with the person, there is collaboration with goals, and the way to the goals jointly determined.

Another approach is to envisage the relationship as a partnership, so you are working with the older person. Together you will walk through the assessment process, identify the pathway to treatment and support, determine the extent to which strategies have been successful, with the entire journey guided by the person (Bernoth et al., 2016; Burmeister et al., 2016). The German philosopher, Heidegger (Horrigan-Kelly et al., 2016) and the nursing theorist Parse, (Parse, 2019) both espouse the concept of 'being with' the person.

It is this 'reality of the other' that drives and sustains the task of caring for or working with the older person with mental health issues. Their approach is consistent with a comprehensive inclusion of the individual, including a **biopsychosocial understanding** of the 'other' (refer to the chapter that looks at assessment in the mental health context). This suggests a number of themes. One is that older people are not a **homogeneous group**. Like any group of individuals, each person is unique in their aims, goals, beliefs, interests, experiences and personality.

Another theme is that effective health professionals do not **pathologise** ageing. Depression, anxiety, dementia, suicide and myriad other mental illnesses are not the inevitable consequence of ageing. Also, it is important to recognise that the older person can be easily excluded from discussions about health care resource allocation, policy initiatives and even their own treatment regimes. It may be the case that older people are not only disadvantaged by their age and the way society views 'being old', but those with a mental illness may also be disadvantaged by the added stigma attached to anyone with mental health problems (Song et al., 2018).

Further, in keeping with the requirement to apprehend the reality of the other, the health professional is urged to see and understand the older person in context. That is, the health professional is encouraged to view the person in terms of their emotional, psychological, physical, sexual and spiritual totality, rather than see them simply as an illness, a diagnosis or as a collection of symptoms. There is a need to acknowledge the meaning of their lives in a truly integrated and comprehensive way (Reich et al., 2020)

Health professionals must also take care to listen to the meaning that is being placed on an experience or event by the other person, rather than place their own interpretation on that experience or event further emphasising the significance of working with the individual. Understanding the experiences of the older person is brought into sharp focus with the problem of delirium. Failure to observe, understand, acknowledge or hear the voice of the older person who has a delirium can have tragic consequences for both the person with a delirium and the health professional. The consequences for the older person with a pre-existing dementia or an already debilitated medical state, an untreated delirium can be fatal (Honan & Green, 2022).

11.2 The impact of ageism

LEARNING OBJECTIVE 11.2 Consider the notion of ageism and the impact on health outcomes for the older person.

In a society that, demographically speaking, is characterised by increasing numbers of older people, ageism exists. Regardless of the current demographics, the phenomenon of discriminating against people based upon their chronological age, first described by Butler (1969), survives and remains a powerful force for shaping perceptions and thus influencing behaviours.

Ageism has a well-established pedigree. Growing old has long been seen as an affliction associated with a deterioration in both mental and physical functioning. The older people have been described in terms such as 'wise', 'slow', ' **senile**', 'ill', 'infirm', 'forgetful', 'frail' and 'decrepit' (Levy et al., 2012). In Western literature, older people have often been convenient caricatures. In William Shakespeare's *As you like it*, Jacques bemoans the inevitable conclusion to the 'strange and eventful history' that is life's journey, which ends in '. . . mere oblivion; sans teeth, sans eyes, sans taste, sans everything' (Act 11, scene 7). Aged character depiction often lurches uneasily from sad and pathetic, as in the folly of Shakespeare's King Lear, to downright evil and repulsive, as with Dickens's Scrooge; '. . . a squeezing, wrenching, grasping, scraping, clutching, covetous old sinner . . . [who] . . . carried his own low temperature always about with him' (Hearn, 2004).

In more recent times, perhaps due in part to mass electronic media, the distinction between being young and being old has come into sharp focus. There appears to be a clear juxtaposition between the (idealised) images of youth, interwoven with cultural ideas and ideals of beauty, sexuality, achievement, strength, vigour and technological sophistication, with a perception, even a fear or revulsion, of the older person with wrinkled, sagging and blotched skin, hunched over and with ponderous mobility, frail and arthritically welded to that icon of ageing — the walking frame. It is not surprising that in recent times there has been an emergent image of the older person who contributes nothing to society yet remains a burden on economic resources, such as medical care, pensions and various welfare programs that drain public monies from more worthwhile endeavours. Despite some attempts at changing attitudes and stereotypes to encourage a recognition of positive ageing, there seems to be a pervasive attitude that sees the older person as somehow not belonging — as a burden to the taxpayer, a drain on social and economic development and thus, somehow as less of a person (van den Heuvel, 2012). In 2020, E-Shien and colleagues, published research linking ageism and poor health outcomes for older individuals.

UPON REFLECTION

Impact of negative attitudes towards ageing on assessment and recovery

It is clear that the negative attitudes of a health professional can have an impact on the way in which they relate to and provide assistance for a patient. Reflection and appropriate clinical supervision are key aspects of a health professional's ability to understand their own values and how they may have an impact on the provision of care.

....

QUESTIONS

1. Do you think that a patient's concept of age would have an impact on their ability to recover from physical or psychological illness? Why?
2. What impact would the attitudes of a health professional have on an older person's recovery?
3. How could ageist attitudes affect the ability to build rapport and developing trust during the assessment and treatment?
4. How do you feel about growing old and what rights do you expect as you enter old age?

Ageist attitudes

Societal norms are pervasive and can easily influence how health professionals generally engage the older person. In the technologically developed West, discussions about ageing often appear to focus on the medical and moral challenges it presents. For example, ageing is often viewed as a process defined by deterioration in a whole range of physical abilities, attributes and aspects, with the task for the older person being to age 'successfully'. Notions of healthy or positive ageing carry the underlying message that one can get ageing wrong; one can fail at it; one can let the side down; or that one can cost the community (the taxpayer) precious resources. To fail at ageing is to court moral censure, so the older person must lift their game and not 'let the side down'. In 2021, Voigt proposed the term 'adaptive ageing' to find an inclusive term to embrace the ageing process.

A combination of ageist social values and an increasing tendency to medicalise ageing sees the ageing process often couched in terms of **cognitive decline** (Aberdeen & Bye, 2013). Ageing is another stage of life (see Erikson, 1959) involving growth, challenges, joys and sadness, frustrations and achievements (Hughes et al., 2022). Health professionals are encouraged to reframe ageing to incorporate positive elements, including notions of wisdom, experience and a 'third (or golden) age', which presents the older person with many new opportunities.

Oliver (2008) notes pervasive ageism among health professionals in the way the older person is so easily labelled in pejorative terms like '**social admission**' and '**acopia**'. He suggests that terms such as these reflect the social judgements of health professionals, rather than any attempt to identify actual physical or psychological disease processes, and they also allow physicians to avoid taking the concerns of the older person seriously. It is recognised that health professionals have a tendency to shy away from caring for older people with a mental illness (Singleton & Douglas, 2012; Walsh & Shutes, 2013). This view is reinforced by recent research by Rayner and colleagues (2022), which reveals that graduate health professionals regard working with older people as boring. Further evidence of dismissing the needs of older people, and demonstrating infantilisation of older patients, is the use of physical and chemical restraints (Thomann et al., 2021). The use of restraint was addressed in the final report of the Royal Commission into Aged Care Quality and Safety (RCACQ&S). Recommendation 17 outlines the changes needed to reduce and regulate restraints (RCACQ&S, 2021, pp. 221–222); however, these relate to residential aged care only. The use of restraints continues to occur in acute care despite the increasing evidence against the use of restraints with vulnerable populations.

Discrimination

Discrimination has many faces. One may be a simple negative attitude towards the older person based upon a fear or dread of ageing (Bishop et al., 2008) and mortality. Another may be the tendency to see the older person as a member of a subgroup primarily defined in terms of their deficits (Horta, 2010). A further act of discrimination includes the practice of seeing all older people — that is, everyone over 65 years — as a member of a homogeneous collection of individuals (van den Heuvel, 2012) with identical needs, wants, ambitions, fears, beliefs and values. Such perceptions are not uncommon. Indeed, ageism is so pervasive that even older people themselves will endorse ageist attitudes and behaviours towards themselves and other older persons (Bryant et al., 2012).

Thus, the first challenge for the health professional working with the older person is to see each individual within the context of their own lives and their own meanings, and to set aside their own preconceived ideas about what should be and what should not be; what is and what is not; and who is deserving of care and who is not. Social images of older people seem to oscillate between the cranky, irritable, cantankerous and intolerant 'grumpy old men' and 'grumpy old women' (there are even television shows by those names) and someone who is a cross between Santa Claus and Agatha Christie's Miss Marple — without any distinctive personality, shapeless and invisible, always pleasant to small children and dogs, without ambition, beliefs, voice or opinion and decidedly asexual. Yet the health professional will be confronted with older people who have a mental illness or dementia, who have sexual relationships, who live independently or who identify as lesbian, gay, bisexual, transgender, gender diverse, intersex, queer, asexual or questioning (LGBTQIA+).

Older people remain in the workforce, are primary carers for grandchildren and other family members, identify as First Nations and other diverse cultures. They may speak several languages and English may or may not be one of them. Realities such as these may challenge the professional's preconceived ideas of what it means to be old; and yet the responsibility of the health professional is to acknowledge the uniqueness of the individual person (Burns et al., 2019). It may be that the health professional's first step towards confronting ageism lies in emotional intelligence — honest and thorough examination of their own attitudes and values — and exploring unconscious cultural bias. Being culturally aware and safe means respectful, informed, sensitive interactions with Aboriginal and Torres Straight Islander peoples and people from diverse cultures. Chontelle Gibson's research (2020) with older First Nations women, provides an invaluable resource for health professionals as a guide for respectful conversations called 'yarning'.

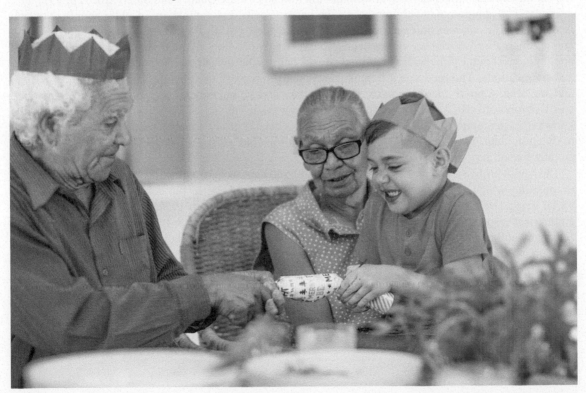

11.3 Assessing the older person

LEARNING OBJECTIVE 11.3 Outline the major aspects of assessing the older person.

The assessment process begins with listening to the story of the person. At one level this 'listening' is just that: listening to the older person's perspective. A person's life is often understood as a series of narratives (Bruner, 2004) — that is, stories about who we are, who we have been and how we have come to this particular point. Just listening to the words of the other person as they tell their particular story — whether it is a story of dementia, depression, suicidal thoughts, chronic mental health issues, grief or loss — is a powerful way for the health professional to build a rapport based upon the existence of the older person as a person. If the ability to confront one's own preconceived ideas about ageing is the first skill of the health professional, then the ability to listen without judgement is the second.

A biopsychosocial approach

On a deeper level, this listening takes on a more profound form of knowing. This facilitates the enactment of the biopsychosocial approach to mental illness and recognises the complexities this involves (Engert et al., 2020). In the past, health professionals have tended to debate the relative merits of nature versus nurture, mind versus body and biology versus environment when it comes to the understanding of cause and process of mental illness (McKay et al., 2012). There is no easy distinction to be made; people are a complex interaction of relationships and interrelationships; there is an 'interplay between environment, physical, behavioural, psychological, and social factors' (Beddoe, 2013, p. 25).

The biopsychosocial model is predicated upon the interaction between the physical, mental and emotional beings, the sorts of relationships people have with others in their lives and the environment we live within.

In terms of the assessment process, the health professional works from the biopsychosocial and person-centred approaches described in the chapter that looks at assessment in the mental health context. In this chapter, these two approaches are combined to be called the **biopsychosocial person-centred approach** to assessment and care. The additional term, 'person-centred', reminds the professional that the person and the care of the person is the rationale for undertaking any form of assessment. 'Quality of life is a measurable outcome of good person-centred care, and good quality of life is shown to have positive impact on clinical outcomes' (Royal Commission into Aged Care Quality and Safety, 2021, p. 95).

Figure 11.1 diagrammatically represents the heterogeneity and complexity of older people. Not only is the person a complex interaction of diverse influences, but also these influences cannot be easily compartmentalised. Variables such as depression can easily fit within all three parts of the model. The same applies to most of the dimensions identified — each has psychological, sociological and biological impacts and implications. The model is a flexible conceptual framework to structure approaches to assessment and ongoing support for the person, their families and communities. As recognised by Santangelo and Dobrohotoff (2022), implementing the biopsychosocial model of care involves the diverse skills, knowledge, perceptions and experience of a range of health professionals to address the specific needs of the individual. To ensure interdependent factors of the older person are addressed, the collaboration of an interdisciplinary team is required.

The health professional who adopts the person-centred approach, recognises that 'personhood is a status or standing which is bestowed upon one human being by others, in the context of relationships and social being [which] implies recognition, respect and trust' (Kitwood, 1977, p. 8). Person-centred care emphasises respect for the individual as a unique human being (Kitwood & Bredin, 1992). In his research, Mack and colleagues (2021) found that person-centredness is based on relationships between all actors in the care giving environment. It may be suggested that the relationship between the person's social being, and their psychological and physical self is one of primus inter pares or first among equals. In whatever way this relationship is conceptualised, the health professional is called upon to consider the person with all their individuality and complexities — revealed through skilled assessment. What does this mean in practice? Questions such as these are discussed in the next section.

FIGURE 11.1 The biopsychosocial person-centred model

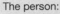

The person:
- An individual
- A social being
- With intrinsic value and rights
- Personal experiences
- Personal history
- Culture and background
- Personal preferences
- Unique abilities
- Personal needs

Aspects of:
- Depression
- Anxiety
- Worries
- Loneliness
- Isolation
- Ageing
- Mortality
- Grief and loss
- Cognition
- Ethnicity
- Delusions
- Hallucinations
- Capacity

Psychological

Sociological

Biological

Aspects of:
- Family
- Friends
- Upbringing
- Education
- Occupation
- Religion/spirituality
- Ethnicity
- Values
- Community
- Hobbies
- Legal
- Sexuality
- Finances

Aspects of:
- Biomedical history
- Current biomedical issues including levels of pain and medications
- Ageing
- Disability
- Mobility
- Diet
- Capacity
- Physical environment

Knowing the person

Knowing a person is a complex process that can be difficult to quantify or qualify. In the health context, it means that the health professional must know the totality of the person and not seek to reduce the older person to a collection of symptoms, an artefact of medical pathology, or a deviation from how older people are often portrayed in society. It means that a systematic approach to knowing the person begins with an understanding of the personal experiences and history of the individual, their relationships with others, the significant events in their lives and the meanings they place on their experiences.

Knowing the older person also means that treatment is collaborative. The idea of 'collaboration' is usually couched within the context of members of the multidisciplinary team working in harmony. This is certainly crucial for optimal outcomes. However, even this form of collaboration is dependent upon a more basic form of engagement: the collaboration of the professional with the older person. The health professional works *with* the older person and does not impose a set of judgements or treatment options *upon* that person.

Getting to know the older person (Anna's story)

At the age of 82, Anna decided that it was time to retire from her work as a community nurse. She was widowed, had raised two children who live some distance away, and she wanted to spend more time visiting them, her adult grandchildren and her friends. Anna also wanted to travel, see her beloved Australia and the world. For the following 5 years, Anna indulged in her passion for life and travel despite increasing restrictions imposed on her by chronic health.

Throughout her adult life, Anna had grappled with the pain and impaired function caused by osteoarthritis and depression, both of which had greater imposts on her life as she grew older. In her early adult years, Anna had been hospitalised for depression and had been subjected to electroconvulsive therapy. Her experiences with depression and the treatments she had endured were only shared with intimate family as it caused her distress to talk about her mental health experiences.

Anna had interrupted sleep patterns because of her many years working night duty and because of the pain of osteoarthritis. She had difficulty getting to sleep and then would not wake until late into the morning. Osteoarthritis made movement increasingly difficult, and her manual dexterity was impaired by the impact on her fingers and hands. She often dropped items she was holding, found it difficult to open jars and impossible to continue to knit.

Sleeping until late, challenges getting dressed and pain all increasingly restricted this previously gregarious woman's life. Anna became increasingly depressed.

Anna's medications are as follows.

Medication	Dose	Frequency
Panadol Osteo	2 tabs	Three times a day
Zoloft	200 mg	In the morning
Nexium	20 mg	Twice daily
Olmesartan	20 mg	Twice daily
Lipitor	40 mg	At night
Panadeine Forte	2 tabs	When needed
Temazepam	2 tabs	When needed

In an attempt to manage her symptoms, Anna also used Fisiocrem and hot packs to relieve her osteoarthritis and St John's Wort to lighten her mood.

As she tried to prepare some lunch, Anna had a fall and was found by a neighbour who heard Anna's cries for help. She was taken by ambulance to the local hospital. On admission, she was confused and could not recall what had happened, could not inform the admitting doctor of her medications nor when she had taken anything for pain.

QUESTIONS

1. Consider how Anna would be feeling physically and mentally on her presentation to the Emergency Department.
2. Identify possible causes for the confusion Anna is experiencing on admission.
3. What are the consequences for Anna if her confusion is assumed to be dementia?
4. What strategies would be essential for the admitting nurse to use to gain Anna's trust and lead to a comprehensive assessment?
5. Link aspects of Anna's case study with the domains of the biopsychosocial model.
6. Identify the relevant health professionals to include on the Interdisciplinary Team to support Anna.

Thinking biopsychosocially

One way of understanding the biopsychosocial approach is to think of the various options the health professional may have in a case such as that described in the previous 'in practice' feature. The health professional may take a strictly biological approach and ask questions such as:

- 'Is Anna physically unwell?'
- 'Has an adverse medication event contributed to the fall?'

- Has Anna experienced falls or other traumas in the past and if so, what were the causes?
- 'Is this confused state unusual for Anna? How will I access this information?'
  If this is the pathway of investigations then other questions might be asked, such as:
- 'What is Anna's pain status?'
- 'Has Anna been feeling depressed and is she currently experiencing depression?'
- 'What assessments need to be undertaken of Anna's environment prior to her discharge to ensure her safety?'

The health professional may also conduct a variety of investigations, being cognisant of atypical presentations of pathology in older people — abdominal emergencies, acute myocardial infarction, elder abuse, sepsis and infection which can all result in the older person experiencing a fall and trauma. Follow-up tests may involve a chest X-ray, blood tests, an ECG, urinalysis and CT scan of the abdomen.

To screen for delirium or dementia, the health professional initially engages in conversation with Anna to gain insight into her level of cognition. Then check with the family about Anna's usual level of cognition asking if her presentation is normal or changed since the fall. As a more formal means of assessment, a simple mini-mental state exam (MMSE) or an Addenbrooke's cognitive examination (ACE), are two simple assessments for cognitive functioning. These can be undertaken through conversations rather than a formal assessment to ensure Anna feels comfortable and the outcomes are a true reflection of cognition.

To embrace a biopsychosocial approach to the assessment, further assessment is undertaken. In terms of the person's psychological needs, the health professional may explore the mental health, emotional or behavioural causes for the person presenting to the health service for assistance, such as the following.
- What is the mood and affect of the person?
- Do they report feelings of depression or anxiety? (Refer to the chapter that looks at caring for a person with depression and anxiety for more information on these conditions.)
- What are their thoughts and behaviours?
- What are their perceptions?

The health professional is aware that both depression and anxiety often go together and, in the older person, this may display as a somatic presentation. The health professional will also explore thoughts of self-harm, asking questions such as the following.
- 'Do you have future plans?'
- 'How have you coped with problems in the past?'
- 'Is there a personal or family history of depression, anxiety, self-harm or even suicide?'
- 'What do you worry about?'
- 'What is your usual sleeping pattern?'

The health professional then asks questions of a more sociological nature. They will take the time to get to know their client as a person, building rapport and trust, so the patient is comfortable and confident in the skills of the person interacting with them. This will involve taking a personal history and ascertaining aspects of their life, such as:
- who they live with, and whether this has changed recently
- where they have moved from
- whether they are married, single, widowed or divorced
- what social supports they have
- what family they have and how much support they have from them
- what their financial situation is
- their educational and occupational background.

This list is by no means exhaustive but, following on from the previous 'In practice' example, a picture soon emerges that reveals a situation far more complex than was first presented.

Anna reveals her history of depression and the multiple interventions and medications she has endured over many years of her adult life. She shares that her pain is getting more difficult to live with and her general practitioner refuses to listen to her concerns and prescribe more effective medications such as Tramadol or morphine. Anna feels his concern is not for her but rather is concerned he will be audited by the regulatory authority. This makes her feel hopeless and helpless, making her depression more pronounced and more difficult to overcome. Anna shares that her sleep patterns are far from healthy as a result of year doing night shift as a nurse. She does not go to sleep until the early hours of the morning, is constantly woken by the pain from her arthritis and then finds it challenging to get up before lunchtime. This impacts her social life as she is unable to get to social events planned for the morning. Recently she had an accident while driving and is reluctant to drive, which restricts her ability to visit her family, who live at a distance.

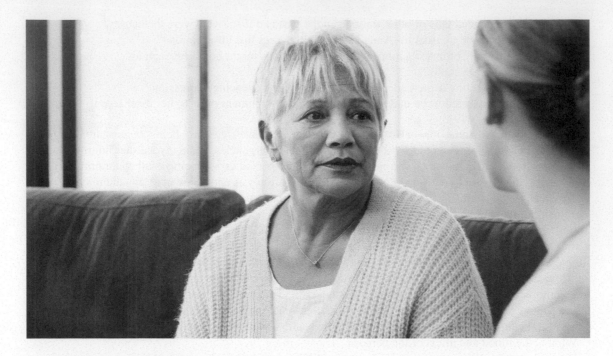

The biopsychosocial approach described is instructive. It suggests that it is imperative for the health professional to know what is happening with the person beyond the physical symptoms that the person may immediately present. It may be that the older person is not willing to divulge sensitive personal material immediately. It may also be that to talk of depression is at odds with their views on resilience and self-esteem. The older person may feel ashamed to suggest they have a mental illness, or they may not, in fact, know they have a mental illness. If the health professional — in this case, the GP — is younger, then the older person may feel uncomfortable about revealing intimate aspects of their lives. Only after they have established a rapport and feel that it is safe to talk may they be willing to divulge relevant information.

'Knowing the person' is at the heart of an assessment of the older person. To focus on one aspect of an assessment is to perhaps miss out on vital information and subsequently implement incorrect treatment. The importance of biology cannot be denied; however, it must be seen through the prism of an enduring psychosocial reality of meaning, context, history and relationships.

Cognitive assessment

In order to provide optimal outcomes for the older person, the health professional is called upon to holistically conceptualise their world. This is itself an undertaking that requires great sensitivity, empathy and effort, and demands the health professional know the totality of the older person. In the following section, the major mental health issues that confront the older person are explored. The answer is the same, whether discussing dementia, depression or delirium: in order to deliver care that reflects best practice, the health professional is called upon to actively know the person for whom they are caring. So far, the chapter has discussed assessment in an informal sense. Some time will now be spent in briefly commenting on a more formal approach to assessment.

The assessment and diagnosis of a mental illness is a sophisticated process that requires a specialist, such as a **psychogeriatrician** or **geriatrician**. This does not mean, however, that health professionals cannot conduct or participate in a structured assessment process. In fact, it is crucial that both these professional groups are aware of appropriate assessment processes, not only to inform their own engagement with the older person, but also to alert other members of the multidisciplinary team.

Mini-mental state exam

One assessment tool is the **mini-mental state exam (MMSE)**, a quick and effective pencil-and-paper test that provides a reliable instrument for dementia screening and identifying delirium in the older person (Folstein et al., 1975). It includes asking the person to count backwards by 7s from 100, to identify common objects (e.g. a pen, a watch), to spell simple words backwards, to write a sentence and to demonstrate that they are oriented today, month and year, as well as town and country. Although there are limitations to this tool — for example, it is not sensitive to mild cognitive impairment, does not provide diagnostic certainty, and does not account for low education level, poor literacy, cultural diversity and lack of English proficiency (Arevalo-Rodriguez et al., 2021; Larner, 2018) — it remains an effective instrument for the health professional to make valid assessments of the older person's cognitive ability. Another important drawback for the health professional to remember is that the MMSE is not sensitive to persons with an executive function disturbance, such as frontotemporal dementia. In this case, the health professional may utilise the **Addenbrooke's cognitive examination (ACE)**.

Addenbrooke's Cognitive Examination (ACE)

The ACE, as it has come to be known, is an effective screening tool 'sensitive to the early stages of dementia, and capable of differentiating subtypes of dementia including Alzheimer's disease, frontotemporal dementia, progressive supranuclear palsy and other parkinsonian syndromes' (Beishon et al., 2019). The tool is used to identify frontotemporal dementia; however, an issue for health professionals is that the ACE may take up to half an hour to administer and, for the very old or frail, this may be tiring. Even so, like the MMSE, it is easy to administer and is based on asking the person a series of questions, the answers to which are then written down by the examiner, and a number of pencil-and-paper tasks completed by the subject. These may be undertaken over time and are more accurate if a rapport is already established and the person is comfortable, not feeling pressured or stressed that they are being judged.

Mental state exam (MSE)

A final formal assessment tool to consider is the mental state exam (MSE). The MSE is described in detail in the chapter that looks at assessment in the mental health context. The advantage of the MSE is that it can be done while the person is being interviewed. It is a subjective assessment of the person's mental state and allows the skilled health professional to make judgements about a person's appearance, behaviour, mood, affect, speech, cognitions, thought patterns and level of consciousness, largely through a face-to-face conversation with the person. The MSE needs to ensure that 'risk' (including content of thought) is comprehensively assessed to ensure that the older person being reviewed is not at risk of suicide.

It is wise to remember that the MSE has at least two caveats. First, successfully administering the MSE requires a great degree of skill and experience. Health professionals unfamiliar with the MSE are advised to seek training and education to become proficient at it rather than simply reading about it. If a less experienced health professional is required to complete the MSE, then it is strongly advised that they seek confirmation of the MSE outcome from a more experienced colleague before implementing any treatments or interventions.

Second, it is important to remember that all effective assessments of older persons depend in large part upon an attitude the health professional has toward them, rather than the tools they use. That attitude has been described in terms of a biopsychosocial person-centred approach, which is based upon an engagement with the person that is antecedent to any particular assessment tool. This approach, which is based on listening to the person, being in touch with the person's reality, hearing the person's experiences and acknowledging the person's meaning, is the bedrock of any assessment of value. Implicit here is also an understanding of the health professional's own values and attitudes toward the elderly and ageing. Without these skills and attitudes, more formal assessments will be of little use.

11.4 Depression in older people

LEARNING OBJECTIVE 11.4 Clarify how to recognise depression in an older person.

The central features of depression are lowered mood and a loss of interest in life and formerly enjoyed activities (Wilkinson et al., 2018). Yet, in the older person, for a variety of reasons, depression may not be acknowledged by the individual or easily identified by the health professional (Choi, et al., 2013). This may be because the older person has little understanding of depression or may see it as a weakness or a moral failure rather than a treatable condition. They may not be open to reflecting psychologically on their wellbeing or feelings and may be reluctant to make an appointment to see a health professional for anything other than clearly identifiable physical ailments. Thus, depression in the older person is often missed.

What constitutes depression?

Depression and its signs and symptoms are detailed in the chapter that looks at depression and anxiety. The following discussion aims to add some quite specific points relating to the older person.

In the past, epidemiologists have tended to define depression in terms of strict diagnostic criteria for a **major depressive episode**, which indicates rates in older people are lower than other populations (Barry et al., 2012). Yet the number of older people who present with depressive symptoms that fall short of fulfilling such rigid criteria suggests much higher rates. Once again, this identifies the limitations of a strict biomedical approach to mental illness. Symptoms of depression, such as despair, sadness, feelings of failure and low self-worth, can be powerfully debilitating. To the person who experiences such feelings, whether they qualify for a diagnosis of major depressive episode is probably not uppermost on their minds. To the health professional, the biopsychosocial person-centred approach demands a focus on the person and the way they experience and interpret their lives rather than on any rigid diagnostic criteria.

As noted in the chapter that looks at depression and anxiety, depression itself is to be distinguished from 'feeling down' or 'upset' or 'having the blues'. While everyone has periods in their lives when they feel sad, miserable or low, perhaps in response to a tragedy or loss, such feelings typically fade as the person comes to terms with the event. Loss and grief are, after all, a normal part of human life and health professionals need to ensure that they do not pathologise common human reactions to stressful situations (refer to the chapter that looks at common reactions to stressful situations). With depression, however, concerns emerge when such feelings are intense in nature and 'have a prolonged course, when they interfere with psychosocial functioning and when they cluster with other symptoms' (Sands, 2001, p. 171). This may include a threat of self-harm and/or suicide.

Depression, at whatever age it is encountered, displays a complex interaction of experiences across a number of dimensions — biological, psychological and social. Not all people who are depressed display these feelings and not all feelings are displayed with the same intensity. Also, the symptoms described do not fit neatly into each respective dimension. Indeed, it is impossible to make clear-cut distinctions between the different dimensions of the symptoms. Decreased libido, for example, may be a biological response to depression, but it has psychological consequences for the person in terms of self-worth and self-esteem, and social consequences in terms of relationships with partners. A similar comment could be made about sleep disturbance, such as early morning wakening, another biological indicator of major depression. In the early hours of the morning, after the person with depression wakes, they may lie in bed and ruminate on negative self-thoughts about how they have wasted their life and how others might be 'better off' without them. Such attitudes may undermine an already vulnerable mental state and render acts of self-harm more likely. Thus, depression is an interaction of a variety of different elements and, consequently, needs to be approached as such.

Knowing and engaging with the person

When engaging the older person who may have depression, the standard principle for the health professional remains the same: first, know and effectively engage with the person. The health professional needs to take time to establish a rapport with the person, listen to their story and ask questions. It may be that they require some form of relationship or rapport with the health professional before they will 'open up' to them. Assessment of another's mental state is an intimate process and needs to be treated accordingly. A general rule of thumb is, when meeting the older person on the first occasion, it is best to concentrate on getting to know them. Listen to the story of their life and experiences and focus on understanding them; validate their accomplishments and the strategies used to overcome adversity. In this way, an assessment is already taking place. The thoughtful health professional will, in many cases, be able to discern whether the person is depressed by simply engaging in conversation.

What does depression look like?

Whereas in the younger person depression may present as a clear sadness, low mood, **nihilistic thoughts** and feelings, social withdrawal and loss of interest in life (refer to the chapter that looks at depression and anxiety) in the older person there is a tendency towards a display of both somatic symptoms and cognitive impairment. In the older person, there may also be a significant element of anxiety; a restless, irritable, agitated quality to their affect. In fact, there is a high degree of comorbid prevalence between depression and anxiety. According to Santangelo and Dobrohotoff (2022), anxiety and depression often co-exist with anxiety disorders masking an underlying depression disorder.

The older person may present to a health professional with a variety of physical complaints, aches and pains, and chronic unexplained physical symptoms, which may be seen as warranting further medical investigation. They may also present with a degree of cognitive impairment suggestive of an underlying dementia (Santangelo & Dobrohotoff, 2022). Given that older people with depression are likely to present with somatic symptoms or cognitive impairment, depression can easily be missed. An incorrect diagnosis of dementia when the real issue is depression, can result in significant negative impacts for the person including a loss of trust in the health professional and attempts to undertake further assessment.

As you read through the following list of symptoms of depression in the older person, consider the extent to which they apply to Anna:

- somatic complaints, aches and pains, reports of feeling unwell
- difficulty with memory and concentration
- lack of energy, but may feel restless, anxious and irritable
- sleep disturbance
- loss of appetite
- a tendency to ruminate and worry
- loss of pleasure and interest in life
- feeling unworthy or a burden on others
- thoughts that life is pointless or not worth living.

Assessment of depression

There are at least two ways the health professional may assess for depression in the older person. The first is to rely on one of the many assessment tools available. A number of these are listed in the chapter that looks at depression, anxiety and perinatal mental health. For the older person, perhaps the most common or useful scale is the Geriatric Depression Scale (Yesavage & Sheikh, 1983). This tool is described in more detail in the following section.

For those older people who may have depression in pre-existing dementia, another useful tool is the Cornell Scale for Depression in Dementia (CSDD) (Alexopoulos et al., 1988). The CSDD is designed for the assessment of depression in older people with dementia who are able to communicate their basic needs. The tool differentiates between the diagnostic categories and severity of depression. Scores are determined by a combination of prior observation and two interviews: 20 minutes with the carer and 10 minutes with the person with dementia.

There is much discussion in the literature about the efficacy of screening tools in terms of their validity and reliability, ease of use and appropriateness with the older population (Maurer et al., 2018). Health professionals who are interested in this area of health care are encouraged to read more about assessment tools in a specialised text. The focus of this chapter and, therefore, this discussion is to familiarise health professionals with notions of depression as a 'lived experience' of the older person. Moreover, there is a danger in relying on specific tools to measure and assess the experience of others. While assessment tools have their place, they can never substitute for the relationship between one person and another.

Geriatric Depression Scale

The **Geriatric Depression Scale (GDS)** (Yesavage & Sheikh, 1983) is widely used as a tool to diagnose depression in the older person. The GDS certainly has its place in the assessment process. It is easy to administer and score, requiring only a 'yes' or 'no' response. Respondents, however, seldom give simple yes/no answers to questions; rather they tend to expand, ponder, reflect upon their circumstances, perhaps even explain or justify their answers, and this can provide valuable insights into their mental and emotional state. It can also begin a discussion between the health professional and the older person and in this way, break down the barriers between both, facilitating a free exchange of shared understanding and thus build a relationship of warmth and trust.

FIGURE 11.2 Geriatric Depression Scale

Patient name: _____   Date: _____

GERIATRIC DEPRESSION SCALE (GDS)

Instructions: Please circle the best answer for how you felt over the past week.

1.	Are you basically satisfied with your life?	Yes	No
2.	Have you dropped many of your activities and interests?	Yes	No
3.	Do you feel that your life is empty?	Yes	No
4.	Do you often get bored?	Yes	No
5.	Are you hopeful about the future?	Yes	No
6.	Are you bothered by thoughts you can't get out of your head?	Yes	No
7.	Are you in good spirits most of the time?	Yes	No
8.	Are you afraid that something bad is going to happen to you?	Yes	No
9.	Do you feel happy most of the time?	Yes	No
10.	Do you often feel helpless?	Yes	No
11.	Do you often get restless and fidgety?	Yes	No
12.	Do you prefer to stay at home, rather than going out and doing new things?	Yes	No
13.	Do you frequently worry about the future?	Yes	No
14.	Do you feel you have more problems with memory than most?	Yes	No
15.	Do you think it is wonderful to be alive now?	Yes	No
16.	Do you often feel downhearted and blue?	Yes	No
17.	Do you feel pretty worthless the way you are now?	Yes	No
18.	Do you worry a lot about the past?	Yes	No
19.	Do you find life very exciting?	Yes	No
20.	Is it hard for you to get started on new projects?	Yes	No
21.	Do you feel full of energy?	Yes	No
22.	Do you feel that your situation is hopeless?	Yes	No
23.	Do you think that most people are better off than you are?	Yes	No
24.	Do you frequently get upset over little things?	Yes	No
25.	Do you frequently feel like crying?	Yes	No
26.	Do you have trouble concentrating?	Yes	No
27.	Do you enjoy getting up in the morning?	Yes	No
28.	Do you prefer to avoid social gatherings?	Yes	No
29.	Is it easy for you to make decisions?	Yes	No
30.	Is your mind as clear as is used to be?	Yes	No

Scoring for the Geriatric Depression Scale (GDS) In scoring the Geriatric Depression Scale, each item is scored 0 or 1 depending upon whether the item is worded positively or negatively. The total score on the scale ranges from 0 to 30. For items 2–4, 6, 8,10–14, 16–18, 20, 22–26, 28 the scoring is:

- Yes = 1
- No = 0

Items 1, 5, 7, 9, 15, 19, 21, 27, 29, 30 are reverse scored as follows:

- No = 1
- Yes = 0

Source: Yesavage & Sheikh (1983).

UPON REFLECTION

Assessing depression in older people

The GDS is the most commonly used screening tool for older people with possible depression. Review the GDS in figure 11.2, specifically focusing on the content of the questions.

QUESTIONS

1. Should all depression screening tools be the same? Discuss your rationale.
2. What makes this tool different (if anything) and why?
3. Would you do this scale in isolation? If not what else would need to be conducted?
4. As a health professional how can you ensure that the older person provides accurate responses to the 30 items?

Of course, there are drawbacks to the GDS. For example, it places minimal emphasis on somatic issues (physically experienced symptoms), which may be common in the older person where depression is masked by numerous medical complaints, and it has no items related to sexuality. This latter fact may sometimes be a positive as such discussion may offend or upset the older person. Also, it does not provide any rating as to the severity of depression, nor does it describe or assess risk of self-harm or suicide. These issues need to be approached directly by the health professional.

QUESTIONS

1. With this information, would it be useful at any time to perform an assessment of risk regarding self-harm or suicide?
2. What other risks may you want to assess for when faced with an older patient?
3. Do you think that sexuality is important in older people?

The interview and clinical judgement

The most effective way to assess for depression is by interviewing the older person. Interviewing skills, however, are not innate, rather, they are learned. Moreover, it can take some years for health professionals to gain the experience, confidence and expertise required to effectively engage an older person, establish a non-threatening environment and build a relationship that enables the older person to talk. Even so, interviewing skills are well worth developing. Further, it must be understood that this assessment and interview process is one that requires collaboration between health professionals who are skilled and educated in working with the elderly, especially those with mental illness (Nizette et al., 2021).

Depression is an emotion, a subjective feeling that a person has about themselves and their world, and the health professional accesses these feelings by making a personal connection with the older person. Human beings are social creatures who engage others in relationships based on trust, empathy and shared understandings. Although there is something artificial and distancing in attempting to quantify the emotional world of the older person, this does not mean that the relationship between the older person and the health professional is unstructured. There are signposts along the way that alert the health professional to the older person's distress and helps make sense of what the older person is experiencing.

Some areas are crucial in alerting the health professional to depression in the older person who may not want to admit such an experience. These areas or signposts include:

- sleep disturbance
- changes in appetite

- feeling tired or worn out
- loss of interest in things formerly enjoyed
- motor activity that may be described as either agitated or reduced
- poor concentration and attention span
- a sense of poor self-esteem or failure
- the prominence of physical complaints that may not have an underlying clear diagnosis (Santagelo & Dobrohotoff, 2022).

Depression — knowing the person

My name is Alan, and I am a 75-year-old Australian male. When I was a kid, my family moved a lot for Dad's work, so I had challenges making friends, and I now realise my learning difficulties were related to undiagnosed dyslexia. These issues meant I was ostracised by the other kids and often chastised by the teachers because I struggled to read and write. Mum spent time in hospital being treated for depression, which, when I was young, was a stigma on her and our family, so we didn't talk about it much. I left school to work with a carpenter.

Over the years, I had times when I was angry and took that out on my wife by verbally abusing her. One night I got so angry, I took the gun from the gun safe and went down into the back paddock of our farm, wanting to stop the misery that I was causing my family. The wife and my girls were terrified and rang the police. That's when I had to confront the fact: I needed help.

For me, admitting I had a mental health issue was tough and even tougher getting help. The GP prescribed anti-depressants, but I couldn't tolerate the side effects. Tricyclic antidepressants caused Meniere's disease, so I couldn't get my head off the pillow without feeling sick. Then Zoloft caused erectile dysfunction, which was confronting to me as a man and a husband. All of this was making me lose hope in treatment strategies. I requested a mental health plan and referral to a psychologist but which psychologist?

My wife asked family and friends for help, and someone suggested a psychologist who was close to my age and a male. Having a health professional who was my gender and age mattered to me. It enabled me to communicate freely. The psychologist did a lot of listening; he was genuinely interested in me and my experiences. Each session, he gave me challenges to undertake and reflections to engage with. I involved my wife in these, we talked about issues and feelings. Over time, I gradually developed insight into my lifelong struggle with depression. To continue to be connected and engaged with other men, I found an Older Men New Ideas group where we meet regularly and support each other. The struggles continue but the strategies I've learnt through therapy certainly help.

Risk factors

These feelings are accessed by listening to the older person tell their story, by asking them directly, by observation and by asking those around them who know them.

The health professional also needs to be alert to the various psychological, social and biological risk factors for depression in older people. Social isolation and loneliness, bereavement, low socio-economic status, being a carer and being female are prominent factors. Other indicators include chronic illness, including cerebrovascular disease, stroke, Parkinson's disease, Alzheimer's disease, diabetes, hypothyroidism and hyperthyroidism, and previous episodes of depression or anxiety (Maier et al., 2021)

There is a high prevalence of depression among residents in aged-care facilities. Rates vary, depending upon the different studies, but the AIHW state that in 2018, the majority (86 per cent) of all aged care residents had at least one diagnosed mental health or behavioural disorder, half (49 per cent) had depression and half (52 per cent) had a diagnosis of dementia. It is estimated that for people with a diagnosis of dementia, there is a 40–50 per cent chance of depression (NHMC, 2019). These figures are pre-COVID-19 which has had a significant impact on the mental and physical health of residents.

Entry into residential aged care can be a challenging experience and the presence of depression can add to this challenge. Older people entering residential aged care with physical comorbidities — such as stroke, heart disease, arthritis, diabetes, cancer and chronic pain — are also at higher risk of depression (Maire et al., 2021). Other high-risk groups include:
- those with dementia, with up to 20 per cent of those diagnosed with Alzheimer's disease having depression (AIHW, 2019)

- older people who are carers for family members who have a chronic illness (Baldwin, 2008)
- older women, who are more likely than older men to experience depression and anxiety disorders (Slade et al., 2009).

It is important that the health professional who works with older people is able to recognise the signs and symptoms and intervene, as appropriate.

Concerns about the rates of depression among residents in aged care facilities were expressed by the National Mental Health Commission (NMHC) in their submission to the Royal Commission in 2019. To support older people with mental health concerns, the NMHC recommended:

'Mental health care for older people needs to be underpinned by a person-centred approach based on the following principles.
- Promote an optimal quality of life for people with mental illness.
- Respect for the rights of older people, their carers and families.
- Respect the needs, culture and traditions of different community groups and ensure their needs are met appropriately.
- Recognise the burden of loss and grief in later life.
- Increase access to non-pharmacological treatments in all aged care settings.
- Promote the quality use of medicines in all aged care settings.
- Increase focus on modifiable risk factors for improving physical and mental health in older age.
- Respond to the needs of older carers as they may also be at risk of developing mental health needs and require additional supports.
- Evaluate access and effectiveness of these services to ensure that older people's needs are being met (NMHC, 2019, p.4).

Suicide

Old age suicide is a complex area and, like depression itself, suicidal ideation is not easily identified. Moreover, a death is not recorded as a suicide until it is identified as such by a coroner and deaths of older people do not always fit within the parameters of a coronal investigation. Social, ethical and religious factors are thus likely to have an impact on such decision making as the legal identification of suicide will have profound implications for the family. Suicide rates for older men and women are higher than for adolescents and young people but the number of attempts at suicide are higher among adolescents (Conejero et al., 2018). Table 11.1 shows the numbers of deaths by self-harm according to age and gender. It shows that in 2020, three in four of the deaths were by males and one in four by females (ABS, 2021) which is 16 per cent of all deaths from intentional self-harm across all age groups.

TABLE 11.1 Deaths of older people (65 and over) from intentional self-harm by sex and age group, 2020

Age group (years)	Men	Women	Total
65–69	106	30	136
70–74	89	31	120
75–79	71	24	95
80–84	52	19	71
85+	74	20	94
Total (all age groups)	2384	755	3139

Source: Adapted from ABS, 2021.

With regard to depression, anxiety and vulnerability to self-harm and suicide, the health professional needs to be aware of the various assumptions about older people that may accompany such problems. Depression, despair, hopelessness, self-harm and suicide are not an inevitable part of the ageing process. Rather, they are mental health conditions, but it is imperative that the health professional has the skills to recognise the vulnerable older person, assess their needs and support them to access treatment. Factors that may predispose the older person to self-harm and suicide include a history of depression or other psychiatric illness, loss of spouse or partner, increased social isolation or a lack of social supports, living alone, loss of autonomy (as in moving into an aged-care facility) or having multiple chronic health conditions. Feeling useless, disconnected from others, psychological distress and physiological pain from chronic conditions are precursors for suicidal thoughts (Conejero et al., 2018). Wand et al. (2018) add that loss of control, attempting to maintain self-identity and a sense of meaninglessness add to vulnerability to self-harm. Being admitted to residential aged care can increase the risk of suicide with maladjustment to residential aged care being the cause of 30 per cent of suicide deaths (Creighton et al., 2016).

Health professionals are encouraged to take a comprehensive or biopsychosocial person-centred approach, rather than stereotype or pre-judge the person based on either ageist attitudes, stereotypes or lack of awareness of the impact of depression on an older person.

As recognised by the Royal Commission, supporting older people is about relationships and social connections so to ensure quality of care for older people, 'physical, social and mental health is maintained, and their lives enriched by engagement with others' (Royal Commission into Aged Care Quality and Safety, 2021, p. 32).

11.5 Dementia

LEARNING OBJECTIVE 11.5 Describe dementia from a person-centred perspective.

Dementia is a syndrome associated with a variety of diseases, characterised by a chronic and progressive cognitive decline involving disturbances of brain function such as memory, thinking, comprehension, abstract thought, language and judgement (van Corven et al., 2021). This cognitive decline reveals itself through increasing functional deficits, such as memory loss, confusion, language disturbance, an increasing inability to self-care, disturbances of executive function, psychiatric pathology (depression and anxiety being the most common) and medical comorbidities (World Health Organization [WHO], 2017). The WHO (2018) differentiates dementia from other mental illnesses by classifying dementia as a neurodevelopmental disorder.

The trajectory of dementia is one of increasing cognitive deficits involving what are called behavioural and psychological symptoms of dementia (BPSD), which can include wandering, pacing, hoarding, verbal and physical aggression, screaming, repetitive vocalisations, delusions and hallucinations, sexual disinhibition and faecal smearing. Typically, dementia ends in permanent dependence in all aspects of care and, ultimately, death (WHO, 2017).

Dementia and ageing

The greatest risk factor for dementia is increasing age, although younger onset dementia, which occurs before age 65, is becoming more frequent. In 2022, there are an estimated 28 800 people with younger onset dementia (Dementia Australia, 2022). Dementia however, remains the most challenging problem confronting the older person, their families and those health professionals who support them. The rates of dementia, in both Australia and worldwide, are having, and will continue to have, a major impact on personal, local and national wellbeing. According to Dementia Australia (2022), the following observations can be made about dementia in Australia.

- Key facts and statistics (Australian statistics from the Dementia Australia website, 2022)
- Dementia is the second leading cause of death of Australians.
- Dementia is the leading cause of death for women.
- In 2022, there are up to 487 500 Australians living with dementia. Without a medical breakthrough, the number of people with dementia is expected to increase to almost 1.1 million by 2058.
- In 2022, there are an estimated 28 800 people with younger onset dementia, expected to rise to 29 350 people by 2028 and 41 250 people by 2058. This can include people in their 30s, 40s and 50s.
- In 2022, it is estimated that almost 1.6 million people in Australia are involved in caring for someone living with dementia.
- Approximately 65 per cent of people with dementia live in the community.
- More than two-thirds (68.1 per cent) of aged care residents have moderate to severe cognitive impairment.

The greatest risk factor for dementia is advancing age. The implications of this are profound both currently and into the future if a cure is not revealed through research. The number of people aged 85 years is growing more rapidly than the general population. The Royal Commission into Aged Care Quality and Safety (2021) reports that the percentage of this group will increase from 2 per cent in 2017 to between 3.6 and 4.4 per cent by 2066. This has major implications for resource allocation directed towards the care of the person with dementia, for support services, institutional placements, medical and psychiatric interventions, the education of carers, and for the inevitable cost of dementia in terms of lost productivity and absenteeism of employees who stay at home to care for a family member (Dementia Australia, 2022).

Types of dementia

A number of diseases can be identified under the umbrella of dementia. Most common is Alzheimer's disease, which accounts for approximately two-thirds of all cases (62 per cent), and vascular dementia (17 per cent), which accounts for about one-quarter of cases. Together these two conditions account for over 86 per cent of all cases of dementia in Australia (CEPAR, 2018). Other major forms of dementia include Lewy body dementia (up to 5 per cent of cases), and frontotemporal dementia (5–10 per cent of cases) although, in those people below age 60, frontotemporal dementia may be as common as Alzheimer's disease (CEPAR, 2018).

Less common types of dementia include:

- dementia in Parkinson's disease
- alcohol-induced dementia
- drug-related dementia
- head injury dementia
- dementia in Huntington's disease
- dementia that develops as a result of human immunodeficiency virus (HIV) or Creutzfeldt-Jakob disease (APA, 2013).

In all, there are thought to be at least 100 different causes of dementia. Table 11.2 identifies the major forms of dementia in terms of clinical course, associated behavioural presentations typically associated with each type of dementia, possible causes and some associated or relevant issues.

TABLE 11.2   **Clinical course and features of the major forms of dementia**

Type of dementia	Clinical course and common associated behavioural displays	Possible causes	Associated issues
Alzheimer's disease	Gradual onset Progressive decline Increasing deficits in memory, recognition of people and objects, ability to self-care, naming familiar people/objects, calculation, visuo-spatial skills and language Deterioration of social skills Emotional unpredictability Emergence of challenging behaviors, such as depression, agitation, aggression and sexually inappropriate behaviour Late in the illness immobility and mutism appear with death from systemic infections related to incapacity	Presence of the APoE4 gene Presence of 'plaques' (protein deposits and dead cells) outside brain cells and 'tangles' (protein deposits) inside brain cells that impair functioning and lead to cell death	Protective factors: • Regular exercise • Intellectual and social activities • Higher education • Moderate alcohol use Risk factors: • Old age • Family history of Alzheimer's disease • Head injury • Smoking • Hypertension • Poor diet

(continued)

TABLE 11.2 *(continued)*

Type of dementia	Clinical course and common associated behavioural displays	Possible causes	Associated issues
Vascular dementia	Slow and steady deterioration or 'step-wise' decline related to type of neurological insults (repeated mini-strokes or a single major event) Impaired executive function Difficulty completing tasks, slowed thinking, poor problem solving, limited ability to focus while memory remains relatively intact Apathy, depression, mood swings, impulsive aggression maybe present Gait disturbances common, frequent falls	Multiple discrete infarcts, strategic single infarcts or diffuse subcortical white matter disease	Protective factors: • Healthy weight • Exercise • Optimal blood pressure • Optimal; cholesterol • Manage stressors • Awareness of family history of cardiovascular disease • Regular health monitoring. Risk factors: • Hypertension • Stroke • Cardiovascular disease • Diabetes • Excessive alcohol use • Smoking • Overweight • Sedentary lifestyle
Frontotemporal dementia	Insidious onset with gradual deterioration Financial vulnerability — gullible and susceptible to exploitation Abstract thinking and higher level cognitive skills impaired Three variants identified: i. behavioural — neglect of hygiene and grooming, lack of social tact, sexual disinhibition, apathy, hyperorality ii. progressive non-fluent aphasia — loss of ability to speak or to speak logically, reduced output of speech iii. semantic — loss of meaning or understanding of words	Possible mutation in tau protein gene on chromosome 17	Occurs early (45–65 years) 50 per cent have a family history with first-degree relatives
Lewy body disease	Gradual onset Progressive decline Fluctuating cognitions Recurrent visual hallucinations Parkinsonism features (rigidity, bradykinesia, unsteady gait and postural instability) Frequent falls Nighttime behavioural disturbances Apathy, depression and paranoid ideas may be present Visuo-spatial disturbance	Presence of abnormal structures (Lewy bodies), within the nerve cell which cause death of nerve cells	Contraindication of antipsychotics in treatment of delusions and visual disturbances raises difficult care issues

Assessment of dementia

The formal diagnosis of dementia is typically performed by a specialist, such as a psychiatrist, geriatrician or psychogeriatrician. But that does not mean that other health professionals have no role to play. Certainly, all health professionals are likely to encounter, in their day-to-day practice, individuals who present with dementia-like symptoms, such as a decline in memory, reasoning and communication, a reduction in the ability to successfully undertake everyday tasks of living and increasing confusion and changes in mood. In such circumstances, when dementia is suspected, it is important for the person to be seen by a specialist to rule out other possible causes of the presentation. For example, forgetfulness, attention difficulties, getting words wrong and slowed thinking processes can be an indication of early-stage dementia or an indication of depression. The formal process of diagnosing dementia may include the use of scans or pencil-and-paper tests such as the mini-mental state examination (MMSE) and Addenbrooke's Cognitive Examination (ACE) which were discussed in the previous section of the chapter.

Dementia can be thought of as a chronic, irreversible, neurological disorder. An important aspect of the condition is that it shows an ongoing deterioration from previous levels of functioning. In the absence of any other diagnosis, a gradual deterioration over time in the person's cognitive ability will suggest a dementia. Power and colleagues (2018) uses the term 'dementia spectrum' as a means of labelling the progression of dementia. This alerts the health professional to an understanding of the importance of being aware of the person's current level of functioning so that information regarding any deterioration can be documented and passed on to those who will ultimately make the diagnosis.

Ethical and legal considerations

Ethical considerations that are specific to people with a mental illness are discussed in the chapter on the legal and ethical context of mental health care. The discussion in this section relates more specifically to the older person. This is because the existence of medical and psychiatric **comorbidities** makes the disease process exceedingly difficult to categorise. Questions that could be asked by the health professionals include the following.

- How does the health professional identify capacity of the person with dementia and their level of involvement in decision making related to health and legal issues; for example, advance care planning, appointing an enduring guardian and power of attorney?
- What signs may indicate restriction of movement and access to care of the person with dementia?
- What signs might alert the health professional to vulnerability to elder abuse and financial manipulation?

The disease process sees increasing deterioration in the person's mental and physical abilities. This in itself raises complex issues, such as the person's ability to care for themselves and make what might be called 'best interest decisions' with regard to their own wellbeing. Again, this gives rise to complex issues of autonomy, self-determination and capacity. It would seem, then, that in addition to all the skills of engagement the health professional requires, an understanding of ethical and legal contexts is vital. In particular, the professional needs to be aware that capacity (i.e. the ability of an individual to make best interest judgements) is a domain-specific rather than a general global construct (Pozgar, 2019). What this means in reality is that while the person with dementia may not have capacity in certain specific areas, such as the ability to trade in stocks and shares or to buy and sell property, or even to understand why they do not have the capacity to consent to treatment, they may very well have the capacity to make judgements about where they live and who they spend time with and what makes them happy and sad.

For this reason, health professionals need to be wary about a **paternalism** that denies a voice of any kind to the person with dementia, and they need also to educate families and other caregivers that a diagnosis of dementia does not mean that the person has no ability at all to make any decisions whatsoever about their lives and how they live their lives. The assessment of whether someone can make decisions about their lives must be approached on a case-by-case and situation-by-situation context (Dementia Australia, 2022) rather than an 'all or none' ability. A reminder of Kitwood's words from 1997 (p. 8) that still are so relevant — 'treat each other with deep respect' irrespective of the challenges confronting either party.

Dementia and medication

As dementia is typically described and conceptualised as a biomedical problem, there is a tendency to respond to challenging behaviours (e.g. verbal and physical aggression, restlessness, screaming, sexual disinhibition) with antipsychotics. Such an approach is problematic on a number of accounts. The use on antipsychotic medications as a first resort means the causative factors of the behaviour have not been assessed. A concerning example is a study by Green et al. (2016) who found that older people with dementia, admitted to acute care following a fractured neck of femur, routinely received antipsychotic medication rather than analgesia.

Antipsychotics do not change the dementia-related behaviours of the person in any meaningful way. Many behaviours derive from the actual experience of dementia or the environment in which the person with dementia is located, rather than resulting from any obvious psychosis. Behaviours that do not respond to antipsychotics include anxiety, depressed mood, hoarding, restlessness, screaming, sexual disinhibition, shadowing, swearing, wandering and the agitation and restlessness that is often seen in the late afternoons or early evenings that carers may describe as 'sundowning' (National Prescribing Service Limited [NPS], 2022). Moreover, evidence suggests that even in situations where antipsychotics may be indicated, such as for treatment of severe aggression, agitation or psychotic symptoms, the effect is at best a minor positive (NPS, 2022).

The introduction of antipsychotics can result in a whole variety of new behaviours that emerge as part of adverse reactions and side effects. Such responses may include cardiovascular problems, uncontrollable movements, sleepiness, urinary symptoms, gait disturbance and dry mouth (Harrison et al., 2018). When present, these will increase the burden of care and markedly reduce the quality of life of the person with dementia. This was a focus of the Royal Commission (2021) where numerous accounts of the inappropriate use of antipsychotic medication were revealed and resulted in Recommendation 17 (p. 221) related to the use of chemical restraints.

Third, there are some severe and life-threatening responses to antipsychotics of which the health professional must be aware. These reactions include delirium, cardiotoxicity and stroke (NPS, 2022). The health professional must be alert to the impact these medications can have on the person with dementia, ensure assessment has been undertaken to identify the cause of any behaviour of concern, use non-pharmacological strategies, continually evaluate outcomes of strategies and reassess when the plan of care is no longer achieving goals.

Previous sections have covered depression and dementia. The next section discusses delirium, highlighting the vital importance of the health professional being able to identify a delirium, which can be a life-threatening condition.

11.6 Delirium

LEARNING OBJECTIVE 11.6 Differentiate between dementia, depression and delirium.

Never assume an older person presenting in a confused state has dementia. Instead, begin a process of investigation — 'are they usually confused?' is an invaluable question to ask the family. According to Wilson et al. (2020), delirium is a syndrome involving an acute deterioration in mental functioning, fluctuating level of awareness, difficulty staying focused and/or the presence of perceptual disturbance caused by a medical condition. It is a common presentation in the older person, particularly those in hospitals and residential care. However, delirium also presents a risk to the individual in the community who is frail, has a chronic illness or has a pre-existing dementia. It is important that all health professionals who work with older people have a detailed understanding of delirium, because delirium in the older person can be life threatening, but also because a delirium has the ability to negatively affect the quality of life of the older person and their family. For example, a delirium will almost certainly make any pre-existing condition, such as dementia or a mental health condition, much worse, and will thus inevitably place an extra burden on carers. If identified and responded to quickly, delirium can be reversed, and much pain and suffering can be reduced. However, if it is left untreated, cognitive function can be irreversibly impacted leading a cascade of inappropriate interventions, poor quality of life and/or death.

Assessment of delirium

The formal diagnosis of a delirium is made by the medical specialist and is based on the results of a variety of assessments, such as blood chemistry, erythrocyte sedimentation rate, ECG, chest X-ray and urinalysis. However, the most effective way of identifying a delirium is through observing a change in the person's behaviour. In fact, any change in the person's usual behaviour must alert the health professional to the possibility that a delirium may be present. This, of course, demands a knowledge of the person's usual behaviour to identify any recent change, reminding the health professional of the importance of knowing the person and involving the family in the assessment process. They are aware of the usual level of cognition whereas the health professional may be meeting the person with the delirium for the first time.

In addition to the health professional observing or identifying changed behaviours, there are also a number of practical tests the health professional can perform to make a reasonable judgement about the presence of delirium. Health services are required to have approaches to screen older people at high risk of delirium (The Australian Commission on Safety and Quality in Health Care [ACSQHC], 2016). Diagnostic screen tools include:

- 4AT
- the confusion assessment method (CAM)
- the delirium symptom interview (DSI)
- the delirium risk assessment tool (DRAT)
- the delirium rating scale.

Assessment for delirium is continuous and changes in behaviour need constant monitoring of those at risk of delirium. Questions to ask as the person is observed are as follows.

- Does the person show a sudden deterioration in their ability to perform the assessment?
- Do they suddenly present as disoriented?
- Is their attention span suddenly affected?
- Can the person count backwards from 10, to say the months of the year backwards, to give their name and address, or to identify the day of the week, the month of the year or the season.

If the result of such an exercise reveals that an older person is suddenly unable to perform such basic mental tasks, then a delirium should be assumed, and action taken immediately to have a detailed medical assessment done.

Characteristics of a delirium

There are a number of central features of a delirium that the health professional needs to commit to memory. These features are outlined below, along with the means of assessment of symptoms.

An easy way to recall some of the causes of delirium is PINCHME:

- Pain
- Infection
- Nutrition
- Constipation
- Hydration
- Medication
- Environment.

Continuously observe the older person for the following.

- *Acute onset and fluctuating presentation.* Determine whether there is a brief or severe change in mental status.
- *Inattention.* Assess whether the individual has trouble focusing and keeping track of the conversation.
- *Disorganised thinking.* Are they incoherent, unpredictable and struggling to form logical thoughts?
- *Altered level of consciousness.* Determine whether the person is drowsy but easily aroused (lethargic), difficult to arouse (stuporous), unable to be aroused (comatose) or overly alert (hypervigilant).

The typical onset of delirium is hours or days, different from the slow insidious onset of dementia or depression. Also, the condition tends to fluctuate; that is, the person may present as well in the morning, yet confused and muddled in the afternoon, or appear better in the evening and have a restless, agitated and disturbed night. This suggests the importance of health professionals talking to each other about an older person's presentation and talking to carers, such as non-professional institutional carers or the family. Further, delirium is characterised by:

- impaired attention
- increased distractibility
- thinking that is muddled, chaotic and confused.

In dementia, and indeed in depression, this is not typically the case, certainly at the outset. Sleep is usually disturbed in delirium, while in dementia, it is not. The person with delirium may also have visual disturbances and mood swings. Fear, anger, irritability or even euphoria may all be present, but the central theme remains the same: have these behaviours and presentations only recently emerged? If so, the health professional must assume a delirium and immediately refer for a medical assessment.

Issues for the health professional may emerge when the person has a pre-existing dementia that is moderate to severe, making a **differential diagnosis** difficult. Here, again, the most important advice is to be aware of any recent change in the person's behaviour. It is far better to assume a delirium might exist and to act accordingly than to assume no delirium and not act. The consequences of missing a delirium for the person may be profound.

Those health professionals who work with the older person who is in hospital, or is expected to be hospitalised, or who is in, or about to go into, residential care, need to remember that between 23 per cent older patients who are admitted to hospital present with delirium and 20 per cent develop delirium post operatively (Wilson et al., 2020).

Types of delirium

There are three identified types of delirium:
1. hyperactive
2. hypoactive
3. a mixed presentation, which involves features of both.

In hyperactive delirium, the person can present as agitated, restless, over-active and hyper-alert (van Velthuijsen et al., 2018). They may be uncharacteristically verbally aggressive, loud, threatening and chaotic in their presentation and may engage in random acts of confused and pointless activity. This type of delirium is easy to identify, perhaps because it is so disruptive and challenging to carers.

The hypoactive presentation, on the other hand, can easily be missed because the person may be withdrawn, insular, isolative and quiet with little motor activity. It is easy to miss such presentations in the hustle and bustle of medical wards, or in the understaffed and poorly trained aged-care sector. Consequently, the outcomes are much worse for this subgroup. In the mixed form of delirium, there are elements of both. Psychotropic medications are contra-indicated for older people with delirium (van Velthuijsen et al., 2018); instead, the focus is on identifying the cause and then treatment is focused on the precipitating factor.

UPON REFLECTION

Distinguishing between dementia and delirium

Many health professionals are unsure of the difference between dementia and delirium, or delirium and mental illness generally. If they observe an older person with symptoms of a delirium, they may perceive this as a dementia process or mental illness.

QUESTIONS

1. Consider the biopsychosocial consequences of not identifying delirium for a hospitalised older person.
2. What skills does the health professional require to be alert for delirium?
3. Consider the impact of workforce shortages and ageist attitudes on recognising and intervening in a situation where a person has hypoactive delirium.
4. What strategies are needed to prevent delirium in older people in the community, in acute care and in residential aged care?

The health professional also needs to be alert to the variety of predisposing factors for delirium so preventative strategies can be implemented. Martins and Fernandes (2012) and Saxena and Lawley (2009) have identified the following as predisposing factors for delirium:
- advanced age
- alcohol abuse
- comorbid conditions
- dehydration and malnutrition
- dementia and depression
- functional dependence
- male gender
- polypharmacy
- visual and/or hearing impairment.

Predisposing factors themselves are a complex dynamic. Inouye and Charpentier (1996) outline the relationship between predisposing and precipitating factors: the former are existing vulnerabilities identified above, whereas the latter identify acute adverse events, such as infection, drugs, indwelling catheters, uncontrolled pain, surgery or fall with a resultant fracture. In particularly old and frail persons, it may only take a relatively minor event to trigger an episode of a delirium.

Responding to a delirium

The principles of management of delirium are focused on identifying the cause. Thorough assessment of the person, establishing trust, listening to concerns and addressing these will provide the best chance of resolving the delirium. Other means of providing support are to reduce stimulation; maintain hydration; reassurance and compassionate intervention to both person and family; reorientate the individual; and facilitate familiar friends and family to remain with the person while ensuring compliance with prescribed medical treatment (Nizette et al., 2021). Measures to achieve these principles of care include:

- maintaining fluid balance, nutrition, elimination and general comfort
- monitoring with regard to changes in vital signs, behaviour and mental status
- providing a quiet, well-lit room with moderate levels of stimulation, while, at night, a dim night light is important in case the person wakes and is frightened or confused
- maintaining orientation through the provision of clocks, calendars, family photos and other personal possessions
- ensuring paid health carers clearly identify themselves. Ideally, the number of different paid health carers must be kept to a minimum. Enlist the support of family members wherever possible
- assess and treat pain
- regular toileting and assistance with activities of daily living
- providing education, support and reassurance to family members
- encouraging family members to stay with the person when possible.

Physical and chemical restraints should be avoided unless the person's safety cannot be maintained by any other means. Physical restraint is an affront to the humanity of the person, causes more distress, causes injury and in some cases, death. Chemical restraint through the use of pharmacological sedation has the potential to cause respiratory depression and hypotension and death (Simpkins et al., 2016). It is dehumanising and extremely distressing to the family to witness their loved one sedated unnecessarily (Royal Commission into Aged Care Quality and Safety, 2021). By recognising a delirium and providing appropriate treatment, health professionals will be well-placed to provide the best possible care to the older person, support the improvement of their health outcomes and enhance their quality of life.

THE BIG PICTURE

Challenges of the twenty-first century

Australia's population has been ageing steadily, and it has been estimated that the proportion of people aged 65 and over will reach 20 per cent (or 4.9 million people) by 2025. Considering this trend, it is clear government policy will require a consistent and comprehensive approach to managing the issues that will arise from the changing age composition of Australia's population. These issues bring with them at least two major challenges and include the development of an appropriate evidence base and consideration of the development of appropriate health care services.

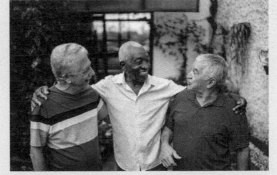

The first challenge is to develop a clear and 'real world' evidence base for the effective treatments of the range of mental health issues affecting older Australians (e.g. depression, dementia and other chronic mental health conditions). Older patients are underrepresented in clinical trials because they are often receiving concurrent medications, have coexisting medical problems or are simply outside of the age cut-off — clearly leaving us with a significant deficit in knowledge of older persons. Data and evidence specifically relating to the efficacy of the range of possible and potential treatments and interventions for the older person are needed because age at diagnosis is a critical factor that significantly modifies prognosis.

For example, some cancers may become more aggressive in the older person when compared to younger cohorts; consequently, effective or optimal treatments can be different in the two age populations. Further, these treatments may have different side effects or consequences that medical practitioners do ▸

not clearly understand, and this may affect significant decisions made relating to the end-of-life care requirements.

The second challenge is to develop responsive and effective health systems that can manage the expected rise in demand by increased populations, and therefore increased severity of illness in our older people. Further, this system will need to provide access to high-quality care and effective and appropriate new technologies (depending on the outcome of the first challenge). A two-tiered health system — where affluent, younger patients obtain effective and up-to-date treatments in the private sector and vulnerable and older patients obtain care in the public sector, with varied funding arrangements — may not be considered tolerable by many and this must be managed in a social context.

It may be a difficult task for the future health care system to provide effective and evidence-based treatments to older persons in rural and remote regions of Australia. In Australia today, effective (and costly) treatments for a range of chronic illnesses are generally provided only in major metropolitan areas; however, as the rural/remote population ages, the provision of care in these areas will need to be reviewed. Despite the recommendations of the Royal Commission in Quality and Safety in Aged Care (2021) for the enhancement of support for older people in regards mental health, the access to geriatricians and psycho-geriatricians in rural and remote areas remains problematic. Distance to assessment, service provision and treatment, despite the use of telehealth, deters the older, rural dwelling, person from engaging in measures that may improve their quality of life.

Source: Adapted from Martin et al. (2012).

SUMMARY

The care of the older person with a mental health problem is an invitation to advocate for the welfare of another human being. Like all meaningful relationships, the provision of this care begins with knowing the person. To know the person demands that the health professional is open to the story of the other and connects with them, their history, meaning, values and experiences. Knowing the person requires going beyond diagnoses, signs and symptoms and biomedical explanations and interpretations to discover the meaning of a life that defies simplistic definition. Knowing another person also means that the health professional must be aware of their own values, meanings and style of interacting, being emotionally intelligent — that is, be aware of what it is the health professional brings to the relationship and then is able to set aside prejudices and preconceived attitudes.

This chapter considers the extent of what it means to care for the older person who occupies a world that is, in many ways, very different to the one inhabited by the health professional. In no small way, the reality of ageism is the first barrier that must be overcome to enter this world. This chapter suggests that a powerful way of both entering and understanding this world is through the biopsychosocial person-centred perspective that sees the older person as very much more than simply a defective or broken-down medical organism, but rather views (or connects with) the person as a valid individual in whatever context they are located. This, in turn, recognises that context — social, personal, historical — is crucial. Through this approach, dementia can be understood as a social construct as much as (or more than) a medical one, and depression and suicide can be seen as a social and personal experience. Perhaps the most powerful example of knowing the person emerges with a discussion of delirium, where knowing and not knowing may in fact be the difference between life and death. Delirium is a salutary lesson for all those who work with the older person.

Often it is assumed that, as health professionals, the care provided to people represents a kind of linear relationship. That is, the health professional does the caring and the person they are helping is the recipient, the beneficiary of care. In reality, however, it is both the health professional and the person who bring uniqueness to the relationship, drawn from their own experiences, values and beliefs, and their own stories with the most effective reached when they work together. As the health professional has an impact on the person, so the person has an impact on the health professional. The health professional needs to be open to know the person — not as a 'patient' or 'client'; not as a person who has a mental illness, a diagnosis of dementia, depression or delirium. They need to know them as a person: a person with a past, culture and relationships; with ambitions, sadnesses, joys and triumphs; with an individual perception of what the complexity of human life means to them. To know the person means knowing them for who they are, not as some mirror image of the health professional, but as a valid and dynamic human being in their own right. From there, and only there, can the healing process begin.

KEY TERMS

acopia A label often used to describe someone who has a low level of coping skills or finds it difficult to cope with life's experiences, usually negative connotation.

Addenbrooke's cognitive examination (ACE) A self-reporting tool for assessing dementia, including the different types of dementia; the tool takes five minutes to complete and test memory.

biopsychosocial person-centred approach an approach that understands the person as a biological, social and psychological being, with the person defined in terms of their relationships and interrelationships at the centre of the matrix of care.

biopsychosocial understanding An approach that considers the biological, psychological and social dimensions of a person's experience.

cognitive decline Deterioration or decline in abilities, such as memory, reasoning, judgement, planning, decision making, language and other aspects of mental or intellectual functioning.

comorbidities the simultaneous presence of two health conditions, illnesses or disorders.

dementia A chronic, irreversible, neurological disorder that sees a progressive deterioration in a person's cognitive, mental and physical abilities.

differential diagnosis Being able to identify which diagnosis, from a number of possible competing diagnoses, is correct.

Geriatric Depression Scale (GDS) A series of 30 questions requiring a yes/no response that gives a rating of the presence or absence of depression.

geriatrician A medical specialist in the physical care of the elderly.

homogeneous group A group with the same or similar characteristics, preferences, needs and lifestyle.

major depressive episode A group of symptoms used to identify depression as a serious clinical mental illness involving profoundly debilitating symptoms, which may include a potential for self-harm or suicide.

mini mental state exam (MMSE) A brief psychological test that enables a health professional to assess a person for and/or differentiate between a dementia, delirium, psychosis and affective disorders.

nihilistic thoughts Negative thoughts that the world or a person's body, mind or self is utterly worthless or does not exist.

paternalism Attitudes or actions by people in positions of power (e.g. government, health professional) that subordinates should be controlled for their own good.

pathologise The tendency for health professionals to place the ordinary human reactions, responses, thoughts, feelings and behaviours of various stages of life into a biomedical frame, label what is happening as a 'condition', and prescribe treatment.

Psychogeriatrician A medical specialist in mental illness of old age.

senile A state where the person may exhibit memory loss or unclear cognitive or mental impairment that is sometimes associated with ageing.

social admission A label often used to describe a patient who has been admitted to hospital to address social needs, rather than a biomedical condition, usually negative in connotation.

REVIEW QUESTIONS

1 What is meant by 'ageism'?
2 How can discrimination of the elderly affect health care delivery?
3 What challenges and opportunities does the Australian health care system face in the coming years, as the population grows older?
4 How does the health professional demonstrate cultural safety when interacting with an Indigenous elder presenting with a cognitive impairment?
5 Describe ways in which a health professional can build rapport with an older person especially with a person from a CALD background?
6 Why is differentiating the type of dementia significant for the quality of life of the older person with a diagnosis of dementia?.
7 Identify the outcomes of the Royal Commission that relate to older people with mental illness.
8 What are the risk factors for depression in an older person?
9 How could we mitigate these risk factors?
10 Describe how you would administer the GDS to ensure responses are
11 Apart from using a screening tool with the older people with a mental health issue, what else needs to be done to ensure a comprehensive assessment?
12 Identify the most important strategies for the management of behaviours of concern.

DISCUSSION AND DEBATE

1 Discuss the possible negative attitudes that a health professional may have in relation to older people and how this could affect the provision of care. List ways in which these negative attitudes can be recognised and managed so that appropriate health care is provided.
2 Suicide in the older person is an issue that is attracting increasing attention in the media. However, in a society that has limited resources, it could be argued that the taxpayer's dollars are better spent on addressing issues of self-harm in young people; the older person has already lived their life. What do you think?
3 Why are older people more vulnerable to experience depression in later life and what factors could contribute to depressive symptoms that may not be common factors in younger people?
4 Person-focused approaches to care are labour intensive. Discuss how the health professional can realistically provide biopsychosocial person-centred care in the current health system in Australia.

---

5 Discuss concepts of caring for a person and working with a person. How do we ensure our interactions are not patronising but rather enhance the autonomy and dignity of the individual?.

6 Identify measures you can use to support an older person with a delirium?

7 Identify current services and strategies that support older people with mental illness both in the community and in residential aged care.

8 Consider the vulnerability of an older person to loneliness with the impact of age related changes and a chronic mental illness. How would you support someone to prevent loneliness?

PROJECT ACTIVITY

Using the 'In practice' case study featuring Anna, complete the following.

1 Discuss how you would form an appropriate rapport with Anna.

2 How would you determine the most important care goals for Anna? Use the biopsychosocial model to prioritise these issues in conjunction with Anna.

3 Complete and rate the GDS as you think Anna may respond.

4 Complete a suicide risk assessment for Anna, listing the key issues that are causing you concern and discuss how you could work with Anna to reduce the risk.

5 Based on your responses to the first four questions, work with Anna to devise an appropriate care plan. In your answer consider how you and Anna may want to involve the family, in any care planning as a significant other.

6 Could Anna benefit from any other community organisations to aid in recovery and ongoing support?

WEBSITES

1 Australian Bureau of Statistics. (2022). National Study of Mental Health and Wellbeing. Australian Government. www.abs.gov.au/statistics/health/mental-health/national-study-mental-health-and-wellbeing/latest-release#self-harm

2 Australian Institute of Health & Welfare. (2021). Older Australians. Australian Government. www.aihw.gov.au/reports/older-people/older-australians/contents/health/health-status-and-functioning

3 Australian Institute of Health & Welfare. (2022). Suicide and Self-harm monitoring. Australian Government. www.aihw.gov.au/suicide-self-harm-monitoring

4 NSW Government. (2022). Older people's mental health. www.health.nsw.gov.au/mentalhealth/Pages/services-opmh.aspx

5 SA Health. (2022). Older people's mental health services. www.sahealth.sa.gov.au/wps/wcm/connect/public+content/sa+health+internet

6 World Health Organization. (2017). Global Action Plan on the Public Health Response to Dementia 2017-2025. WHO. https://apps.who.int/iris/bitstream/handle/10665/259615/9789241513487-eng.pdf?sequence=1

7 World Health Organisation. (2022). International Classification of Disease. (ICD-11). www.who.int/standards/classifications/classification-of-diseases

REFERENCES

Aberdeen, L., & Bye, L. (2013). Challenges for Australian sociology: Critical ageing research-ageing well? *Journal of Sociology*, 49, 3–21.

Alexopoulos, G. S., Abrams, R. C., Young, R. C., & Shamoian, C. A. (1988). Cornell scale for depression in dementia. *Biological Psychiatry*, 23(3), 271–284.

American Psychiatric Association. (2013). *Diagnostic and statistical manual of mental health disorders*. (5th ed).

Arevalo-Rodriguez, I., Smailagic, N., Roque-Figuls, M., Ciapponi, A., Sanchez-Perez, E., Giannakou, A., Pedraza, O. L., Cosp, X. B., & Cullum, S. (2021). Mini-Mental State Examination (MMSE) for the early detection of dementia in people with mild cognitive impairment (MCI). *Cochrane Database of Systematic Reviews*, 7(7).

Australian Bureau of Statistics. (2019). *Disability, ageing and carers, Australia: Summary of findings, 2018*. Australian Government.

Australian Bureau of Statistics. (2021). *Causes of death, Australia*. Australian Government. www.abs.gov.au/statistics/health/causes-death/causes-death-australia/latest-release

Australian Commission on Safety and Quality in Health Care. (2016). *Delirium Clinical Care Standard*. ACSQHC. www.safetyandquality.gov.au/our-work/clinical-care-standards/delirium-clinical-care-standard

Australian Institute of Health & Welfare. (2018). *Australia's Health, 2018*. Australian Government. https://doi.org/10.25816/5ec1e56f25480

Australian Institute of Health & Welfare. (2018). *GEN fact sheet 2017–18: People's care needs in aged care*. AIHW.

Australian Institute of Health and Welfare. (2019). *Dementia in Australia*. AIHW

Australian Institute of Health & Welfare. (2021). *Older Australians*. Australian Government. www.aihw.gov.au/reports/older-people/older-australians/contents/health/health-status-and-functioning

Australian Institute of Health & Welfare. (2022). *Dementia in Australia*. Australian Government. www.aihw.gov.au/reports/dementia/dementia-in-aus/contents/summary

Barry, M. J., & Edgman-Levitan, S. (2012). Shared decision making — The pinnacle patient-centered care. *The New England Journal of Medicine*, *366*(9), 780–781. https://doi.org/10.1056/NEJMp1109283

Baldwin, R. (2008). Mood disorders: Depressive disorders. In R. Jacoby, C. Oppenheimer, T. Denning & A. Thomas (Eds.) *Oxford textbook of old age psychiatry* (4th ed.). Oxford University Press

Beddoe, L. (2013). 'A profession of faith' or a profession: Social work, knowledge and professional capital. *New Zealand Sociology*, *28*(2), 44–63. www.researchgate.net/publication/257139303_'A_Profession_of_Faith'_or_a_Profession_Social_Work_Knowledge_and_Professional_Capital

Beishon, L. C., Batterham, A. P., Quinn, T. J., Nelson, C. P., Panerai, R. B., Robinson, T., & Haunton, V. J. (2019). Addenbrooke's cognitive examination III (ACE-III) and mini-ace for the detection of dementia and mild cognitive impairment. *Cochrane Database of Systematic Reviews*, *12*(12). https://doi.org/10.1002/14651858.CD013282.pub2

Bernoth, M., Burmeister, O. K., Morrison, M., Islam, M. Z., Onslow, F., & Cleary, M. (2016). The impact of a participatory care model on work satisfaction of care workers and the functionality, connectedness, and mental health of community-dwelling older people. *Issues in Mental Health Nursing*, *37*(6), 429–435. https://doi.org/10.3109/01612840.2016.1149260

Bernoth, M., & Montayre, J. (2022). The impact of physiological changes on older people; implications for nursing practice. In M. Bernoth & D. Winkler, *Healthy ageing and aged care* (2nd ed.). Oxford University Press

Bishop, J. L., Roden, B. K., Bolton, A. C., & Wynn, R. V. (2008). *An assessment of the relationships among attitudes toward the elderly, death anxiety, and locus of control*. Psychology Program, Department of Behavioral and Social Science, University of Montevallo, Montevallo, Presentation Dominican University of California.

Bruner, J. (2004). Life as narrative. *Social Research*, *71*(3), 691–710. https://ewasteschools.pbworks.com/f/Bruner_J_LifeAsNarrative.pdf

Bryant, C., Bei, B., Gibson, K., Komiti, A., Jackson, H., & Judd, F. (2012). The relationship between attitudes to ageing and physical and mental health in older adults. *International Psychogeriatrics*, *24*(10), 1674–1683. https://doi.org/10.1017/S1041610212000774

Burmeister, O. K., Bernoth, M., Dietsch, E., & Cleary, M. (2016). Enhancing connectedness through peer training for community-dwelling older people: A person centred approach. *Issues in Mental Health Nursing*, *37*(6), 406–411. https://doi.org/10.3109/01612840.2016.1142623

Butler, R. N. (1969). Age-ism: Another form of bigotry. *The Gerontologist*, *9*, 243–246. https://doi.org/10.1093/geront/9.4_part_1.243

Centre of Excellence in Population Ageing Research. (2018). *Cognitive ageing and decline: Insights from recent research*. UNSW.

Choi, N. G., Kunik, M. E., & Wilson, N. (2013). Mental health service use among depressed, low-income homebound middle-aged and older adults. *Journal of Aging and Health*, *25*(4), 638–655. https://doi.org/10.1177/0898264313484059

Conejero, I., Olié, E., Courtet, P., & Calati, R. (2018). Suicide in older adults: Current perspectives. *Clinical Interventions in Aging*, *13*, 691. https://doi.org/10.2147/CIA.S130670

Creighton, A. S., Davison, T. E., & Kissane, D. W. (2016). The prevalence of anxiety among older adults in nursing homes and other residential aged care facilities: A systematic review. *International Journal of Geriatric Psychiatry*, *31*(6), 555–566. https://doi.org/10.1002/gps.4378

Dementia Australia. (2022). *Dementia statistics*. www.dementia.org.au/statistics

Engert, V., Grant, J. A., & Strauss, B. (2020). Psychosocial factors in disease and treatment—A call for the biopsychosocial model. *JAMA Psychiatry*, *77*(10), 996–997. https://doi.org/10.1001/jamapsychiatry.2020.0364

Erikson, E. (1959). *Identity and the life cycle*. International University Press.

E-Shien, C., Kannoth, S., Levy, S., Shi-Yi, W., Lee, J. E., & Levy, B. R. (2020). Global reach of ageism on older persons' health: A systematic review. *PLoS One*, *15*(1), 1–24. https://doi.org/10.1371/journal.pone.0220857

Folstein, M. F., Folstein, S. E., & McHugh, P. R. (1975). "Mini-mental state": A practical method for grading the cognitive state of patients for the clinician. *Journal of Psychiatric Research*, *12*(3), 189–198. https://doi.org/10.1016/0022-3956(75)90026-6

Gibson, C., Crockett, J., Dudgeon, P., Bernoth, M., & Lincoln, M. (2020). Sharing and valuing older Aboriginal people's voices about social and emotional wellbeing services: A strength-based approach for service providers. *Aging & Mental Health*, *24*(3), 481–488. https://doi.org/10.1080/13607863.2018.1544220

Graffigna, G., & Barello, S. (2018). Spotlight on the Patient Health Engagement model (PHE model): A psychosocial theory to understand people's meaningful engagement in their own health care. *Patient Preference and Adherence*, *12*, 1261. https://doi.org/10.2147/PPA.S145646

Green, E., Bernoth, M., & Nielsen, S. (2016). Do nurses in acute care settings administer PRN analgesics equally to patients with dementia compared to patients without dementia? *Collegian*, *23*(2), 233–239. https://doi.org/10.1016/j.colegn.2015.01.003

Harrison, S. L., Bradley, C., Milte, R., Liu, E., Kouladjian O'Donnell, L., Hilmer, S. N., & Crotty, M. (2018). Psychotropic medications in older people in residential care facilities and associations with quality of life: A cross-sectional study. *BMC Geriatrics*, *18*(1), 1–8. https://doi.org/10.1186/s12877-018-0752-0

Hearn, M. P. (2004). *The Annotated Christmas Carol: A Christmas Carol in prose by Charles Dickens*. W.W. Norton & Company.

Honan, B., & Green, E. (2022). The older person in acute care. In M. Bernoth & D. Winkler (Eds.), *Healthy ageing and aged care*. Oxford University Press.

Horrigan-Kelly, M., Millar, M., & Dowling, M. (2016). Understanding the key tenets of Heidegger's philosophy for interpretive Phenomenological Research. *International Journal of Qualitative Methods*, *15*(1). https://doi.org/10.1177/1609406916680634

Horta, O. (2010). Discrimination in terms of moral exclusion. *Theoria: Swedish Journal of Philosophy*, *76*, 346–364. https://doi.org/10.1111/j.1755-2567.2010.01080.x

Hughes, C., Stirling, C., & Harvey, R. (2022). The opportunities and challenges of ageing in Australia. In M. Bernoth & D. Winkler (Eds.), *Healthy ageing and aged care*. Oxford University Press.

Inouye, S.K., & Charpentier, P.A. (1996). Precipitating factors for delirium in hospitalised elderly persons. Predictive model and interrelationships with baseline vulnerability. *Journal of the American Medical Association, 275*(11), 852–857. https://pubmed.ncbi.nlm.nih.gov/8596223

Kitwood, T. (1997). *Dementia reconsidered: The person comes first*. Open University Press.

Kitwood, T., & Bredin, K. (1992). Towards a theory of dementia care: Personhood and well-being. *Ageing Society, 12*, 269–287. https://doi.org/10.1017/s0144686x0000502x

Larner, A. J. (2018). Mini-mental state examination: Diagnostic test accuracy study in primary care referrals. *Neurodegenerative Disease Management, 8*(5), 301–305. https://doi.org/10.2217/nmt-2018-0018

Levy, B. R., Slade, M. D., Murphy, T. E., & Gill, T. M. (2012). Association between positive age stereotypes and recovery from disability in older persons. *Journal of the American Medical Association, 308*(19), 1–5. https://doi.org/10.1001/jama.2012.14541

Mack, S., Bernoth, M., & Biles, J. (2021). Researching aged care during COVID: Adapting to the unexpected: the use of an online medium while conducting qualitative interviews in residential aged care during COVID-19. In *The 54th AAG Conference: Innovations in ageing for the future*. https://researchoutput.csu.edu.au/en/publications/researching-aged-care-during-covid-adapting-to-the-unexpected-the

Maier, A., Riedel-Heller, S. G., Pabst, A., & Luppa, M. (2021). Risk factors and protective factors of depression in older people 65+. A systematic review. *PLoS One, 16*(5), e0251326. https://doi.org/10.1371/journal.pone.0251326

Martins, S., & Fernandes, L. (2012). Delirium in elderly people: A review. *Frontiers in Neurology, 3*, 101. https://doi.org/10.3389/fneur.2012.00101

Maurer, D. M., Raymond, T. J., & Davis, B. N. (2018). Depression: Screening and diagnosis. *American Family Physician, 98*(8), 508–515. https://pubmed.ncbi.nlm.nih.gov/30277728

McKay, R., McDonald, R., Lie, D., & McGowan, H. (2012). Reclaiming the best of the biopsychosocial model of mental health care and recovery for older people through a person-centred approach. *Australasian Psychiatry, 20*(6), 492–495. https://doi.org/10.1177/1039856212460286

Moyle, W., Jones, C. J., Murfield, J. E., Thalib, L., Beattie, E. R., Shum, D. K., O'Dwyer, S. T., Cindy Mervin, M., & Draper, B. M. (2017). Use of a robotic seal as a therapeutic tool to improve dementia symptoms: A cluster-randomized controlled trial. *Journal of the American Medical Directors Association, 18*(9), 766–773. https://doi.org/10.1016/j.jamda.2017.03.018

National Mental Health Commission. (2019). *Submission to the Royal Commission into Aged Care Quality and safety*. Australian Government. Submission AWF.001.04486.02_0 https://agedcare.royalcommission.gov.au/system/files/2020-07/AWF.001.04486.02_0.pdf

National Prescribing Service MedicineWise. (2022). *Older people with dementia*. https://www.nps.org.au/search?q=older+people+with+dementia&scope=all

Nizette, D., McAllister, M., & Marks, P. (2021). *Stories in mental health* (2nd ed.). Elsevier Health Sciences.

Oliver, D. (2008). 'Acopia' and 'social Admission' are not diagnoses: Why older people deserve better. *Journal of the Royal Society of Medicine, 101*(4), 168–174. https://doi.org/10.1258/jrsm.2008.080017

Parse, R. R. (2019). Nurses and person-centered care. *Nursing Science Quarterly, 32*(4), 265–265. https://doi.org/10.1177/0894318419864335

Power, M. C., Mormino, E., Soldan, A., James, B. D., Yu, L., Armstrong, N. M., Bangen, K., Delano-Wood, L., Lamar, M., Lim, Y., Nudelman, K., Zahodne, L., Gross, A., Mungas, D., Widaman, K., & Schneider, J. (2018). Combined neuropathological pathways account for age-related risk of dementia. *Annals of Neurology, 84*(1), 10–22. https://doi.org/10.1002/ana.25246

Pozgar, G. D. (2019). *Legal and ethical issues for health professionals*. Jones & Bartlett Learning.

Rayner, J. A., Fetherstonhaugh, D., Beattie, E., Harrington, A., Jeon, Y. H., Moyle, W., & Parker, D. (2022). "Oh, older people, it's boring": Nurse academics' reflections on the challenges in teaching older person's care in Australian undergraduate nursing curricula. *Collegian*. https://doi.org/10.1016/j.colegn.2022.08.009

Reich, A. J., Claunch, K. D., Verdeja, M. A., Dungan, M. T., Anderson, S., Clayton, C. K., Goates, M. C., & Thacker, E. L. (2020). What does "successful aging" mean to you?—systematic review and cross-cultural comparison of lay perspectives of older adults in 13 countries, 2010–2020. *Journal of Cross-Cultural Gerontology, 35*(4), 455–478. https://doi.org/10.1007/s10823-020-09416-6

Remm, S., Halcomb, E., Hatcher, D., Frost, S. A., & Peters, K. (2021). Understanding relationships between general self-efficacy and the healthy ageing of older people: An integrative review. *Journal of Clinical Nursing*. 10.1111/jocn.16104. Advance online publication. https://doi.org/10.1111/jocn.16104

Royal Commission into Aged Care Quality & Safety. (2021). *Final report: Care, dignity and respect*. Australian Government. https://agedcare.royalcommission.gov.au/sites/default/files/2021-03/final-report-volume-1_0.pdf

Sands, R.G. (2001). *Clinical social work practice in behavioural mental health: A postmodern approach to practice with adults* (2nd ed.). Allyn and Bacon.

Santangelo, P., & Dobrohotoff, J. (2022). Maintaining mental health through the ageing experience. In M. Bernoth & D. Winkler (Eds.), *Healthy ageing and aged care*. Oxford University Press.

Saxena, S., & Lawley, D. (2009). Delirium in the elderly: A clinical review. *Postgraduate Medical Journal, 85*(1006), 405–413. https://doi.org/10.1136/pgmj.2008.072025

Simpkins, D., Peisah, C., & Boyatzis, I. (2016). Behavioral emergency in the elderly: A descriptive study of patients referred to an Aggression Response Team in an acute hospital. *Clinical Interventions in Aging, 11*, 1559. https://doi.org/10.2147/CIA.S116376

Singleton, A., & Douglas, D. H. (2012). Ageism among health care providers and interventions to improve their attitudes towards older adults. *Journal of Gerontological Nursing, 38*(5), 26–35. https://doi.org/10.3928/00989134-20120307-09

Slade, T., Johnston, A., Teesson, M., Whiteford, H., Burgess, P., Pirkis, J., & Saw, S. (2009). *The mental health of Australians 2: Report on the 2007 National Survey of Mental Health and Wellbeing*. Department of Health and Ageing. www.research gate.net/publication/236611613_The_Mental_Health_of_Australians_2_Report_on_the_2007_National_Survey_of_Mental_Health_and_Wellbeing

Song, J., Mailick, M. R., & Greenberg, J. S. (2018). Health of parents of individuals with developmental disorders or mental health problems: Impacts of stigma. *Social Science & Medicine*, *217*, 152–158. https://doi.org/10.1016/j.socscimed.2018.09.044

Thomann, S., Zwakhalen, S., Richter, D., Bauer, S., & Hahn, S. (2021). Restraint use in the acute-care hospital setting: A cross-sectional multi-centre study. *International Journal of Nursing Studies*, *114*, 103807. https://doi.org/10.1016/j.ijnurstu.2020.103807

van Corven, C. T., Bielderman, A., Wijnen, M., Leontjevas, R., Lucassen, P. L., Graff, M. J., & Gerritsen, D. L. (2021). Defining empowerment for older people living with dementia from multiple perspectives: A qualitative study. *International Journal of Nursing Studies*, *114*, 103823. https://doi.org/10.1016/j.ijnurstu.2020.103823

van den Heuvel, W. J. A. (2012). Discrimination against older people. *Reviews in Clinical Gerontology*, *22*, 293–300. https://doi.org/10.1017/S095925981200010X

van Velthuijsen, E. L., Zwakhalen, S. M., Mulder, W. J., Verhey, F. R., & Kempen, G. I. (2018). Detection and management of hyperactive and hypoactive delirium in older patients during hospitalization: A retrospective cohort study evaluating daily practice. *International Journal of Geriatric Psychiatry*, *33*(11), 1521–1529. https://doi.org/10.1002/gps.4690

Voigt, T. (2021). *AAG Discussion Paper: 'Adaptive Ageing' versus 'Successful or Positive ageing. Draft for member consultation*. Australasian Association of Gerontology.

Walsh, K., & Shutes, I. (2013). Care relationships, quality of care and migrant workers caring for older people. *Ageing and Society*, *33*(3), 393–420. https://doi.org/10.1017/S0144686X11001309

Wand, A. P. F., Peisah, C., Draper, B., & Brodaty, H. (2018). Understanding self-harm in older people: A systematic review of qualitative studies. *Aging & Mental Health*, *22*(3), 289–298. https://doi.org/10.1080/13607863.2017.1304522

Wilkinson, P., Ruane, C., & Tempest, K. (2018). Depression in older adults. *BMJ*, *363*. https://doi.org/10.1136/bmj.k4922

Wilson, J. E., Mart, M. F., Cunningham, C., Shehabi, Y., Girard, T. D., MacLullich, A. M., Slooter, A. J., & Ely, E. (2020). Delirium. *Nature Reviews Disease Primers*, *6*(1), 1–26. https://doi.org/10.1038/s41572-020-00223-4

World Health Organization. (2017). *Global action plan on the public health response to dementia 2017–2025*. https://apps.who.int/iris/bitstream/handle/10665/259615/9789241513487-eng.pdf?sequence=1

Yesavage, J. A., & Sheikh, J. I. (1986). 9/Geriatric depression scale (GDS) recent evidence and development of a shorter version. *Clinical Gerontologist*, *5*(1-2), 165–173. https://doi.org/10.1300/J018v05n01_09

ACKNOWLEDGEMENTS

Extract: © National Mental Health Commission. (2019). *Submission to the Royal Commission into aged care quality and safety.* Submission AWF.001.04486.02_0. Licensed under CC BY 3.0.

Photo: © Lisa-S / Shutterstock.com

Photo: © shapecharge / Getty Images

Photo: © JulieanneBirch / Getty Images

Photo: © FG Trade / Getty Images

Mental health service delivery

LEARNING OBJECTIVES

This chapter will:

12.1 consider current approaches to the delivery of mental health services in Australia

12.2 describe the importance of primary health care services, including approaches to mental health promotion and illness prevention across the lifespan, and early intervention services for young people

12.3 outline the role of acute mental health facilities, mental health consultation-liaison teams in hospitals, community mental health teams and other secondary-level mental health services

12.4 explain the main characteristics of tertiary-level health services, such as forensic mental health services and dual disability services.

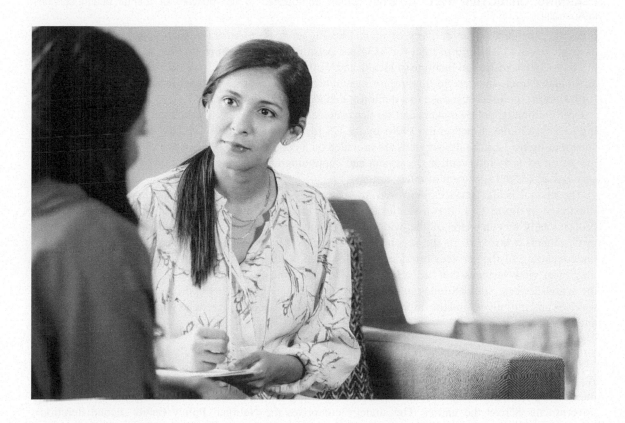

Introduction

Mental health services provided in contemporary Australia differ from those available before deinstitutionalisation. Since the 1980s, the number, type, range and settings of services for children, young people, adults and older people, including individuals, families, groups and communities, have expanded substantially. There is a need for health professionals to be aware of the many different services available, so they can inform consumers of the various options to support mental health Recovery. Awareness of the different services can also help health professionals assist carers who are seeking help and support.

This chapter describes some of the main mental health services available in Australia, focusing on the primary, secondary and tertiary contexts. The categorisation of services can be arbitrary because some services span the primary, secondary and tertiary sectors. Additionally, there are differences in how the services operate, depending on their location. Even so, categorising the services provides a useful way of considering their scope and function, enabling health professionals to understand these differences.

The chapter begins by examining the importance of national strategies for mental health promotion, mental illness prevention, and early intervention. Following this is an outline of various secondary-level health services, including consultation-liaison services, community mental health teams, inpatient services, and mental health services for children, adolescents and older persons. The chapter concludes with a description of tertiary-level mental health services, including forensic mental health services and dual disability services, and a consideration of the role of the National Disability Insurance Scheme (NDIS) in supporting people with chronic and severe mental illness.

12.1 Approaches to mental health service delivery in Australia

LEARNING OBJECTIVE 12.1 Consider current approaches to the delivery of mental health services in Australia.

Funding expended in the delivery of mental health services in Australia each year is substantial. For example, over $11 billion in total (or $431 per Australian) was spent to provide mental health services in 2019–2020 (Australian Institute of Health and Welfare [AIHW], 2022b). Since 2015–16, there has been an annual average increase in funding for mental health services of 3 per cent in real terms (i.e., adjusted for inflation), in direct response to a demonstrated need (AIHW, 2022c).

Conventionally, policy makers and service providers worldwide classify mental health services according to a system developed in the 1990s by the US Institute of Medicine (Mrazek & Haggerty, 1994). As shown in figure 12.1, health services are provided on a continuum that begins with illness prevention and moves on to early intervention, treatment and continuing care. Health promotion activities underpin all services across the spectrum of interventions.

The mental health services delivered in Australia today occur across the spectrum of interventions illustrated in figure 12.1. It is essential to highlight this spectrum of interventions because many health professionals are unaware of the wide-ranging nature of these health services. For example, health professionals who work in the secondary and tertiary sectors, such as hospitals, may have a limited understanding of the services provided outside of the acute hospital setting. These health professionals may even view services that are delivered in the community as lower in status than those delivered in the acute services. Such attitudes suggest a lack of understanding of the importance of primary health care services and initiatives, and the improved health outcomes and cost efficiencies generated by these services and initiatives.

National standards for health services

As noted in the chapter on mental health care in Australia, the **National Mental Health Strategy** guides the development, planning, implementation and delivery of mental health services by state and territory governments across the nation. The strategy comprises the National Policy (in its second iteration), National Plan (in its fifth iteration), roadmap for national mental health reform, National Statement of Rights and Responsibilities and various national health care agreements (Department of Health and Aged Care, 2022a). Associated initiatives include the National Digital Mental Health Framework, which guides the development of digital mental health services across Australia (Department of Health and Aged Care, 2022c).

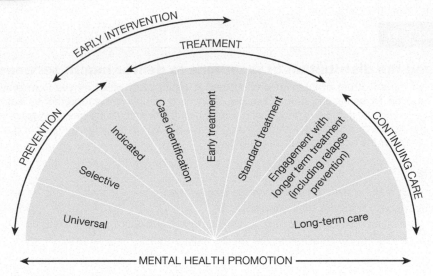

Source: Adapted from Mrazek and Haggerty (1994); Emerging Minds (2022)

The specific aims of the National Mental Health Strategy are to:
- promote the mental health of the Australian community
- prevent the development of mental disorders
- reduce the impact of mental disorders on individuals, families and the community
- assure the rights of people with a mental illness (Department of Health and Aged Care, 2022d).

These aims are achieved through various mental health organisations and services located across Australia, with the quality of these organisations and services guided by the set of national standards developed and implemented by the Australian Government in 2010.

The **National Standards for Mental Health Services** are an essential component of the National Mental Health Strategy and comprise 10 standards (Department of Health, 2010). The key principles informing the standards are as follows.
- Mental health services promote an optimal quality of life and support sustained Recovery for people with mental illness.
- Participation by consumers and carers is integral to the development, planning, delivery and evaluation of mental health services.
- Treatment, care and support must be tailored to meet the person's specific needs and impose the least personal restriction on the rights and choices of the consumer.
- Consumers should be involved in all decisions regarding their treatment and care and, as far as possible, have the opportunity to choose the types of interventions utilised and the location of where they receive them.
- Consumers have the right to have their nominated carer(s) involved in all aspects of their care.
- The roles, needs and requirements of carers, which are different and separate from those of consumers, must also be supported (Department of Health, 2010, p. 5).

These principles frame all of the services described in this chapter. In addition, mental health services must align with the annual general reforms for all health services across Australia (e.g. AIHW, 2022d). For this reason, mental health services have a primary health care focus, promote social inclusion, and enable people and communities to be self-supporting.

State or territory variations

It would be difficult to list all of the many diverse services operating in Australia across the continuum illustrated in figure 12.1. This difficulty is compounded by the Australian health system's multiple layers at the national, state or territory, and local levels. For example, similar service types may have a different structure or appearance in Western Australia compared to service types in New South Wales or Tasmania.

Likewise, services provided in capital cities may differ from those provided in rural Australia. All services must conform to the National Mental Health Strategy and National Standards; nevertheless, local, regional and jurisdictional differences are inevitable. Hence, the services described in this chapter are broad, providing health professionals with a starting point to explore further.

12.2 Primary health care services

LEARNING OBJECTIVE 12.2 Describe the importance of primary health care services, including approaches to mental health promotion and illness prevention across the lifespan, and early intervention services for young people.

As explained in the chapter on mental health care in Australia, primary health care focuses on health rather than illness, prevention rather than cure, and communities rather than hospitals (AIHW, 2021). Primary health care services are the first point of contact for someone experiencing mental health issues. Generally, no referral is needed to access these services. Primary health care services comprise health professionals from multiple practice backgrounds and include services, resources and information to promote healthy lifestyles within communities, to support communities (Raphiphatthana et al., 2020; Wranik et al., 2019). Primary health care services aim to support consumers to take ownership of the services they receive.

Mental health promotion and disease prevention

The World Health Organization's (WHO) *Ottawa charter for health promotion* (1986) was described in the chapter that looked at delivering culturally appropriate mental health care. The Ottowa Charter presented an action plan to enable 'health for all' by 2000 by addressing the social **determinants** of health, such as peace, shelter, education, food, income, a stable ecosystem, sustainable resources, social justice and equity. The *Jakarta declaration* (1997) built on the Ottawa charter and identified the urgency for further investment in health, especially for disadvantaged groups such as women, children, older people, Indigenous populations, those living in poverty and other marginalised populations. The key components of these two initiatives include strategies to safeguard health and improve the outcomes of individuals, communities and larger population groups across the lifespan (Thompson et al., 2018). These strategies provide direction for Australian policy on delivering primary health care services.

The place of **health promotion** and **illness prevention actions** is central to delivering health services across Australia (Australian Health Promotion Association, 2021; O'Hara et al., 2018). The aims and objectives of related activities include building on the existing strengths of people and communities to reduce the extent and severity of ill-health. Health promotion and illness prevention activities are the responsibility of all health professionals, not just those involved in research, policy development, community action and program activity.

Mental health promotion and **mental illness prevention** activities are a subset of mainstream health promotion and illness prevention. They are an integral part of the mental health continuum identified in figure 12.1, with services aimed at enhancing the capacity of people and communities to understand and respond appropriately to people with mental health issues (Graham et al., 2019). As with health promotion more broadly, mental health promotion is about improving the quality of life and potential for health, rather than alleviating symptoms or improving the deficits caused by ill-health. Similarly, mental illness prevention involves the action or activities to support the development of optimal social and emotional environments and, thereby, support the best possible levels of mental health and wellbeing of the person, communities, and various population groups (WHO, 2022).

Conventionally, there are three different ways to approach the prevention of mental illness:

1. universal prevention, which targets general populations
2. selective prevention, which targets individuals or subgroups whose risk of developing a mental disorder is greater than the general population
3. indicated prevention, which targets people at high risk of mental health issues. Indicated prevention places less emphasis on assessing or addressing environmental influences or community values (Bährer-Kohler, 2017).

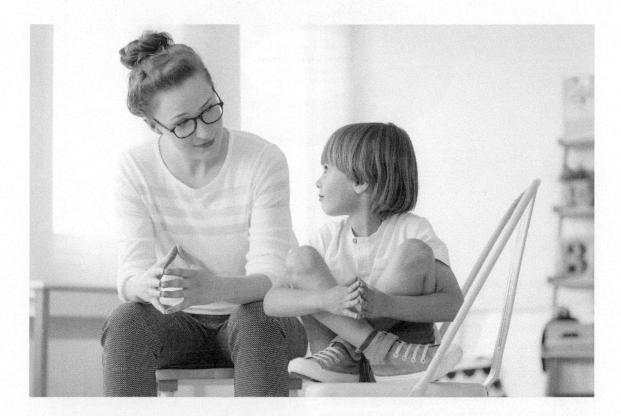

These three approaches are depicted in figure 12.1 as early interventions.

Another way of conceptualising the promotion of the mental health and wellbeing of populations, communities and individuals is provided in figure 12.2. This flowchart illustrates the broad contextual principles and other factors involved in mental health promotion and illness prevention activities, regardless of location and social and economic determinants. For example, for mental health promotion and illness prevention strategies to succeed, whole communities rather than individuals must be engaged (Milstein et al., 2020). These strategies present a range of challenges for health professionals.

For example, if whole-of-community engagement is to occur, it must be accompanied by a major philosophical shift in how health services are provided and resources are allocated (Hickie, Scott et al., 2019). Perhaps most notably, the greatest proportion of health-related resources is currently directed towards secondary and tertiary health services (particularly hospitals). Yet, the health needs of the majority of people fall into the primary health care category. True equity of service delivery and better mental health outcomes will only ever be achieved when there is a balanced allocation of resources across the entire spectrum of health service delivery (Alves-Bradford et al., 2020).

FIGURE 12.2   The Prevention First Framework

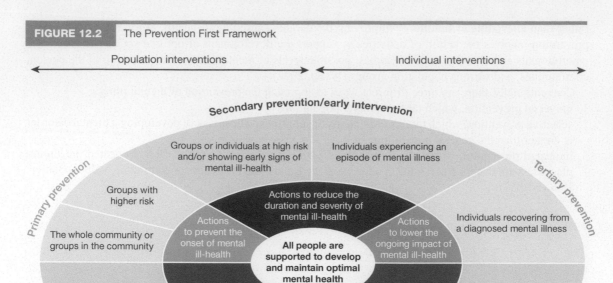

Source: Everymind (2017).

Australian Men's Shed Association

In Australia, males are three times more likely than females to take their own lives (AIHW, 2022f). Moreover, men tend to be more reluctant to discuss their emotions or to ask for help, and more likely to drink alcohol, take risks and experience isolation, loneliness and depression than women (McKenzie et al., 2018, Peltier et al., 2019). Relationship breakdown, loss of access to children following divorce, retrenchment or early retirement, and physical or mental illness are also problems faced by many men, with men reporting that they don't have the knowledge or skills to overcome the challenges involved (Loxton et al., 2018).

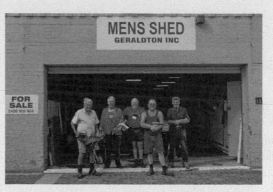

The Men's Shed movement is an excellent example of a primary health care initiative (Wilson et al., 2019). A man's shed has long figured in the Australian culture as a place where he can be himself. The Men's Shed movement has used this cultural icon to provide men with a place to go to participate in a variety of community activities that are meaningful to men from all cultures, while at the same time supporting one another (Cavanagh et al., 2022).

The Australian Men's Shed Association (AMSA) considers good health to be the result of many factors, including feeling good about oneself, being productive and valuable to one's community, connecting to friends, and maintaining an active body and active mind (Misan et al., 2017). According to the organisation, Men's Shed membership:

> provides a safe and busy environment where men can find many of these things in an atmosphere of old-fashioned mateship. And, importantly, there is no pressure. Men can just come and have a yarn and a cuppa if that is all they're looking for (AMSA, 2017).

> The movement seeks to involve men from all backgrounds — what they all have in common is spare time with which they would like to do something meaningful. A Men's Shed should have:
>
> > a Management Committee that has developed a safe and happy environment where men are welcome to work on community projects, specific Men's Shed projects or a project of their choice in their own time and where the only 'must' is to observe safe working practices. All in a spirit of mateship.
> >
> > The Men's Shed movement has become a powerful tool in addressing health and wellbeing and helping men to once again become valued and productive members of our community (AMSA, 2017).

A key aspect of mental health promotion and illness prevention is working to minimise risk factors for developing mental illness, and building or supporting the protective factors that prevent mental illness. All health professionals, regardless of where they work, need an understanding of these risk and protective factors so they can identify the potential for mental health issues to develop and work with individuals, families, groups or communities to build resilience (see the chapter on mental health care in Australia). Risk and protective factors are the focus of the next section.

Risk and protective factors

Many different factors contribute to a person developing a mental health issue. As explained in the chapter focusing on depression, anxiety and perinatal mental health care, a variety of biological, psychological and social factors contribute to a person developing depression, including genetics and family history, physical illness and pain, trauma and substance use (Black Dog Institute, 2022). With so many possible factors involved, the causes of depression are often described as multifactorial.

Traditionally, distinctions have been made between the factors that influence health and illness, with these distinctions based on the relationship between causes and health outcomes. A **cause** is an external agent that results in ill-health. For example, soldiers in a combat zone who experience highly stressful and traumatic situations may develop post-traumatic stress disorder (PTSD). The cause of the PTSD in soldiers is most often combat-related stress, while the outcome is a mental health problem.

Causes can be linked to the determinants of health. A **determinant** is a factor that operates at the social, community or systems level to affect the likelihood that a person will develop a particular health condition (WHO, 2016). For example, the social determinants of health, as discussed in the chapter on culturally appropriate mental health care, include peace, shelter, education, food, income, a stable ecosystem, sustainable resources, social justice and equity. In light of these determinants, it is often argued that certain population groups — such as refugees, survivors of natural disasters, or those who have experienced large-scale social upheaval, injustice or economic inequity — are more likely to develop health issues, including mental health issues (Rees et al., 2019, Schweitzer et al., 2018).

However, not everyone who experiences a traumatic event will go on to develop a mental health problem. For example, less than 10 per cent of people exposed to highly stressful or traumatic events develop PTSD (Phoenix Australia, 2019). This statistic raises questions about why some people develop mental health issues while others who are exposed to similar experiences or events do not. Answers to these questions partly lie with a person's risk and protective factors.

UPON REFLECTION

Risk factors and refugees or asylum seekers

People who come to Australia as refugees or asylum seekers have often experienced high levels of stress or trauma prior to and/or during migration. Stress and trauma are significant risk factors contributing to refugees or asylum seekers developing mental health issues in the short term or long term (Blackmore et al., 2020).

Many refugees and asylum seekers have no family in Australia and find it difficult to find appropriate social support upon arrival. Social isolation presents another risk factor contributing to poor health outcomes for refugees and asylum seekers.

▶

QUESTIONS

1. Identify possible risk and protective factors for refugees or asylum seekers in Australia.
2. If you were responsible for planning and developing health services for newly arrived refugees or asylum seekers, what would be your top five priorities? Why?
3. What primary-level mental health services are available for refugees and asylum seekers who live in the same region as you?

Risk factors and **protective factors** are similar to the determinants of health, but tend to operate at the level of individuals or groups. Risk factors increase the likelihood that an individual or group will develop a disorder; protective factors reduce the likelihood of developing a disorder (Substance Abuse and Mental Health Services Administration [SAMHSA], 2019). These factors account for why one person may develop health issues when exposed to particular events or experiences, while the next person does not. Table 12.1 provides examples of some of the risk and protective factors contributing to a person developing a mental illness. The table includes individual attributes and behaviours, environmental factors, and social and economic circumstances. A person's risk factors may be reduced by their protective factors — and vice versa.

TABLE 12.1   **Examples of protective factors and risk factors for mental health and wellbeing**

Examples of protective factors	Examples of risk factors
Safe, secure and positive physical environment and shelter	Physical environment and shelter that is unsafe, insecure, crowded and/or unstable
Strong community and/or cultural (including religious or spiritual) inclusion and engagement	Experiences of community and/or cultural (including religious or spiritual) exclusion and disengagement
Access to appropriate educational opportunities with good levels of education	Minimal access to or fragmented opportunities for education and/or low levels of education
Access to acceptable and affordable health care and/or support services	Limited access to affordable health care and/or support services
Opportunities for and experiences of appropriate employment and level of income that meet the person's needs	Limited opportunities for or experiences of employment and poor level of income
Positive childhood experiences and good family connections	Poor childhood experiences and family connections
Good personal resilience and physical health	Poor levels of personal resilience and physical health
Low levels of risk-taking behaviours (e.g. substance abuse, anti-social activity)	High levels of risk-taking behaviours (e.g. substance abuse, anti-social activity)
Limited or no family history of mental illness	Family history of mental illness

Source: Adapted from Beyond Blue (2020); Cruwys et al. (2019); Haines et al. (2018); SAMSHA (2019); WHO (n.d.).

It is worth reiterating that although risk factors are associated with poorer mental health outcomes, it cannot always be presumed that people who have experienced or identify with one or more of these factors will inevitably develop a mental health issue. Some people will not be affected by risk factors; moreover, for others, a so-called risk factor may actually serve as a protective factor. For this reason, the risk factors in table 12.1 must be viewed as a guide only. The list does not consider the notion of **resilience**, discussed in the chapter on mental health care in Australia. Nor does the list include how health professionals can work with individuals or groups to strengthen their ability to cope with stress or manage their life experiences.

Finally, there is a need to ponder the degree to which the determinants of health, and risk and protective factors lie outside the control of health professionals. Of course, this does not negate the need for health professionals to undertake health promotion and illness prevention activities; however, it does highlight the complexity of the situation. Long-term sustained effort is required to improve the various determinants of health. In the meantime, health professionals can support at-risk people with early intervention services and strategies.

Early intervention

Early intervention occurs when there is early recognition of a mental health issue, and the person affected is provided with timely and appropriate treatment and support (Iorfino et al., 2019). Early intervention strategies support the person experiencing the issue and their family or significant others (Coates, Wright et al., 2019).

To ensure a person or group of people is provided with appropriate early interventions, all health professionals must be able to recognise early warning signs or symptoms. In general, the early warning signs or symptoms of a mental health issue are:

- fewer than those required to diagnose a disorder
- present for a shorter period than is required to diagnose a disorder
- less intense and disruptive than those of a diagnosable disorder (Gaskin & Dagley, 2018, Mrazek & Haggerty, 1994).

The more common early warning signs for conditions that occur across the lifespan — such as depression, anxiety or psychosis — include changes in feelings, thinking and behaviour. Table 12.2 provides a list of the more common early warning signs.

TABLE 12.2   Common early warning signs for mental health issues

Changes in feelings	Changes in thinking	Changes in behaviour
Feeling anxious or worried	Difficulty concentrating or remembering things	Isolating from others, not wanting to go outside
Feeling tense or restless	Difficulty making decisions	Increased or decreased appetite
Feeling irritable or quick to become angry	Racing thoughts or thinking that is slow or jumbled/confused	Increased or decreased sleep
Feeling depressed or unhappy	Thoughts that are overly negative or pessimistic	Increased risk-taking/dangerous behaviour (e.g. alcohol or illicit drug use)
Feeling unsafe or threatened	Hearing voices that are not coming from other people	Increase in emotional outbursts (e.g. crying, laughing or yelling)
Feeling paranoid (e.g. thinking that others are talking about you)	Thinking about harming yourself	Reduced energy levels and/or motivation to participate in activities and interests
	Dwelling on past events	Difficulty in looking after personal appearance and living environment

Source: Adapted from Beyond Blue (2019) and Parekh (2018).

The origins of or reasons for these early warning signs are mostly non-specific. They can be caused by, or be symptomatic of, several different health conditions; they can be transitory, making them very difficult to identify. Even so, people who develop a mental illness often report prior changes — non-specific in nature — in their thoughts, behaviours or physical being.

In psychosis, early warning signs or an 'at risk mental state' can be called the 'prodromal period'. As explained in the chapter focusing on serious mental illness, the prodromal period is a retrospective concept, because until there is an established psychotic illness, the prodromal period does not exist. The prodromal period has been described as a time when 'something is not quite right' (Ohwovoriole, 2022). Symptoms include changes in perception, beliefs, cognition, mood, affect and behaviour. Because these signs and symptoms are non-specific, health professionals must:

- be aware that any change, however subtle, needs to be documented
- consider referring the person for a full assessment (Gaskin & Dagley, 2018).

These early intervention strategies enable the best possible outcomes for the person.

Some people who experience early warning signs are reluctant to use conventional health services such as general practitioners (GPs) or the emergency department of a hospital, especially if they think they have a mental health problem (Iorfino et al., 2019). Alternatively, some may present to a service complaining of trouble sleeping, tiredness or chest pain (Cabrieto et al., 2019). Others may not be aware of an underlying mental health issue, or they may feel uncomfortable talking about their concerns and use related issues, such as headaches or other physical problems, as a 'cry for help' (Coates, Saleeba et al., 2019). Reasons for such reluctance to report mental health problems may be the social stigma associated with mental illness or the self-stigma some people attach to the symptoms they experience (see the chapter on mental health care in Australia). Social stigma is one of the reasons why many early intervention services have been integrated into the community as 'just another health service' and located where people live, work or learn (Hickie, Davenport et al., 2019).

Risk factors, early warning signs and front-line health professionals

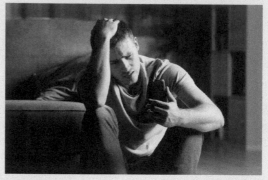

Tadhg, 20 years old, commenced studying full-time at the local university 18 months ago. He still lives at home with his mother Aoife, 53, who works at a nearby supermarket. She is very proud that Tadhg has made it to university and is keen to support him in completing his course.

Over the last couple of months, Aoife has begun to feel worried about Tadhg. His patterns of behaviour have changed. For example, his personal hygiene has deteriorated and he often appears dishevelled. His bedroom is a total mess but he refuses to allow her access to clean it. Also, he doesn't seem to be sleeping and instead paces the house at night, muttering to himself. When Aoife asks Tadhg if he is okay, he explains that he is worried about some assessment tasks, which is not uncommon for students. But Aoife still feels that something is not quite right.

Things come to a head when Tadhg begins to insist that they keep the curtains at the front of the house closed, day and night. He tells Aoife that this is necessary to stop people from spying on them. He explains that he is pretty sure they are under surveillance by Australia's secret service as he has seen an unmarked car containing two men parked across the street on several occasions. This suggestion doesn't make sense to Aoife — they have done nothing to invite surveillance from the secret service and she has not seen a suspicious car containing two men hanging around outside the house at any time. What's more, it is impossible to see inside the house from the street; there are too many shrubs.

Aoife decides it is time to insist they open the curtains to let in some light. Her insistence, however, led Tadhg to become irrationally angry, telling her that she didn't understand the seriousness of the situation. Opening the curtains could mean the end of the world as they know it! Tadhg was so visibly upset and fearful that Aoife decided not to talk anymore about the curtains.

In the privacy of her bedroom, however, Aoife rings the local hospital's emergency department to ask for advice. The health professional to whom Aoife speaks asks her if the matter is an emergency. Aoife explains that she was not sure it was an emergency, but it was certainly very distressing for her. The health professional suggests to Aoife that if she fears for her safety, she should ring the police and stop wasting the emergency department's time. The health professional terminates the call.

....

QUESTIONS

1. What are the risks and protective factors for Tadhg?

2. What are Tadhg's possible early warning signs of deteriorating mental health?

3. How could the health professional in the emergency department have better dealt with the call from Aoife?

4. What are some of the primary health care services or resources that Aoife could access, in the short and medium term, to help her manage this situation?

Early intervention services for young people

The best approaches to preventing or minimising the impact of mental health issues across the lifespan commence with children and adolescents. Mental health problems in young people can have far-reaching effects on a person's physical wellbeing and educational, psychological and social development (Emerging Minds, 2022; Iorfino et al., 2019). Children who are healthy, both physically and mentally, are better able to:

• learn

• experience stronger relationships with teachers, family members and peers

- negotiate challenges, including the transition into adolescence and then adulthood
- achieve long-term education and career goals
- enjoy a better quality of life.

If the early signs or symptoms are ignored, there is the potential for mental health issues to become more serious for the young person, who may go on to develop a mental illness (Hickie, Scott et al., 2019).

A comprehensive approach to early interventions must be taken when working with children and adolescents because the social determinants of health have a much greater potential to affect the health outcomes of children. For example, adolescents with mental health issues are less likely to complete secondary school or go on to further study and find employment (McGorry & Mei, 2018). Children and adolescents with mental health issues are more likely to develop long-term mental and physical health issues, impacting families, friends and the community (Bhullar et al., 2018). For this reason, all services and service providers, including early childhood services, social services, schools, parents and families, and health services, must make it their business to co-operate to achieve the best possible outcome (Read et al., 2018).

Research into risk and protective factors reveals that several groups of young people with particular mental health needs are at an increased risk of developing mental health issues. Attention and support for these groups can potentially prevent mental health problems from developing in the long term. These groups include:

- children and young people from Indigenous Australian cultures
- children affected by significantly adverse life events such as severe trauma, loss or grief
- children of parents with a mental illness.

Children of parents with a mental illness are particularly at risk (Children of Parents with a Mental Illness (COPMI), 2021). Services provided to this group are described later in this chapter.

The increase in mental health promotion and illness prevention campaigns over the past two decades has increased the number of young people who access services (Hoare et al., 2020). Even so, there is room for improvement, particularly in decreasing the delay between when the young person first experiences symptoms and when they actually receive help (Beckwith et al., 2021). Because most young people don't regularly visit, or necessarily feel comfortable with, conventional medical or community health services, it is more difficult to provide them with information or inform them about early warning signs or how to seek help (Shatkin, 2019). For this reason, the government has funded custom-made services for young people, such as headspace and the Be You program. A number of these services are outlined in figure 12.3.

FIGURE 12.3   Early intervention services for young people

Youth intervention programs

- *Early Psychosis Prevention & Intervention Centre (EPPIC)* (http://oyh.org.au/our-services/clinical-program/continuing-care-teams/eppic-early-psychosis-prevention-intervention) is operated by Orygen Youth Health (OYH) (www.oyh.org.au). Orygen, a Melbourne-based youth mental health organisation, has three main components: a specialised youth mental health clinical service, a research centre, and an integrated training and communications program.

  EPPIC works with young people with psychotic disorders by facilitating early identification and treatment to reduce any disruption to the young person's functioning and psychosocial development. Services include case management and home visits; support to families and carers; specialised treatments, including psychological therapy, medication and family work; and psychosocial recovery programs.

- *headspace* (www.headspace.org.au) provides personal mental health wellbeing support, information and services to people aged 12–25 and their families. There are many headspace 'shop fronts' across Australia, all staffed by youth-friendly health professionals who can help people with general health concerns; provide general counselling, education, employment and other services; and offer alcohol and other drug services. Online information and services are also offered by headspace.

- *ReachOut* (www.au.reachout.com) is an online mental health organisation for young people and their parents. It provides practical support, tools and tips to help young people deal with everyday issues or difficulties they may encounter as a part of life. Likewise, the website supports parents, providing information they may need to guide their children or teenagers through life's challenges. ReachOut is accessed by people more than 1.5 million times each year.

▶

- The *Beyond Blue* 'Be You' program provides educators with the knowledge, resources and strategies to help children and young people achieve their best possible level of mental health (https://beyou.edu.au).

   The Be You program supports educators with:
   - professional learning
   - handbooks, handbooks, tools and guides
   - events
   - support for suicide prevention and response (Be You, 2022).

   The school structure offers a systematic means of identifying children at the highest risk or who are already showing early warning signs, then intervening early and engaging the children in early treatment. Schools are uniquely placed to provide information and support to parents and families regarding their child's mental health and wellbeing. The Be You program has been developed to work through educators as part of the school structure.

- *MoodGYM* (https://moodgym.anu.edu.au) is an online, interactive program offering a range of modules to help people to gauge how they feel, understand why they feel the way they do, and change the way they think, know what makes them upset, and be assertive. People may use MoodGYM at home and at their own pace. MoodGYM has achieved many positive outcomes and provides an accessible means through which young people with mental health concerns can access primary health care support (Twomey & O'Reilly, 2017).

The examples in figure 12.3 highlight the diversity of mental health services operating in primary health settings. The service providers for young people include schools and universities, employment agencies and social services (e.g. Centrelink). All those who work in these diverse areas must be aware of the different types of early warning signs, how to identify them, and how to provide appropriate and timely interventions. Similarly, there is a need for mental health services across Australia to continue to develop partnerships and build connections with non-government and community service organisations; departments of housing, education, disabilities and community services; together with the ambulance and police services. Such collaborators enable diverse service providers to work together towards the common goal of improving the mental health of young people in Australia.

Children of parents with a mental illness

In Australia, over a million children have at least one parent with a mental illness (Emerging Minds, 2021). These children face many challenges that can negatively impact their development and wellbeing (von Doussa et al., 2022). Various services and programs have been established to support children of parents with a mental illness in Australia, funded under the national Children of Parents with a Mental Illness (COPMI) initiative, including the Be You initiative, already mentioned in a previous section (Be You, 2022).

The main aim of the COPMI initiative is to develop information to support children of parents with a mental illness as well as the parents, partners of parents, carers, family and friends. With knowledge about mental health and illness, available services, and how to access these services, all those involved are more able to make informed choices about the services (Karibi & Arblaster, 2019). The information generated by the COPMI initiative complements the online training courses developed for professionals supporting families. In addition, COPMI programs facilitate community support groups, educators, service organisations and the media — to produce resources that aim to:

- build resilience and foster better mental health outcomes for children of parents with a mental illness
- reduce stigma associated with parental mental illness
- help friends, family and workers in a range of settings respond to the needs of the children and their families
- respond to the needs of the children and their families where a parent has a mental illness.

These resources are developed under the guidance of people who have experienced living in a family where a parent has a mental illness, leading researchers and service providers in the mental health field (Be You, 2022, COPMI, 2021). You can read more about COPMI services in the chapter focusing on mental health assessment.

Mental health literacy

A significant part of mental health promotion and illness prevention is **mental health literacy**. This term is described briefly in the chapters that cover mental health care in Australia and culturally appropriate mental health care. Mental health literacy involves increasing the awareness or knowledge of mental health issues in individuals and communities (Stanton et al., 2019).

Key aspects of mental health literacy are:

- raising community awareness of the social and emotional wellbeing of communities, and how this can be affected by issues related to mental health and ill-health
- providing information on mental health and ill-health, including risk factors, self-treatment and where to go for professional help
- promoting attitudes that improve recognition and appropriate help-seeking
- assisting with community recognition of specific disorders.

Activities designed to improve mental health literacy include the ongoing education of people of all ages and a continuous flow of information between service providers and community organisations (Tully et al., 2019). An Australian initiative that has worked effectively to increase the mental health literacy of various populations is the Mental Health First Aid (MHFA) course (www.mhfa.com.au). Professor Tony Jorm and Betty Kitchener, a mental health consumer, developed the program to help people provide first-response support to someone with a mental health issue. The course has been rolled out across Australia and has been taken up internationally (Jorm & Kitchener, 2018). Outcomes of the MHFA program include increases in mental health knowledge, reductions in mental health stigma, and increases in the community support provided to people with mental health issues (Maslowski et al., 2019).

The program has several aims, many similar to conventional first aid courses. For example, the MHFA program aims to:

- preserve life when the person is a danger to themselves or others
- help prevent a mental health problem from becoming a mental illness
- promote the Recovery approach to achieving good mental health
- provide comfort to a person experiencing mental distress
- develop the skills needed to help people deal with a mental health crisis (MHFA, 2019).

Mental health crises may involve situations in which a person is feeling suicidal, is having a panic attack, has had a recent traumatic experience, is acutely psychotic and perceived to be threatening violence, or has taken an overdose of medication or some other substance. Actions to take are listed under the acronym ALGEE.

- **A**ssess risk of suicide or harm.
- **L**isten non-judgmentally.
- **G**ive reassurance and information.
- **E**ncourage the person to get appropriate professional help.
- **E**ncourage self-help strategies (MHFA, 2019).

Several population group-specific MHFA courses are available, including culturally and linguistically modified courses, Aboriginal and Torres Strait Islander courses for urban and rural Indigenous community members, and courses suitable for adults working with adolescents. Increasingly, MHFA training is recommended for those employed in occupations with greater potential for contact with people with mental health problems. This includes generalist health professionals such as counsellors, dieticians or nutritionists, GPs, Indigenous health workers, nurses or midwives, occupational therapists, paramedics, physiotherapists, psychologists or social workers. More information about MHFA courses can be found at www.mhfa.com.au.

UPON REFLECTION

Digital Mental Health Promotion

The Australian government's Department of Health and Aged Care provides a range of digital mental health promotion resources from trusted service providers to improve the mental health literacy of people and communities across Australia on their Head of Health website. These resources include those related to natural disaster support, anxiety and stress, eating well, mental health wellbeing, the connection between physical and mental health and supporting children. You can access the Head to Health resources at http://beta.headtohealth.gov.au.

QUESTIONS

1. In your view, how useful are the resources provided on the Head to Health website for improving people's mental health literacy? Justify your answer.
2. How can people, including health professionals, know if the information they access on the internet is trustworthy?

In addition to undertaking an MHFA course, health professionals who work in generalist health services have many other options for learning more about mental health and mental illness. These options include the following.

- *Mental Health Professionals Online Development (MHPOD)*. This Australian government initiative supports the development of knowledge about mental health and illness. MHPOD is a learning resource for health professionals and draws on evidence-based research for mental health treatment, care and contemporary practice. The program aims to support health professionals by improving access to evidence-based educational programs. Practitioners, consumers, carers and educators across the country have contributed to MHPOD, which can be found at www.mhpod.gov.au.
- *Black Dog Institute*. Health professionals from any discipline can access education and training on mental health and illness, focusing on mood disorders, through the Black Dog Institute. Resources include case-based workshops, webinars, online training and podcasts, and toolkits to assist with assessment and intervention. Information about this training can be found at www.blackdoginstitute. org.au/education-training/health-professionals.
- *The National Education Alliance for Borderline Personality Disorder.* This not-for-profit service aims to raise public awareness and understanding of borderline personality disorder by providing access to research and information. The organisation delivers an education series to support health professionals learn the principles for diagnosing and treating borderline personality disorder. These free courses are available at www.bpdaustralia.org/free-online-course-for-professionals.
- *headspace*. Various free and accredited online training modules are available from headspace for allied and other health professionals who work with young people. These modules are available online, and links to clinical resources and interviews with experts in the field are provided. Information about this training can be found at https://headspace.org.au/professionals-and-educators/health-professionals/online-training.

Early treatment

When framed by an early intervention approach, early treatment differs from more conventional mental health treatments (Fisher, 2021). Mental health issues often develop over time and are episodic or recurring. Consequently, early treatment services must have a long-term perspective and focus more on the determinants of a person's mental state (Wolf et al., 2022). Early treatment involves identifying ways of reducing the impact of the person's risk factors and supporting or strengthening the person's protective factors (see table 12.1). For this reason, it is unlikely that early intervention will be a one-off or short-term activity.

Early treatment, like early intervention, is not usually delivered by mental health professionals or mental health services (Moritz et al., 2019). Instead, early treatment is provided by general health services, educational institutions, housing or employment services, or not-for-profit organisations (see the section on not-for-profit organisations later in this chapter). Strategies include teaching the person coping skills and developing their personal strengths (Knopf, 2018). Improving access to social support and building a sense of connectedness within the community is particularly important to enhance resilience (McDonald & Cotter, 2019). Early treatment may also involve referral to specialist mental health services, with the referral's aim to strengthen protective factors rather than provide conventional treatment.

Another aim of early treatment is to improve the knowledge of mental health and illness in a person who is showing the early signs and symptoms of mental illness. Informed people can make better choices about their health (Cowdrey et al., 2018). Awareness of the signs and symptoms of a mental health problem, and what these signs and symptoms may indicate, can give a person reason to seek help earlier and improve outcomes. Likewise, there is a need to provide information and support to families or carers, as they spend more time with the person than the health professional and so will have a close interest in the choices made by the person (Knopf, 2018). Approaches to support families or carers are discussed in more detail in the next section.

Mental health literacy for culturally diverse populations

Embrace: Multicultural Mental Health is run by Mental Health Australia and funded by the Australian government's Department of Health. Embrace: Multicultural Mental Health offers many different resources for community members and service providers in multiple languages. The website provides:

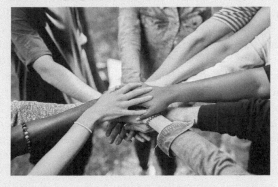

- personal stories from people about mental health and illness, multilingual information on mental health and wellbeing
- a list of culturally sensitive mental health services and community organisations in locations across Australia
- resources for community leaders
- resources for service providers, including webinars, a knowledge hub, policies, and information on best practice (Embrace Multicultural Mental Health, n.d.).

The Framework for Mental Health in Multicultural Australia is a free, nationally available online resource to support organisations and individual practitioners in evaluating and enhancing their cultural responsiveness. The framework is mapped against national standards to help organisations meet their existing requirements. The framework provides free access to a wide range of support and resources to assist organisations and practitioners in building their knowledge and skills in providing culturally responsive health services. The resources and supporting information include good practice examples, a knowledge exchange and links to useful policy documents and websites, and five key concept sheets on:

- cultural responsiveness
- risk and protective factors
- culturally responsive practice
- consumer and carer participation
- Recovery and cultural diversity (Embrace Multicultural Mental Health, n.d.).

Much of what is known about mental health and illness relates to the general Australian population, with the specific mental health needs of culturally and linguistically diverse communities largely unknown (Embrace Multicultural Mental Health, n.d.). Improving the mental health literacy of all Australians about the mental health of diverse populations is essential; likewise, there is a need to develop the mental health literacy of diverse populations. Access the Embrace Multicultural Mental Health website to answer the following questions.

QUESTIONS

1. How well do the 'How', 'What', 'When', 'Who' and 'Why' of the Framework for Mental Health in Multicultural Australia enable services and organisations to meet the needs of culturally diverse communities? Justify your answer.
2. What culturally inclusive policies, practices and programs have your employers implemented to build a culturally responsive workforce?
3. What steps can you take, as a health professional, to help improve your mental health literacy in relation to culturally and linguistically diverse populations?
4. What steps can you take, as a health professional, to help improve the mental health literacy of the general community on the mental health needs of culturally and linguistically diverse populations?
5. What steps can you take, as a health professional, to help improve the mental health literacy of culturally and linguistically diverse populations?

Consumer and carer networks

Consumer and carer participation in the planning, implementation and delivery of health services is now an expectation of governments across Australia, so it is not surprising that consumer and carer networks have a high profile. A **consumer** is a person who uses or has previously used a mental health service (Health Consumers NSW, n.d.). As explained in the chapter focusing on mental health care in Australia, the term 'consumer' was developed as part of the consumer movement to empower people with mental illness. The expression 'mental health consumer' connotes ideas of choice for individuals in the treatment or services they utilise.

A **carer** is a person who, through a family relationship or other relationship, provides unpaid support to a person with a disability, mental illness, chronic condition, terminal illness, an alcohol or other drug issue, or who is frail aged (Carers Australia, 2022). As explained in the chapter on serious mental illness, a carer can be a member of the consumer's family, a legal guardian or another person who is significant to the consumer (Mental Health Carers Australia, 2019).

Consumers and carers often have quite different voices and needs. Consequently, health professionals need to listen and respond to the stories and experiences of both groups. The health professional spends a comparatively short time with the consumer. In contrast, the consumer spends considerable time with their carers, partner, family members, friends or community members. Moreover, the relationship between the consumer and carer can significantly impact health outcomes. For example, people with mental illness supported by family or carers achieve better outcomes than those with no or limited family or carer support (Javed & Harrman, 2017). Additionally, consumers and carers often share and negotiate a lifestyle between them. The role of the carer in the Recovery journey of the consumer, then, is central.

Yet, many carers feel they lack the skills or capacity to adequately support the person exhibiting symptoms of mental illness (Hielscher et al., 2019). Carers, therefore, look to health professionals for support and information on how to develop the skills they need. The type of support and information the health professional provides will depend on the needs and preferences of the carers (Olasoji et al., 2017).

Health professionals must consider how they can better support the mental health of carers. Caring (especially long-term) can be very stressful (Visa & Harvey, 2019). Caring for a person with a chronic illness, such as a mental illness, is a risk factor for carers, who may develop a mental health problem of their own if they are not adequately supported. Finally, if the person caring for the consumer at home becomes unwell or develops a stress-related illness, the consumer will be affected, often detrimentally (Liu et al., 2020). For this reason, delivering comprehensive health care by a health professional to a consumer must include supporting or assisting the carer.

Consumer and carer networks and/or support groups operate in all states and territories across Australia. Health professionals are encouraged to provide the groups' contact details to consumers and carers. For example, organisations such as Carers Australia (www.carersaustralia.com.au) or Mental Health Carers Australia (www.mentalhealthcarersaustralia.org.au) support consumers and carers to achieve Recovery and empowerment, with services such as home-based and intensive outreach services, Recovery care programs and flexible respite options.

Another key organisation that supports consumers and carers is the National Mental Health Consumer and Carer Forum (www.nmhccf.org.au), which provides the means for consumers and carers to actively participate in developing mental health policy and service development in Australia. This forum aims to:

- utilise the lived experience of its members and their unique expertise in mental health, to identify what does and does not work in the mental health sector
- identify innovative ways to bring about positive change within the mental health system
- be a powerful, respected, combined national voice for mental health consumers and carers.

This organisation also provides consumers and carers with a united and national conduit through which they can create a more responsive system to improve their quality of life.

Not-for-profit organisations

Many hundreds of **not-for-profit organisations (NPOs)** operate across Australia, and the large majority of these organisations provide a crucial means of supporting people in their communities (LifeinMind, 2022; Mind, 2019). The activities of these organisations include community and capacity building, the promotion of social inclusion, and activities more specifically related to mental health promotion and illness presentation (Hungerford et al., 2016; Luzia et al., 2019).

Lifeline (www.lifeline.org.au) is a well-known example of an NPO in Australia that provides easily accessible primary-level mental health services. In particular, Lifeline offers a range of mental health services, including a 24-hour, 7-days-a-week telephone service staffed by trained volunteer telephone counsellors who take calls from people with concerns or mental health issues, from anywhere in Australia. Lifeline answers around 450 000 calls per year from people needing emotional support. All health professionals are advised to memorise the Lifeline phone number (13 11 14) so they can immediately provide it to people in need.

Community-managed organisations (CMOs) are NPOs that play a central role in supporting the mental health of individuals, families and communities (Taylor et al., 2018; Mental Health Coordinating

Council [MHCC], n.d.). CMOs are administered, managed and operated independently of the government. They may include charitable or social organisations, clubs or other associations.

The core purpose of CMOs is the welfare or wellbeing of the community. This purpose is reflected in the nature of the activities undertaken by the CMOs, which contribute to supporting or building the capacity of communities. For example, Rotary International (www.rotary.org/en) is a worldwide movement with clubs located in districts or communities worldwide and members working to 'make the world a better place'. Rotary Australia (www.rotaryfoundationaustralia.org.au) coordinates diverse Australian-specific programs and projects, such as drought and bushfire recovery projects, to support communities in rebuilding after experiencing natural disasters. It undertakes to fundraise for health-related organisations like the Royal Flying Doctor Service. Additionally, CMOs such as Lions and Apex play an active role in supporting communities, including the health of those communities. While these and similar community clubs are not ordinarily viewed as health-related, their contribution to supporting improvements in the social determinants of health highlights their capacity to work alongside health services to improve health outcomes.

CMOs include religious or faith-based organisations located across Australia. For example, the Salvation Army (www.salvos.org.au) is a Christian, community-based organisation that offers a wide range of front-line and support services across the lifespan. These services include aged care, children's services, youth services, community services, court and prison services, crisis and support accommodation, disability services, emergency services, employment services, financial counselling, professional counselling, Recovery services and support for those who may be feeling suicidal. This list demonstrates the diversity and inclusive approach taken by some faith-based organisations in supporting the health and wellbeing of people and communities.

Non-government organisations (NGOs) are similar to CMOs because they are operated independently of governments. However, NGOs generally have a broader focus than CMOs. The purpose and function of NGOs vary considerably. Examples of NGOs include organisations that provide human rights advocacy or group social welfare initiatives, relief responses and natural disaster responses. Some NGOs serve as a 'check-and-balance' for governments to minimise the possibility of corruption or discrimination. Other NGOs can provide the means by which government initiatives are rolled out (Department of Foreign Affairs and Trade, n.d.). NGOs are generally more global in orientation than CMOs.

In Australia, many of the services provided by CMOs and NGOs are supported financially by the National Disability Insurance Agency, which implements the NDIS (n.d.) to provide disability support funding across the nation. This funding source is typically augmented by resources from state or territory mental health budgets. CMOs across Australia now receive an increasingly large proportion of the mental health budget, as they can provide services more efficiently than the public health care system.

In response to increases in government funding, a coalition of community mental health peak bodies in all Australian states and territories has been established. For example, the MHCC represents community mental health organisations in New South Wales, aiming to build a viable and sustainable mental health sector and promote the value and outcomes delivered by community-managed mental health services based on a philosophy of Recovery and social inclusion (MHCC, 2021). The types of Recovery-oriented services provided by CMOs include, without being limited to:
- housing, accommodation and residential support (e.g. Housing and Accommodation Support Initiative (HASI) and Community Living Support (CLS), which is a partnership program funded by the NSW government and CMOs that links government housing with specialist support for people with mental illness)
- day-to-day supported living (e.g. One Door Mental Health)
- activities of daily living and employment (e.g. Clubhouse Australia)
- Recovery coaching, support coordination, social and community participation and community access (e.g. Mental Illness Fellowship Australia, with state-level specific organisations available in each of the states and territory)
- integrated community services for people with complex issues, such as mental illness, homelessness, family and domestic violence, and forensic issues (e.g. Ruah Community Services, WA)
- respite care for families and consumers (e.g. Carers Australia)
- generic counselling services (e.g. Anglicare, Centacare, Relationships Australia)
- Post and Antenatal Depression Association (PANDA)
- step-up/step-down facilities as an alternative to inpatient admission or for a period of transition after hospital discharge, with clinical input from the local community-based clinical service (e.g. Wellways).

Although services like these generally deliver social and emotional interventions rather than clinical treatment, some CMOs and NGOs provide access to specialist mental health clinical care, usually through GPs. This specialised mental health care includes the Better Access Initiative, NDIS support, private counsellors or psychotherapists or public mental health services. A number of these services are described in subsequent sections.

UPON REFLECTION

Community-managed organisations and Indigenous Australians

Indigenous communities across Australia are successfully managing programs and services to improve the health and wellbeing of their communities. Key components for this success include community ownership of and control over decision making; ensuring that local Indigenous Elders, culture and history are given a central place in the organisation; enabling the employment of local Indigenous staff to work in a program or service; and maintaining good relationships with partners (Mental Health Commission of NSW, 2022; HealthInfoNet, n.d.).

QUESTIONS

1. In light of the social determinants of health, what difference can successful CMOs make to the mental health of Indigenous Australians?
2. In light of the principles of self-determination, what difference can effective community-managed organisations make to the mental health of Indigenous Australians?

Better Access to Mental Health Care Initiative

The Better Access to Mental Health Care Initiative (Better Access Initiative) provides accessible and focused psychological interventions to people with mild-to-moderate mental health problems (Department of Health and Aged Care, 2022a). The Australian government established the Better Access Initiative as a primary healthcare option for people with short-term mental health issues. Treatment received under this initiative is subsidised by Medicare Australia, the national government agency that delivers a range of health-related payments and services to the Australian community. The Better Access Initiative is provided by allied health workers, including psychologists, clinical psychologists and social workers. Most people who access services funded under the Better Access Initiative have a mood or behavioural disorder rather than chronic symptoms of mental illness (Rosenberg & Hickie, 2019). Since its implementation, the initiative has been utilised far beyond expectations, demonstrating the need and demand for this type of service in the community (Judd & Davis, 2019).

Accessing a consultation with an allied health professional via the Better Access Initiative requires a GP, psychiatrist or paediatrician to complete a detailed mental health assessment, prepare a mental health treatment plan, and refer the person to the allied health professional (Department of Health and Aged Care, 2022a). Eligible people can receive a number of subsidised individual or group therapy services in one calendar year.

While the long-term outcomes of the initiative are debatable (Rosenberg & Hickie, 2019), its high utilisation suggests that this initiative provides a means by which people can readily access specialist mental health support and interventions. More information about the Better Access Initiative is available on the Australian government's Department of Health and Aged Care website (www.health.gov.au) or the Australian Psychological Society website (www.psychology.org.au).

Disaster services

The chapter describing common reactions to stressful situations explained that Australia is known for its challenging environments. State and national governments across Australia have implemented health promotion and injury prevention programs to educate people and communities on how to manage a range of disasters, including storms, cyclones and floods, bushfires and heat events (e.g. Department of Health and Aged Care, 2022b; Department of Premier and Cabinet, 2021). Such programs include encouraging people to prepare for possible disasters by storing water, food and other consumables, and an emergency kit; and to consider how they will stay connected with other people during such times (Ingham et al., 2021). Emergency personnel play a key role in supporting the health of people and communities during disasters, including assisting all those caught up in traumatic or life-threatening events (Travers et al., 2022).

Disaster-related education programs include information for emergency workers who may be exposed to environmental health risks in a disaster or other emergency event. Preparations involve environmental risk reductions, vaccinations, prevention of mosquito bites and the management of abrasions and simple wounds (Australian Institute of Disaster Resilience, n.d.). By accessing the information on disaster preparedness and management, emergency personnel can minimise the potential for injury and death due to a disaster and support achieving the best possible outcomes for people and communities.

Online or digital mental health services

The age of information and technology has witnessed significant advances in the development of digital and other online health services, including mental health services. These primary sector health care services are easily accessed by people, regardless of their location, and require no referral. These benefits were leveraged during the COVID-19 pandemic, when many health services, particularly mental health services, were forced to move to online or virtual environments with good outcomes (Mahoney et al., 2021).

Post-COVID-19, Australian and overseas-based online services continue to be available for people to access, without the need for a referral from medical or other health professionals. These services include government-funded services or initiatives, and services set up by private providers, including online counselling, psychotherapy and mental health information services.

Two well-known government-funded Australian-based online services are the following.
- *Beyond Blue* (www.beyondblue.org.au) — an Australian initiative that can be accessed via the internet. As well as providing national leadership on mental health issues, Beyond Blue offers web-based support and outreach programs, and a telephone information line.
- *Black Dog Institute* (www.blackdoginstitute.org.au) — an educational, research, clinical and community-oriented facility offering specialist expertise in mood disorders, including depression and bipolar disorder. The Institute is attached to the Prince of Wales Hospital in New South Wales and is affiliated with the University of New South Wales.

These examples illustrate how organisations across Australia are working together to raise awareness about mental health issues, and provide information to specific and general population groups to change attitudes in the community and support people and populations with services.

IN PRACTICE

Services for veterans

The Royal Commission into Defence Veteran Suicide (2022) identified that up to 18 per cent of Australian veterans experience mental health and wellbeing issues within one year of entering military service. The rate of suicide among Australian veterans is higher than that of the general population.

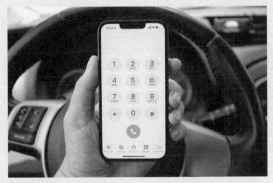

Phoenix Australia (2022) works closely with veterans and military populations to understand issues such as post-traumatic stress disorder (PTSD), its impact on individuals and families, and the influence of military culture on the decisions made by veterans and military populations. Such understanding is central to developing a positive relationship and delivering effective treatment. Phoenix Australia also provides a range of resources for those working with veterans and the military, developed from rigorous research findings.

A key clinical service for veterans and military personnel is Open Arms – Veterans and Family Counselling, which delivers free counselling (24-hour access), treatment programs and workshops for mental health literacy and resilience building, community and peer programs, and self-help tools to veterans and family members. Many of the services provided are online. Moreover, Open Arms' workers are trained in supporting military personnel and veterans, who have their own unique experiences and understanding of the world.

For example, Dan is a 35-year-old male who was medically discharged from the military after sustaining significant injuries to one of his legs when an improvised explosive device was detonated nearby while he was on patrol in Afghanistan. One of Dan's mates was killed in the incident. Dan experiences flashbacks to what happened, can't sleep and ruminates over whether he could have done more to save his mate. Additionally, Dan is in chronic pain as a result of his injury. As well as taking his prescribed medications to help manage this pain, Dan uses alcohol to excess and cannabis to help him to manage his moods.

Dan feels rejected and angry that the army medically discharged him — he devoted the best years of his life serving, and it's like he is now being cast away. He feels like a fish out of water in the civilian world — no one understands what he's been through and he doesn't want to try to explain it. Worst of all, he is unable to work because of his injuries, so he feels useless and bored.

Dan punches walls at home or yells at his wife when his feelings get too much. It sometimes seems like she and the kids seem to spend most of their time crying. Dan hates what he is doing, but he feels unable to stop himself.

When his wife starts talking about leaving, Dan wonders if everyone would be better off if he, too, had died in Afghanistan. At least he'd be a hero instead of half the man he used to be.

Dan starts to plan his suicide. He drives to an out-of-the-way location with a piece of rope he has purchased for a noose. He reaches for his wallet and the family photo he carries around to say his goodbyes. As he looks at the photo, taken in better times, he suddenly wonders if he is doing the right thing, leaving his daughters like this. He doesn't want them to remember him like this.

He finds an Open Arms business card, with the crisis line, in his wallet. He glances at his phone lying on the seat next to him and wonders if he should give his life one more chance.

QUESTIONS

1. Dan is experiencing many issues. What are they?

2. How could digital mental health services help Dan at this time?

3. How could a peer support worker (i.e. someone who has been in the military and experienced mental health issues) help Dan?

Primary care nurses

Primary care nurses work in various settings, including community health, general practice, aged care, schools, correctional health, Aboriginal community-controlled health, refugee health, private practice and other primary care settings (Australian Primary Health Care Nurses Association 2022). Primary care nurses can be registered nurses (RNs) or enrolled nurses (ENs) who may or may not be mental health specialists. Regardless of their background, primary care nurses provide various primary health services to individuals and groups across the lifespan, including people with mental health issues. Mental health support provided by primary care nurses can include:

- mental health promotion and illness prevention activities
- mental health screening and assessment
- clinical care, including pharmacological and non-pharmacological interventions
- ongoing support and maintenance.

Primary health nurses require a broad knowledge of the resources available within the community and health sectors to facilitate care to individuals/groups and the skills to communicate and educate (Heaslip & Nadaf, 2019). The role requires the nurse to work collaboratively with other members of the multidisciplinary team — internal and external to the general practice — and to promote health services focused on individuals and groups (Coffey, 2019).

Primary Health Networks

The Australian government established the Primary Health Networks (PHNs) in 2015 with the main objective of increasing the efficiency and effectiveness of medical services, including mental health services, for people at risk of poor health outcomes (Department of Health and Aged Care, n.d.). The PHNs, located in local communities, focus mainly on the 'commissioning' of services, which involves deciding where services or health care interventions are provided and who should provide them (Bates et al., 2022). These services aim to improve the coordination of care for those with health needs within their communities and ensure people receive the right care at the right time in the right place (Piper et al., 2022).

Examples of health services commissioned by the PHNs to meet the needs of communities or populations include health promotion programs, support for those who provide primary care (e.g. private practices) and continuing education.

Public health for mass gatherings post–COVID-19

The WHO has published key public health considerations for mass gatherings of people (Endericks et al., 2015). These considerations include psychosocial issues, such as crowd behaviour and its impact on individuals. Physical health considerations include those related to the environment (e.g. heat-related illness, dehydration, lack of food and water, hypothermia, inclement weather, fire, overcrowding), infection control (e.g. spread of disease, poor sanitation), and trauma and injury (e.g. stampede, crush, stretched medical services).

With the advent of the COVID-19 pandemic, perceptions of the public health safety of mass gatherings took on new meaning. Initially, many sporting, musical, religious and recreational mass gatherings were cancelled. After the mass vaccinations of populations worldwide, mass gatherings were re-instituted with strict public health measures. The effectiveness of these measures is mixed (Walsh et al., 2022).

QUESTIONS

1. How did the COVID-19 pandemic change how all people, including health professionals, view mass gatherings?

2. How safe do you feel — physically and psychosocially — at a mass gathering, since the COVID-19 pandemic?

12.3 Secondary health care services

LEARNING OBJECTIVE 12.3 Outline the role of acute mental health facilities, mental health consultation-liaison teams in hospitals, community mental health teams and other secondary-level mental health services.

The delivery of mental health services at the secondary level is complex and varies across the states and territories as well as the urban, rural and remote settings (AIHW, 2022c). As noted in the chapter on mental health care in Australia, generally, a person can only access secondary sector health services when a health professional refers them. The obvious exception to this is self-presentation to a hospital emergency department.

This section provides an overview of a selection of secondary sector mental health services, which comprise:
- child and adolescent mental health services
- community mental health teams
- consumer and carer consultants
- inpatient services
- mental health consultation-liaison services
- perinatal mental health services
- older persons' mental health services.

Health professionals aware of how these services operate can provide appropriate advice or referral to people in need. It is recommended that health professionals obtain information about these services specific to their local area.

Child and adolescent mental health services

According to the Australian Government, around 14 per cent of all children and adolescents (those aged up to 17 years) have a mental disorder (AIHW, 2022a). There is a range of secondary sector child and adolescent mental health services (CAMHS) across Australia to meet the needs of younger consumers. Many CAMHS are related to the early intervention and treatment services described earlier in this chapter under 'Primary health care services'. In addition, specific community services are available for children and adolescents who require ongoing treatment and care (Pajer et al., 2022).

CAMHS focus on providing assessment and treatment for children and young people less than 18 years of age who are experiencing mental health issues (Lu et al., 2022). CAMHS funded by state governments have both a secondary and tertiary healthcare focus and therefore require a referral from a health professional such as a GP or a school counsellor before a full assessment can be conducted and appropriate interventions recommended (Foster & Smedley, 2019).

The type of mental health issues experienced by children and adolescents have some similarities to those experienced by adults. Diagnoses may include depression, anxiety and phobias, psychosis, bipolar affective disorder, suicidal thoughts and behaviours, self-harming behaviours, behavioural and conduct disorders, and eating disorders (Hickie, Scott et al., 2019).

Also important are the early intervention and treatment provided for children with conditions on the autism spectrum; however, funding arrangements for these conditions lie outside the mental health budget in Australia, and come from the Department of Social Services and the NDIS (Churruca et al., 2019). Even though autism spectrum disorder is now in the *Diagnostic and Statistical Manual of Mental Disorders* (DSM-5), in Australia, the condition continues to be viewed as a disability (Autism Awareness Australia, 2021). Consequently, a somewhat artificial boundary limits CAMHS services to young people with this diagnosis. It is recommended that health professionals assist parents or carers of children with autism spectrum disorder by referring them to the appropriate NDIS or other government services.

CAMHS teams are generally multidisciplinary and, alongside assessment and treatment, provide:
- personal and family counselling
- outreach or drop-in services, which young people attend for personal or group therapy
- consultation-liaison with other services, including GPs
- family and carer support
- adolescent therapeutic and educational day programs
- residential programs for young people who are either stepping down from inpatient mental health care, or stepping up from community care to more intense care that is not inpatient care
- community education and training
- perinatal consultation for parents.

Through these secondary-level services, CAMHS provides complementary support to the primary health care services for young people described in the first section of this chapter.

Community mental health teams

Community mental health teams (CMHTs) are part of Australia's public health care system and play an integral role in delivering mental health services to people with serious mental illness. The most common diagnosis for people who access the services provided by CMHTs is schizophrenia, accounting for just over 22 per cent of all contacts, followed by depressive episodes (just under 7 per cent) and schizoaffective disorder (just over 6 per cent) (AIHW, 2022c).

Community mental health teams comprise Aboriginal and Torres Strait Islander mental health workers, medical practitioners, nurses, psychologists, social workers, occupational therapists and peer support workers, and are usually located in community health or mental health centres (Ehrlich et al., 2020). The community-based location is central to their effectiveness (Fehily et al., 2020). For example, health professionals are located in the community rather than on a hospital campus to become an integrated part of local service networks. The community location fosters a primary health care approach, including promoting ideas of social inclusion and enabling access to other services such as housing, employment and recreation (Williams & Smith, 2019).

The responsibilities of a CMHT can include the delivery of ongoing care to people who are required by law to receive treatment in a community setting (see the chapter on the legal and ethical context of mental health care). Most CMHTs work with people who voluntarily receive health interventions without needing a psychiatric order. The main services provided are case management, care-coordination and casework (Arya, 2020).

The role of health professionals in CMHTs varies from service to service and location to location. For example, community mental health professionals in rural and remote areas provide many different services from satellite locations rather than offices in large regional centres (Lecamwasam et al., 2022). In general, CMHTs provide at least one of the following services:
- acute and continuing care, including clinical and medication management and Recovery planning
- acute assessment and treatment provided on a mobile basis at extended hours, 7 days a week (e.g. Mobile Intensive Treatment Teams)
- intensive or crisis treatment, sometimes called assertive outreach teams or crisis and assessment treatment teams, is provided on an outreach basis and available on an extended hours basis, 7 days a week, for people with ongoing or recurrent serious mental ill-health and associated disabilities
- telephone triage, often utilising an 1800 telephone number — available 24 hours a day, 7 days a week — to triage consumers and refer them to the most appropriate service

- consultation or shared care with local GPs, psychiatrists and other primary health care practitioners
- telehealth, comprising a two-way telecommunication linkup that enables specialist mental health professionals to provide advice, consultation, peer support, education and training services
- residential rehabilitation in community settings with round-the-clock on-site staff
- ongoing advice and **psychoeducation** to carers and significant others
- tertiary-level clinical care for specific groups such as forensic mental health clients.

Community mental health teams work closely with relevant acute inpatient services (Williams & Smith, 2019). For example, a mental health professional who works for a CMHT may visit a consumer in a hospital if that consumer is usually case-managed in the community and requires inpatient treatment for some reason. The mental health professional in the hospital ensures the consumer is discharged in a timely way. This collaboration promotes what is known as a 'seamless continuity of care' between inpatient and community services, with this seamlessness describing the process whereby a person moves from community to inpatient and back to community care without disruption to their treatment, care or Recovery journey (Jørgensen et al., 2021).

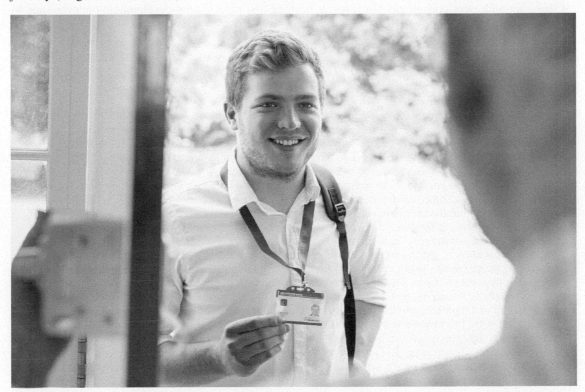

Consumer consultants, peer workers and carer consultants

In many secondary-level public mental health services across Australia, consumer consultants and carer consultants are employed to assist with the delivery of services (Piccone, Moodie et al., 2018). Consumer consultants are sometimes called consumer representatives or consumer advocates.

A **consumer consultant** in the mental health sector is a person who has used a mental health service, is well along in their Recovery journey and works within the mental health service to support and assist people experiencing symptoms of mental illness. A consumer consultant may work from a community health centre or a hospital (Scholz et al., 2017).

Peer support workers are sometimes mistaken for consumer consultants. However, the role of peer workers is different — for example, the focus of the role of a consumer consultant is to advise health professionals about consumer issues and consult with consumers. The role of the peer support work is to work as part of the multidisciplinary team to support the consumer (Ehrlich et al., 2020). Peer support workers are becoming a key component of the mental health workforce. You can read more about peer support workers in the chapter focusing on mental health care for people with serious mental illness.

A **carer consultant** is someone who, first, has cared for a family member or significant other who has experienced a mental illness; and secondly, is employed to provide resources and support to other carers. Carer consultants are sometimes called carer representatives, carer advocates or carer workers.

Like consumer consultants, many carer consultants operate from community health centres or hospitals in various roles that support carers of people with mental illness to access the services they need (Ng et al., 2020).

Health professionals work closely with consumer and carer consultants to ensure that the consumer and carer perspective is considered in their decision-making (Piccone, Sanderson et al., 2018). Consumer and carer consultants provide a vital means of improving service responsiveness by involving themselves with the direct experience of mental health service delivery, so they are often able to promote or advocate for change more quickly than if they were in an administrative position only (Piccone, Moodie et al., 2018). Generally, consumer and carer consultants are involved in:

- ensuring consumer and carer perspectives are included in all aspects of the planning, delivery and evaluation of mental health services
- advocating for the needs of consumers and carers to the service
- communicating consumers' broad views on mental health services and other relevant services, such as housing or accommodation, Centrelink, employment and need.

Consumer and carer consultants also provide training and professional development opportunities to health professionals and other workers.

LIVED EXPERIENCE

On being a Peer Support Worker

It took me a long time on my rocky Recovery journey to reach the stage where I was able to think about what I could do to help others. For me, the most obvious thing to do was to work toward being a Peer Support Worker. I could see great value in someone with the lived experience of mental illness supporting other people with mental illness to negotiate some of the pitfalls in the mental health system. I also figured that people with mental illness would be more likely to listen to someone who had 'been there, done that'. But most of all, I was keen to try to make some changes to how acute mental health services operate. I looked back at how some health professionals treated me when I was acutely unwell — with little regard for me as a person and sometimes with downright contempt — and I wanted to make sure that kind of thing never happened to someone else. Being treated badly got in the way of my Recovery and did nothing for my self-esteem or the way I saw myself.

It took me a while to get the training I needed to take on the role. Then I had to work my way 'up' to a role in an acute mental health facility; they kept telling me that I needed more experience, but I didn't know what they meant. I was a mental health consumer and felt that was the only experience I needed.

Once I finally achieved my goal and commenced work there, I soon realised what they meant. When I was a patient in a mental health facility, I didn't understand the kinds of stresses the health professionals have to deal with: the responsibility, the pressure to meet deadlines, the documentation, the fast pace, and the anger and aggression from the consumers. I remember the first time I was assaulted. I was so shocked! All I could think was, 'But I'm here to help you!' I wasn't hurt — but I was very very upset.

I soon accepted that the health system is complex, mental health services are complex, and people with a mental illness have many different presentations. Their experiences are not just like mine. On the other hand, there are some commonalities including the barriers people with mental illness face on their Recovery journey.

So, despite the challenges, I continued to see it as a privilege to help bridge the divide between consumers, health professionals, community members, and government and non-government organisations. I play a big role in encouraging consumers to give feedback about the challenges they face, including what it's like to negotiate the system, so we can work together to bring about change. This work is important to meet the unique needs of each and every person with a mental illness who comes to the health service for help.

Inpatient services

In Australia, there are many types of inpatient or bed-based services, including acute, subacute, older persons, forensic, perinatal, child and adolescent, young persons, rehabilitation and extended care services (AIHW, 2022c). These services may be voluntary or involuntary. Involuntary facilities are known as 'gazetted' facilities, where people are provided with health care when they have been constrained under the mental health legislation of the state or territory in which they are located. Gazetted acute inpatient facilities accept voluntary admissions; only about one-third of all people who stay overnight in a gazetted inpatient facility are admitted involuntarily (AIHW, 2022c). Involuntary or gazetted facilities are most often locked or have sections within them that are locked, which means that entry into, and exit out of, the facility or locked section is restricted. This practice ensures the safety of the consumer, the community and the staff working in these facilities.

Mental health facilities function similarly to any other hospital facility or ward. As with conventional bed-based facilities, some mental health facilities are part of the public health care system, while others are private facilities that provide mental health services to people who can pay through their private health insurance or personal resources.

Acute mental health inpatient facilities

Most hospitals in metropolitan or large regional cities have one or more acute mental health facility(ies) or unit(s) (AIHW, 2022c). The majority of these facilities are for adults. The more specialised facilities (such as adolescent, perinatal or forensic inpatient facilities) are generally located in metropolitan areas and viewed as tertiary-level services.

Acute adult mental health inpatient facilities are hospital-based and staffed by a multidisciplinary team of consultant psychiatrists, psychiatry registrars, other medical officers, RNs and ENs, Aboriginal and Torres Strait Islander mental health workers, occupational therapists, peer support workers, psychologists, social workers and welfare officers (Healthdirect, 2022; Mackean et al., 2020). This team provides:

- clinical assessment and treatment of the acute symptoms of mental illness experienced by the consumer
- care planning, including medication management and related psychoeducation
- psychological, social, and occupational or functional interventions, individually or in groups
- support and psychoeducation for carers
- **care coordination**, with the team working closely with carers and families, community mental health teams and community organisations to ensure consumers receive the appropriate level of care and support once they are discharged into the community.

In light of the primary health care model that is central to service delivery across Australia, and the principle of least restrictive care espoused by the National Standards for Mental Health Services, people are only admitted involuntary to a mental health facility when they cannot be treated safely or appropriately in the community (Fletcher et al., 2019). The average stay in an acute inpatient unit is just over 15 days; however, this number of days is dependent on a wide range of factors, including location, resourcing and the consumer's diagnosis (AIHW, 2022c).

Rehabilitation and extended care facilities

While most people with chronic and severe mental illness live in the community in social or other housing, a small number of rehabilitation or long-stay inpatient mental health facilities continue to operate in major cities across Australia (AIHW, 2022c). These facilities generally house people who experience severe symptoms of mental illness, are being treated involuntarily, and require a higher degree of psychosocial support than those provided in acute mental health facilities or in the community setting (Curtin & Hitch, 2018; Evans et al., 2020). Secure extended stay facilities are for people with mental illness who are being held for criminal behaviour and require custodial care.

The average length of stay in a rehabilitation facility can be six to 18 months (Mental Health Commission of Western Australia, n.d.). As with acute inpatient facilities, rehabilitation or long-stay inpatient mental health facilities are staffed by a multidisciplinary team of allied health, medical and nursing professionals (Thomas & Rusten, 2019). This team can provide one or more of the following services, depending on the policy(ies) of the organisation:

- life skills education, including cooking, paying bills and maintaining employment
- psychoeducation, including managing behaviours and the side effects of medications
- extended care for those who are having issues with finding appropriate accommodation and support in the community
- respite care to enable carers to have some short-term respite from the primary responsibility of caring for people who have high support needs
- care coordination, where the health professional coordinates the care and treatment provided to the consumer. The work includes the health professional engaging directly with the consumer; managing the overall care process, including the development and communication of the treatment or care plan to all relevant stakeholders; and ensuring that all treatment and care is delivered to meet the quite particular needs of the consumer and their carer.

The focus of care in rehabilitation and extended care facilities is Recovery-oriented and aimed at providing the person with the skills to live a full and meaningful life in the community (Maxwell et al., 2019).

Mental health consultation liaison services

As has been noted throughout this text, around 46 per cent of Australians aged 16–85 years have or will experience a mental health problem in their lifetime (AIHW, 2022c), including adults being treated by health professionals for a physical condition in a hospital or community setting. This means that one in five of the adults cared for by any health professional is likely to have a coexisting or comorbid mental health issue. Moreover, other people may develop mental health problems during their hospital stay or treatment in the community (Lele et al., 2021).

Of further concern is the significant number of people with a chronic physical illness who experience symptoms of depression, anxiety or other psychological distress, but do not receive any mental health treatment or interventions for these conditions (Valdés-Stauber & Kendel, 2021). One reason for this high percentage is that many health professionals do not recognise mental health issues. Another reason is that some health professionals feel unequipped to provide appropriate treatment (see the chapter that looks at caring for a person with a serious mental illness). This situation is problematic as it means the person with the comorbid condition is not receiving the care they need.

Mental health consultation-liaison services, enable appropriate care and treatment for people with co-occurring conditions or issues. **Mental health consultation-liaison (CL)** is a generic term that applies to various mental health services delivered in a range of practice settings that involve mental health professionals consulting and liaising with generalist health professionals about a person with a comorbid mental health issue (AIHW, 2019). In Australia, CL teams or workers can be found in both urban and rural settings; in general hospitals, including wards and emergency departments; or in community teams that provide support and advice to health professionals (e.g. GPs) in primary care settings, the emergency services or community service organisations. The CL team comprises a range of health disciplines, including allied health professionals with a mental health specialty, psychiatrists, other medical practitioners and nurses (Wand et al., 2018). Health professionals who work in health settings that focus on physical conditions are encouraged to seek the help of the CL team for support or assistance when working with someone with a comorbid mental health issue (Asuquo et al., 2022).

The role of the CL team

The role of the mental health CL team is to support people who exhibit symptoms of mental illness in physical health settings by engaging in consultation or liaison activities with health professionals in these settings (Toynbee et al., 2021). Services provided by the CL team include:

- mental health assessment
- risk assessment and management
- brief psychological interventions and advice on medication management
- mental health promotion
- advice on mental health treatment and care
- clinical supervision
- education to health professionals, consumers or carers regarding mental health issues
- connection between the general hospital and mental health services.

The assistance provided by the CL team is collaborative, with mental health CL professionals working alongside health professionals located in general settings to ensure that the mental health needs of the consumer are identified and addressed (Oldham et al., 2019).

Consultation-liaison teams may work across various health settings, but the most common settings include those where acute stress or chronic illness frequently occurs, such as emergency departments, renal units and cancer units (Sharpe et al., 2020). Reasons health professionals refer a person to the CL team may include:

- self-harm or suicidal ideation
- mood disorders, including depression, anxiety or bipolar disorder
- acute stress reactions
- disturbed, aggressive or 'bizarre' behaviour
- problems associated with excessive alcohol and illicit drug use
- confused states and dementia.

This list is by no means exhaustive or exclusive. Health professionals who work in any context and are troubled about the mental health status of a person should not hesitate to contact their local mental health CL service for advice. They can do this by accessing the website of their local health service.

Referral to the CL team

Sometimes it may be difficult to decide when or why a referral needs to be made to the CL team (Lele et al., 2021). A referral may be generated for no reason other than the health professional's uncertainty about what is needed to help the person. As already noted, a valuable aspect of the mental health CL team is the provision of advice, information and guidance before problems become severe or entrenched. For this reason, a referral should always be made, even if the health professional is not sure it is necessary.

There may be times when more formal referrals are required (Valdés-Stauber & Kendel, 2021). In these instances, referrals should be considered in the same way as referrals to other specialist teams. Some conditions, including delirium, acutely disturbed behaviour, agitation or uncooperative behaviour, can lead the health professional to assume the person is exhibiting symptoms of a mental illness. In fact, these behavioural symptoms are more frequently associated with an underlying physical cause. The most common physical symptoms that may be mistaken for a mental health problem are outlined in table 12.3. Common side effects of medications that may be mistaken for a mental health issue are outlined in table 12.4. All possible underlying causes of unusual behaviour must be excluded and treated before a formal referral is made to the CL team.

TABLE 12.3 Physical causes of issues commonly associated with mental ill-health

Symptom	Possible physical cause
Depression	Cancer Infections Electrolyte imbalance (e.g. low sodium level) Endocrine disorders (e.g. hypothyroidism) Neurological disorders (e.g. epilepsy, Parkinson's disease, dementia, stroke) Addison's disease Autoimmune disease (e.g. systemic lupus erythematosus, rheumatoid arthritis)
Anxiety	Endocrine disorders (e.g. hyperthyroidism) Substance withdrawal (e.g. sudden cessation of benzodiazepines, sudden cessation of alcohol) Hypoglycaemia Pheochromocytoma Neurological disorders
Fatigue	Anaemia Sleep disorders (e.g. sleep apnoea) Chronic infections Diabetes Endocrine disorders (e.g. hypothyroidism, Addison's disease, Cushing's syndrome) Cancer Radiotherapy
Weakness	Autoimmune disease (e.g. myasthenia, rheumatoid arthritis) Peripheral neuropathy Neurological disorders (e.g. Parkinson's disease)
Headache	Migraine Brain tumours Temporal arteritis

TABLE 12.4 Medications with side effects that may be mistaken for mental ill-health

Side effect	Medication
Acute confusion (i.e. delirium)	Central nervous system depressants (e.g. hypnotics, sedatives, antidepressants, antihistamines) Antimuscarinics (e.g. procyclidine) Beta-blockers Digoxin Cimetidine

(continued)

TABLE 12.4 *(continued)*

Side effect	Medication
Psychotic symptoms	Appetite suppressants Beta-blockers Corticosteroids Levodopa Indometacin
Depression	Antihypertensives Oral contraceptives Antipsychotics Anticonvulsants Corticosteroids Levodopa
Elated mood	Antidepressants Corticosteroids Antimuscarinics (e.g. benzhexol)
Behavioural disturbance	Anaesthetic agents Benzodiazepines Antipsychotics Lithium toxicity

The referral process to access assistance from the mental health CL team varies from service to service and team to team. Health professionals are advised to identify their local CL operational policy, which should clearly identify the role and function of the CL team in their area. However, before initiating a referral, it is vital that all members of the treating team have been consulted (Oldham et al., 2019). Best-evidence practice in this area includes:

- discussing reasons for a mental health referral with the treating team
- understanding the role of the CL team and answering questions or concerns about the need for a referral
- discussing the need for a mental health review with the person being referred — wherever possible, the views and consent of the person should be obtained. Discussion with family members or significant others is also advisable
- ensuring that the relevant history and background information is available and accessible before making the referral (e.g. contacting the person's GP, obtaining collateral information from significant others, community health teams or other community services)
- being clear about what is expected of the CL team (e.g. anticipated outcome of the assessment); this may include obtaining specialist advice regarding treatment or care, participating in discharge planning by arranging mental health follow-up or identifying ongoing risk
- being open-minded and receptive to the ideas or advice offered by the CL team.

By taking a consumer-centred approach to care, the skills of mental health professionals can be utilised proactively to improve the person's experience (Asuquo et al., 2022). Good preparation stands in contrast to a 'tick-box' approach, where mental health referrals are viewed as a task that needs to be completed with little impact on the health outcomes of the person receiving the treatment.

CL services are a key part of health services in Australia and have enabled the integration of physical and mental health treatment and care. By working with the CL team, health professionals can ensure that the person receives comprehensive health care that addresses all of their biopsychosocial needs. Health professionals can enable the person to achieve the best possible outcomes.

IN PRACTICE

Mental health consultation-liaison team and e-health services in rural Australia

Nellie is a 64-year-old Indigenous Australian woman. She lives in rural Queensland, in a town with no specialist mental health clinician; a mental health nurse and psychologist drive in and out of the town only once a week to provide services.

Nellie's family is worried about her as she seems to be becoming increasingly depressed about life. Nellie is one of the Stolen Generation and has told her family that the older she gets, the more she ruminates about what happened to her as a child.

When Nellie began to talk about suicide, her family decided it was time to do something. They called an ambulance, which transported Nellie to the small local hospital.

After assessing Nellie and talking to her family, the local GP decided he didn't have the knowledge or skills to determine her level of risk. He decided to talk to Nellie's family about contacting the mental health CL team in the city, via the telehealth services, to discuss the best way forward.

QUESTIONS

1. How could the first responders (e.g. paramedics) best support Nellie and her family upon arriving at her home?
2. How could the health professionals in the local hospital best support Nellie while she is awaiting assessment by the GP?
3. What are the benefits and challenges of accessing the mental health CL team via telehealth?

Perinatal mental health services

Perinatal mental health issues have a high profile across Australia (AIHW, 2019a). As noted in the chapter on depression, anxiety and perinatal mental health care, about 9–21 per cent of women will experience symptoms of anxiety and/or depression during the perinatal period (McLeish & Redshaw, 2017). Puerperal or postnatal psychosis is less common, affecting one to two women in every 1000 (del Corral Serrano, 2019), with the condition presenting a serious risk to the mother and baby. Early and effective assessment helps to identify potential problems and allows for interventions and treatment (Chambers et al., 2018).

A new mother, her partner, or other family members may not be aware that there is a problem because perinatal mental health issues can present with ambiguous signs and symptoms (Biggs et al., 2019). For example, the arrival of a baby is always a time of great change and can generate stress, so unusual behaviours may be rationalised as 'just a stage' the woman is experiencing.

Generally, the symptoms for women with perinatal mental health issues include marked changes in mood; prolonged lack of interest or pleasure in routine activities; and persistent feelings of anxiety or inadequacy, failure, hopelessness, guilt and shame (see the chapter on depression, anxiety and perinatal mental health). Treatment options include psychological and/or pharmacological interventions (RANZCP, 2021).

Perinatal mental health services are now a common feature of mental health services (Lim et al., 2022). These services are collaborative and include midwives, maternity and child health nurses, GPs, mental health nurses, psychologists and psychiatrists. The structure of these services varies from jurisdiction to jurisdiction (Irvine, 2018). Most often, perinatal mental health services offer the assessment, diagnosis and treatment of women who experience mental health issues during the preconception, antenatal and postnatal periods, rather than clinical management or counselling. Care coordination is also necessary, as multiple services may be required to meet the complex needs of the woman, baby, partner and family unit (Bohren et al., 2019). Other services a health professional may recommend to a woman with perinatal mental health issues include:

- *Post and Ante Natal Depression Association (PANDA)*, which provides support groups for both women and men experiencing depression and anxiety related to pregnancy, birth and early parenting (www.panda.org.au)
- *Australian Breastfeeding Association*, which provides information and education on perinatal mental health and ill-health (www.breastfeeding.asn.au).

Women at risk of postnatal depression or other issues who are identified during pregnancy or as early as possible after birth can receive effective psychological and social interventions as soon as possible. This can reduce the impact of the woman's issues and prevent illness (Harvey et al., 2018).

Older person's mental health services

According to the WHO (2017), over 20 per cent of older adults experience a mental illness or neurological disorder, accounting for over 6 per cent of all disabilities. The most common mental illnesses and neurological disorders in older people are depression (7 per cent of the world's older population, respectively). Anxiety disorders affect almost four per cent of the older population, and substance use problems affect almost 1 per cent. Approximately a quarter of deaths from self-harm are among older people (WHO, 2017).

It is alarming that mental health problems are under-identified by health professionals. The stigma surrounding these conditions makes older people reluctant to seek help. The good news is that specialised services to support older people with mental health problems are now the norm in Australia.

Key aspects of providing a health service to older people with mental health issues are discussed in the chapter that looks at caring for an older person with a mental illness. Mental health service delivery for people in this population group is highly specialised because the older person often has more than one comorbid and/or chronic issues that add layers of complexity to their care (Kelly et al., 2019; Loxton et al., 2018). Older person's community mental health teams, older person's mental health inpatient units and older person's mental health residential services all form part of the services provided to older people across Australia (AIHW, 2022e). Other, more specific initiatives or programs implemented by the states and territories are described in figure 12.4, and provide insight into the breadth of services that are now provided in this significant area of health service provision.

FIGURE 12.4	Mental health initiatives for older people

Mental health care for older people

Examples of mental health initiatives that have been developed for older people across Australia include the following.

- In South Australia, a range of services specific to the mental health of older people are available, provided in conjunction with community, ageing and primary health care sectors, aimed at reducing the incidence or escalation of mental health issues among older persons (South Australia Health, 2022). This includes community teams, transition care services, acute inpatient services, non-acute bedded services and country older persons mental health services. In particular, a country liaison service allows for direct clinical assessments of people in their usual place of residence, e-health assessments of people, assistance to service providers with formulating management plans, a remote consultation service for service providers, and education for service providers and the community as a whole on topics relating to the mental health issues of older people. This service also seeks to address the lower life expectancy of Aboriginal and Torres Strait Islander peoples, who may be referred from 45 years of age.
- In New South Wales, the Department of Health has a 10-year Older People's Mental Health Services Service Plan (2017–27) to support the systematic development of specialist mental health services for older people (OPMH) (NSW Health, 2022). This plan was required to support the ageing population and the increasing number of older people with complex mental health problems. The services provide integrated assessment and management of older people with severe, complex behavioural disturbance in partnership with aged care services and services established with residential aged care providers.
- Neuroscience Research Australia (NeuRA) is an independent, not-for-profit research institute based in Sydney that aims to prevent, treat and cure conditions of the brain and nervous system. A crucial focus of this institute is the mental health and wellbeing of older Indigenous Australians, including finding the best ways to promote healthy ageing and ensuring older Indigenous Australians gain access to the health services they need. More information about this initiative can be accessed at www.neura.edu.au/health/aboriginal-ageing.

More generally:

- The Australian government provides a directory of services across Australia for older people. This can be found at www.myagedcare.gov.au
- Beyond Blue provides information and links to resources for older people with mental health issues, particularly the more common issues, such as depression, grief and loss, financial stress, changing living arrangements and increasing social isolation (www.beyondblue.org.au/who-does-it-affect/older-people)
- Dementia Australia offers a range of support and information services for people diagnosed with dementia, carers, family members and others affected by a diagnosis of dementia, whatever its cause. Dementia Australia provides information and education for health professionals (www.dementia.org.au).

In light of the ageing population in Australia, health professionals must be aware of the variety of services available. This knowledge will help them to advise older consumers and their carers so they can access more appropriate mental health services. Read more about the services provided to support older people's mental health in the chapter focusing on the care of older people with mental health concerns.

Substance use by older people

Substance misuse and substance use disorders can be overlooked in older populations (WHO, 2017). Alcohol, tobacco and prescription medications are more likely to be misused by older people than illicit drugs (Choi et al., 2022). Additionally, some 25 per cent of older people are consuming up to five different prescribed medications simultaneously for multimorbidity, with many of these interacting with one another or with alcohol or benzodiazepines. There is a need to design programs for older adults to meet the complex needs of those with mental health and/or substance use problems and to incorporate innovative service delivery models that can improve older adults' access.

QUESTIONS

1. How can substance misuse affect the mental health of older people? How can the mental health of older people after the way older people misuse substances?
2. Why are specialised services required for older people with substance use issues?

12.4 Tertiary health care services

LEARNING OBJECTIVE 12.4 Explain the main characteristics of tertiary-level health services, such as forensic mental health services and dual disability services.

As noted in the chapter on mental health care in Australia, tertiary sector services are characterised by high specialisation, which suggests they are most often located in larger service centres. Many different tertiary-level mental health services are available, such as forensic mental health services, duality disability services, dual diagnosis services (for people with both mental health and substance use issues), eating disorder clinics and specific services for people with a diagnosis of borderline personality disorder. This section describes the first two services.

Forensic mental health services

Forensic mental health refers to the mental health services provided to people who have been or are at risk of being involved in the criminal legal system in some way and exhibit symptoms of mental ill-health (Barr et al., 2019). Forensic mental health is a fast-developing area of mental health service delivery in Australia, with a high incidence of mental health issues in the forensic population (Ellis, 2020). For example, forensic populations have a higher rate of mental illness and substance use than the general population, with rates of serious mental illnesses, such as schizophrenia and depression, three to five times higher in the forensic population than in the general community (AIHW, 2022b; Royal Australian and New Zealand College of Psychiatrists (RANZCP), 2017). This situation has been attributed to a range of factors, including limited access to mental health services in the forensic system, the intolerance of many societies for complex behaviours leading to high rates of incarceration, and the failure to promote treatment, care and rehabilitation for all populations groups (Senneseth et al., 2022).

The commitment by the federal and state/territory governments across Australia to provide systematic mental health assessment, appropriate treatment, and ongoing support to the forensic population is timely (Davidson et al., 2017). Not only will such services enable equitable health outcomes for this group of people; they may assist in diverting people from the forensic system to be more appropriately supported by mental health services (Davey et al., 2020).

Forensic services

A person may be referred to forensic mental health services for assessment by a health professional, the police, courts or corrections personnel. A diverse range of forensic mental health services currently exists across Australia — in the community, the hospital and the forensic system (Ellis, 2020). These services include assessment of the person's capacity to make a plea in court, assessment of the person's state of mind at the time of the offence and provision of ongoing treatment to the person (Spencer & Dean, 2019). Support and treatment may be provided in the community or prison, or the person may require hospitalisation in a secure facility (RANZCP, 2017), as per the following examples.

- *Court assessment and liaison services.* In these programs, mental health professionals, including allied health workers and mental health nurses, assist the courts by conducting assessments, obtaining information about prior contact with mental health services and connecting people with a mental illness who are coming before the courts with mental health service providers.

- *Detainee or prison services* provide tertiary mental health care to alleged offenders, remandees and sentenced prisoners, including mental health assessments of people entering the custodial environment. Health professionals may provide mental health services to people with mental health issues in the prison system, with mental health professionals working alongside other health service providers in that location. Detainee or prison services usually involve screening on entry into the forensic system, ongoing assessment, crisis intervention, acute care or rehabilitation and planning for release.

- *Secure inpatient facilities* provide ongoing treatment to people with serious mental illness who have committed crimes. These facilities are operated according to the legislation of the state or territory in which they are located. There are stand-alone facilities, facilities co-located with prisons and facilities co-located with major hospitals. One of the main challenges for health professionals working in these facilities is balancing the requirements of the prison system with therapeutic approaches.

- *Community outreach services or integration team*s provide pre- and post-release and offer a continuum of care for those with emerging or serious mental illness and/or alcohol and drug dependence. Given that relapses in mental illness can contribute to deterioration and ultimately re-offending, information about an offender's mental health needs should be shared with parole authorities so that appropriate conditions may be attached to parole to help ensure that offenders receive mental health services when released from custody.

- *Youth services.* Younger people access youth services, which are similar to early intervention and treatment services described in the first section of this chapter. The earlier a young person at risk is identified and appropriate intervention provided, the greater the likelihood of positive health outcomes.

- *Drug and alcohol services* can include a diversion program for offenders dependent on or addicted to alcohol or drugs, aimed at reducing the person's symptoms, or compulsory drug treatment programs that are court mandated.

Further development of these services could assist in lowering the incidence of mental health problems in the forensic system and improve overall health outcomes of people with mental illness who have been detained in jail.

UPON REFLECTION

Are jails the new psychiatric institutions?

Some suggest that the widespread closure of mental health institutions in Australia created more problems than it solved. Many people who had previously lived in institutions — where they were provided with food, clothes and a roof over their head — became homeless when those institutions were closed. Another challenge is statistics that indicate that almost half of prison entrants (49 per cent) report that a health professional has told them that they have a mental health disorder, and more than one in four (27 per cent) are currently on medication for a mental health disorder (AIHW, 2019d). Some commentators suggest prisons have become the psychiatric institutions of the twenty-first century.

QUESTIONS

1. What are the benefits of deinstitutionalisation for people with mental illness in the latter part of the 1900s?

2. What do you see are the challenges of deinstitutionalisation?

3. How would you respond to those who suggest that our prisons are 'the new institutions' of the twenty-first century for people with a mental illness?

Dual disability services

Many states and territories provide dual disability services — that is, services for people who experience symptoms of mental illness and have an intellectual disability or developmental delay (Man & Kangas, 2019). Services are available for their carers. **Intellectual disability** is a developmental disorder that a person most often experiences from an early age. People with an intellectual disability have difficulty learning new things, solving problems, understanding concepts, concentrating and remembering (Sutton & Gates, 2020). They need additional support to live full and contributing lives.

According to the *Diagnostic and Statistical Manual of Mental Disorders* (DSM-5), there are three criteria for intellectual disability:

1. significant intelligence limitations, including limited capacity for reasoning, problem solving, planning, abstract thinking, judgement, academic learning and learning from experience, with an intelligence quotient (IQ) of about 70 or less as measured on a standardised intellectual assessment. It should be noted that such tests can be problematic, as people from diverse backgrounds who have experienced a wide range of issues can have low IQ for reasons other than limitations in intelligence
2. significant limitations in the skills needed to live and work in the community — including difficulties with communication, self-care, social skills, safety and self-direction
3. limitations in intelligence and living skills that are evident before the person turns 18 years of age.
   All three criteria must be present for a person to be considered to have an intellectual disability.

Causes of intellectual disability

Quite often, there is no clear reason for a person's intellectual disability or developmental delay. However, some of the more common causes or reasons are:

- genetic conditions, such as Down syndrome or Rett syndrome
- problems during pregnancy, including infections or exposure to toxins
- problems during birth, such as lack of oxygen
- health problems, such as measles or meningitis
- environmental factors, such as inadequate medical care or exposure to poisons, such as lead or mercury.

Specific identification of a cause or reasons for a disability can sometimes be useful if it helps health professionals to work with the person and their families to more effectively identify the best intervention or way to manage the disability.

Intellectual disability or mental illness?

Some people argue that the difference between mental illness and intellectual disability is quite clear; for example, mental illness is a medical condition with a biological basis, while intellectual disability results from problems with the structure or working of the brain. Mental illness can be treated and the symptoms reduced, while intellectual disability is characteristically static and needs to be managed (Vinquist et al., 2022). However, there is an overlap in the challenges for health professionals working with people with a mental illness and intellectual disability (Man et al., 2018). Such challenges include stigma, unemployment, homelessness, reduced capacity to maintain relationships or manage money, and sometimes exhibiting (South Australia Department of Human Services, 2022). There are commonalities in the broad approaches to addressing these problems, including providing psychosocial support and educational, vocational and recreational assistance (Araten-Bergman & Werner, 2017).

Challenges for service delivery

Perhaps the most significant challenge concerning service delivery for people with an intellectual disability and a mental illness is determining which issue — such as challenging behaviours — is a consequence of the person's intellectual disability and which issue is the result of the person's mental illness (Madden & Bundy, 2019). Once this determination has been made, the next challenge is identifying the most appropriate referral service.

The different ways in which intellectual disability and mental illness have been viewed in the past have led to differences in the approaches taken by service providers (Leitner et al., 2019). For example, one of the principles guiding the development of disability services is 'normalisation'. People with an intellectual disability are encouraged and supported to lead a 'normal' life, with the same choices and opportunities as the larger population. Consequently, a case manager who works for disability services will assist consumers in accessing services through regular channels rather than directly providing these services (Werner, 2019). The approach taken by those who work for disability services stands in contrast to that of health professionals who provide direct treatment or therapeutic interventions to people (Sundar et al., 2018). Consequently, some health professionals may presume that disability services are the same as health services when, in fact, a disability worker is more of a care coordinator who enables the person with a disability to access the services they need.

Intellectual disability and mental illness

People with an intellectual disability are far more likely to experience mental illness than people who do not have an intellectual disability. There are many reasons for this, including the fact that people with intellectual disabilities have fewer friends or support networks, have experienced more loss and rejection, have less control over their life, have experienced bullying or abuse, and have trouble learning the skills needed to manage their stress or solve their problems (South Australia Department of Human Services, 2022). The challenges in diagnosing mental illness in a person with an intellectual disability are of particular concern because communication difficulties can make it more difficult for them to describe their feelings, perceptions or experiences.

Take, for example, Marie, a 22-year-old woman with an intellectual disability, who is brought into the emergency department by her parents with cuts to her wrists and legs. One of these cuts requires stitches. Marie's parents state that her mental health seems to have deteriorated since she had been allocated a new care worker three months before, but Marie was unable or unwilling to tell them what was worrying her.

QUESTIONS

1. When helping people with disabilities and their carers, what steps can health professionals take to ensure the health care they give is 'accessible'?

2. When helping people with disabilities and their carers, what steps can health professionals take to ensure the health care they give is 'equitable'?

Impact of dual disability

There are consequences of the different philosophical underpinnings of health and disability services. One of these consequences is that a person with an intellectual disability may be inadvertently excluded from receiving a mental health service (Werner, 2019). For example, specialist health professionals may have the skills to assess and work with people with a mental illness but not people with an intellectual disability, and vice versa. This situation can result in mental health professionals sometimes saying, 'This is not our responsibility; the person has an intellectual disability!', while the disability workers will respond with 'But the person has a mental illness, they need help!', giving rise to a 'lose–lose' for the person with an intellectual disability (Leitner et al., 2019).

Another unforeseen outcome of the philosophy of normalisation is the assumption that 'normal' or mainstream health services can provide adequate treatment to people with an intellectual disability when, in reality, specialist health services are required. For example, people with a dual disability can present with complex issues, which are often beyond the experience or expertise of the GP or other generalist health professional (Schwartz et al., 2020). The divide between health services and disability services means that many health professionals and disability workers have a limited understanding of the other's work. The wise health professional will make it their business to bridge this gap at the individual level and encourage managers to develop links and protocols at the organisational level. People with a dual disability must be supported to access the most appropriate specialist health services. A collaborative and consultative approach is required between all involved, including health professionals, disability workers, carers, families and other agencies (Man et al., 2018).

The National Disability Insurance Scheme

The NDIS aims to provide long-term, high-quality support for the approximately half a million Australians who have a permanent disability (including chronic and severe mental illness) that significantly affects their communication, mobility, self-care or self-management (NDIS, 2019). The scheme focuses on supporting people to access early interventions and long-term support and providing information and care coordination for, or referral to, mainstream, disability and community services. The NDIS enables people to plan beyond their immediate needs to consider what is required across their lifespan, with particular emphasis placed on giving people choice and control and encouraging social and economic participation (Lloyd et al., 2020).

People with a dual disability are eligible to apply for assistance through the NDIS. Despite the issues that have been identified with the NDIS in terms of 'red tape' (Barr et al., 2021), the scheme is a significant step forward for this consumer group, who can seek support to develop an individual plan, obtain an individually funded package, and access information about the different supports and services available in the community and from government programs that relate to health, employment and education (Collings et al., 2019). Information about NDIS and its services is provided by the Australia Department of Human Services, is available at www.ndis.gov.au.

Mental health and the NDIS

Some people with mental illness have a psychosocial disability — that is, a disability that arises from the way a person's life is affected due to mental illness. Examples include the challenges encountered by people with mental illness to set goals, make plans, engage in education or employment, or participate in cultural activities.

If a person with mental illness can prove the permanency of their psychosocial disability, they may be eligible to receive help through the NDIS for services that help them to:

- set and achieve aims or goals in life
- increase participation in community activities, including gaining confidence in using public transport or going shopping
- develop personal skills and confidence
- access support services, such as health, housing and family support.

QUESTIONS

1. Why must people be supported psychosocially?

2. What links do you see between psychosocial disability and the social determinants of health?

3. As a health professional, how can you work with the NDIS to support the health and wellness of people with chronic illness and disability?

SUMMARY

This chapter described the major approaches to mental health service delivery in Australia and how this service delivery is structured. The description commenced with an overview of the National Mental Health Strategy, which frames how all mental health services in Australia are delivered.

Consideration was given to the differences between primary, secondary and tertiary health services and the different approaches taken by each. It was shown how mental health promotion and illness prevention strategies fit with the WHO's *Ottawa charter for health promotion* and the *Jakarta declaration on leading health promotion into the 21st century*. A particular focus of the first section of the chapter was the risk and protective factors that contribute to people developing a mental illness and early intervention strategies and treatment interventions that can be employed to reduce the impact of mental illness.

Following this was an overview of secondary mental health services provided across Australia, including community and hospital-based services funded by state and territory governments and private providers. It was noted that utilisation of these services can occur only with a referral from a medical practitioner or other health professional. Highly specialised or tertiary-level services were outlined, including those provided in the forensic environment and to people with an intellectual disability.

The need to understand these different kinds of services was explained in light of the need for health professionals to support the choices made by individuals, families and communities. Mental illness is one of Australia's most prevalent health issues, significantly affecting the social and emotional wellbeing of the community. To address the effects of mental illness throughout the community, health professionals must work together to support the health reforms that continue to be rolled out in Australia. Health professionals must work closely and collaboratively with all stakeholders to improve access, enable the implementation of early interventions when required, ensure integrated service delivery and support pathways to Recovery.

KEY TERMS

care coordination An activity undertaken by an advanced practice health professional who manages and coordinates the overall care process of the consumer.

carer A person who has a close relationship or a caring role with a consumer. Some carers suggest that they have their own experiences of mental illness, by virtue of this relationship.

carer consultant A person employed to represent the interests of carers and advocate for their needs.

cause In health, an agent or event that results in an illness or disorder; the illness or disorder is a direct consequence of the cause.

community-managed organisations (CMOs) Organisations that provide services to, and are administered or operated by, the community.

community mental health teams Multidisciplinary teams of health professionals employed by the public health care system to provide services to consumers who live in the community.

consumer A person who is currently using, or has previously used, a mental health service.

consumer consultant A person employed to represent the interests of consumers and advocate for their needs.

determinant A factor that operates at the social, community or systems level and influences the likelihood that a person or group will develop a health condition.

early intervention Strategies that target individuals who are displaying the early signs and symptoms of a health issue.

forensic mental health Mental health services that are provided to people who are, or have been, involved with the criminal legal system.

health promotion The process of enabling people to increase control over their health, to improve their health.

illness prevention The measures taken to prevent the occurrence of disease, such as risk factor reduction, arresting the progress of disease or reducing the consequences of the diseases once established.

intellectual disability A developmental disorder that involves the person experiencing difficulty in learning new things, solving problems, understanding concepts, concentrating and remembering.

mental health consultation-liaison (CL) Mental health services that are consultative in nature and delivered by specialist mental health professionals in a range of health settings.

mental health literacy The knowledge and understanding about mental health and illness that assists people to recognise, manage or prevent mental health issues.

mental health promotion Process or actions aimed at maximising mental health and promoting social and emotional wellbeing across entire populations, for groups and individuals.

mental illness prevention Activities that occur before the initial onset of a mental health issue, aimed at preventing the development of that mental health issue.

National Mental Health Strategy The national long-term approach guiding the development, planning, implementation and delivery of mental health services in Australia, produced and articulated by the Australian Government in collaboration with key stakeholders.

National Standards for Mental Health Services An Australian Government document that describes 10 standards for mental health services that must be met by all organisations who provide these services in Australia.

non-government organisations (NGOs) Organisations that provide services to the communities and population groups that are administered or operated by non-government bodies.

not-for-profit organisations (NPOs) Voluntary sector organisations that seek to promote and/or represent the interests of members and the community.

protective factors Factors that decrease the likelihood that an individual or group of people will develop a condition or illness; they are measured in terms of consequence and likelihood.

psychoeducation An approach that involves the provision of information to consumers and their carers or significant others regarding signs, symptoms, clinical management, Recovery planning and discharge related to mental health and mental ill-health.

resilience The psychological and emotional strengths, assets, stamina and endurance of a person to adapt to changed circumstances.

risk factors Factors that increase the likelihood that an individual or group of people will develop a condition or illness; they are measured in terms of consequence and likelihood.

REVIEW QUESTIONS

1 Why is it imperative to have national standards for mental health services?

2 What is the difference between primary, secondary and tertiary health services? Provide an example of each from your local area.

3 What are five risk factors and five protective factors that affect the likelihood of people developing a mental health issue?

4 Recognising the early warning signs of mental illness and implementing early interventions achieves better outcomes for people with a mental illness, particularly young people. Explain how.

5 What is mental health literacy and how can health professionals develop this kind of literacy in themselves and others?

6 List and describe five early warning signs for mental health conditions.

7 What is the Better Access Initiative and how does it work? Who can utilise this service?

8 As a health professional, how could you use mental health consultation-liaison services?

9 Describe the range of older persons' mental health services available in the community. How can these services be accessed?

10 What are consumer and carer consultants in the health care system? What role do they play in supporting health professionals in caring for people with a mental illness?

11 Name six different types of services available to people in the forensic health system.

12 What is the difference between a mental illness and an intellectual disability? How important is this difference? What role does the NDIS in supporting people with a dual disability?

DISCUSSION AND DEBATE

1 Although our current health system tends to emphasise treating illness and disease, crucial progress has been made in the past and continues to be made in the present in promoting health and preventing illness. Identify at least two notable improvements in the mental health of communities in Australia over the past two decades. How were these outcomes measured and achieved?

---

2 Discuss how first responders or emergency personnel can best support people who present to them with symptoms of mental illness, including their social and mental health needs?

3 There are many different primary health care services available to support people who are affected by symptoms of mental illness. Discuss the strategies you could use to become familiar with these services to ensure consumers and carers can access the services they need.

4 The average length of stay for people admitted to an acute mental health facility is around 2 weeks. The focus of their admission is stabilisation and then discharge back into the community. How are people who are discharged from an acute mental health facility followed up in the community?

5 Whose responsibility is it to identify if someone with a physical illness is experiencing a mental health problem? What strategies can you employ to determine, in the course of your work, if someone with a physical illness is experiencing mental health problems?

6 Discuss the notions of care coordination and continuity of care, including their importance for consumers and carers.

7 There is an overrepresentation of people with mental illness in the criminal justice system. Discuss why and consider the role of the justice and forensic mental health services.

8 There will be times when a person with a dual disability is hospitalised for treating a physical condition. Discuss the management strategies that could be used to support this person should they exhibit behavioural disturbances.

PROJECT ACTIVITY

Identify a primary health care service that is physically located in your local community. This service cannot be an online or 'virtual' service.

The service may be one that you have read about in this textbook or another service that has been established to meet the particular mental health needs of consumers or carers in your locality. Examples of such services include (but are not limited to):

- Men's Shed
- headspace
- Aboriginal Medical Service
- Flourish Australia.

Once you have identified the service, undertake the following activities.

1 Read about the service via their webpage, or other information you have accessed, and write down some questions or comments about the service.

2 Contact the service, introduce yourself, explain that you are conducting a small project and respectfully ask if it would be possible to arrange a time to visit the service to learn more about what they do. Most organisations are keen to promote their services and will welcome your visit.

(a) Negotiate a suitable time.

(b) Ring to confirm the day before — and ensure you attend on time.

(c) Take your list of questions or comments on the day.

(d) After the visit, write a short summary of what you learned.

(e) Email the service after your visit and thank them for their time.

WEBSITES

1 Open Arms – Veterans and Family Counselling is a primary mental health service for veterans and their families. The services provides counselling, treatment programs and workshops for mental health literacy and resilience building, community and peer programs, and self-help tools. Services can be accessed without referral, in person or face-to-face. www.openarms.gov.au

2 The Butterfly Foundation is primary mental health services that operates online, specialising in eating disorders. According to the website, over a millions Australians are currently experience an eating disorder, with less than a quarter of these people getting treatment of support. The Butterfly Foundations aims to help to address the services gap. https://butterfly.org.au

3 The Children of Parents with a Mental Illness website provides information for family members where a parent has a mental illness and for people who care for and work with them. The organisation works with the media, researchers, educators, service organisations, consumers, carers and others: www.cop mi.net.au

4 Mental Health First Aid (MHFA) provides training and information to people in the community about mental health, mental health issues and ways of supporting family, friends or people in the community with mental health problems: www.mhfa.com.au

5 Open Doors is a project aimed at changing the way people living with disabilities, their families, carers and support workers are represented in the media, and develop a body of media reporting about issues affecting the disability sector. Open Doors developed resources and guides for people living with disability about their rights when engaging with media. https://projectopendoors.org

6 Flourish Australia is a not-for-profit organisation that supports people with chronic and severe mental illness. Many of the services they provide are funded through the NDIS, and include a primary care psychiatric liaison service, mental health peer worker program, a physical and mental health program, daily support, social support, accommodation assistance and employment assistance: www.flourishaustralia.org.au

7 ACSO (Australian Community Support Organisation) is a community support organisation that assists some of the most highly disadvantaged members of our community, in particular those with complex presenting issues or offending history: www.acso.org.au

REFERENCES

Alves-Bradford, J., Trinh, N., Bath, E., Coombs, A., & Mangurian, C. (2020). Mental health equity in the twenty-first century: Setting the stage. *The Psychiatric Clinics of North*, *43*(3), 415–428. https://doi.org/10.1016/j.psc.2020.05.001

Araten-Bergman, T., & Werner, S. (2017). Social workers' attributions towards individuals with dual diagnosis of intellectual disability and mental illness. *Journal of Intellectual Disability Research*, *61*(2), 155–167. https://doi.org/10.1111/jir.12300

Arya, D. (2020). Case management, care-coordination and casework in community mental health services. *Asian Journal of Psychiatry*, 50. https://doi.org/10.1016/j.ajp.2020.101979

Asuquo, S., Goodman, M., Gaynes, B., & Nakamura, Z. (2022). A proactive consultation-liaison psychiatry implementation framework for the management of medical and surgical inpatients with psychiatric comorbidities. *General Hospital Psychiatry*, *74*, 149–151. https://doi.org/10.1016/j.genhosppsych.2021.09.010

Australian Health Promotion Association. (2021). *Health promotion and illness prevention: Policy position statement*. https://www.phaa.net.au/documents/item/2880

Australian Institute for Disaster Resilience. (n.d.). *Australian institute for disaster resilience*. https://www.aidr.org.au

Australian Institute of Health and Welfare (AIHW). (2022a). *Australia's children*. Australian Government. https://www.aihw.gov.au/reports/children-youth/australias-children/contents/health/children-mental-illness

Australian Institute of Health and Welfare (AIHW). (2022b). *Health of prisoners*. Australian Government. https://www.aihw.gov.au/reports/australias-health/health-of-prisoners

Australian Institute of Health and Welfare (AIHW). (2022c). *Mental health services in Australia*. Australian Government. https://www.aihw.gov.au/reports/mental-health-services/mental-health-services-in-australia

Australian Institute of Health and Welfare (AIHW). (2022d). *National healthcare agreement 2022*. Australian Government. https://meteor.aihw.gov.au/content/725844

Australian Institute of Health and Welfare. (2021). *Primary health care*. Australian Government. https://www.aihw.gov.au/reports-data/health-welfare-services/primary-health-care/overview

Australian Institute of Health and Welfare. (2022e). *Older people*. Australian Government. https://www.aihw.gov.au/reports-data/population-groups/older-people/overview

Australian Institute of Health and Welfare. (2022f). *Suicide and self-harm monitoring: Suicide and intentional self-harm*. Australian Government. https://www.aihw.gov.au/suicide-self-harm-monitoring/summary/suicide-and-intentional-self-harm

Australian Institute of Health and Welfare (2019a) *The health of Australia's prisoners 2018*. www.aihw.gov.au/reports/prisoners/health-australia-prisoners-2018/summary

Australian Men's Shed Association(AMSA). (2017). *About Men's sheds*. https://mensshed.org/what-is-a-mens-shed

Australian Primary Health Care Nurses Association. (2022). *What is primary health care nursing?* https://www.apna.asn.au/profession/what-is-primary-health-care-nursing

Autism Awareness Australia. (2021). *NDIS and funding*. https://www.autismawareness.com.au/funding

Bährer-Kohler, S. (2017). Introduction to the book: Global mental health: Promotion and prevention. In S. Bährer-Kohler & F. J. Carod-Artal (Eds.), *Global mental health: Prevention and promotion* (pp. 1–8). Springer.

Barr, L., Wynaden, D., & Heslop, K. (2019). Promoting positive and safe care in forensic mental health inpatient settings: Evaluating critical factors that assist nurses to reduce the use of restrictive practices. *International Journal of Mental Health Nursing*, *28*(4), 888–898. https://doi.org/10.1111/inm.12588

Barr, M., Duncan, J., & Dally, K. (2021). Parent experience of the national disability insurance scheme (NDIS) for children with hearing loss in Australia. *Disability & Society*, *36*(10), 1663–1687. https://doi.org/10.1080/09687599.2020.1816906

Bates, S., Wright, M., & Harris-Roxas, B. (2022). – Early View). Strengths and risks of the primary health network commissioning model. *Australian Health Review*, *19*. https://doi.org/10.1071/AH21356

Be You. (2022). *Growing a mentally health generation*. https://beyou.edu.au

Beckwith, D., Briggs, L., Shapiro, M., & Carrasco, A. (2021). Engaging young people in early psychosis services – a challenge for social work. *Social Work in Mental Health*, *19*(2), 105–125. https://doi.org/10.1080/15332985.2021.1884636

Beyond Blue. (2019). *Suicidal warning signs*. www.beyondblue.org.au/the-facts/suicide-prevention/feeling-suicidal/suicidal-warning-signs

Beyond Blue. (2020). *What causes mental health conditions?* https://healthyfamilies.beyondblue.org.au/pregnancy-and-new-parents/maternal-mental-health-and-wellbeing/what-causes-mental-health-conditions

Bhullar, G., Norman, R., Klar, N., & Anderson, K. (2018). Untreated illness and recovery in clients of an early psychosis intervention program: A 10-year prospective cohort study. *Social Psychiatry & Psychiatric Epidemiology, 53*(2), 171–182. https://doi.org/10.1007/s00127-017-1464-z

Biggs, L., McLachlan, H., Shafiei, T., Liamputtong, P., & Forster, D. (2019). 'I need help': Reasons new and re-engaging callers contact the PANDA — Perinatal Anxiety and Depression Australia National Helpline. *Health & Social Care in the Community, 27*(3), 717–728. https://doi.org/10.1111/hsc.12688

Black Dog Institute. (2022). *Causes of depression.* https://www.blackdoginstitute.org.au/resources-support/depression/causes

Blackmore, R., Boyle, J., Fazel, M., Ranasinha, S., Gray, K., Fitzgerald, G., Misso, M., & Gibson-Helm, M. (2020). The prevalence of mental illness in refugees and asylum seekers: A systematic review and meta-analysis. *PLOS Medicine, 17*(9), e1003337. https://doi.org/10.1371/journal.pmed.1003337

Bohren, M., Berger, B., Munthe-Kaas, H., & Tunçalp, Ö. (2019). Perceptions and experiences of labour companionship: A qualitative evidence synthesis. *Cochrane Database of Systematic Reviews, 3*, CD012449. https://www.cochranelibrary.com/cdsr/doi/10.1002/14651858.CD012449.pub2/full

Cabrieto, J., Adolf, J., Tuerlinckx, F., Kuppens, P., & Ceulemans, E. (2019). An objective, comprehensive and flexible statistical framework for detecting early warning signs of mental health problems. *Psychotherapy & Psychosomatics, 88*(3), 184–186. https://doi.org/10.1159/000494356

Carers Australia. (2022). *Who is a carer?* www.carersaustralia.com.au/about-carers/who-is-a-carer

Cavanagh, J., Pariona-Cabrera, P., & Bartram, T. (2022). Culturally appropriate health solutions: Aboriginal men 'thriving' through activities in Men's Sheds/groups. *Health Promotion International, 37*(3). https://doi.org/10.1093/heapro/daac066

Chambers, G., Randall, S., Mihalopoulos, C., Reilly, N., Sullivan, E., Highet, N., Morgan, V. A., Croft, M. L., Chatterton, M. L., & Austin, M. P. (2018). Mental health consultations in the perinatal period: A cost-analysis of Medicare services provided to women during a period of intense mental health reform in Australia. *Australian Health Review, 42*(5), 514–521. https://doi.org/10.1071/AH17118

Children of Parents with a Mental Illness (COPMI). (2021). *What is COPMI? Emerging Minds.* https://www.copmi.net.au/

Choi, N., Namkee, G., & DiNitto, D. M. (2022). Characteristics of mental health and substance use service facilities for older adults: Findings from U.S. National Surveys. *Clinical Gerontologist, 45*(2), 338–350. https://doi.org/10.1080/07317115.2020.1862381

Churruca, K., Ellis, L., Long, C., Pomare, C., Wiles, L., Arnolda, G., Ting, H. P., Woolfenden, S., Sarkozy, V., de Wet, C., Hibbert, P., Braithwaite, J., & CareTrack, Kids Investigative Team. (2019). The quality of care for Australian children with autism spectrum disorders. *Journal of Autism & Developmental Disorders, 49*(12), 4919–4928. https://doi.org/10.1007/s10803-019-04195-7

Coates, D., Saleeba, C., & Howe, D. (2019). Mental health attitudes and beliefs in a community sample on the Central Coast in Australia: Barriers to help seeking. *Community Mental Health Journal, 55*(3), 476–486. https://doi.org/10.1007/s10597-018-0270-8

Coates, D., Wright, L., Moore, T., Pinnell, S., Merillo, C., & Howe, D. (2019). The psychiatric, psychosocial and physical health profile of young people with early psychosis: Data from an early psychosis intervention service. *Child & Youth Services, 40*(1), 93–115. https://doi.org/10.1080/0145935X.2018.1553613

Coffey, S. (2019). Reducing liability and risk for the advanced practice nurse. Part 2. *AAACN Viewpoint, 41*(5), 14–13. https://www.proquest.com/docview/2309764099/fulltextPDF/874D7E1FCF464CBDPQ/1?accountid=14844

Collings, S., Dew, A., & Dowse, L. (2019). 'They need to be able to have walked in our shoes': What people with intellectual disability say about National Disability Insurance Scheme planning. *Journal of Intellectual & Developmental Disability, 44*(1), 1–12. https://doi.org/10.3109/13668250.2017.1287887

Cowdrey, F., Hogg, L., & Chapman, K. (2018). Is there a choice to make? A pilot study investigating attitudes towards treatment in an early intervention for psychosis service. *Mental Health Review Journal, 23*(2), 110–120. https://doi.org/10.1108/MHRJ-09-2017-0038

Cruwys, T., Saeri, A., Radke, H., Walter, Z., Crimston, D., & Ferris, L. (2019). Risk and protective factors for mental health at a youth mass gathering. *European Child & Adolescent Psychiatry, 28*, 211–222. https://doi.org/10.1007/s00787-018-1163-7

Curtin, J., & Hitch, D. (2018). Experiences and perceptions of facilitators of The WORKS. *Work, 59*(4), 607–616. https://doi.org/10.3233/WOR-182701

Davey, Z., Jackson, D., & Henshall, C. (2020). The value of nurse mentoring relationships: Lessons learnt from a work-based resilience enhancement programme for nurses working in the forensic setting. *International Journal of Mental Health Nursing, 29*(5), 992–1001. https://doi.org/10.1111/inm.12739

Davidson, F., Heffernan, E., Greenberg, D., Butler, T., & Burgess, P. (2017). Key performance indicators for Australian mental health court liaison services. *Australasian Psychiatry, 25*(6), 609–613. https://doi.org/10.1177/1039856217711052

del Corral Serrano, J. (2019). Puerperal psychosis. In M. Sáenz-Herrero (Ed.), *Psychopathology in women: Incorporating gender perspective into descriptive psychopathology* (2nd ed., pp. 581–594). Springer Nature Switzerland.

Department of Foreign Affairs and Trade. (n.d.). *Working with Non-government organisations (NGOs): Effective development partners statement.* https://www.dfat.gov.au/development/who-we-work-with/ngos/non-government-organisations-effective-development-partners-statement

Department of Health and Aged Care. (2022a). *Better access initiative.* Australian Government. https://www.health.gov.au/initiatives-and-programs/better-access-initiative

Department of Health and Aged Care. (2022b). *Bushfires and floods.* Australian Government. https://www.health.gov.au/health-topics/emergency-health-management/what-were-doing/bushfires-and-floods

Department of Health and Aged Care. (2022c). *National digital mental health framework.* Australian Government. https://www.health.gov.au/resources/publications/national-digital-mental-health-framework

Department of Health and Aged Care. (2022d). *What we're doing about mental health.* Australian Government. https://www.health.gov.au/health-topics/mental-health-and-suicide-prevention/what-were-doing-about-mental-health

Department of Health and Aged Care. (n.d.). *Primary health networks.* Australian government. https://www.health.gov.au/initiatives-and-programs/phn

Department of Health. (2010). *National mental health standards 2010.* Australian Government. https://www.health.gov.au/sites/default/files/documents/2021/04/national-standards-for-mental-health-services-2010-and-implementation-guidelines-national-standards-for-mental-health-services-2010.pdf

Department of Premier and Cabinet. (2021). *State emergency management plan.* Government of South Australia. https://www.dpc.sa.gov.au/responsibilities/security-emergency-and-recovery-management/state-emergency-management-plan

Ehrlich, C., Slattery, M., Vilic, G., Chester, P., & Crompton, D. (2020). What happens when peer support workers are introduced as members of community-based clinical mental health service delivery teams: A qualitative study. *Journal of Interprofessional Care, 34*(1), 107–115. https://doi.org/10.1080/13561820.2019.1612334

Ellis, A. (2020). Forensic psychiatry and mental health in Australia: An overview. *CNS Spectrums, 25*(2), 119–121. https://doi.org/10.1017/S1092852919001299

Embrace Multicultural Mental Health. (n.d.). *Welcome.* https://embracementalhealth.org.au/welcome

Emerging Minds. (2021). *COPMI: About COPMI. Children of Parents with a Mental Illness Initiative.* https://www.copmi.net.au/about-copmi-2/

Emerging Minds. (2022). *In focus: Prevention and early intervention.* https://emergingminds.com.au/resources/in-focus-prevention-and-early-intervention/

Endericks, T., McCloskey, B., Vincent, E., Llamas, A., & Berns, S. (2015). *Public health for mass gatherings: Key considerations.* World Health Organization. https://www.who.int/publications/i/item/public-health-for-mass-gatherings-key-considerations

Evans, A., Quinn, C., & McKenna, B. (2020). The governance of sexuality in a Recovery-oriented mental health service: Psychosis, consumers and clinical approaches. *Journal of Psychiatric and Mental Health Nursing, 27*(2), 194–202. https://doi.org/10.1111/jpm.12569

Everymind. (2017). *Prevention first: A prevention and promotion framework for mental health. Version, 2.* https://everymind.org.au/resources/prevention-first

Fehily, C. M. C., Bartlem, K. M., Wiggers, J. H., Wye, P. M., Clancy, R. V., Castle, D. J., Wilson, A., Rissel, C. E., Wutzke, S., Hodder, R. K., Colyvas, K., Murphy, F., & Bowman, J. A. (2020). Effectiveness of embedding a specialist preventive care clinician in a community mental health service in increasing preventive care provision: A randomised controlled trial. *Australian & New Zealand Journal of Psychiatry, 54*(6), 620–632. https://doi.org/10.1177/0004867420914741

Fisher, H. (2021). 'The early bird catches the worm'—the need for even earlier intervention and targeted prevention for mental illnesses. *Journal of Child Psychology & Psychiatry, 62*(4), 369–371. https://doi.org/10.1111/jcpp.13407

Fletcher, J., Hamilton, B., Kinner, S., Sutherland, G., King, K., Tellez, J., Harvey, C., & Brophy, L. (2019). Working towards least restrictive environments in acute mental health wards in the context of locked door policy and practice. *International Journal of Mental Health Nursing, 28*(2), 538–550. https://doi.org/10.1111/inm.12559

Foster, C., & Smedley, K. (2019). Understanding the nature of mental health nursing within CAMHS PICU: Identifying nursing interventions that contribute to the recovery journey of young people. *Journal of Psychiatric Intensive Care, 15*(2), 87–102. https://doi.org/10.20299/jpi.2010.012

Gaskin, C., & Dagley, G. (2018). *Recognising signs of deterioration in a person's mental state.* Australian Commission on Safety and Quality in Health Care https://www.safetyandquality.gov.au/sites/default/files/migrated/Recognising-Signs-of-Deterioration-in-a-Persons-Mental-State-Gaskin-Research-Final-Report.pdf

Graham, A., Brooker, J., Hasking, P., Clarke, D., & Meadows, G. (2019). Receipt and perceived helpfulness of mental illness information: Findings from the Australian National Survey of Mental Health and Wellbeing. *Health Communication, 34*(1), 39–45. https://doi.org/10.1080/10410236.2017.1384355

Haines, A., Brown, A., Javaid, S., Khan, F., Noblett, S., Omodunbi, O., Sadiq, K., Zaman, W., & Whittington, R. (2018). Assessing protective factors for violence risk in U.K. General Mental Health Services Using the structured assessment of protective factors. *International Journal of Offender Therapy & Comparative Criminology, 62*(12), 3965–3983. https://doi.org/10.1177/0306624X17749449

Harvey, S., Bennett, J., Burmeister, E., & Wyder, M. (2018). Evaluating a nurse-led community model of service for perinatal mental health. *Collegian, 25*(5), 525–531. https://doi.org/10.1016/j.colegn.2017.12.005

Health Consumers NSW. (n.d.). *Who is a health consumer? And other definitions.* www.hcnsw.org.au/consumers-toolkit/who-is-a-health-consumer-and-other-definitions

Healthdirect. (2022). *Australian mental health services.* Australian Government. https://www.healthdirect.gov.au/australian-mental-health-services#inpatient

HealthInfoNet. (n.d.). *Social and emotional wellbeing: Organisations.* Perth, Edith Cowan University. https://healthinfonet.ecu.edu.au/learn/health-topics/social-and-emotional-wellbeing/organisations

Heaslip, V., & Nadaf, C. (2019). Diversity and health inequalities: The role of the practice nurse. *Practice Nursing, 30*(12), 596–599. https://doi.org/10.12968/pnur.2019.30.12.596

Hickie, I., Davenport, T., Burns, J., Milton, A., Ospina-Pinillos, L., Whittle, L., Ricci, C. S., McLoughlin, L. T., Mendoza, J., Cross, S. P., Piper, S. E., Iorfino, F., & LaMonica, H. M. (2019). Project synergy: Co-designing technology-enabled solutions for Australian mental health services reform. *Medical Journal of Australia, 211*(7), S3–S39. https://doi.org/10.5694/mja2.50349

Hickie, I., Scott, E., Cross, S., Iorfino, F., Davenport, T., Guastella, A., Naismith, S. L., Carpenter, J. S., Rohleder, C., Crouse, J. J., Hermens, D. F., Koethe, D., Leweke, F. M., Tickell, A. M., Sawrikar, V., & Scott, J. (2019). Right care, first time: A highly personalised and measurement-based care model to manage youth mental health. *Medical Journal of Australia, 211*(9), S1–S46. https://doi.org/10.5694/mja2.50383

Hielscher, E., Diminic, S., Kealton, J., Harris, M., Lee, Y., & Whiteford, H. (2019). Hours of care and caring tasks performed by Australian carers of adults with mental illness: Results from an online survey. *Community Mental Health Journal, 55*(2), 279–295. https://doi.org/10.1007/s10597-018-0244-x

Hoare, E., Thorp, A., Bartholomeusz-Raymond, N., McCoy, A., Butler, H., & Berk, M. (2020). Be You: A national education initiative to support the mental health of Australian children and young people. *Australian & New Zealand Journal of Psychiatry, 54*(11), 1061–1066. https://doi.org/10.1177/0004867420946840

Hungerford, C., Hungerford, A., Fox, C., & Cleary, M. (2016). Recovery, non-profit organizations and mental health services: 'Hit and miss' and 'dump and run'? *International Journal of Social Psychiatry*, *62*(4), 350–360. https://doi.org/10.1177/0020764016634384

Ingham, V., Islam, M., Hicks, J., & Burmeister, O. (2021). Guide for community leaders to meet the challenges of personal preparation in the event of a disaster. *Australian Journal of Rural Health*, *29*(4), 502–511. https://doi.org/10.1111/ajr.12753

Iorfino, F., Scott, E., Carpenter, J., Cross, S., Hermens, D., Killedar, M., Nichles, A., Zmicerevska, N., White, D., Guastella, A. J., Scott, J., McGorry, P. D., & Hickie, I. B. (2019). Clinical stage transitions in persons aged 12 to 25 years presenting to early intervention mental health services with anxiety, mood, and psychotic disorders. *JAMA Psychiatry*, *76*(11), 1167–1175. https://doi.org/10.1001/jamapsychiatry.2019.2360

Irvine, A. (2018). Enhancing perinatal and infant mental health through an innovative integrated and collaborative partnership. *International Journal of Integrated Care*, *18*(S1), 11. https://www.ijic.org/articles/abstract/10.5334/ijic.s1011/

Javed, A., & Herrman, H. (2017). Involving patients, carers and families: an international perspective on emerging priorities. *BJPsych International*, *14*(1), 1–4. https://doi.org/10.1192/s2056474000001550

Jørgensen, K., Rasmussen, T., Hansen, M., & Andreasson, K. (2021). Recovery-oriented intersectoral care between mental health hospitals and community mental health services: An integrative review. *The International Journal of Social Psychiatry*, *67*(6), 788–800. https://doi.org/10.1177/0020764020966634

Jorm, A., & Kitchener, B. (2018). The truth about mental health first aid training. *Psychiatric Services*, *69*(4), 492–492.

Judd, F., & Davis, J. (2019). Better Access — necessary but not sufficient. *Australian & New Zealand Journal of Psychiatry*, *53*(3), 256–257. https://doi.org/10.1176/appi.ps.201800006

Karibi, H., & Arblaster, K. (2019). Clinician experiences of 'Let's Talk about Children' training and implementation to support families affected by parental mental illness. *Journal of Mental Health Training, Education & Practice*, *14*(4), 201–211. https://doi.org/10.1108/JMHTEP-08-2018-0044

Kelly, J., Jayaram, H., Bhar, S., Jesto, S., & George, K. (2019). Psychotherapeutic skills training for nurses on an acute aged mental health unit: A mixed-method design. *International Journal of Mental Health Nursing*, *28*(2), 501–515. https://doi.org/10.1111/inm.12555

Knopf, A. (2018). First-episode psychosis: Early treatment is effective. *Brown University Child & Adolescent Behavior Letter*, *34*(7), 9–10. https://doi.org/10.1002/cbl.30310

Lecamwasam, D., Gupta, N., & Battersby, M. (2022). An audit of mental health care plans in community mental health services for older persons in rural communities in a state in Australia. *The Journal of Behavioral Health Services & Research*, *49*(2), 162–189. https://doi.org/10.1007/s11414-021-09775-z

Leitner, R., Son, J., Debono, D., Lenroot, R., & Johnson, J. (2019). Pass the parcel: Service provider views on bridging gaps for youth with dual diagnosis of intellectual disability and mental health disorders in regional areas. *Journal of Paediatrics & Child Health*, *55*(6), 666–672. https://doi.org/10.1111/jpc.14266

Lele, K., Cartoon, J., & Griffiths, A. (2021). Increased referrals to an Australian Consultation Liaison Psychiatry service during the COVID-19 pandemic. *Australasian Psychiatry*, *29*(3), 340–343. https://doi.org/10.1177/1039856221992937

LifeinMind. (2022). *Organisations. Everymind*. https://lifeinmind.org.au/organisations

Lim, I., Newman-Morris, V., Hill, R., Hoehn, E., Kowalenko, N., Matacz, R., Paul, C., Powrie, R., Priddis, L., Raykar, V., Wright, T., Newman, L., & Sundram, S. (2022). You can't have one without the other: The case for integrated perinatal and infant mental health services. *The Australian and New Zealand Journal of Psychiatry*, *56*(6), 586–588. https://doi.org/10.1177/00048674221083874

Liu, Z., Heffernan, C., & Tan, J. (2020). Caregiver burden: A concept analysis. *International Journal of Nursing Science*, *7*(4), 438–445. https://doi.org/10.1016/j.ijnss.2020.07.012

Lloyd, J., Moni, K., Cuskelly, M., & Jobling, A. (2020). Engaging with national disability insurance scheme planning: Perspectives of parents of an adult with intellectual disability. *Journal of Intellectual & Developmental Disability*, *45*(3), 254–263. https://doi.org/10.3109/13668250.2019.1654275

Loxton, D., Dolja-Gore, X., Byles, J., D'Este, C., & Blyth, F. (2018). Differences in use of government subsidised mental health services by men and women with psychological distress: A study of 229,628 Australians aged 45 years and over. *Community Mental Health Journal*, *54*(7), 1008–1018. https://doi.org/10.1007/s10597-018-0262-8

Lu, Z., Geus, H., Roest, S., Payne, L., Krishnamoorthy, G., Littlewood, R., Hoyland, M., Stathis, S., Bor, W., & Middeldorp, C. M. (2022– Early View) . *Early intervention in Psychiatry*. https://doi.org/10.1111/eip.13275

Luzia, M., Agnes, O., Aline, B., Fabiane, M., & Wetzel, C. (2019). Intersectoral actions for mental health: An integrative review. *Revista de Pesquisa: Cuidado e Fundamental*, *11*(3), 763–777. https://doi.org/10.9789/2175-5361.2019.v11i3.763-770

Mackean, T., Withall, E., Dwyer, J., & Wilson, A. (2020). Role of aboriginal health workers and liaison officers in quality care in the Australian acute care setting: A systematic review. *Australian Health Review*, *44*(3), 427–433. https://doi.org/10.1071/AH19101

Madden, R., & Bundy, A. (2019). The ICF has made a difference to functioning and disability measurement and statistics. *Disability & Rehabilitation*, *41*(12), 1450–1462. https://doi.org/10.1080/09638288.2018.1431812

Mahoney, A., Elders, A., Li, I., Haskelberg, H., Guiney, H., & Millard, M. (2021). A tale of two countries: Increased uptake of digital mental health services during the COVID-19 pandemic in Australia and New Zealand. *Internet Interventions*, *25*, 100439. https://doi.org/10.1016/j.invent.2021.100439

Man, J., & Kangas, M. (2019). Service satisfaction and helpfulness ratings, mental health literacy and help seeking barriers of carers of individuals with dual disabilities. *Journal of Applied Research in Intellectual Disabilities*, *32*(1), 184–193. https://doi.org/10.1111/jar.12520

Man, J., Kangas, M., Trollor, J., & Sweller, N. (2018). Clinical practices and barriers to best practice implementation of psychologists working with adults with intellectual disability and comorbid mental ill health. *Journal of Policy & Practice in Intellectual Disabilities*, *15*(3), 256–266. https://doi.org/10.1111/jppi.12256

Maslowski, A., LaCaille, R., LaCaille, L., Reich, C., & Klingner, J. (2019). Effectiveness of mental health first aid: A meta-analysis. *Mental Health Review Journal*, *24*(4), 245–261. https://doi.org/10.1108/MHRJ-05-2019-0016

Maxwell, A., Tsoutsoulis, K., Menon, T., Zivkovic, F., & Rogers, J. (2019). Longitudinal analysis of statistical and clinically significant psychosocial change following mental health rehabilitation. *Disability & Rehabilitation, 41*(24), 2927–2939. https://doi.org/10.1080/09638288.2018.1482505

McDonald, C., & Cotter, D. (2019). Special Issue: Psychosis from early intervention to treatment resistance. *Irish Journal of Psychological Medicine, 36*(4), 239–241. https://doi.org/10.1017/ipm.2019.40

McGorry, P., & Mei, C. (2018). Early intervention in youth mental health: Progress and future directions. *Evidence Based Mental Health, 21*(4), 182–184. https://doi.org/10.1136/ebmental-2018-300060

McKenzie, S., Collings, S., Jenkin, G., & River, J. (2018). Masculinity, social connectedness, and mental health: Men's diverse patterns of practice. *American Journal of Men's Health, 12*(5), 1247–1261. https://doi.org/10.1177/1557988318772732

McLeish, J., & Redshaw, M. (2017). Mothers' accounts of the impact on emotional wellbeing of organised peer support in pregnancy and early parenthood: A qualitative study. *BMC Pregnancy Childbirth, 17*, 28. https://doi.org/10.1186/s12884-017-1220-0

Mental Health Carers Australia. (2019). *What is a Mental Health Carer?* https://www.mentalhealthcarersaustralia.org.au/

Mental Health Commission of NSW. (2022). *Aboriginal communities.* https://www.nswmentalhealthcommission.com.au/content/aboriginal-communities

Mental Health Commission of Western Australia. (n.d.). *Residential services for mental health.* Government of Western Australia. https://www.mhc.wa.gov.au/getting-help/residential-mental-health-services/

Mental Health Coordinating Council. (2021). *What we do.* https://mhcc.org.au/who-we-are/what-we-do/

Mental Health Coordinating Council. (n.d.). *About the sector.* https://mhcc.org.au/who-we-are/about-the-sector/

Mental Health First Aid Australia (MHFA). (2019). *What do we do at Mental Health First Aid.* https://mhfa.com.au/about/our-activities/what-we-do-mental-health-first-aid

Milstein, G., Palitsky, R., & Cuevas, A. (2020). The religion variable in community health promotion and illness prevention. *Journal of Prevention & Intervention in the Community, 48*(1), 1–6. https://doi.org/10.1080/10852352.2019.1617519

Mind. (2019). *Mental health sector organisations.* www.mindaustralia.org.au/resources/mental-health-sector-organisations

Misan, G., Oosterbroek, C., & Wilson, N. J. (2017). Informing health promotion in rural men's sheds by examination of participant health status, concerns, interests, knowledge and behaviours. *Health Promotion Journal Of Australia, 28*(3), 207–216. https://doi.org/10.1071/HE16081

Moritz, S., Gawęda, L., Heinz, A., & Gallinat, J. (2019). Four reasons why early detection centers for psychosis should be renamed and their treatment targets reconsidered: We should not catastrophize a future we can neither reliably predict nor change. *Psychological Medicine, 49*(13), 2134–2140. https://doi.org/10.1017/S0033291719001740

Mrazek, P., & Haggerty, R. (1994). *Reducing risks for mental disorders: Frontiers for preventive intervention research.* Institute of Medicine, National Academy Press.

National Disability Insurance Scheme (NDIS). (n.d.). *What is the NDIS. National disability insurance authority.* https://www.ndis.gov.au/understanding/what-ndis

Ng, F., Townsend, M., Jewell, M., Marceau, E., & Grenyer, B. (2020). Priorities for service improvement in personality disorder in Australia: Perspectives of consumers, carers and clinicians. *Personality and Mental Health, 14*(4), 350–360. https://doi.org/10.1002/pmh.1485

NSW Health. (2022). *Older People's Mental Health (OPMH) services.* NSW Government. www.health.nsw.gov.au/mentalhealth/Pages/services-opmh.aspx

O'Hara, L., Taylor, J., & Barnes, M. (2018). The invisibilization of health promotion in Australian public health initiatives. *Health Promotion International, 33*(1), 49–59.

Ohwovoriole, T. (2022). *What is the prodromal phase in schizophrenia? Verywellmind.* https://www.verywellmind.com/the-prodromal-phase-in-schizophrenia-5203945

Olasoji, M., Maude, P., & McCauley, K. (2017). Not sick enough: Experiences of carers of people with mental illness negotiating care for their relatives with mental health services. *Journal of Psychiatric & Mental Health Nursing, 24*(6), 403–411. https://doi.org/10.1093/heapro/daw051

Oldham, M., Chahal, K., & Hochang, B. (2019). Collaborative care meets hospital medicine proactive consultation-liaison psychiatry. *Psychiatric Times, 36*(11), 25–27. https://www.psychiatrictimes.com/view/collaborative-care-meets-hospital-medicine-proactive-consultation-liaison-psychiatry

Pajer, K., Pastrana, C., Gardner, W., Sivakumar, A., & York, A. (2022). – Early View). A scoping review of the Choice and Partnership Approach in child and adolescent mental health services. *Journal of Child Health Care.* https://doi.org/10.1177/13674935221076215

Parekh, R. (2018). *Warning signs of mental illness.* American Psychiatric Association. www.psychiatry.org/patients-families/warning-signs-of-mental-illness

Peltier, M., Verplaetse, T., Mincur, Y., Petrakis, I., Cosgrove, K., Picciotto, M., & McKee, S. (2019). *Sex differences in stress-related alcohol use. Neurobiology Stress.* https://doi.org/10.1016/j.ynstr.2019.100149

Phoenix Australia. (2019). *Australian PTSD Guidelines.* www.phoenixaustralia.org/australian-guidelines-for-ptsd

Phoenix Australia. (2022). *Supporting veteran mental health.* www.phoenixaustralia.org/treatment-and-support/supporting-veteran-mental-health

Piccone, J., Moodie, K., Sanderson, L., Bond, M., & DeGraeve, G. (2018). Sharing wisdom II: Integrated care in partnership — designing youth mental health services in Queensland, Australia. *International Journal of Integrated Care, 18*(s2), 103. https://doi.org/10.5334/ijic.s2103

Piccone, J., Sanderson, L., Moodie, K., & Kimber, J. (2018). Sharing wisdom: Integrated care — a work in progress. *International Journal of Integrated Care, 18*(S1), A93. https://doi.org/10.5334/ijic.s1093

Piper, D., Jorm, C., Iedema, R., Goodwin, N., Searles, A., & McFayden, L. (2022). Relational aspects of building capacity in economic evaluation in an Australian Primary Health Network using an embedded researcher approach. *BMC Health Services Research, 22*(1), 813. https://doi.org/10.1186/s12913-022-08208-7

Raphiphatthana, B., Sweet, M., Puszka, S., Dingwall, K., & Nagel, T. (2020). Evaluation of a three-phase implementation program in enhancing e-mental health adoption within Indigenous primary healthcare organisations. *BMC Health Services Research*, *20*(1), 1–16. https://doi.org/10.1186/s12913-020-05431-y

Read, H., Roush, S., & Downing, D. (2018). Early intervention in mental health for adolescents and young adults: A systematic review. *American Journal of Occupational Therapy*, *72*(5), 1–8. https://doi.org/10.5014/ajot.2018.033118

Rees, S., Fisher, J., Steel, Z., Mohsin, M., Nadar, N., Moussa, B., Hassoun, F., Yousif, M., Krishna, Y., Khalil, B., Mugo, J., Tay, A. K., Klein, L., Mres, H., & Silove, D. (2019). Prevalence and risk factors of major depressive disorder among women at public antenatal clinics from refugee, conflict-affected, and Australian-born backgrounds. *JAMA Network Open*, e193442–e193442. https://doi.org/10.1001/jamanetworkopen.2019.3442

Rosenberg, S., & Hickie, I. (2019). Making better choices about mental health investment: The case for urgent reform of Australia's Better Access Program. *Australian & New Zealand Journal of Psychiatry*, *53*(11), 1052–1058. https://doi.org/10.1177/0004867419865335

Royal Australian and New Zealand College of Psychiatrists (RANZCP). (2021). *Perinatal mental health services*. Position statement. https://www.ranzcp.org/news-policy/policy-and-advocacy/position-statements/perinatal-mental-health-services

Royal Australian and New Zealand College of Psychiatrists (RANZCP). (2017). *Involuntary mental health treatment in custody*. RANZCP. www.ranzcp.org/news-policy/policy-and-advocacy/position-statements/involuntary-mental-health-treatment-in-custody

Royal Commission into Defence and Veteran Suicide. (2022). *Overview of roundtable discussions – November and December 2021*. https://defenceveteransuicide.royalcommission.gov.au/publications/overview-roundtable-discussions-november-and-december-2021

Scholz, B., Gordon, S., & Happell, B. (2017). Consumers in mental health service leadership: A systematic review. *International Journal of Mental Health Nursing*, *26*(1), 20–31. https://doi.org/10.1111/inm.12266

Schwartz, A., Kramer, J., Rogers, E., McDonald, K., & Cohn, E. (2020). Stakeholder-driven approach to developing a peer-mentoring intervention for young adults with intellectual/developmental disabilities and co-occurring mental health conditions. *Journal of Applied Research in Intellectual Disabilities*, *33*(5), 992–1004. https://doi.org/10.1111/jar.12721

Schweitzer, R., Vromans, L., Brough, M., Asic-Kobe, M., Murray, K., Correa-Velez, I., & Lenette, C. (2018). Recently resettled refugee women-at-risk in Australia evidence high levels of psychiatric symptoms: individual, trauma and post-migration factors predict outcomes. *BMC Medicine*, *16*(1). https://doi.org/10.1186/s12916-018-1143-2

Senneseth, M., Pollak, C., Urheim, R., Logan, C., & Palmstierna, T. (2022). Personal recovery and its challenges in forensic mental health: Systematic review and thematic synthesis of the qualitative literature. *BJPsych Open*, *8*(1), e17. https://doi.org/10.1192/bjo.2021.1068

Sharpe, M., Toynbee, M., & Walker, J. (2020). Proactive integrated consultation-liaison psychiatry: A new service model for the psychiatric care of general hospital inpatients. *General Hospital Psychiatry*, *66*, 9–15. https://doi.org/10.1016/j.genhosppsych.2020.06.005

Shatkin, J. (2019). Mental health promotion and disease prevention: It's about time. *Journal of the American Academy of Child & Adolescent Psychiatry*, *58*(5), 474–477. https://doi.org/10.1016/j.jaac.2019.01.012

South Australia Department of Human Services. (2022). *Intellectual disability and mental illness*. South Australian Government. www.sa.gov.au/topics/care-and-support/disability/health/intellectual-disability-and-mental-illness

South Australia Health. (2022). *Older persons mental health services*. Government of South Australia. https://www.sahealth.sa.gov.au/wps/wcm/connect/public+content/sa+health+internet/services/mental+health+and+drug+and+alcohol+services/mental+health+services/older+persons+mental+health+services

Spencer, S., & Dean, K. (2019). Involuntary psychiatric treatment in custody — to be unequivocally opposed or supported with safeguards and significant service improvements? *Australian & New Zealand Journal of Psychiatry*, *53*(9), 839–840.

Stanton, R., Rebar, A., & Rosenbaum, S. (2019). Exercise and mental health literacy in an Australian adult population. *Depression & Anxiety*, *36*(5), 465–472. https://doi.org/10.1177/0004867419847765

Substance Abuse and Mental Health Services Administration (SAMSHA). (2019). *Risk and protective factors*. US Department of Health & Human Services. www.samhsa.gov/sites/default/files/20190718-samhsa-risk-protective-factors.pdf

Sundar, V., O'Neill, J., Houtenville, A., Phillips, K., Keirns, R., Smith, A., & Katz, E. (2018). Striving to work and overcoming barriers: Employment strategies and successes of people with disabilities. *Journal of Vocational Rehabilitation*, *48*(1), 93–109. https://doi.org/10.3233/JVR-170918

Sutton, P., & Gates, B. (2020). Narrating personal experience of living with learning disabilities and mental health issues in institutional and community settings: A case study. *British Journal of Learning Disabilities*, *48*(4), 323–331. https://doi.org/10.1111/bld.12338

Taylor, C., Gill, L., Gibson, A., Byng, R., & Quinn, C. (2018). Engaging 'seldom heard' groups in research and intervention development: Offender mental health. *Health Expectations*, *21*(6), 1104–1110. https://doi.org/10.1111/hex.12807

Thomas, M., & Rusten, K. (2019). Trial implementation of CIRCuiTS cognitive remediation therapy for people with schizophrenia in Orange, New South Wales. *Australian Journal of Rural Health*, *27*(5), 463–468. https://doi.org/10.1111/ajr.12578

Thompson, S., Watson, M., & Tilford, S. (2018). The Ottawa Charter 30 years on: Still an important standard for health promotion. *International Journal of Health Promotion & Education*, *56*(2), 73–84. https://doi.org/10.1080/14635240.2017.1415765

Toynbee, M., Walker, J., Clay, F., Hollands, L., van Niekerk, M., Harriss, E., & Sharpel, M. (2021). The effectiveness of inpatient consultation-liaison psychiatry service models: A systematic review of randomized trials. *General Hospital Psychiatry*, *71*, 11–19. https://doi.org/10.1016/j.genhosppsych.2021.04.003

Travers, C., Rock, M., & Degeling, C. (2022). Responsibility-sharing for pets in disasters: Lessons for One Health promotion arising from disaster management challenges. *Health Promotion International*, *37*(1), daab130. https://doi.org/10.1093/heapro/daab130

Tully, L., Hawes, D., Doyle, F., Sawyer, M., & Dadds, M. (2019). A national child mental health literacy initiative is needed to reduce childhood mental health disorders. *Australian & New Zealand Journal of Psychiatry*, *53*(4), 286–290. https://doi.org/10.1177/0004867418821440

Twomey, C., & O'Reilly, G. (2017). Effectiveness of a freely available computerised cognitive behavioural therapy programme (MoodGYM) for depression: Meta-analysis. *Australian & New Zealand Journal of Psychiatry, 51*(3), 260–269. https://doi.org/10.1177/0004867416656258

Valdés-Stauber, J., & Kendel, U. (2021). The differences between referred and non-referred patients to a psychiatric consultation-liaison service in a general hospital. *International Journal of Psychiatry in Medicine, 56*(6), 389–407. https://doi.org/10.1177/0091217420982102

Vinquist, K., Walters, S., Fiedorowicz, J., & Tate, J. (2022). Specialized inpatient unit for adults with co-morbid mental illness, intellectual disability and challenging behavior. *Journal of Health & Human Services Administration, 45*(1), 24–44. https://doi.org/10.37808/jhhsa.45.1.2

Visa, B., & Harvey, C. (2019). Mental health carers' experiences of an Australian Carer Peer Support program: Tailoring supports to carers' needs. *Health & Social Care in the Community,27*(3), 729–739. https://doi.org/10.1111/hsc.12689

von Doussa, H., Hegarty, M., Sanders, B., Cuff, R., Tivendale, K., McLean, S., & Goodyear, M. (2022). Early View). Peer support for children of parents with mental illness (copmi). In Australia: Responses from children, parents and facilitators of the champs peer support program. *Advances in Mental Health.* https://doi.org/10.1080/18387357.2022.2075411

Walsh, K. A., Tyner, B., Broderick, N., Harrington, P., O'Neill, M., Fawsitt, C. G., Cardwell, K., Smith, S. M., Connolly, M. A., & Ryan, M. (2022). Effectiveness of public health measures to prevent the transmission of SARS-CoV-2 at mass gatherings: A rapid review. *Reviews in Medical Virology, 32*(3), e2285. https://doi.org/10.1002/rmv.2285

Wand, A., Sharma, S., Carpenter, L., & Gatsi, M. (2018). Development of an operational manual for a consultation-liaison psychiatry service. *Australasian Psychiatry, 26*(5), 503–507. https://doi.org/10.1177/1039856218758563

Werner, S. (2019). Service use and perceptions of service effectiveness by parents of individuals with intellectual disabilities: Comparing Jewish and Arab Israeli parental caregivers. *Journal of Intellectual Disability Research, 63*(8), 957–968. https://doi.org/10.1177/1039856218758563

Williams, T., & Smith, G. (2019). Laying new foundations for 21st century community mental health services: An Australian perspective. *International Journal of Mental Health Nursing, 28*(4), 1008–1014. https://doi.org/10.1111/inm.12590

Wilson, N., Cordier, R., Parsons, R., Vaz, S., & Ciccarelli, M. (2019). An examination of health promotion and social inclusion activities: A cross-sectional survey of Australian community Men's Sheds. *Health Promotion Journal of Australia, 30*(3), 371–380. https://doi.org/10.1002/hpja.217

Wolf, R. T., Puggaard, L. B., Pedersen, M. M. A., Pagsberg, A. K., Silverman, W. K., Correll, C. U., Plessen, K. J., Neumer, S. P., Gyrd-Hansen, D., Thastum, M., Bilenberg, N., Thomsen, P. H., & Jeppesen, P. (2022). Systematic identification and stratification of help-seeking school-aged youth with mental health problems: A novel approach to stage-based stepped-care. *European Child & Adolescent Psychiatry, 31*(5), 781–793. https://doi.org/10.1007/s00787-021-01718-5

World Health Organization. (2016). *Health impact assessment: The determinants of health.* WHO. https://www.who.int/tools/health-impact-assessments

World Health Organization. (2017). *Mental health of older adults.* https://www.who.int/news-room/fact-sheets/detail/mental-health-of-older-adults

World Health Organization. (2022). *Mental health: Strengthening our response.* WHO. https://www.who.int/news-room/fact-sheets/detail/mental-health-strengthening-our-response

World Health Organization. (n.d.). *Social determinant of health.* WHO. https://www.who.int/health-topics/social-determinants-of-health

Wranik, W., Price, S., Haydt, S., Edwards, J., Hatfield, K., Weir, J., & Doria, N. (2019). Implications of interprofessional primary care team characteristics for health services and patient health outcomes: A systematic review with narrative synthesis. *Health Policy, 123*(6), 550–563. https://doi.org/10.1016/j.healthpol.2019.03.015

ACKNOWLEDGEMENTS

Figure 12.2: © Everymind (2017). Prevention First: A Prevention and Promotion Framework for Mental Health. Version 2. Newcastle, Australia. Reproduced with permission from Everymind.

Extract: © Australian Men's Shed Association (AMSA) (2017) *About Men's Sheds.* Retrieved August 30, 2022 from https://mensshed.org/what-is-a-mens-shed.

Photo: © SDI Productions / Getty Images

Photo: © KatarzynaBialasiewicz / Getty Images

Photo: © Rob Walls / Alamy Stock Photo

Photo: © Antonio Guillem / Shutterstock.com

Photo: © Roman Chazov / Shutterstock.com

Photo: © DenPhotos / Shutterstock.com

Photo: © Monkey Business Images / Shutterstock.com

INDEX